Bone and Joint Disorders
of the Foot and Ankle

A Rheumatological Approach

Springer

Paris
Berlin
Heidelberg
New York
Barcelona
Budapest
Hong Kong
London
Milan
Santa Clara
Singapore
Tokyo

Bone and Joint Disorders of the Foot and Ankle

A Rheumatological Approach

Editor
Maurice Bouysset

Preface by **Jean-Charles Gerster**
Foreword by **Karl Tillmann**

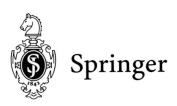 Springer

Dr Maurice Bouysset
Rhumatologist
Attaché des Hôpitaux de Lyon
138, rue Philippe Héron
69400 Villefranche-sur-Saône
France

Original French edition
Le pied en rhumatologie
© Springer-Verlag France, Paris, 1998

Coordinators of «Le pied en rhumatologie»: André Bardot, Michel Bonnin, Maurice Bouvier, Bernard Daum, Francois Eulry, Christophe Piat

ISBN: 3-540-63992-6
Springer-Verlag Berlin Heidelberg New York

Library of Congress Cataloging-in-Publication Data
Pied en rhumatologie. English.
    Bone and joint disorders of the foot and ankle / editor, Maurice Bouysset ; with the collaboration of Andre Bardot ... [et al.].
        p.   cm.
ISBN 3-540-63992-6 (hardcover ; alk. paper)
1. Podiatry.   I. Bouysset, Maurice, 1946- . II. Bardot, Andre.   III. Title.
[DNLM: 1. Foot--pathology.   2. Ankle--pathology.   3. Bone Diseases.   4. Joint Diseases.   WE 880 P613b 1997a]
RD563.P5313 1997
617.5'85--dc21
DNLM/DLC
for Library of Congress   97-42750
                                                                                    CIP

© Springer-Verlag Berlin Heidelberg 1998

Printed in France

The use of general descriptive names, registered names, trademarks, etc. in this publication does not imply, even in the absence of a specific statement, that such names are exempt from the relevant protgective laws and regulations and therefore free for general use.

Product liability: The publishers cannot guarantee the accuracy of any information about the application of operative techniques and medications contained in this book. In every individual case the user must check such information by consulting the relevant literature.

SPIN: 10663606   Printed on acid-free paper

The authors

Dr Didier Acker, Certifié de Podologie de l'Université René Descartes, Attaché à l'Hôpital Lariboisière (Chirurgie orthopédique), à l'Hôpital Saint-Louis (Diabétologie), à la polyclinique de l'Hôpital Corentin Celton, 15-17 avenue Simon Bolivar, 75019 Paris

Pr André Bardot, Professeur h.onoraire des Universités, Chirurgien orthopédiste, 17A boulevard de l'Avenir, 13012 Marseille

Dr Abdelssamad Belmouhoub, Centre Hospitalier d'Aubenas, Service de Méfdecine interne, 07205 Aubenas

Dr Jacques Bernard, Médecin en Chef, Médecin des Hôpitaux, Chef de Service, Service de Médecine Interne, CHA H. Larrey, 24 Chemin de Pouvourville, 31998 Toulouse Armées

Dr Monique Bonjean, Centre des Massues, 92 rue E. Locard, 69322 Lyon Cedex 05

Pr François Bonnel, Professeur à la faculté, Chirurgien des Hôpitaux, Service d'Orthopédie, Hôpital Lapeyronie, Avenue Gaston Giraud, 34000 Montpellier

Dr Michel Bonnin, Chirurgien Orthopédiste, Clinique Charcot, 51-53 rue du Commandant Charcot, 69110 Sainte-Foy-Les-Lyon

Pr Maurice Bouvier, Professeur à la Faculté Lyon-Sud, 165 chemin du Grand Revoyet, 69310 Pierre Bénite

Dr Maurice Bouysset, Rhumatologue, 138 rue Philippe Héron, 69400 Villefranche-sur-Saône.
Attaché des Hôpitaux de Lyon, Hôpital Édouard Herriot, Service du Pr Meunier, 69003 Lyon

Dr Eric Butin, Praticien Hospitalier, Service de Chirurgie A, Centre Hospitalier, Avenue Winston Churchill, 62000 Arras

Dr François Canovas, Praticien Hospitalier, Laboratoire d'Anatomie, Faculté de Médecine, Hôpital Lapeyronie, Avenue Gaston Giraud, 34000 Montpellier

Dr Moussa Chamoun, Chirurgie Orthopédique et Traumatologique, CHU Lapeyronie, 34059 Montpellier

Dr Paul Chauvot, Chef de Service, Centre Régional Léon Bérard, Département de Médecine Nucléaire, 28 rue Laënnec, 69373 Lyon Cedex 08

Dr Thierry Conrozier, Praticien hospitalier, Rhumatologue, 8 place Bellecour, 69002 Lyon

Dr Arnaud Constantin, Médecin Aspirant, Interne des Hôpitaux, Service de Médecine Interne, CHA H. Larrey, 24 Chemin de Pouvourville, 31998 Toulouse Armées

Pr Georges Curvale, Professeur des Universités, Chirurgien orthopédiste des Hôpitaux, Service de Chirurgie orthopédique et Traumatologique, Hôpital de la conception, 130005 Marseille

Pr Dr Jean Dequeker, Rhumatologue, Chef de Service, Rhumatologie Universitaire Ziekenhuizen, Katholieke Universiteit Leuven, Weligerveld 1, 3212 Pellenberg, Belgium

Dr Patrice François Diébold, Chirurgie Orthopédique, 34 rue Gambetta, 54000 Nancy

Dr Isabelle Durieu, Chef de Clinique, Service de Neurologie C, CHRU, Hôpital Roger Salengro, Boulevard du Pr Leclercq, 59037 Lille Cedex

Pr François Eulry, Professeur au Val de Grâce, Médecin des Hôpitaux des Armées, Chef du Service de Rhumatologie, Hôpital d'instruction des Armées Bégin, 69 avenue de Paris, 94163 Saint-Mandé Cedex

Carol Frey, MD, Orthopaedic Foot and Ankle Center, 1200 Rosecrans, Suite 208, Manhattan Beach, CA 90266, USA

Dr François Gaillard, Ancien Chef de Clinique Assistant, Rhumatologue, 22 rue Simon, 51100 Reims

Dr Francisco Giammarile, Centre Léon Bérard, 28 rue Laënnec, Service de médecine nucléaire, 69373 Lyon cedex 08

Pr Daniel Goutallier, Professeur des Universités, Chirurgien des Hôpitaux, Hôpital Henri Mondor, 94000 Créteil

Pr Pierre Groulier, Professeur des Universités, Chirurgien des Hôpitaux, Service de Chirurgie Orthopédique et Traumatologie, Hôpital de la Conception, 147 boulevard Baille, 13385 Marseille Cedex 5

Dr Geneviève Guaydier-Souquières, Rhumatologue, Praticien Hospitalier, Service de Rhumatologie, CHU, avenue de la Côte de Nacre, 14033 Caen Cedex

Pr William G. Hamilton, 345 West 58th street, New-York, NY 10019, USA

Dr Claudine Huber-Levernieux, Rhumatologue, 31 avenue des États-Unis, 78000 Versailles. Hôpital Lariboisière, Paris. Hôpital Henri Mondor, Créteil

Dr Françoise Lapeyre-Gros, Spécialiste en Rééducation Fonctionnelle, Centre d'Appareillage de Lyon, 53 rue de Créqui, 69412 Lyon Cedex 06

Dr Carlos Maynou, Praticien Hospitalier, Service d'Orthopédie Traumatologique, CHRU, 59037 Lille Cedex

Pr Henri Mestdagh, Professeur à la Faculté de Médecine de Lille, Chef du Service d'Orthopédie Traumatologie D, CHRU, 59037 Lille Cedex

Dr Raoul Meyer, Rhumatologue, 22 avenue de la Paix, 67000 Strasbourg

Dr Éric Noël, Praticien Hospitalier, Service de Rhumatologie, Hôpital Édouard Herriot, place d'Arsonval, 69003 Lyon

Dr Christophe Piat, Ancien Chirurgien des Hôpitaux. Hôpital Henri Mondor, 51 avenue De Lattre de Tassigny, 94000 Créteil

Dr Frédéric Picard, Chirurgien Orthopédiste, Chirurgien des Hôpitaux, CHU de Grenoble, Hôpital Sud, 38042 Grenoble Cedex 09

Pr Gérard Rémy, Professeur de Maladies Infectieuses, Hôpital Robert Debré, CHU Reims, rue Alexis Carrel, 51100 Reims

Dr Alexandre Rochwerger, Chirurgien orthopédiste, Service de Chirurgie Orthopédique et Traumatologie, Hôpital de la Conception, 147 bd Baille, 13385 Marseille Cedex 5

Pr Jacques Rodineau, Hôpital National de Saint-Maurice, Service de Rééducation et Traumatologique du Sport, 14 rue du Val d'Osne, 94410 Saint-Maurice

Pr Dominique Saragaglia, Professeur des Universités, Service de Chirurgie Orthopédique et de Traumatologie du Sport, CHU de Grenoble, Hôpital Sud, 38042 Grenoble Cedex 09

Thierry Serpollet, Technicien au Centre de grand appareillage, Ministère des anciens combattants, 53 rue de Créqui, 69412 Lyon Cedex 06

Dr Thierry Tavernier, Radiologue, Clinique de la Sauvegarde, Avenue Ben Gourion 69261 Lyon Cedex 09

Dr Alain Thomas, Médecin Aspirant, Service de Médecine Interne, CHA H. Larrey, 24 Chemin de Pouvourville, 31998 Toulouse Armées

Dr Patricia Thoreux, Chirurgien orthopédiste, Hôpital Avicenne, 125 rue de Stalingrad, 93000 Bobigny

Prof. Dr Karl Tillmann, Facharzt für Orthopädie, Rheumaklinik Bad Bramstedt, Postfach 1448, 24572 Bad Bramstedt, Germany

Dr Yves Tourné, Chirurgien Orthopédiste, Chirurgien des Hôpitaux, CHU de Grenoble, Hôpital Sud, 38042 Grenoble Cedex 09

Pr Patrick Vexiau, Service de Diabétologie, Endocrinologie, Nutrition, Hôpital Saint-Louis, 1 avenue Claude Vellefaux, 75475 Paris Cedex 10

Dr Denis Vial, Centre de Rééducation et Réadaptation Fonctionnelles, Villa Richelieu, rue Philippe Vincent, 17028 La Rochelle Cedex

Anthony B. Ward, BSc, MD, FRCP (Ed), FRCP (Lond), North Stafforrdshire Rehabilitation Centre, The Haywood, High Lane, Burslem, Stoke-on-Trent, Staffordshire, ST6 7AG

Dr René Westhovens, Rhumatologue, Chef de Service, Rhumatologie Universitaire Ziekenhuizen, Katholieke Universiteit Leuven, Weligerveld 1, 3212 Pellenberg, Belgique

Dr Laurent Zabraniecki, Médecin Aspirant, Interne des Hôpitaux, Service de Médecine Interne, CHA H. Larrey, 24 Chemin de Pouvourville, 31998 Toulouse Armées

Preface

This encyclopedia on the pathology of the foot is to some extent a response to the wishes expressed in 1978 by the organizers of the "Premières Journées Européennes de Podologie" in Paris; in effect, they advocated a close collaboration between the diverse specialities of medicine and orthopedics in the field of the study and treatment of affections of the foot with a view to an ever closer collaboration for the well-being of the patients. An increasing number of patients seek the help of the rheumatologist or orthopedist for disorders of the feet, the clinician is then confronted either with a diagnostic problem when the foot is the organ primarily affected, or a therapeutic problem when a sufferer from a well-defined rheumatic disease is led to consult him for persistent pain.

Even if the pathology of the feet has often been neglected by the medical profession, whereas the hands have received every attention, many European rheumatologists and orthopedic surgeons have for long addressed this problem. The names of some of the pioneers in this subject during the 1950s and 60s will be familiar: EGL Bywaters and A St Dixon in Great Britain, WS Vainio in Finland, K Tillmann in Germany, AS Denis and S Braun in France. Further, one should not ignore the considerable contribution to our knowledge of podology provided by the Monographies de podologie published by Masson under the supervision of Lucien Simon and his team at Montpellier: some ten volumes in all.·

Medicine advances rapidly and its practitioners are increasingly urged to act not only effectively but also economically, The concept of "evidence-based medicine" has a particular application to the locomotor system. Can there be any better method of succeeding than to provide a manual that is encyclopedic to the point of being up-to-date while discussing the diverse disorders of the foot in detail? Is not this organ the meeting-place of various clinicians: rheumatologists, neurologists, angiologists and their orthopedic surgical colleagues? Before planning treatment to relieve a fore- or hind-foot condition, the diagnosis must be based primarily on the clinical experience that the practitioner can refresh as required by an attentive reading of the various chapters of this book. The methods of auxiliary investigation, especially imaging, which are many, should, as pointed out by M Bouysset and M Bonnin in Chapter 6, be judiciously and economically selected with the aim of resolving the relevant problem.

It is clear that this work covers the field of the pathology of the adult foot, and that it studiously avoids the pediatric field; similarly, it does not deal with traumatic fractures, a subject that is the province of a very distinct speciality.

The clarity of the subjects discussed in each of the 34 sections and the quality of the illustrations contained in this book lead me quite naturally to congratulate Maurice Bouysset and his collaborators; they have understood that "obscurity is the kingdom of error" as Vauvenargues, a moralist of the 18th century wrote; they cast a new and original light on a large chapter in the pathology of the locomotor system.

This volume, written mostly by European authors, and published in the English language, will become without any doubt a reference work for many doctors, physiotherapists, occupational therapists and podologists at the dawn of the year 2000 and for many years to come

Professor Jean-Charles Gerster
Professor of Rhumatology,
Centre Hospitalier Universitaire Vaudois,
1011 Lausanne, Switzerland

Foreword

At the moment, there is growing, worldwide, medical interest in the subject of the foot and its disorders. This is reflected in the increasing number of scientific magazines and specialized scientific societies. Since the specialized literature concerning the medical aspects of the foot is growing, one has to have very good reasons to add a new publication to the list of the good and up-to-date books which are already available.

This book is indeed special and unique. It reflects the most recent knowledge of foot pathology, clinical and imaging diagnosis, present possibilities of conservative as well as surgical therapy, and it includes the rheumatological view. This is what gives it practical significance and special character.

Maurice Bouysset is the most competent person I know to succeed in this demanding mission, because of his outstanding knowledge and experience and his special gift to co-operate and stimulate co-operation from others. His clear organization of the book and his selection of authors are the best preconditions for the success of this work.

This book is written to inform those rheumatologists who are more interested in patients than in theory or laboratory investigations. But, because of its balance of authors: rheumatologists, surgeons and co-disciplinary members, it is also relevant to a wide orthopaedic audience, not only to arthritic surgeons.

When I read the proofs, the approach from the standpoint of rheumatologists, unusual as it was for me, was fascinating. The more detailed information of basic research in conservative treatment (including ortheses and shoes) was most enjoyable. There was also sufficient additional surgical information. I believe this new experience will be extremely useful for any orthopaedic surgeon engaged in foot problems, at least it was for me.

The more marginal subject matters such as neuropathies, septic arthritis, diabetes, metabolic diseases and traumatological disorders and their sequelae are essential with respect to differential diagnosis and furthermore these "excursions" make the book attractive for anyone who has to manage foot problems at all.

Last but not least, one can recognize the French origin of this book in spite of its respect for the international "state of the art". France has indeed a great tradition in foot medicine that shines through this substantial work.

Thanks and congratulations to the editor. Best wishes for the book!

Prof. Dr. Karl Tillmann

Acknowledgements

To Claudine, Cécile, Raphaël and Claire.

With specific aknowledgements to Professor M Bouvier, Professor PJ Meunier and Doctor E Noël; without their help this book would not have been possible.

And for their help, a special gratitude to
. Corinne Gauthier, secretary
. Professor Jacques Tebib, Professor PD Delmas, Professor P. Miossec

David LeVay, Mark Gelpke, Michel Bonnin, Nina Crowte, Rachid Belmouhoub and Heidi Schell gave extra help with the translation in English.

Editors of the book "Le pied en rhumatologie" : Andre Bardot, Michel Bonnin, Maurice Bouvier, Bernard Daum, Francois Eulry, Christophe Piat.

The following people are also thanked for their direct or indirect participation in the making of this book :

Didier Acker, Cécile Aloin, Nadine Biffy, Paule Bonnevie, Richard Bonnevie, Hélène Bonnin, Michel Bochu, Alain Bouysset, Céline Bouysset, Yves Bouysset, Roland Chapard, Jean-Pierre Duivon, Alain Fraisier, Kitty Guglielmi, Jocelyne Jalby, Fred Jouhaud, Françoise Jouhaud, André-Louis Lanier, Bernard Lanier, Gabrielle Lanier, Françoise Lapeyre, Linda Lee, Guy Lorca, Philippe Magnin, Alain Marcot, Marcel Pacaud, Raymond Paulat, Solange Perret, Michelle Pradel, Patricia Sibaud, Catherine Tavernier, Karl Tillmann, Jeanne Tovar, Claire Vasseur, Elisabeth Vianey, Jean-Claude Vianey, Éric Vignon, Nicole Walch.

Contents

1 Anatomy of the foot and ankle 1
F. Bonnel, F. Canovas, M. Bonnin,
M. Chamoun and M. Bouysset
Bones, ligaments, joints 1
  Talocrural joint 2
  Subtalar joint (talocalcaneal joint) 5
  Talonavicular joint 5
  Calcaneocuboid joint 5
  Tarsometatarsal joint 6
  Metatarsophalangeal joints 6
  Interphalangeal joints 6
  Metatarsosesamoid joint 6
  Accessory bones 6
Muscles 7
  Extrinsic muscles 7
    Muscles of the anterior compartment 7
      Tibialis anterior muscle 7
      Fibularis tertius muscle 7
      Extensor hallucis longus muscle 7
      Extensor digitorum longus muscle 8
    Lateral compartment muscles 8
      Fibularis brevis muscle 8
      Fibularis longus muscle 8
    Muscles of the posterior compartment 8
      Tibialis posterior muscle 8
      Flexor digitorum longus muscle 8
      Flexor hallucis longus muscle 9
      Triceps surae muscle 9
  Intrinsic muscles 9
    Extensor digitorum brevis muscle 9
    Flexor digitorum brevis muscle 9
    Flexor hallucis brevis muscle 9
    Quadratus plantae muscle 9
    Abductor hallucis muscle 9
    Abductor digiti minimi muscle 10
    Adductor hallucis muscle 10
    Dorsal interosseous muscles 10
    Plantar interosseous muscles 10
Plantar aponeurosis 10
Innervation 11
Vascularization 11
Bursae and synovial tendon sheaths 12
  Calcaneal area 12
  Retromalleolar area 12
  The instep 12
  Intercapito-metatarsal spaces 12

Adhesion function to the ground 12
Topographic areas 13
  Medial part: tibio-talo-calcaneal
      or tarsal tunnel 13
  Lateral part: fibular tunnel 13
  Intercapito-metatarsal space 14

2 Clinical examination of the foot and ankle . . . 15
C. Frey

3 Radiography of the foot 21
M. Bouysset and T. Tavernier
Radiographic views of the foot 21
Angular and axial relationships of the foot 21
  Dorsoplantar view in weight-bearing 22
  Lateral view in weight-bearing 22
  Frontal view of the ankle, calcaneal
     deviation in the frontal plane:
     measurement 24
  Load-bearing bifocal radiography
     of the entire foot 24

4 Sectional imaging of the foot and ankle:
  CT and MRI 27
T. Tavernier
Techniques and processing 27
  CT 27
  MRI 30
Normal CT and MR images of the foot and ankle 32
Advantages and disadvantages
     of both techniques 46
CT and MRI performances related
     to the pathology 46
  Bone pathology 46
    Fractures 46
    Occult fractures, microfractures,
      stress fractures 47
    Osteochondral injuries of the talar dome . 49
    Osteonecrosis 50
    Algodystrophy 50
    Loose bodies 50
    Synostosis and synchondrosis 50
    Osteitis, osteomyelitis, arthritis 50
    Bone tumors 51
  Soft tissue pathology 51
    Calcaneal tendon (Achilles tendon) 51

Other tendons 51
  Tenosynovitis 51
  Tendinopathies 52
  Ruptures 52
  Longitudinal fissures 52
  Subluxation and dislocation 52
Ligamentous lesions 52
Plantar aponeurosis 54
Morton's neuroma 54
Accessory muscles 54
Soft tissue tumors 54

5 Nuclear medicine in foot pathology 57
P. Chauvot and F. Giammarile
Tracers 57
Techniques 57
"Normal scintigraphy" 57
Indications 58
  Infectious 58
  Injuries and stress fractures 58
  Vascular disorders, necrosis
    and osteochondritis 58
  Neoplastic or degenerative diseases,
    dysplasia 59
  Particular orthopedic problems 59

6 Correct use of auxiliary investigations in foot
   and ankle disorders 61
M. Bouysset, M. Bonnin and T. Tavernier
In current practice 61
  Clinical assessement 61
When these first investigational stages
    are negative 62
Auxiliary investigations 63
  Bone scintigraphy 63
  Computed tomography 63
  Arthrography with CT 63
  Tenography with CT 63
  MRI 63
  Ultrasonography 63
  Electromyography 65
  Other procedures 65
  Biopsy-arthroscopy of the ankle 65
The procedure varies with every
    diagnostic possibility 65

7 The neuropathic foot 67
A. Bardot, A. B. Ward and G. Curvale
Pathophysiology 67
  Neurological 67
  Biomechanical 68
    Kinetics 68
      Muscle imbalance in the sagittal plane 68

Muscle imbalance in
    the frontal plane 69
Muscle imbalance in
    the horizontal plane 69
Deformities of the neuropathic foot 69
  Hindfoot deformities 69
  Midfoot deformities 69
  Forefoot deformities 69
  Equinus and calcaneocavus foot 70
  Clawed toes 70
A general guide to the examination. 70
  Past history and etiologic enquiry
    at the first consultation 70
  General assessment 71
  Neurologic examination 71
    Peripheral nerve pathology 71
    CNS pathology 71
  Orthopedic examination 71
  Trophic and vascular assessment 71
  Functional assessment 71
Therapeutic measures 72
  Medication 72
  Physical medicine 72
  Neuroablative procedures 74
    Chemical neurolysis or blockade 74
    Neuroablative surgical procedures 74
  Orthopedic surgery 74
Clinical forms and principles of treatment 75
  The peripheral neuropathic foot 75
    Clinical pictures 75
    Principles of treatment 76
      Flail foot 76
      Foot drop. Equinus foot 76
      Paralytic valgus foot 77
      Paralytic varus foot 77
      Paralytic calcaneocavus foot 77
      Pes cavus 78
  The neurodegenerative foot 78
    Clinical features 78
      Charcot-Marie-Tooth disease 78
      Friedreich's ataxia 79
    Principles of treatment 79
  The central neuropathic foot 79
    Clinical features and treatment 79
      The paraplegic foot 79
      Cerebral palsy foot 80
      The foot in adult cerebral lesions 81
      The hemiplegic foot 81

8 Septic arthritis of the foot and ankle 85
F. Gaillard and G. Rémy
  Frequency 85
  Diagnosis 85

Bacteriologic diagnosis 85
Several factors explain the particular
    features of foot lesions 86
  The anatomy 86
  The origin 86
  The history 86
  The infected joint 87
  Particular diagnostic problems
    in septic arthritis of the foot 87
Treatment 88
  Antibiotics 88
  Immobilization 88
  Drainage 88
  Particular problems 88
  The criteria for stopping the treatment 89
Course and prognosis 89

9 The diabetic foot 91
P. Vexiau, D. Acker and A. Belmouhoub
Epidemiology 91
  Generalities 91
  Complications 91
  Trophic risks in diabetics 92
Physiopathology 92
  Arteriopathy 92
  Neuropathy 92
  Infections 93
    Mycoses 93
    Bacterial infections 93
Clinical examination 93
  Clinical examination of the foot 93
  General examination 95
Auxiliary examinations 95
  X-rays without preparation 95
  Vascular examination 96
  Additional examinations searching
    for infective lesions 96
Treatment 97
  Preventive treatment 97
  Treatment 97
  Treatment of lesions 98
  Surgery 98
  Plantar orthoses 99
  Toe orthoses 99
  Shoes 99
  The role of rehabilitation 100
  Treatment of mycosis 100
  Treatment of diabetes 100
  Antibiotherapy 101
  Anticoagulant treatment 101
  Treatment of neuropathy 101
  Treatment of arteriopathy 101
  Treatment of other risk factors 101

10 Metabolic arthropathies of the foot 105
R. Westhovens, Th. Conrozier, and J. Dequeker
Gout 105
Hydroxyapatite crystal arthropathy 107
Chondrocalcinosis 107
Other crystal arthropathies 107
Hyperlipidemia 108
Hemochromatosis and Wilson's disease 108
Thyroid acropachy 108
Acromegaly 108
Hereditary storage disorders 108

11 The rheumatoid foot 111
M. Bouysset
General remarks 111
Pathomechanics 111
  Hindfoot deformities 112
  Forefoot deformities 113
    Deformities of the toes 113
Clinical features 115
  At the onset 115
  The established state 116
  Radiography 118
  Additional imaging techniques 119
  Other rheumatoid features 120
  Course 121
Treatment 121
  Nonoperative treatment 121
  Therapeutic indications 123
  General indications 123

12 Surgery of the rheumatoid foot: indications . 129
K. Tillmann
General considerations 129
Preventive surgery 129
Reconstructive procedures 130
  Tendon repair 130
  Osteotomy 130
  Arthrodesis 131
  Arthroplasty 131
Endoprosthetic replacement 132

13 Foot involvement in spondylarthropathies . . 135
F. Eulry
General pathophysiology 135
  Pathology 135
  Pathogenesis 136
Diagnostic criteria of spondylarthropathies 136
Involvement of the foot joints
    in the spondylarthropathies 137
  Hindfoot involvement 137
  Forefoot involvement 139
  Other joint disorders in the foot 140

Skin involvement in spondylarthropathies 140
  Keratoderma palmaris and plantaris
       of Vidal-Jacquet 141
  Pustulosis palmaris et plantaris 141
  Psoriasis 141
Diagnostic difficulties 142
Problems of prognosis and treatment 143
  The treatment of local inflammation 143
  Prevention of the deformities 144
  Obtaining normal walking 144
  Treatment of local complications 144

14 Algodystrophies of the foot and ankle 149
F. Eulry
Physiopathology 149
Etiology 150
Clinical study 150
  Articular features 150
  Vasomotor disturbances and
      trophic symptoms 150
  Clinical syndromes 151
Complementary investigations 151
  Radiologic features 151
  99mTc bone scan 152
  Magnetic resonance imaging 152
Diagnostic difficulties 152
Clinical course 153
Treatment 154
  Systemic drugs against vasomotor
      disturbances 154
  General analgesics 154
  Local and loco-regional treatment 154
  Management of treatment 154
  Does a preventive treatment exist? 155

15 Valgus flat foot and tarsal fusions 157
Ch. Piat and D. Goutallier
Definition 157
Characteristics 157
Pathomechanics 159
Clinical examination 160
Radiographic investigation 161
Functional signs 164
  Medial pain syndrome 164
  The painful contracted flat foot 165
  Pain of the subtalar and
      midtarsal center of rotation 165
  Failure of compensatory mechanisms
      in the forefoot 165
  Evolution of symptoms with age 166
  Treatment 166

Conservative treatment 166
  Plantar orthoses 166
  Functional rehabilitation 166
  Tarsal fusions 166
Surgical treatment 167
  Soft tissue procedures 167
  Bone and joint procedures 167
  Indications 168

16 Pes cavus in the adult 173
H. Mestdagh, C. Maynou, E. Butin and I. Durieu
Pathologic anatomy 173
Pathophysiology 174
  Muscle dysfunction 174
    Dysfunction of the long plantar
      flexor muscles 174
    Loss of balance between the anterior
      and posterior muscles 174
    Dysfunction of the intrinsic muscles
      of the foot 174
  Capsular and ligamentous contracture 174
Etiology 175
  Muscular conditions 175
  Peripheral neuron diseases 175
    Trunk lesions 175
    Polyneuropathies 175
    Hereditary motor and
      sensory neuropathy 175
    Cauda equina root lesions 176
    Anterior horn lesions of the
      spinal cord 176
    Hereditary spinocerebellar
      degenerative diseases 176
    Acquired non-hereditary pyramidal conditions
      of the central nervous system 176
  Primary pes cavus 176
Clinical diagnosis 176
  Reasons for consultation 176
  Clinical examination 176
  Radiology 177
Treatment 178
  Treatment with orthoses (insoles) 178
  Surgical treatment 178
    Operations on the soft tissues 178
      Lengthening of the achilles-plantar
       system 178
      Tendon transplantation 179
    Bone operations 179
      Anterior pes cavus 179
      Posterior pes cavus 179
  Therapeutic indications 180

17 **Pathology of the first ray** 183
A. Hallux valgus
Y. Tourné, F. Picard and D. Saragaglia
Anatomy of the first ray 183
   Descriptive anatomy 183
     The metatarsophalangeal joint
      of the hallux 183
     The cuneiform-metatarsal joint 183
     Intrinsic muscles of the first ray 183
     Extrinsic muscles of the first ray 184
   Functional anatomy 184
   Morphotypes of the foot 184
Anatomy and pathology of hallux valgus 184
   The osteo-articular lesions 184
   Muscular dysfunction 185
   Associated lesions 185
Etiology and pathogenesis of hallux valgus 186
   The role of shoes 186
   Predisposing anatomic factors 186
Clinical considerations 187
   Reasons for consultation 187
     Exostosis 187
     Pain 187
     Problems with footwear 187
   Anatomic and radiographic studies 187
     Osteo-articular axial deviation 188
     Morphotypes of the foot 190
     Associated lesions 190
       Overloading of the middle rays 190
       Foot statics 190
   Reducing deformities of the first ray 191
Treatment 191
   Objectives 191
   Conservative treatment 191
   Surgical treatment 192
     Bunionectomy 192
     Conservative methods 192
       Recentering the sesamoid sling 192
       McBride's procedure 192
       Shortening the proximal phalanx 192
       Metatarsal osteotomies 192
       Osteotomy of the base of
        the metatarsal 193
       Distal osteotomies 193
       Bipolar osteotomy 193
       Diaphysial osteotomies 193
       Operations on the
        cuneo-metatarsal joint 194
     Radical methods 194
       Implanted prostheses:
        the Swanson prosthesis 194
       Interposition prostheses 194
       Resurfacing prostheses 194

     Metatarsophalangeal arthrodesis 194
   Surgical indications 195
     Congenital static hallux valgus 195
     Acquired static hallux valgus with
      healthy articular cartilage 195
     Cartilaginous lesions 195
   Treating surgical complications 195
     Trophic disturbances 195
     Metatarsophalangeal joint stiffness
      of the hallux 195
     Complications linked to osteotomy . . 195
     Relapses 196
     Overcorrection 196
     Postoperative metatarsalgia 196
   Treatment of associated lesions 196

17 **Pathology of the first ray** 199
   B. Hallux rigidus
D. Saragaglia, Y. Tourné and F. Picard
Physiopathology 199
Pathogenesis 199
Clinical observations 200
Treatment 200

18 **Disorders of the sesamoid bones** 203
F. Gaillard
Anatomy and physiology 203
Clinical features 203
   Static or microtraumatic pathology 203
   Necrosis of the sesamoids 204
   Reflex sympathic algodystrophy (RSD) . . . 204
   Fractures of the sesamoids 204
   Arthritis 205
   Microcrystalline pathology 205
   Septic pathology 205
   Other pathologies 205

19 **Some reflections on the first ray** 207
P. Groulier and A. Rochwerger

20 **Static pathology of the forefoot** 209
   (Morton syndrome excluded)
P. Diébold, R. Meyer and M. Bonjean
Biomechanical considerations 209
Clinical examination 211
Etiology 211
   First ray insufficiency 212
   Second ray syndrome 212
     Course 213
     Treatment 213
   Freiberg's disease 214
     Clinical features 214
     Course 214

Radiographic signs 215
Diagnosis 215
Treatment 216
The round forefoot or anterior round foot . . 216
Mechanism 216
Clinical features 216
Treatment 217
Surgical Treatment 217
Insufficiency of a middle metatarsal 218
Congenital shortness of the metatarsals . . 218
Iatrogenic metatarsal insufficiency 218
Metatarsal insufficiency of
neurologic origin 219
Treatment of metatarsal insufficiency . . . 219
Intractable plantar hyperkeratosis 219
Lateral plantar overloading with
secondary pathology 219
Lateral bursitis of the 5th metatarsal head . . 220
Clinical features 220
Radiographic features 220
Conservative treatment 220
Surgical treatment 221
Metatarsalgia: conclusion 221
Toe disorders (excluding the first ray) 221
Pathogenesis of clawed toes 221
Clinical features 222
General treatment of clawed toes 223
Total clawing 223
Clinodactyly 224
Suppradductus of the second toe 224
Quintus varus supradductus 224

21 Morton's metatarsalgia 227
C. Huber-Levernieux
Pathologic anatomy 228
Diagnosis 228
Treatment 229
Conservative treatment 229
Surgical treatment 230

22 Painful heel syndromes of mechanical origin 233
G. Guaydier-Souquières
Anatomic review 233
Physiologic review 234
Clinical presentation 234
Clinical examination 234
Supplementary investigations 235
Clinical forms 236
Acute form 236
Forms related to a specific terrain 236
Etiologies 236

Differential diagnosis 237
Inflammatory rheumatic diseases 237
Other systemic disorders 237
Bone lesions 237
Soft tissue lesions 238
Nerve lesions 238
Arterial lesions 238
Treatment 238
Rest 238
Heel supports 238
Advice on footwear 238
Other therapeutic measures 239
Surgery 239

23 Tendinopathy of the calcaneal tendon 241
M. Bouysset
Pathology 241
Predisposing and precipitating factors 241
Clinical features and supplementary tests 242
Anatomo-clinical types 243
Peritendinitis 243
Tendinopathy of the tendon itself 243
Tendinopathies secondary to inflammatory,
infectious or metabolic diseases . . . 243
Rupture of the calcaneal tendon 243
Differential diagnosis 244
Treatment 244
Surgical treatment 244
Treatment of tendon rupture 245

24 Ankle tendon pathology 247
(excluding calcaneal tendon disorders)
M. Bonnin
Tibialis posterior tendon pathology 247
Anatomy 247
Biomechanics 248
Ruptures of the tibialis posterior tendon . . . 248
Pathogenesis 248
Clinical features 249
Treatment 251
Dislocation of the tibialis posterior tendon . . 252
Fibular tendon pathology 252
Anatomy 252
Split lesions of the fibularis
brevis tendon 253
Pathology of the fibularis longus tendon 253
Extrinsic pain in the fibular tendons 255
Dislocation of the fibular tendons 255
Pathology of the tendon of the flexor hallucis
longus muscle (FHL) 256
Pathology of the tendon of the tibialis
anterior muscle 256

25 Entrapment neuropathies 259
(excluding Morton's neuroma)
G. Guaydier-Souquières
Tarsal tunnel syndrome 259
Anatomic and physiologic review 259
Clinical features 260
Physical examination 260
Supplementary investigations 261
Etiology 261
Differential diagnosis 261
Treatment 262
Nerve branch entrapment distal to
the tarsal tunnel 262
Nerve to the abductor digiti minimi muscle . 262
Lateral plantar nerve 263
Medial plantar nerve 263
Superficial fibular nerve entrapment 263
Symptoms 264
Etiology 264
Differential diagnosis 264
Treatment 265
Deep fibular nerve entrapment 265
Symptoms 265
Etiology 265
Differential diagnosis 266
Treatment 266
Sural nerve entrapment 266
Symptoms 266
Etiology 266
Differential diagnosis 267

26 Stress fractures of the foot and ankle 269
*J. Bernard, L. Zabraniecki, A. Constantin
and A. Thomas*
Pathophysiology 269
Risk factors 269
Circumstances of occurrence 270
Increased physical activity 270
Changes in load distribution 270
Clinical features 270
Methods of diagnosis 270
Clinical 270
Conventional radiology 271
Bone scintigraphy 271
Modern imaging techniques 271
Bone densitometry 271
Frequency and distribution of stress fractures .. 272
Fracture sites and characteristics 273
Clinical forms 274
Differential diagnosis 274
Clinical course 274

Treatment 276
Prevention 276

27 Sprains of the ankle 279
J. Rodineau and P. Thoreux
Lateral ankle sprains 280
Interrogational data 280
Physical examination 281
Imaging 281
Standard films 281
Films in forced positions 282
Ultrasound 282
Treatment 282
Anterior ankle sprains 284
Pathologic anatomy 284
Clinical assessment 284
Radiographic assessment 284
Treatment 284
Medial ankle sprains 284
Pathologic anatomy 284
Clinical assessment 285
Radiographic assessment 285
Treatment 285
Rehabilitation of ankle sprains 285
Countering residual edema 285
Countering painful phenomena 286
Improving the range of movement 286
Restoration of full function 286

28 Ankle sprain sequelae 287
(excluding reflex sympathetic
algodystrophy)
M. Bonnin
Laxity of the talocrural joint 288
Biomechanics 288
Diagnosis 289
Treatment 291
Subtalar laxity 291
Biomechanics 291
Clinical features 292
Treatment 293
Anterolateral impingement 293
Osteochondral lesions of the talar dome 293
Treatment 295
Tibiofibular syndesmosis injuries 295
Anatomy and biomechanics 295
Clinical features 296
Sinus tarsi syndrome 297
Occult fractures 297
Anterior impingement syndrome 298
Pathology of the posterolateral
talar tuberosity 298

29 Current concepts in the treatment of acute and chronic lateral ankle instability 303
W. G. Hamilton
The modified Brostrom procedure for
symptomatic lateral ankle instability 306

30 Bone tumors, dystrophies and rare bone lesions of the foot 309
M. Bouvier
Bone Tumors 309
Cystic lesions which simulate tumors 309
Idiopathic cyst 309
Aneurysmal cyst 310
Tumors with exclusive or predominant
bone differentiation 311
Osteoid osteoma 311
Osteoblastoma 312
Osteosarcoma 312
Tumors with exclusive or predominant
cartilaginous differentiation 313
Exostoses 313
Chondromas 313
Solitary chondroma 313
Enchondroma 314
Juxtacortical chondroma 314
Multiple chondromas or
enchondromatosis 314
Chondrosarcoma 314
Benign chondroblastoma 315
Chondromyxoid fibroma 315
Giant-cell tumor 315
Vascular tumors 316
Angioma or hemangioma 316
Angiosarcoma or hemangioendothelioma ... 316
Lipoma 316
Bone marrow tumors 316
Ewing's sarcoma 316
Solitary plasmocytoma of the bone 317
Distal metastases 318
Bone dystrophies 319
Paget's disease 319
Fibrous dysplasia 319
Rare bone lesions 319
Constitutional osteopetroses 319
Genetic bone diseases with
excessive bone transparency 320

31 Overuse syndromes of the foot during running 323
M. Bouysset, E. Noël and M. Bonnin
Etiology 323
Intrinsic factors 323
Malalignment syndromes 323

Limb-length discrepancy 324
Muscle weakness 325
Other factors 325
Extrinsic factors 325

32 Foot orthoses 329
*D. Acker, M. Bouysset, G. Guaydier-Souquières,
D. Vial and F. Lapeyre-Gros*
*with the help in making the orthoses of Mr Kieffert,
Mr Lavigne, Mr Menou and Mr Gérard*
Different types of orthoses 329
Materials 330
Composition of the orthosis 330
Clinical assessment before prescribing
foot orthoses 331
Examples of foot orthoses 332
Metatarsalgia 332
Varus pes cavus 334
Hallux rigidus 334
Hallux valgus 335
Flatfoot 335
Static flatfoot in adults 335
Hypermobile flatfoot in children 335
Talalgia 336
Rheumatoid arthritis 337
Neurotrophic feet 338
Toe orthoses 338
Legislation regarding foot orthoses in France .. 338

33 General ideas about footwear 341
F. Lapeyre-Gros and T. Serpollet
History 341
The shoe 341
Basic requirements of proper shoes 343
The last 344
The different units of measurement 344
Different types of shoes: advantages
and drawbacks 344

34 The orthopedic shoe 347
F. Lapeyre-Gros and F. Gaillard
*With the technical support of P. Vernay,
technician at the Centre d'Appareillage de Lyon*
The different parts of the orthopedic shoe
and manufacturing principles 347
The inner orthosis (or orthotic cork sole) ... 347
The upper and support pieces 347
The sole 348
Indications 348
Rheumatologists and the orthopedic shoe 350

Index 351

1.

Anatomy of the foot and ankle

F Bonnel, M Bonnin, F Canovas, M Chamoun and M Bouysset

The foot represents a structure which has to adapt in static fashion to support the body-weight and in dynamic fashion to permit walking. There is a mechanical compromise between a rigid framework, represented by the osteo-ligamentous system, and the structures that allow motion and engage the musculo-tendinous elements. Actually, the tendons not only have propulsive function, but also a permanent role in joint stability. Without them, the joint is exposed to mechanical instability and structural damage. Here we discuss only some basic details of the anatomy of the foot. This allows, if needed, a better comprehension of pathology and imaging, but it cannot replace some important studies mentioned in the references.

Bones, ligaments, joints

[2, 4, 7, 13, 14, 15]

The bony frame includes 28 bones, which are from the rear to the forefoot: talus, calcaneus, navicular, cuboid, 3 cuneiforms, 5 metatarsals, 5 proximal, 4 middle and 5 distal phalanges, one lateral and one medial sesamoid. Accessory bones may be found (figs. 1.1-1.4).

There are five rays. Each one includes a metatarsal bone and three phalanges (2 for the hallux). The three medial metatarsal bones articulate proximally with the cuneiform bones and the two lateral ones with the cuboid. The navicular is situated between the head of the talus and the cuneiforms.

In the sagittal plane, there are two arches: the medial arch includes the talus, cuneiforms and the

three medial metatarsals. The lateral arch includes the calcaneus, the cuboid bone, and the two lateral metatarsals. The heads of the metatarsals constitute a frontier zone. The foot is like a "vault", resting on the tuberosity of the calcaneus posteriorly and on the metatarsal heads anteriorly. We consider classically that the five metatarsal heads form an arch in

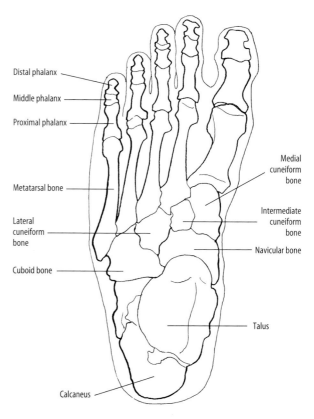

Fig. 1.1. Dorsal view of the foot skeleton

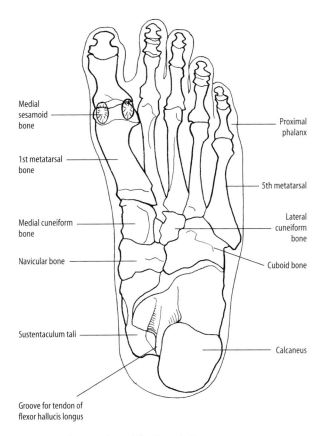

Medial sesamoid bone

1st metatarsal bone

Medial cuneiform bone

Navicular bone

Sustentaculum tali

Groove for tendon of flexor hallucis longus

Proximal phalanx

5th metatarsal

Lateral cuneiform bone

Cuboid bone

Calcaneus

Fig. 1.2. Plantar view of the foot skeleton

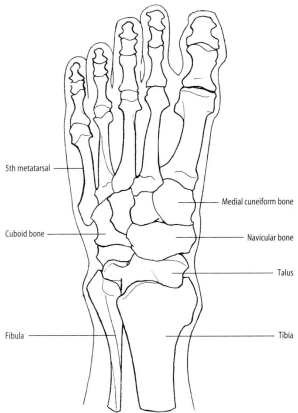

5th metatarsal

Cuboid bone

Fibula

Medial cuneiform bone

Navicular bone

Talus

Tibia

Fig. 1.3. Anterior view of the ankle and dorsal view of the foot skeleton

the coronal plane, whose summit is situated at the second metatarsal head. This arch disappears in weight-bearing and there is a global loading of the metatarsal heads, with two weight units for the first metatarsal head and one unit for each of the other metatarsal heads.

The foot includes three groups of joints. Hindfoot, midfoot and forefoot. The hindfoot includes the talus and calcaneus. The midfoot includes the three cuneiforms, the cuboid and the navicular. It is separated from the hindfoot by the midtarsal joint (transverse joint of the tarsus). The forefoot includes the 5 metatarsal bones and 14 phalanges. It is separated from the midfoot by the tarsometatarsal joint (of Lisfranc).

Talocrural joint (ankle joint, tibiotarsal joint)

The ankle joint brings into contact the domed area of the talus and the inferior aspects of the tibia and fibula (figs. 1.3, 1.5, 1.7). The distal tibia has a hori-

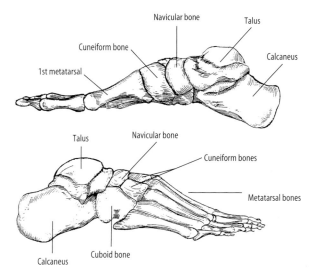

Navicular bone

Talus

Cuneiform bone

Calcaneus

1st metatarsal

Talus

Navicular bone

Cuneiform bones

Metatarsal bones

Calcaneus

Cuboid bone

Fig. 1.4. Lateral and medial views of the foot skeleton

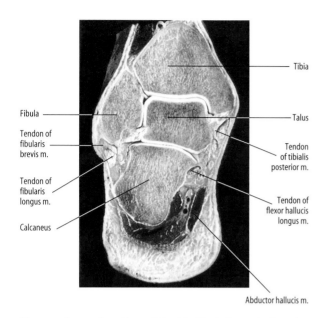

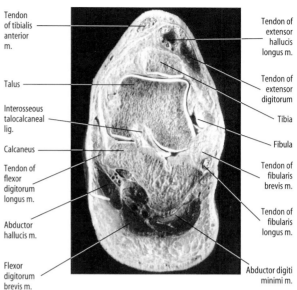

Fibula

Tendon of tibialis anterior m.

Talus

Tibia

Talus

Tendon of fibularis brevis m.

Tendon of fibularis longus m.

Calcaneus

Tendon of tibialis posterior m.

Tendon of flexor hallucis longus m.

Interosseous talocalcaneal lig.

Calcaneus

Tendon of flexor digitorum longus m.

Abductor hallucis m.

Flexor digitorum brevis m.

Tendon of extensor hallucis longus m.

Tendon of extensor digitorum

Tibia

Fibula

Tendon of fibularis brevis m.

Tendon of fibularis longus m.

Abductor digiti minimi m.

Abductor hallucis m.

Fig. 1.5. Coronal section of the hindfoot through the talo-crural and subtalar joints

Fig. 1.6. Coronal section through the subtalar joint with the interosseous talocalcaneal ligaments

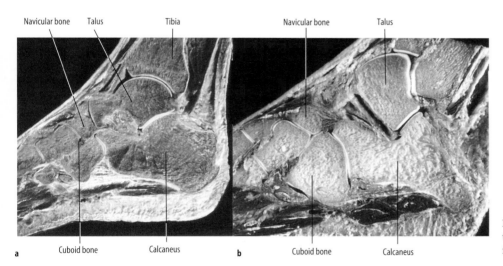

Navicular bone   Talus   Tibia

Navicular bone   Talus

a   Cuboid bone   Calcaneus

b   Cuboid bone   Calcaneus

Fig. 1.7. Sagittal section through the tibia, hind-foot and midfoot

zontal articular area which is oblique posteriorly and broader anteriorly. It is continuous medially with the medial malleolus, and posteriorly with the posterior tibiofibular ligament. The distal fibula (lateral malleolus) is connected with the distal tibia by the anterior and posterior inferior tibiofibular ligaments and by the interosseous ligament.

The superior articular area of the talus forms a pulley convex antero-posteriorly with a curvature of 20 mm radius. The anterior edge is 4 to 6 mm

broader than the posterior [15, 17]. The lateral aspect of the talus is articular; the medial aspect includes an articular area for the medial malleolus, and an extra-articular area where the deep tibiotalar ligament is attached.

The ankle joint is strengthened by two ligamentous systems (figs. 1.8 & 1.9):
- **the lateral ligament with three parts;**
  - anterior talofibular ligament,
  - calcaneofibular ligament,

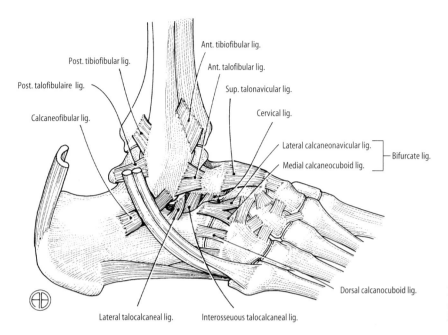

Fig. 1.8. The ligaments of the talocrural, subtalar and midtarsal joints: lateral view (drawing M. Bouysset)

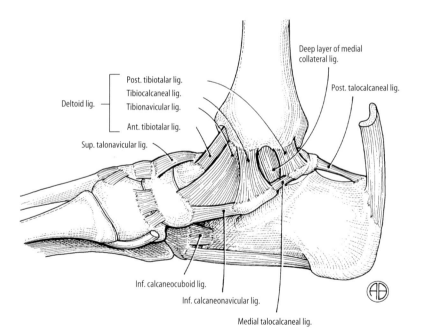

Fig. 1.9. The ligaments of the talocrural, subtalar and midtarsal joints: medial view (drawing M. Bouysset)

- posterior talofibular ligament.
• **the medial ligament** with two layers, deep and superficial, with several bands for each layer. The superficial layer, or deltoid ligament, includes four ligaments;
  - tibionavicular,
  - anterior tibiotalar,
  - tibiocalcaneal,
  - posterior tibiotalar.

The deep layer includes two tibiotalar ligaments. The ankle is more stable medially then laterally; the stability increases in dorsiflexion because of the geometry of the articular surfaces.

Subtalar joint (talocalcaneal joint)

The subtalar joint includes the plantar aspect of the talus and the superior aspect of the calcaneus (figs. 1.5-1.7).

The calcaneal aspect includes two articular surfaces, one convex postero-laterally in the transverse plane and the other concave in the antero-posterior plane. This antero-medial articular surface can be divided into two separate parts: anterior and middle. The corresponding articular surfaces of the talus are symmetric, with one concave posterior and one convex antero-medial surface divided into two surfaces. Between the antero-medial and posterolateral surfaces there is a groove, or sinus tarsi which gives insertion for the interosseous ligaments.

The stability of the subtalar joint is ensured by three ligamentous groups (figs. 1.8 & 1.9):
• the **interosseous talocalcaneal ligament**, situated in the sinus tarsi. It includes three parts: posterior, which is a capsular duplication, medial and antero-lateral or "cervical" ligament.
• the **calcaneofibular ligament**, the lateral talocalcaneal ligament and the extensor retinaculum stabilize the joint laterally.
• the **medial tibiocalcaneal ligament** makes a bridge over the talocrural and subtalar joints.

Talonavicular joint

This is a spheroidal joint. The convex head of the talus fits into the posterior concave aspect of the navicular, and the dorsal antero-medial aspect of the calcaneus and over the inferior calcaneonavicular ligament. Three ligaments strengthen this joint (figs. 1.7-1.9):
• the **inferior** (or plantar) **calcaneonavicular ligament**, or spring ligament, constitutes with its deep layer the glenoidal ligament. Its superficial thick and dense layer is a concave fibrous sheet, between the lateral process of the calcaneal tuberosity and the inferior surface and medial extremity of the navicular bone. It has an important role in the maintenance of the plantar arch in weight-bearing and during walking [16];
• the **superior talonavicular ligament** stretches from the dorsal surface of the talar neck to the posterior aspect of the superior navicular edge. It is strengthened by the anterior fibers of the deltoid ligament;
• the **lateral calcaneonavicular ligament** represents the medial part of the Y or bifurcate ligament. It is

attached to the dorsal surface of the medial process of the calcaneal tuberosity posteriorly, then it becomes broader anteriorly where it is attached over the lateral extremity of the navicular bone. Its inferior edge is in close contact with the plantar calcaneonavicular ligament and they are sometimes fused together. The synovium of the talonavicular joint is distinct from that of the calcaneocuboid joint but is continous with that of the anterior talocalcaneal joint.

Calcaneocuboid joint

This involves the anterior surface of the calcaneus and the posterior surface of the cuboid. The cuboidal articular surface of the calcaneus occupies the entire anterior surface. It is orientated from in front to medially. Triangular, with an inferior base, it is convex horizontally and concave vertically. It is overhung by a bony prominence, the beak or rostrum of the calcaneus. The posterior articular surface of the cuboid bone is entirely articular, triangular with a medial base. It has a double curvature in the vertical plane, opposite to the calcaneal articular surface. The articular capsule inserts near the periphery of the cartilage on the medial parts of both bones. On the lateral side, its insertion is 3 to 4 mm distant from the articular surfaces. It is tight medially and lax laterally.

There are three ligaments (fig. 1.8):
• the **medial calcaneocuboid ligament**, corresponding to the lateral part of the Y ligament, disposed horizontally between the dorsal surface of the medial process of the calcaneal tuberosity and the dorsal surface of the cuboid near its postero-medial angle.
• the **dorsal calcaneocuboid ligament** is a thin fibrous flat sheet extending from the medial process of the tuberosity of the calcaneus to the dorsal surface of the cuboid bone. It strengthens the supero-lateral part of the capsule;
• the **inferior** (or plantar) **calcaneocuboid ligament** is a strong, fibrous, pearly white structure, attached posteriorly to the inferior surface of the calcaneus between the medial and lateral processes of the tuberosity; anteriorly, the fibers are attached partly to the cuboid crest and partly to the base of the four lateral metatarsal bones, after passing like a bridge over the groove for the tendon of the fibularis (peroneus) longus m.

Tarsometatarsal joint

This includes three joints which are distinct anatomically and functionally. They bring into contact, for the medial joint, the medial and lateral cuneiform bones with the first, second, and third metatarsal bones; and for the lateral joint, the anterior surface of the cuboid with the bases of the fourth and fifth metatarsals. Overall, the tarsometatarsal joint articulates the anterior tarsus with the metatarsal bases and is oblique from medial to lateral, from above down and from front to back. The general obliquity of this axis in flexion-extension of the metatarsals participates in eversion-inversion motion.

The global joint organization, with the embedding of the second metatarsal bone, restricts the mobility of the entire joint. In the sagittal plane, during passive movements, there is no extension of the first and fifth metatarsal bones at the tarsometatarsal joint, though extension is possible proximally. The maximal passive flexion of the first metatarsal is about 10 to 15° and that of the fifth metatarsal bone 15 to 20°. Usual movements of the first and fifth tarsometatarsal joints are never isolated in a single plane [3].

Metatarsophalangeal joints

These joints are subjected to considerable mechanical constraints, because of their situation in a frontier mechanical zone of great importance. Their dorsiflexion movement is limited by a dense layer of fibrous tissue: the plantar plate. They include the convex metatarsal head articular surfaces and the glenoidal elliptic cavities of the bases of the proximal phalanges. Their sagittal mobility is 90° in extension and 45° in flexion. In the horizontal plane, the mobility necessary to maintain balance of the forefoot is slight, because of the tightness of the interosseous and interdigital spaces. Their vertical stability is strengthened by a thick plantar ligament. This ligament is connected to the neighbouring ligament by the thick transverse intermetatarsal ligament, which creates with the plantar fascia a fibrous tunnel for the flexor tendon.

Interphalangeal joints

The interphalangeal joints have only one movement axis, orientated in the sagittal plane. They are stabilized by a plantar plate and two collateral ligaments.

Metatarsosesamoid joint

The metatarsosesamoid joint undergoes considerable mechanical constraints because of its functional situation between the static hindfoot and dynamic forefoot. The head of the first metatarsal has two articular surfaces; the first, antero-superior, for the phalangeal articular recess, and the other, plantar-inferior, for the superior gleno-sesamoid surface; the latter is convex, divided in two by a sagittal ridge which separates the medial and lateral sesamoid facets. The sesamoids are situated between the first metatarsal and the ground [1, 10].

At the midline, the tendon of the flexor hallucis longus m. passes between the sesamoids before it inserts at the base of P2. The articular capsule is covered by a fibrocartilage, which includes the sesamoids, to form an articular floor over which the head of the first metatarsal bone glides. This is the sesamoid plate (or glenoid ligament) [12]. In front, it faces the plantar edge of the glenoid fossa of the proximal phalanx, and is separated from it by a deep furrow. Posteriorly, there is the inferior edge of the head of M1. On either side, the collateral ligaments of the metatarsophalangeal joint are thick and resistant. Their inferior edges are connected with the glenoid ligament, while some glenoid bundles stemming from the lateral ligaments cross below the head of the first metatarsal, and connect with those stemming from the opposite lateral ligament. The sesamoids receive the terminal insertions of some of the plantar muscles. The medial sesamoid receives the tendon of the abductor hallucis m. and the medial insertion of the flexor hallucis brevis m. The lateral sesamoid receives the tendon of the adductor hallucis m. and the lateral insertion of the tendon of the flexor hallucis brevis m.

Accessory bones [9, 15]

Several accessory bones may be seen in the foot.
• A tibial bone (accessory navicular) is frequent. It is found in 4 to 10% of feet, situated on the medial aspect of the navicular bone;
• the os trigonum prolongs the postero-lateral tuberosity of the talus. It is found in 2 to 8% of feet and is often bilateral;
• an intermetatarsal bone is observed in 8 to 10% of feet, between the medial cuneiform and the bases of the first two metatarsals;

• a sustentacular bone on the posterior aspect of the sustentaculum tali is rare;
• a secondary calcaneal bone at the level of the beak of the tuberosity in 2% of feet;
• the vesalian bone is rare, situated at the level of the base of M5.

Muscles

There are two muscular systems: extrinsic and intrinsic. The extrinsic muscles arise from the leg skeleton but their tendons act on the foot. The intrinsic muscles are situated entirely within the foot [6].

Extrinsic muscles

The aponeuroses of the leg define three compartments: anterior, posterior and lateral. The muscles of the anterior compartment are innervated by the deep fibular (peroneal) nerve and produce dorsiflexion of the foot. The muscles of the posterior compartment are innervated by the tibial n. and are plantarflexors. The muscles of the lateral compartment are innervated by the superficial fibular (peroneal) nerve and are plantarflexors and abductors of the foot.

Muscles of the anterior compartment (fig. 1.10)

Tibialis anterior muscle

This arises from the superior two-thirds of the lateral surface of the tibia, the adjacent part of the interosseous membrane and superiorly from the leg aponeurosis. It descends along the anterior surface of the distal extremity of the tibia, and enters the foot under the extensor retinaculum, medial to the extensor muscles. Its tendon runs obliquely anteriorly and medially toward the medial edge of the foot and inserts at the medial surface of the first cuneiform and the base of the first metatarsal. The tibialis anterior m. is a dorsiflexor of the ankle, and an invertor, adductor and supinator of the foot.

Fibularis tertius muscle

This muscle arises from the medial surface of the distal fibula and the adjacent parts of the interos-

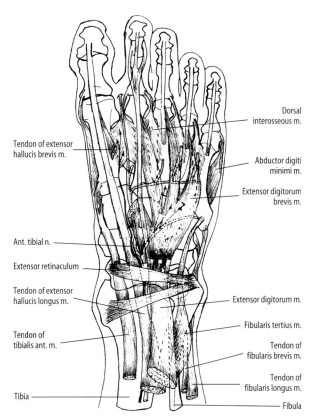

Fig. 1.10. Dorsal view of foot with tendinous and neurovascular structures

Dorsal interosseous m.

Tendon of extensor hallucis brevis m.

Abductor digiti minimi m.

Extensor digitorum brevis m.

Ant. tibial n.

Extensor retinaculum

Tendon of extensor hallucis longus m.

Extensor digitorum m.

Fibularis tertius m.

Tendon of tibialis ant. m.

Tendon of fibularis brevis m.

Tendon of fibularis longus m.

Tibia

Fibula

seous ligament and anterior septum. It crosses the external sling of the extensor retinaculum with the extensor digitorum longus m. and passes over the lateral aspect of the foot to insert on the dorsal aspect of the base of the fifth metatarsal. It is an ankle dorsiflexor and evertor and an abductor and pronator of the foot.

Extensor hallucis longus muscle

This arises from the medial surface of the middle part of the fibula and the adjacent anterior surface of the interosseous membrane. It descends and travels under the extensor retinaculum between the tibialis anterior m. medially and the extensor digitorum longus m. laterally. It passes anteriorly and medially toward the hallux and ends on the dorsal aspect of the bases of its two phalanges. It is a dorsiflexor of the first phalanx on the metatarsal bone. It is also an ankle dorsiflexor and foot invertor.

Extensor digitorum longus muscle

This arises from almost the entire length of the medial surface of the fibula, lateral to the preceding muscle and above the fibularis (peroneus) tertius m. It also arises from the leg aponeurosis and ascends as far as the lateral tuberosity of the tibia. It descends and crosses under the extensor retinaculum. On the dorsal side of the foot, it gives off four tendons, and inserts at the dorsal surface of the bases of the first phalanges. The other tendons join those of the extensor digitorum brevis m. at the level of the metatarsal heads. It is a dorsiflexor, particularly of the first four metatarsophalangeal joints.

Lateral compartment muscles (figs. 1.8 & 1.11)

Fibularis brevis muscle

This arises from the lateral surface of the middle part of the fibula and travels downwards, covered by the muscular body of the fibularis (peroneus) longus m. Its tendon passes behind the lateral malleolus where it bends and goes toward the lateral edge of the foot, to insert at the tuberosity of the fifth metatarsal bone. It is a plantarflexor of the ankle and evertor of the foot.

Fibularis longus muscle

This arises from the lateral surface of the upper half of the fibula and the lateral tuberosity of the tibia, also from the anterior and lateral intermuscular septa and the fascia of the leg. Its tendon descends behind that of the fibularis (peroneus) brevis m., passes in a fibrous groove against the lateral surface of the calcaneus, and glides under the cuboid bone to reach the plantar side of the base of the first metatarsal bone. It is a plantarflexor of the ankle and foot evertor like the other fibular muscles.

Muscles of the posterior compartment (fig. 1.11)

Tibialis posterior muscle

This arises from the tibia and the fibula and the back of the interosseous membrane. Its origin is situated between those of the flexor digitorum longus m. medially and the flexor hallucis longus m. laterally. On the posterior aspect of the distal tibia, it crosses anterior and medial to the flexor digitorum longus m. so that its tendon is situated medial to those of the flexor mm. in the posterior groove of the medial

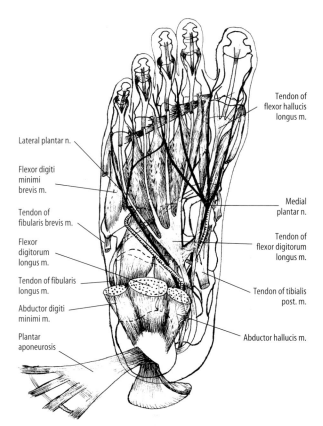

Fig. 1.11. Plantar view of foot with muscular, tendinous, arterial and nervous structures

malleolus. It bends at the medial malleolus, enters the tarsal tunnel in front of and above the two other tendons and goes toward the medial side of the foot. It arises from the navicular tuberosity. It is a plantarflexor of the ankle and a foot invertor.

Flexor digitorum longus muscle

Its area of origin is situated on the posterior surface of the tibial diaphysis, distal to that of the popliteus m. and lateral to the tibialis posterior m. Its tendon is crossed by that of the tibialis posterior m. and on the posterior aspect of the distal tibia it is situated between the tendon of the tibialis posterior medially and the tendon of the flexor hallucis longus laterally. Between these two tendons, it enters the tarsal tunnel, medial to the lateral process of the calcaneal tuberosity. It passes round the medial edge of the foot under the tendon of the flexor hallucis longus, to which it connects by a band. It receives the quadratus plantae m. on the plantar aspect of the foot, which orientates it in the metatarsal axes. It is divided into four tendons whose borders are the origins of the lumbrical muscles in the interosseous spaces. Each tendon, the so-called "perforator", crosses between the slips of the flexor digitorum brevis m. and ends on the base of the third phalanx.

This muscle is a plantarflexor of the outer four toes and plantarflexor and invertor of the foot.

Flexor hallucis longus muscle

This arises from the posterior aspect of the fibula and the lateral intermuscular septum. It is situated lateral to the tibialis posterior m. Because of the crossing of the tendons of the tibialis posterior and flexor digitorum longus, it travels with the former within the tarsal tunnel. It then passes under the medial side of the foot, crossed by the tendon of the flexor digitorum longus, which passes laterally. An expansion connects both tendons to the plantar aspect of the foot. It inserts at the base of the second phalanx of the hallux. It is a plantarflexor of the hallux and ankle; it is also an invertor of the foot.

Triceps surae muscle

This includes the two gastroenemius mm. and the soleus m.:
• the medial gastrocnemius m. arises from the superior pole of the medial femoral condyle and its medial surface between the adductor tubercle and the tibial attachment of the medial collateral ligament of the knee. It descends laterally to join the lateral gastrocnemius with which it fuses.
• the lateral gastroecnemius m. has a symmetric origin comparable to the former. It arises from the superior pole of the lateral femoral condyle and its lateral surface just above the fibular attachment of the lateral collateral ligament, and more distally from the popliteus m. It descends medially to rejoin its medial homolog. Their junction becomes the calcaneal tendon, which inserts on the medial process of the calcaneal tuberosity;
• the soleus m., situated in front of the gastrocnemius, arises from a superior and lateral oblique line which marks the posterior tibial surface under the attachment of the popliteus m. Its origin continues medially on the middle part of the medial side of the tibia and laterally on the posterior part of the fibular head and neck. Between the tibia and fibula, there is a tendinous arcade under which passes the tibial n. and the posterior tibial a. From this broad line of origin the muscular body narrows, becomes flat but thick, and descends to join the calcaneal tendon and the calcaneus.

Intrinsic muscles (figs. 1.10 & 1.11)

Extensor digitorum brevis muscle

This is the only intrinsic muscle situated on the dorsal aspect of the foot. It arises from the tuberosity of the calcaneus, at the level of the lateral foramen of the sinus tarsi. The muscular body extends anteriorly, passing under the tendons of the extensor digitorum longus m., and its tendons insert on the articular capsule of the first, second, third and fourth metatarsophalangeal joints. It is innervated by a branch of the deep fibular n. Its most medial portion is usually designated as the extensor hallucis brevis m.

Flexor digitorum brevis muscle

This arises from the posterior tuberosity of the inferior surface of the calcaneus and travels anteriorly, giving four fascicles whose tendons end on the lateral four toes. These tendons are perforated by those of the flexor digitorum longus m. and end at the lateral sides of the second phalanges. This muscle is a plantarflexor of the second phalanges. Its most medial portion is usually designated as the flexor hallucis brevis m.

Flexor hallucis brevis muscle

This arises from the plantar surface of the cuboid and lateral cuneiforms and the tibialis posterior tendon to form two heads inserted at the medial and lateral sides of the proximal phalanx of the great toe and its sesamoids. It is a flexor of the metatarsophalangeal joint of the great toe.

Quadratus plantae muscle

This muscle is deeper than the former. It arises from the lateral side of the inferior surface of the calcaneus, and travels anteriorly to end on the lateral side of the tendon of the flexor digitorum longus m. By pulling on the flexor digitorum longus m., this muscle is a plantarflexor of the third phalanx on the second and it corrects the axial deviation of the tendons of the flexor digitorum longus which run obliquely medially.

Abductor hallucis muscle

From the postero-medial tuberosity of the inferior surface of the calcaneus it goes anteriorly along the medial arch. It ends at the medial sesamoid and the medial tuberosity of the base of the first phalanx of the hallux. It is an abductor of the hallux and thus participates in lateral stabilization of the foot. It is also a plantarflexor of the hallux, acting during the step impulse.

Abductor digiti minimi muscle

This arises from the postero-lateral tuberosity of the inferior surface of the calcaneus and passes anteriorly along the lateral arch. It ends at the lateral tuberosity of the base of the first phalanx of the fifth toe. It is, like the above, a lateral stabilizer of the foot and also a plantarflexor of the first phalanx of the fifth toe. These two muscles complement the dorsal interosseous muscular system, laterally and medially.

Adductor hallucis muscle (oblique head)

This arises from the inferior surface of the cuboid, third cuneiform and the plantar surface of the bases of the third and fourth metatarsal bones, passing obliquely forward and medially. It ends in a common tendon with the transverse head on the lateral sesamoid bone and the lateral tubercle of the first phalanx of the hallux. It is an adductor of the hallux in relation to the axis of the foot. It stabilizes the hallux laterally, opposing the abductor. It is also a flexor of the first phalanx like the abductor.

Adductor hallucis muscle (transverse head)

This arises from the plantar surface of the capsule of the lateral three metatarsophalangeal joints. It runs transversely and medially along the anterior arch, following the heads of the metatarsal bones. It ends by joining the preceding muscle. It is an adductor of the hallux.

Dorsal interosseous muscles

There are four interosseous muscles. Each arises from the adjacent surfaces of the two metatarsal bones, which border an interosseous space occupied by the muscular body. Anteriorly, each muscle provides a tendon which approaches the foot axis and ends at the lateral tubercle of the first phalanx nearest to this axis. It also sends a dorsal expansion to the tendon of the extensor digitorum longus m. The dorsal interosseous mm. deviate the toes away from the foot axis. They flex and stabilize the toes laterally. As the first and fifth toes are not governed by these muscles, the system is completed laterally by the hallucis and digiti minimi abductor muscles which have the same function.

Plantar interosseous muscles

There are three interosseous mm, occupying the lateral three spaces. They arise from the lateral and medial surfaces of the three lateral metatarsal bones. Their tendons go anteriorly away from the foot axis to end on the medial and lateral sides of the first phalanges of the three lateral toes. They send a dorsal expansion on the same side as their dorsal equivalent muscles. They adduct the lateral three toes toward the foot axis. They are flexors of the lateral three toes and also participate in lateral stabilization of the metatarsophalangeal joints.

● Plantar aponeurosis

This is triangular, with an anterior base and a posterior apex. It is attached transversely to the plantar surface of the calcaneus and extends horizontally, becoming broader at the base of the toes. Thick and compact in its posterior part, it widens anteriorly and develops some thickenings which constitute subtendinous bundles at the level of the tendons of the flexor muscles.

Plantar sagittal extensions: the lateral and medial sides of the plantar aponeurosis are prolonged by the lateral and medial intermuscular septa.

The medial intermuscular septum is attached, from behind forward, to the plantar aspect of the calcaneus, navicular, second cuneiform bone and first metatarsal.

The lateral septum is attached, from behind forward, to the plantar aspect of the calcaneus, the cuboid and the fifth metatarsal.

On each side, the plantar aponeurosis is bordered by a narrow aponeurotic band: the lateral plantar aponeurosis which covers the abductor digiti minimi m. and the medial plantar aponeurosis which covers the abductor hallucis m.

The superposition of talus and calcaneus and the presence of a postero-anterior calcaneo-metatarsal arch require passive reinforcing structures which relax the muscular elements. There are two reinforcing structures: the plantar calcaneocuboid ligament in contact with the bony vault, and more superficially by the plantar aponeurosis. At the level of the metatarsal heads, the plantar aponeurosis and transverse ligament prevent excessive separation of the metatarsals and, through the action of the transverse head of the adductor hallucis m., allow great elasticity in the zone of transition between the posterior static and anterior dynamic triangles. The intrinsic plantar muscle attachments to the medial and lateral septa, and also to the deep surface of the medial and lateral plantar aponeurosis, contribute to the rigidity of these reinforcing structures.

Innervation

Five nerves provide the innervation of the foot (figs. 1.10 & 1.11).
• The **sural nerve** from the popliteal fossa, travels along the lateral surface of the calcaneal tendon in the subcutaneous cellular tissue, passes 10 to 15 mm under the tip of the lateral malleolus, and reaches the base of the fifth metatarsal bone where it divides into two terminal branches. It is a sensory nerve.
• The **superficial fibular (peroneal) nerve** supplies the two peroneal mm. in the lateral compartment of the leg. It becomes subcutaneous at the inferior third of the leg and divides into three terminal sensory branches, distributed on the dorsal side of the foot.
• The **deep fibular (peroneal) nerve** (anterior tibial n.) supplies the muscles of the anterior compartment of the leg. At the midtarsal joint level, it passes under the extensor retinaculum with the anterior tibial artery and divides into two terminal branches, medial and lateral. The medial branch innerves the extensor digitorum brevis m.
• The **saphenous nerve** is a terminal branch from the femoral nerve. It is a satellite of the great saphenous vein in the medial premalleolar area. It is sensory and supplies the medial surface of the foot.
• The **tibial nerve** (posterior tibial n.) supplies the muscles of the posterior compartment of the leg and reaches the foot through the tarsal tunnel. It divides in this tunnel into two terminal branches: the medial plantar and the lateral plantar nn. It supplies all the plantar intrinsic muscles of the foot and gives some sensory branches. The **medial plantar n.** provides the plantar digital n. for the hallux and the plantar digital common nn. for the first, second and third intermetatarsal spaces. The **lateral plantar n.** gives rise to the lateral digital plantar n. to the fifth toe and the common plantar digital n. to the fourth intermetatarsal space.

At the level of the tarsal tunnel, the tibial nerve gives off the calcaneal nerve, which provides sensory innervation to the heel, and the nerve to the abductor digiti minimi m.

Vascularization

Three arteries supply the foot (figs. 1.10 & 1.11).
• The **anterior tibial a.** passes under the extensor retinaculum at the level of the instep and becomes the dorsalis pedis artery. At this level, it gives off the lateral tarsal a. and continues as the medial tarsal a. The later reaches the first intermetatarsal space, gives off the arcuate a., and divides into the first dorsal metatarsal a. for the first space and the deep plantar a. which reaches the deep plantar arch.
• The **posterior tibial a.** passes through the tarsal tunnel where it divides into a medial plantar a. and a lateral plantar a. The medial plantar a. divides into branches for the first, second and third interdigital spaces and the hallux at the level of the base of the first metatarsal bone. Sometimes it forms a superficial plantar arch. The lateral plantar a. becomes the deep plantar arch which gives off the plantar metatarsal aa.
• The **fibular (peroneal) a.** reaches the foot at the level of the posterior surface of the tibiofibular syndesmosis and is distributed in the postero-lateral zone of the ankle. It sends an anterior branch perforating the interosseous membrane which anastomoses with the anterior lateral malleolar branch of the anterior tibial a.

The venous circulation includes a deep and a superficial network. The deep network resembles the arterial one. The superficial network supplies the cellular subcutaneous tissues and is gathered into the saphenous vein.

The great saphenous vein is the medial marginal v. in front of the medial malleolus. It ascends on the medial surface of the leg and ends in the femoral v. The small saphenous v. travels as the lateral marginal v. back to the lateral malleolus. It ascends lateral to the calcaneal tendon and ends in the popliteal v. in the popliteal fossa.

Bursae and synovial tendon sheaths

Calcaneal area

In front of the calcaneal tendon there are two connective tissue bursae which are not connected. The first is rudimentary, above the calcaneus, formed by a cellulo-fatty tissue. The other is lower, localized in the achilleo-calcaneal space between the anterior aspect of the tendon and the postero-superior tuberosity of the calcaneus which is outflanked by the bursa for about 8 to 10 mm. It is formed of a very differentiated connective tissue, identical to synovium. These bursae fill the empty space which appears when the calcaneus is elevated by the tendon of the triceps surae muscle. In the inferior calcaneal zone, between the deep subcutaneous layer and the aponeurosis, opposite the medial process of the tuberosity of the calcaneus, there may also be some bursal tissue.

Retromalleolar area (figs. 1.12 & 1.13)

In the lateral retromalleolar area, the tendons of the fibular muscles have a common sheath; then progressively, in the lateral submalleolar area, the two tendons separate and each has its own sheath.

On the medial side, the synovial sheath of the tendon of the tibialis posterior m. begins 7 cm above the upper border of the flexor retinaculum and is prolonged on the medial side of the foot to 1 cm from its navicular insertion. The synovial sheath of the tendon of the flexor hallucis longus m. is the longest, since it goes from the distal insertion of the tendon to the upper edge of the tibio-talo-calcaneal tunnel. The sheath of the tendons of the flexor digitorum longus m. extends from the middle of the sole of the foot to the upper edge of the calcaneal tunnel [18].

The instep

At the anterior aspect of the instep, the reflexions of the tendons of the fibularis tertius m., the extensor

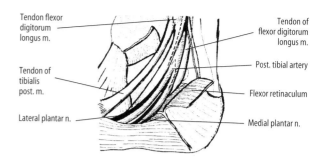

Fig. 1.12. Medial retromalleolar gutter and tarsal tunnel

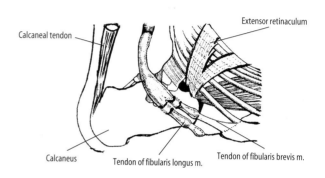

Fig. 1.13. Lateral view of calcaneal canal with fibular tendons

digitorum longus, extensor hallucis longus and tibialis anterior mm. have synovial sheaths and travel in an osteofibrous groove roofed by an extensor retinaculum, arranged transversely in a V or Y shape.

Intercapito-metatarsal spaces

In these spaces, the contact between the metatarsal heads leads to the formation of a bursa. This is the intercapito-metatarsal bursa, which has a sagittal long axis and a vertical small axis. Its general shape is oval. In the normal state, its two surfaces are in contact to allow intermittent gliding between the metatarsal heads.

Adhesion function to the ground

To ensure a better transmission of traction and gliding forces, there exists between the plantar aponeurosis and the deep dermis a vertical septum of connective tissue which strengthens them [17].

Topographic areas

Medial part: tibio-talo-calcaneal or tarsal tunnel (fig. 1.12)

This passage area contains neurovascular and tendinous structures. The upper limit is defined as the area where the tendon of the flexor hallucis longus m. enters into contact with the back of the tibia. The inferior limit corresponds to the inferior edge of the tendon of the abductor hallucis brevis m. The tunnel has 3 segments: the proximal segment corresponds to the posterior surface of the tibia, the intermediate segment is tibio-talar and the distal segment is calcaneal [11].

Proximal segment

In this segment, the structures are arranged in the frontal plane; it has a prismatic triangular form. The anterior bony surface corresponds to the tibial surface, with a well marked gutter for the tendon of the tibialis posterior m. and a less pronounced lateral one for the tendon of the flexor digitorum longus m. The lateral surface is bounded by the medial edge of the calcaneal tendon. The medial subcutaneous surface is closed by a resistant aponeurotic layer formed by the fusion of the superficial and deep leg aponeuroses. Within this space, the tendon of the tibialis posterior m., the tendon of the flexor digitorum longus m., the neurovascular bundle with the posterior tibial artery, vein and nerve, and the tendon of the flexor hallucis longus m. [19] are arranged on the posterior aspect of the tibia, in that order, from medial to lateral side.

Intermediate segment

Relations are chiefly between osseous and ligamentous structures. In front are the posterior surface of the medial malleolus, the medial surface of the talus and the posterior fibers of the tibio-talar ligament. Laterally, we find the adipocellular precalcaneal space and the medial side of the calcaneal tendon. Medially and posteriorly, the retinaculum of the tendons of the flexor mm. ensures stability of the tendons. The neurovascular bundle is in contact with the retinaculum. At this level, the tibial nerve divides into two branches: the lateral and medial plantar nn. All the tendinous and neurovascular structures lie in a posteriorly and laterally oblique plane.

Distal segment

The lateral surface includes: the talus, navicular, sustentaculum tali, calcaneus and deltoid ligament. The antero-superior surface is limited by the medial edge of the sustentaculum tali. The medial surface is in relation with the tendon of the abductor hallucis m. The structures are situated in a sagittal plane.

The tendons are fixed by fibrous septa arising from the intermediate layer of the plantar aponeurosis.

They are, from above to down, the tendon of the tibialis posterior m. facing the talus, the tendon of the flexor digitorum longus m. facing the talocalcaneal articular space, and the tendon of the flexor hallucis longus m. which travels through a groove under the lateral prominence of the sustentaculum tali.

The posterior tibial artery divides into two branches, accompanied by the corresponding plantar nerves. The medial plantar neurovascular bundle is situated between the tendons of the flexor digitorum longus and the tibialis posterior mm. and the lateral plantar bundle above the tendon of the flexor hallucis longus m.

Lateral part: fibular tunnel (fig. 1.13)

The lateral compartment is centered by the passage of the fibularis (peroneus) longus and brevis mm. This area of passage is divided into three parts:
• a lateral supra- and retromalleolar area with the tendon of the fibularis brevis m., which lies against the posterior surface of the fibula and the fibularis longus tendon posteriorly;
• a submalleolar area, where the fibularis brevis tendon changes direction and lies horizontally above the fibularis longus tendon. In this part, the two tendons are plastered against the lateral surface of the calcaneus by their retaining retinaculum;
• in the third or premalleolar part, the fibularis longus tendon crosses the inferior side of the fibularis brevis tendon, which goes toward the posterior edge of the fifth metatarsal tuberosity.

The gliding synovial sheath of the tendons of the fibular muscles

The sheath of the tendon of the fibularis longus m. is localized in the mid-plantar and latero-plantar areas. Behind and below the lateral malleolus it is the same as that of the tendon of the fibularis brevis m. The group of fibular muscle sheaths forms an inverted Y with the stem situated below the retromalleolar part. The sheath of the tendon of fibularis brevis extends toward the dorsal and lateral surfaces of the foot.

Intercapito-metatarsal space

This is situated at the level of the metatarsal heads, with a plantar floor and a dorsal roof.

The mechanical work of each metatarsal head is facilitated by the presence of a gliding connective tissue bursa: the intercapito-metatarsal bursa. The plantar or intercapito-metatarsal fibrous canal is limited above by the transverse intercapito-metatarsal ligament and below by the transverse fibers of the superficial plantar aponeurosis, and the interdigital ligament.

The subtendinous flexor sheaths send two lateral strips at the level of each metatarsophalangeal joint, which pass sagittally on either side of the flexor tendons, perforate the transverse intermetatarsal ligament, and end on the dorsal fascia. These fibers, constituting the lateral walls of the intercapito-metatarsal fibrous tunnel, form between them two kinds of transverse fibrous arches. The digital arches are situated below each metatarsophalangeal joint, in close contact with the corresponding flexor tendon. The interdigital arches, between the preceding arches, form the floor of the fibrous canals.

The anterior edge of the transverse intermetatarsal ligament is situated about 5 mm behind the metatarsophalangeal joint, while the posterior edge of the interdigital ligament projects about 8 to 10 mm in front of the joint. The bifurcation of the common plantar digital nerve into collateral nerves is always accomplished in front of the anterior edge of the transverse intermetatarsal ligaments of the second, third and fourth spaces, at a variable distance of about 5 to 10 mm. Most often, the interdigital n. crosses the anterior edge of the intermetatarsal ligament, behind the metatarsophalangeal joint, and then bifurcates into collateral nerves which cross in front of the joint, the posterior edge and then the deep surface of the interdigital ligament.

In each of these canals, after removal of the corresponding fat pad, the plantar neurovascular bundle and the lumbrical m. may be observed. The plantar metatarsal arteries, which after division give off the proper digital aa. for the toes, arise from the deep plantar arch and pass under the transverse ligament. The satellite artery is situated over this nerve.

There are four lumbrical muscles. Their origins are from the tendons of the flexor digitorum longus m. These muscles are more superficial than the transverse metatarsal ligament, which separates them from the interosseous mm. In the dorsal floor, over the transverse intermetatarsal ligament, there is a bursa which allows gliding and intermittent contact between the metatarsal heads (intermetatarso-phalangeal bursa).

References

1. Bo WJ, Wolfman N, Krueger WA, Meschan I (1989) Basic Atlas of Cross Sectional Anatomy - A Clinical Approach, 2nd edn. W.B. Saunders, Philadelphia
2. Brizon L, Castaing P (1970) Feuillets d'Anatomie IV. Maloine, Paris, pp 38-40
3. Cook JM, Galorenzo R, Gold RH (1981) Lisfranc's joint dislocation: a review and case report. J Am Podiatr Assoc 71 : 611
4. Crafts RC (1985) Textbook of Human Anatomy, 3rd edn. Wiley, New York,
5. Crouch JE (1985) Functional Human Anatomy, 4th edn. Lea Febiger, Philadelphia
6. Daseler ED, Anson BJ (1943) The plantaris muscle : An anatomical study of 750 specimens. J Bone Joint Surg 25 : 82
7. Draves DJ (1986) Anatomy of the Lower Extremity. Williams et Wilkins, Baltimore
8. Elftman H (1934) A cinematic study of the distribution of pressure in the human foot. Anat Rec 59 : 481
9. Ferguson AB (1932) A rare accessory bone of the foot. J Bone Joint Surg 14 : 382
10. Hamilton WJ (1976) Texbook of Human Anatomy, 2nd edn. Mosby Co, St. Louis
11. Kuritz HM, Sokolof TH (1975) Tarsal tunnel syndrome. J Am Podiatr Assoc 65 : 825
12. Mc Carthy DJ, Grode S (1980) The anatomical characteristics of the first metatarsophalangeal joint. J Am Podiatr Assoc 70 : 493
13. Mc Carthy DJ, Saunders MM, Herzberc AJ (1983) The surgical anatomy of the rearfoot : part 1, the greater tarsus. J Am Podiatr Assoc 73 : 607
14. Rouvière H (1977) Anatomie Humaine, tome 3. Masson, Paris, pp 439-440
15. Sarrafian SK (1983) Anatomy of the Foot and Ankle. JB Lippincott, Philadelphia
16. Sawyna CJ, Diemer J, Rubinlicht J (1981) Unilateral Chopart's joint subluxation. J Am Podiatr Assoc 71 : 512
17. Testut L (1931) Traité d'Anatomie Humaine, 3e edn. Doin, Paris
18. Warwick R, Williams P (1973) Gross Anatomy, 36th edn. WB Saunders Co, Philadelphia
19. Williams L, Warwick R (eds) (1980) : Gray's Anatomy, 36th British edn. Churchill Livingstone, Edinburgh
20. Yale JF (1973) Surgical and biomechanical approach to the talonavicular joint. J Am Podiatr Assoc 63: 247

2.

Clinical examination of the foot and ankle

C Frey

The clinical examination of the foot and ankle should begin with an evaluation of the entire musculoskeletal system for systemic and general conditions which can affect the foot and ankle. The function and structure of the foot and ankle may then be evaluated using observation, palpation, and manipulation. When performing the physical examination, the practitioner should be systematic and follow a routine. Furthermore, the foot should be evaluated as part of the entire body, as part of the locomotor system, and during unloaded and loaded conditions.

The examination of the foot should begin with observation of the color, turgor, moisture, appearance, hair distribution, and any calluses present on the skin (fig. 2.1). Note should be made of any vari-

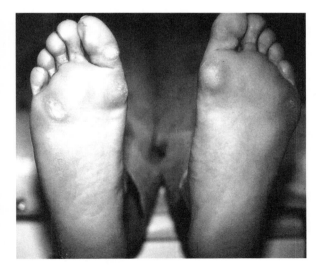

Fig. 2.1. Examination of the foot and ankle should begin with observation of the color, turgor, moisture, appearance, hair distribution and any calluses present on the skin

cosities, swelling or induration. The nails should be examined for thickness, color, quality, and whether or not they are ingrown.

Palpation of the foot should note areas of swelling, induration, warmth, crepitus, bony prominence and condition of the fat pads. Temperature can be evaluated by moving the back of the examiner's hand over the surface of the skin. The skin surface is usually cooler over a joint than over muscles [3]. Palpation should be performed on the anterior tibial artery which is located lateral to the extensor hallucis longus and the posterior tibial artery, which is located just posterior to the tibialis posterior and flexor digitorum longus tendons. The capillary refill after compressing a nail-bed should be noted. Palpation of the nerves in the foot should include the posterior tibial (in the tarsal tunnel), deep fibular, superficial fibular, sural, saphenous, and interdigital nerves to determine if there is any tenderness, hypersensitivity, or mass present. Sensation should be evaluated for light touch, pinprick and vibratory sensation.

The examination of the bones, joints, ligaments and tendons begins with the establishment of the neutral position (the position in which the talonavicular joint is congruous). This examination can be accomplished with the patient sitting on the examination table with the knees flexed at 90°, or with the patient prone with knees flexed at 90°. The foot is positioned into neutral by palpating the talonavicular joint with the thumb and with the other hand manipulating the distal structures until the navicular and the talus are congruous. Normally, the weight-bearing line will pass through the second metatarsal, with the foot being neither abducted or adducted.

The relationship of the forefoot to the hindfoot is then noted. The examiner can now determine if there is forefoot varus (lateral border of foot is more plantarflexed), forefoot valgus (medial border of the foot is more plantarflexed), or if the forefoot is neutral in relation to the calcaneus. This relationship between the forefoot and hindfoot may be flexible or rigid. A fixed varus or valgus of the forefoot will cause the foot not to be plantigrade when the hindfoot is made neutral.

Passive and active range of motion (ROM) is evaluated beginning with the neutral position. Active ROM is evaluated when the patient actively contracts the muscles. The motion that occurs during this should be evaluated and compared to the passive ROM. Muscle strength and possible presence of pain produced are evaluated when active motion is performed by individual muscles (table 2.1).

The transverse midtarsal joint is evaluated by moving the forefoot into adduction and abduction while holding the calcaneus in neutral. The normal finding is that adduction has twice the range of abduction. Forefoot inversion and eversion motion in the frontal plane should be equal (fig. 2.2).

Table 2.1. The extrinsic and intrinsic muscles of the foot

Muscles	Function
Extrinsic muscles	
tibialis anterior	dorsiflexion, adduction, inversion of the foot
extensor hallucis longus	extension at the distal phalanx of the great toe
extensor digitorum longus	extension of the lesser toes
fibularis tertius	dorsiflexion and eversion of the foot
gastrocnemius/soleus	plantarflexion of foot
flexor hallucis longus	flexion of the terminal phalanx of the great toe
flexor digitorum longus	flexion of the terminal phalanges of the lesser toes
tibialis posterior	adduction, inversion and plantarflexion of the foot
fibularis longus	abduction and eversion of the foot and plantarflexion of the first metatarsal
fibularis brevis	eversion, abduction and plantarflexion of the foot
Intrinsic muscles	
extensor hallucis brevis	extension of the great toe from the base of the proximal phalanx
extensor digitorum brevis	extension of the lesser toes 2-4, abduction and flexion of the great toe
flexor digitorum brevis	flexion at the proximal interphalangeal (PIP) joints of the small toes
abductor digiti minimi	abduction and flexion of the little toe
quadratus plantae	adjusts the alignment of the flexor digitorum longus joint to the long axes of the phalanges
lumbricals	flexion at the metatarsophalangeal joints and extension of the interphalangeal joints of the lesser toes
flexor hallucis brevis	flexion at the proximal phalanx of the great toe
adductor hallucis	adduction of the great toe and flexion at the metatarsophalangeal joint
flexor digiti minimi	flexion of the little toe at the metatarsophalangeal joint
plantar interossei	adduction of the lesser toes towards the second toe, flexion of the lesser toes at the metatarsophalangeal joints and extension at the PIP joints
dorsal interossei	abduction of the lesser toes from the line of the second toe, flexion of the lesser toes at the metatarsophalangeal joints and extension at the PIP joints

SUPINATION   PRONATION

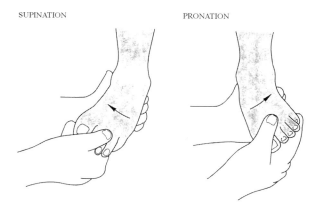

Fig. 2.2. The transverse midtarsal joint: the normal finding is that adduction has twice the range as abduction. Forefoot inversion and eversion in the frontal plane should be equal

The amount of subtalar motion may vary. Generally, the heel can be everted and inverted with inversion two to three times greater than eversion. Although 10° of eversion and 20° of inversion are commonly thought of as average, Isman et al found a range of 20-60° of subtalar motion in cadavers [2].

The motion may be evaluated by rotating the heel and allowing the rest of the foot to move passively. Subtalar joint motion may be examined with the patient sitting on the examination table and

the leg over the side. The examination should begin with the calcaneus in line with the tibia. The heel is then everted and inverted (fig. 2.3).

The position of the first metatarsal is evaluated by placing one thumb beneath the first metatarsal and the other thumb beneath the lateral four metatarsals. If the first metatarsal is in line with the others, it is in the normal position. If it is not, it may be abnormally plantar- or dorsiflexed. Normal motion of the first metatarsal at the tarsometatarsal joint is equal in dorsi- and plantarflexion from the neutrally aligned position.

The toes are examined for position and motion. With a normal foot, the toes will be straight. There will be no contracture of any of the joints and they are supple. The metatarsophalangeal joint of the great toe has dorsiflexion to about 80-90° and plantarflexion to about 45°. Interphalangeal joint motion of the great toe is 0-90°. The metatarsophalangeal joints of toes 2-5 move between about 90° of dorsiflexion and about 45° of plantarflexion with individual variations (fig. 2.4). ROM of the interphalangeal joints is also variable and should be comparable to the other foot [1].

The windlass mechanism of the plantar fascia is evaluated by dorsiflexing the toes. This action usually increases the tension through the plantar fascia and causes the medial longitudinal arch to

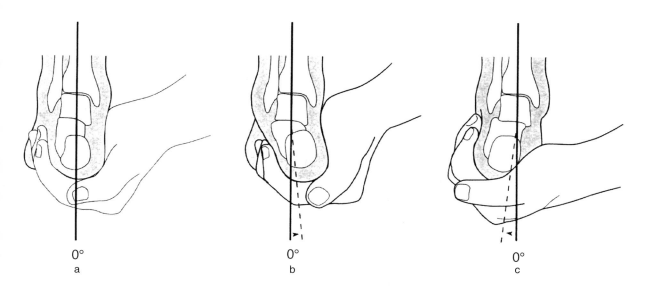

0°   0°   0°
a   b   c

Fig. 2.3. a Subtalar joint motion is evaluated by rotating the heel and allowing the rest of the foot to move passively. This can be done with the patient prone and the knee flexed to 90° (as in this figure) or with the patient sitting on the examination table and the knee flexed to 90°. **b** Inversion and **c** eversion. The amount of subtalar motion may vary. Generally, the range of inversion is two to three times that of eversion

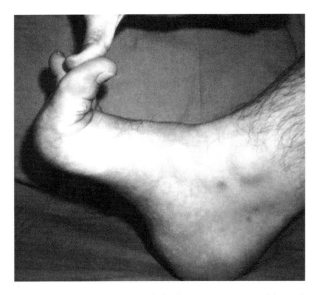

Fig. 2.4. Range of motion of the lesser toes is variable and should be compared to the opposite foot

rise. Chronic and severe pes planus may cause the mechanism to be disrupted (fig. 2.4).

The ankle joint is a single axis joint having approximately 20° of extension and 50° of flexion (fig. 2.5). The axis of the talocrural joint can be approximated by palpating the distal aspects of the medial and lateral malleoli. Depending on the axis, dorsiflexion and plantarflexion may cause some lateral or medial deviation of the foot. The extension should be performed with the knee flexed and extended to determine the effect of the triceps surae on the range of ankle dorsiflexion (fig. 2.5).

The ligaments of the ankle, the deltoid, anterior talofibular ligament (ATFL), calcaneofibular ligament (CFL) and syndesmosis should be palpated for tenderness and evaluated for laxity. One should keep in mind that the position of the ankle influences the results of laxity tests. In plantarflexion, more stress is placed on the ATFL and in dorsiflexion more stress is placed on the CFL. The most common clin-

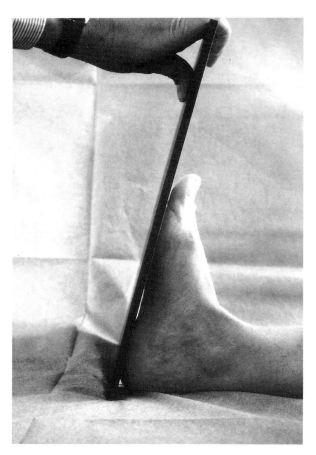

a

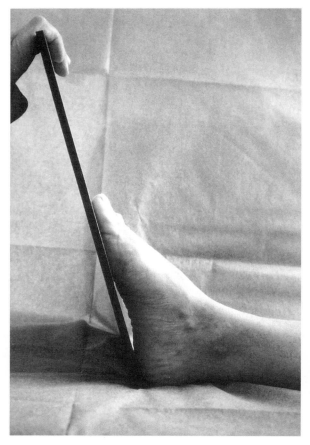

Fig. 2.5. Range of motion of the ankle joints; **a** extension, approximately 20°; **b** flexion, approximately 50°

ical test for ankle laxity is the anterior drawer test, which is performed with the ankle in plantarflexion. The tibia is stabilized and the talus is pushed forward. Another method of performing this test involves stabilising the foot in one hand and pushing the tibia posteriorly with the other. Anterior subluxation of the talus in the mortice is consistent with laxity or rupture of the ATFL.

Clinical evaluation of the injured ankle should also include a varus stress test. This test should be performed on both the injured and uninjured ankles, with the foot held in neutral position. Significant differences between the two sides indicates a possible injury to the CFL [4].

The syndesmosis can be evaluated by comparing posterior displacement of the fibula. Normally there is some displacement but this may be increased with a syndesmosis injury (especially compared to the uninjured side) and the movement will elicit pain.

The relationship of the foot and ankle to the remainder of the lower extremity and trunk should be determined. In weight-bearing, the axis of the lower limb may be compared to the hindfoot axis, which may be in varus-inversion (fig. 2.6) or valgus-eversion (fig. 2.7). The relative alignment of the leg, thigh, hip and knee joints must be evaluated as well as their ranges of motion. Clinical leg lengths should be measured. These factors are important to determine how the foot functions throughout gait.

Finally, the gait is observed with and without shoes. The patient should be evaluated walking to and from the examiner. The gait can be correlated with earlier physical findings. During the early part of the stance phase in the normal foot, the heel everts and the foot becomes supple. Later, in stance and with toe-off, the foot converts to a rigid lever with heel inversion. A limp may be observed which can represent and be characteristic of specific pathologic disorders.

The shoulders usually rotate 180° out of phase with the pelvis. There should be a symmetric arm swing. If symmetry is not noted, this may be because lesions in the lower extremities have upset pelvic rotation.

During gait, the heel should strike the ground first. The foot should be flat on the ground after 7% of the gait cycle. Heel-rise should begin at about 35% into the cycle, at the time that the opposite leg is swinging through [3]. During the swing phase, the leg and foot internally rotate about 15°. At heel-strike the foot should follow the line of progression and at

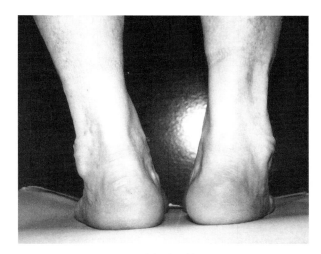

Fig. 2.6. Varus-inversion of the hindfoot

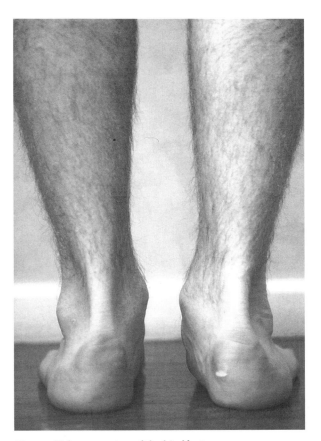

Fig. 2.7. Valgus-eversion of the hindfoot

toe-off the foot and leg are somewhat externally rotated. Normal variations in this pattern may be observed, but the pattern should essentially be as described above. During the first half of stance the hindfoot will evert to varying degrees. It is important to note whether the heel inverts at heel-rise as it should. If the patient's foot remains in eversion with heel-rise this may indicate pathology of the tendon of the tibialis posterior muscle.

Leg lengths may be evaluated by looking for pelvic tilt. This is done by having the patient stand with his back to the examiner. The examiner places his index fingers on the iliac crests and observes the gluteal folds. Both of these anatomic landmarks should be level. Any leg length inequality is evidenced if they are not level.

The patient's shoes should be evaluated and can often give clues to gait patterns and pathology. Wear patterns on the bottom of the shoe can indicate areas of weight-bearing and slippage. Wear patterns on the inner sole (sock liner) of the shoe can indicate areas of increased pressure and bony prominence. Wear patterns on the upper of the shoe may indicate poor fit or bony prominence. The examiner may place the shoes on a table and look at them from behind. If the shoes roll in or out too much without the patient in them, this may indicate excessive pronation or supination with a resultant wearing-down of the heel counter.

References

1. Heck CV, Hendryson IE, Rowe RC (1965) Joint Motion: Method of Measuring and Recording. American Academy of Orthopaedic Surgeons, Chicago, Illinois
2. Isman RE, Inmann VT (1969) Anthropometric studies of the human foot and ankle. Bull Prosthet Res 10-11:97
3. Mann R (1993) Principles of examination of the foot and ankle. In Mann R, Coughlin M (ed) Surgery of the Foot and Ankle. Mosby Yearbook Inc, St Louis
4. Ouzounian T (1993) Ankle instability. In: Frey C, Pfeffer G (eds) Current Practice in Foot and Ankle Surgery. Mac Graw-Hill Inc., New-York

3.

Radiography of the foot

M Bouysset and T Tavernier

As a basic additional examination in foot pathology, radiography allows us to analyse the bone structure and to identify possible deformations. As anatomic and biomechanic knowledge allows better diagnostic interpretation of the X-ray, so treatment becomes more appropriate. The following text merely sets out some essential notions about the subject and cannot take the place of more detailed presentations [9, 12].

In foot pathology many radiographic views are made in weight-bearing. Some authors emphasize two points: on the one hand, the patient must stand in the angle of gait (the angle formed between the axis of the foot and the direction of walking, generally 10 to 15° of external rotation); on the other hand, the conventional distance between the right and left medial malleoli during walking must be respected (approximately 5 cm), which is the basis of gait [6, 10, 11, 16].

● Radiographic views of the foot

Three basic views in weight-bearing must be considered [4, 8, 9, 12].
• **The dorso-plantar view** mainly displays the metatarsal bones (shafts and heads), phalanges and forefoot deformation.
• **The lateral view** emphasizes the first metatarsal bone, medial tarsus, calcaneus and profile of the ankle; most of the cuboid can be seen. Data concerning static disorders of the foot are given.

These last two views are easy to perform and are important for evaluation of biomechanic disorders of the foot [20].
• **The anteroposterior (frontal view of the ankle)** evaluates the talocrural structures. Metal markers allow assessment of hindfoot valgus but accurate performance of this view seems to be difficult and inconstant (see below) [8].

This radiographic evaluation must generally be bilateral.

Some supplementary views may be useful and easy to perform in current practice: they are made in the weight-bearing or non-weight-bearing position:
• **lateral oblique view** of the foot, which gives a better evaluation of the tarsus than the views already described;
• **axial sesamoid view** in non-weight-bearing, which demonstrates the sesamoid bones and plantar aspect of the metatarsal bones, or in weight-bearing which in addition evaluates asymmetric sesamoid bones.

The advantages of many other radiographic views have decreased since the common use of CT [5]; some of them are described in the chapters of pathology.

● Angular and axial relationships of the foot

The measurement of radiographic angles clarifies the relationships between some of the bones. Some examples are presented here of weight-bearing dorso-plantar and lateral views of the foot and the frontal view of the ankle. Some faults are due to technical errors in measurement; in other cases, it is the positioning of the patient during projection which produces faults and care is required when interpreting the results obtained, which differ with varied positioning of the foot [10, 18]. For instance, flexing the weight-bearing knee with internal rotation of the trunk and leg causes depression of the medial arch height of 7.5 mm [18]; indeed, this last position is not rare in pathology, particularly in rheumatoid patients with an involved knee. Another example of an error may be cited: for a foot in weight-bearing in lateral view, if the values of the talar pitch (declination of the talus) in different positions are compared, this decreases by 6 to 8° in supination and increases by 12 to 14° in pronation (the neutral position of the subtalar joint is the one from which there is one-third of the total range of the joint in the direction of pronation and two-thirds of the total range in the direction of supination) [1, 10]. These remarks stress the importance of a permanent clinical and radiologic confrontation that must be kept in mind.

Dorsoplantar view in weight-bearing

• The hallux abductus angle is the one formed by the axis of the first phallanx and the axis of the first metatarsal (mean value 8 to 12°) (fig. 3.1).
• The intermetatarsal angle (metatarsus primus adductus, M1M2 angle) is defined by bisection of the first and second metatarsals (mean value 5°) (fig. 3.1).
• The angle defined by the axes of the first and fifth metatarsals evaluates the spreading of the forefoot (mean value 15-20°) (fig. 3.1).

Lateral view in weight-bearing

• First metatarsal pitch: this is formed between the axis of the first metatarsal (line parallel to the upper cortical surface passing through the center of the first metatarsal head) and the surface of support (fig. 3.2) (mean 18-25°) [12, 14];
• talar pitch [1]: this is the angle between the axis of the talus and the horizontal created by contact of the foot with the ground (mean value 20 to 25°) (fig. 3.3) [10, 12];
• the talo-naviculo-cuneo-metatarsal line is observed by means of several references, particularly the line of Meary (fig. 3.4) and the line of Schade: the first metatarsal pitch and the talar pitch are normally joined and define the line of Meary. In a flat foot these two pitches form an angle open upward; there is a cavus angle when the two pitches determine an angle open downward. These angles are difficult to define when flat or cavus deviations are minor (angles less than 5°) (fig. 3.4) [2, 12];
• calcaneal pitch (fig. 3.5): the antero-inferior and lowest points of the calcaneus are used to form a line which, with the horizontal, defines the calcaneal pitch. This angle is high if over 30°, medium if between 20° and 30°, and low if between 10 and 20° [1, 9];
• Boehler's angle (fig. 3.6) is formed by two lines: the first is defined by the highest anterior and posterior points of the articular surface of the calcaneus; the second is defined by the upper anterior and posterior points of the calcaneal tuberosity (normally 25 to 40°) [11, 12];

• the medial arch angle [8] is formed by the intersection of two lines: the first joins the inferior pole of the medial sesamoid and the lowest point of the talonavicular joint; the second is formed by joining

---

Fig. 3.1. Forefoot angles. M1P1: hallux abductus angle (mean 8-12°), M1M2: intermetatarsal angle (mean 5°), M1M5: angle between first and fifth metatarsals (mean 15-20°)

Fig. 3.2. First metatarsal pitch (mean 18-25°)

Fig. 3.3. Talar pitch (mean 20-25°)

Fig. 3.4. Talo-naviculo-cuneo-metatarsal line

Fig. 3.5. Calcaneal pitch (mean 20-30°)

Fig. 3.6. Boehler's angle (mean 25-40°)

Fig. 3.7. Medial arch angle (mean 120-130°)

Fig. 3.8. Talocrural joint, frontal view with metal markers on the ground

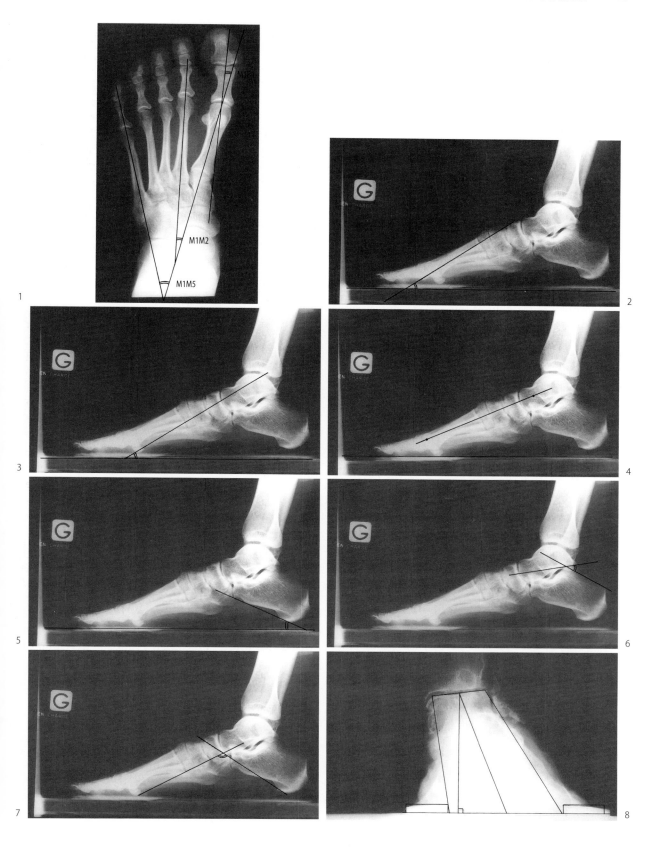

this and the lowest point of the calcaneus. If this angle exceeds 130° the foot is rather flat, and below 120° the foot is rather cavus (fig. 3.7) [2, 8].

Frontal view of the ankle, calcaneal deviation in the frontal plane: measurement

To determine calcaneal deviation by radiograph, metal markers are placed on the ground against the skin, over the inner and outer borders of the heel, and perpendicular to the malleoli. The incident beam passes horizontally in the axis of the fourth metatarsal with the patient standing in weight-bearing on both feet. It is now possible to construct the weight-bearing quadrilateral of the foot, which is defined by four points: the upper medial border of the talus, the upper lateral border of the talus and the inner and outer borders of the skin of the heel in contact with the ground. The axis passing through the middle of the bases makes an angle V with the vertical which allows us to determine the calcaneal valgus (fig. 3.8) [8]. For precise measurement, the direction of the incident beam should be in line with the anteroposterior axis of the calcaneus. The axis of the fourth metatarsal is usually also a reference. In theory, as these two axes do not always correspond, load-bearing bifocal (double exposure) radiography of the entire foot should first be carried out, to determine the calcaneal axis. The direction of the incident beam will thus be defined by the direction of the metatarsal, which is the same as the calcaneal axis [3, 8].

Meary's method

It uses a plumbline around the heel [12]. A radio-transparent heel lift (3-4 cm) is used. The tibial axis normally passes at the junction (N) between the medial 1/3 and lateral 2/3 of the weight-bearing area (defined by the horizontal part of the plumbline under the heel). When the tibial axis passes medial to the N point there is a calcaneal valgus; when the tibial axis passes lateral to the N point there is calcaneal varus (fig. 3.9).

Load-bearing bifocal radiography of the entire foot

This view displays the forefoot and the posterior part of the tarsus in the same radiograph. However, this

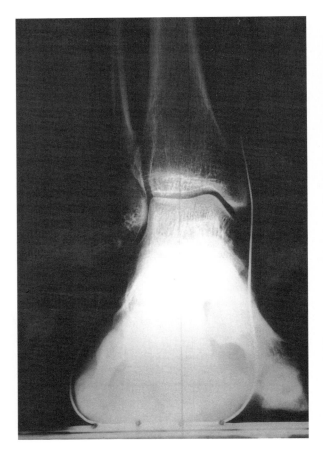

Fig. 3.9. Talocrural joint, frontal view with plumbline around the heel (Meary's method)

procedure appears difficult to perform in practice [7, 10]. Faults in measurement are therefore possible. Moreover, this view inevitably shows a distorted appearance of the posterior tarsus [12]. The main advantage of this view is to pinpoint the axis of the calcaneus in relation to the different metatarsal axes (cf above) and to allow measurement of the angle between the axis of the talus and that of the calcaneus, which is the angle of medial deviation of the neck of the talus (mean value 15 to 25°).

References

1. Altman MI, D.P.M (1968) Sagittal Plane Angles of the Talus and Calcaneus in the Developing Foot. J Am Podiatr Assoc 58: 463-470
2. Bouysset M, Bonvoisin B, Lepiller Ph, Schnepp J, Lejeune E, Bouvier M (1984) Empreinte plantaire encrée et profil radiologique du pied dans la polyarthrite rhumatoide. Lyon Médical 251: 497-501

3. Bouysset M, Bonvoisin B, Lejeune E, Bouvier M (1987) Flattening of the rheumatoid foot in tarsal arthritis on X-ray. Scand J Rheumatol 16: 127-133

4. Braun S (1993) Mesures utiles de la clinique à la radiologie. Rhumatologie pratique.103: 1-4

5. Chemla N, Chevrot A, Langer-Cherbit A, Vacherot B, Dupont AM, Godefroy D (1994) L'exploration radiologique standard. In: Hérisson C, Borderie P, Simon L (eds). La pathologie de l'articulation sous-astragalienne. Monographies de Podologie 15. Masson, Paris, pp 14-29

6. Christman RA (1991) Radiology. In: Kominsky SJ (ed) Yearbook of podiatric medicine and surgery. Mosby-Year Book, Saint louis, p 241

7. DiGiovanni JE, Smith SD (1976) Normal Biomechanics of the Adult Rearfoot: a Radiographic Analysis. J Am Podiatr Assoc 66: 812-824

8. Djian A, Annonier Cl, Denis A et Baudoin P (1967) Radiopodométrie (principes et résultats). Société Française d'Électroradiologie Médicale, pp 769-772

9. Gamble FO, Yale I (1966) Clinical Foot Roentgenology. Williams & Wilkins, Baltimore, pp 151-160, 163-183 & 246-252

10. Hlavac HF (1967) Differences in X-ray Findings with Varied Positioning of the Foot. J Am Podiatr Assoc 57: 465-471

11. Johnson RE (1991) Podiatric radiology. In: Leonard A, Levy (eds) Principles and pratice of podiatric medicine. Churchill Livingstone, New-York, pp 231-271

12. Montagne J, Chevrot A, Galmiche JM (1980) Techniques radiographiques - repères et mesures. In: Atlas de radiologie du pied. Masson, Paris, pp 44-55

13. Montagne J, Chevrot A, Galmiche JM (1987) Examen radioclinique du pied. Doint, Paris

14. Resnick D (1974) Radiology of the talocalcaneal articulations. Anatomic considerations and Arthrography. Radiology 111: 581-586

15. Schnepp J (1981) Physiologie du pied (remarques et applications pratiques en vue de la médecine et de la chirurgie du pied). In: Claustre J, Simon L (eds) Pied normal et méthodes d'exploration du pied. Masson, Paris, pp27-35.

16. Seltzer SE, Weissman BN, Braunstein EM, Adams DF, Thomas WH (1984) Computed Tomography of the Hindfoot. J Comput Assist Tomogr 8: 488-497

17. Sgarlato TE (1965) The Angle of Gait. J Am Podiatr Assoc 55: 645-650

18. Shereff MJ, Di Giovanni L, Bejjani FJ, Hersh A, Kummer FJ (1991): A comparison of Nonweight-Bearing and Weight-Bearing Radiographs of the Foot. In: Kominsky SJ (ed). The Yearbook of Podiatric Medicine and Surgery. Mosby-Year Book, St Louis, pp 240-241

19. Venning P, Hardy RH (eds) (1951) Sources of error in the production and measurement of standard radiographs of the foot. Br J Radiol 24: 18-26

20. Vito G, Kalish S (1990) Biomechanical radiographic evaluation. In: Donatelli R (ed) The biomechanics of the foot and ankle. F.A Davis, Philadelphia, pp 98-130.

21. Wu KK (1990) Foot orthoses, sport shoes and sports medicine. Williams & Wilkins, Baltimore, 380 p

4.

Sectional imaging of the foot and ankle: CT and MRI

T Tavernier

Sectional imaging, first by computed tomography (CT) and more recently by magnetic resonance imaging (MRI), has proved to be of major importance in diagnostic evaluation of different foot pathologies. The origin of this slice imaging was the conventional tomogram, the indications for which have now almost disappeared.

CT was obviously originally applied to bone pathology, specifically traumatic [7, 11, 26]. Subsequently, it was used for study of the soft tissues (tendons, ligaments, etc.) [14, 19, 34]. The combination of CT and other techniques has contributed to further improvements: CT arthrography for cartilage and ligament studies, CT tenography for tendons and their sheaths. More recently, MRI has been of great help in foot scanning, in bone pathology and particularly in soft tissue pathology, thanks to the fact that MRI provides greater soft tissue contrast than any other imaging modality [12, 13], as well as its potential for multiplanar imaging.

These two techniques each have their advantages and disadvantages and are complementary. Today they are an essential complement to clinical examination and conventional radiography. This chapter has two aims: first, a better understanding of CT and MRI indications by the clinician and second, to assist his interpretation of these examinations.

Techniques and processing of the different examinations

CT [7, 11, 14, 18, 19, 25-28, 34]

First, we have to stress that a good ankle or foot CT scan requires the radiologist to have a precise idea about the pathology to be found and/or the part to be explored. Indeed, as for all osteoarticular pathology, CT of the foot must be done in thin slices and therefore cannot be an exhaustive examination but, on the contrary, focussed and segmental [19]. A detailed and precise report from the clinician as to his questioning and clinical examination is essential before starting the CT procedure.

Position of the patient

The patient is examined in the supine position, with both feet in a symmetric position for bilateral and comparative study. This comparison with the asymptomatic foot is often useful to diagnose obscure pathologies [14] or to differentiate reliably between normal variants and pathologic images.

At least two sectional planes must be performed. In most cases (thoracic, abdominal, pelvic, spinal exploration) the only possible slice plane in CT is the axial plane. In peripheral articulations like the hand and foot it is possible to make CT slices in different anatomic planes and it is useful to take advantage of this. Indeed, some authors perform slices in one plane and make reconstructions in other planes [11, 14, 26]. But such reconstructions, generated from contiguous 2D CT images through the use of computed programs, are less qualitative than slices performed in a similar plane. Therefore, we use them only rarely (for instance when direct sagittal slices

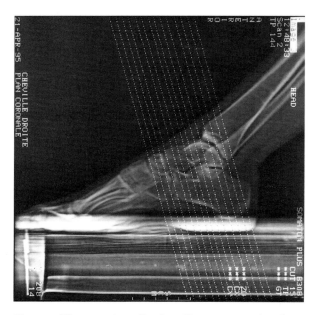

Fig. 4.1. CT scout view allowing slice programming, here oblique coronal slices

are not possible). The two slice planes mostly used are the axial and coronal planes.

• Axial plane (synonym: transverse, horizontal): slices parallel to the sole. Both legs are stretched close together, heels on the table, feet in neutral anatomic position.

• Coronal frontal plane: slices perpendicular to the sole. Knees are bent, close together, soles on the table. In this position the ankles are obviously in extension.

According to the pathology sought and the clinical state of the patient, other slice planes can (more seldom) be performed:

• Sagittal plane: profile slices of ankle or foot. The position is uncomfortable, the patient stands on the table, the examination can only be unilateral.

• Oblique coronal plane: eg., in the long axis of the sinus tarsi, for a better examination of the interosseous talocalcaneal ligament.

• Transverse oblique plane: eg., in the long axis of the calcaneus for a better examination of the talus and talocalcaneal joint.

Slice orientation

Two methods are available to select the slice level to start the examination. A topogram (or scout view) (fig. 4.1), a kind of digitalized foot radiograph made by CT, can be used to orientate slices on the screen. This topogram is especially useful when one wishes to orientate the slices in a particular plane (calcaneal long axis, etc.). Alternatively, if this is not the case, the level of the first slice can be found directly with a light center.

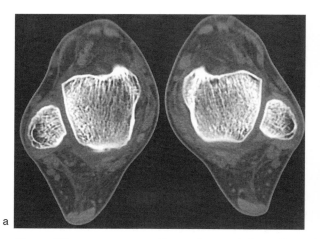
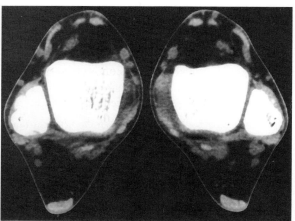

a   b

Fig. 4.2. CT appearances according to chosen window. **a** Bone window, **b** soft tissue window

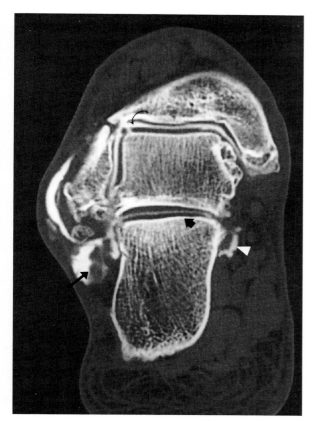

Fig. 4.3. CT arthrography of ankle. Injection into ankle joint shows non-pathologic communications with talocalcanean joint (▶) and flexor hallucis longus tendon sheath (▶). However, communication with the fibular tendon sheath (→) indicates a calcaneofibular ligament rupture. Note cartilage defect of talar dome (⌒)

Technical parameters

Thin slices are absolutely necessary in osteo-articular pathology, especially where the foot is concerned. 1 or 2 mm thick slices are satisfactory. According to the segment to be explored and to the pathology, these slices can be contiguous or spaced (every 3 or 4 mm). Although thick slices (over 3 mm) are often used [11, 14, 26] they reduce spatial resolution, giving an unclear aspect to the anatomic structures.

Double-window examination

CT images are based on a gray range (Hounsfield Units = HU) which can vary in width (W) and level (L) depending on the anatomic structure to be analysed. In the foot, CT slices must be printed both in bone-window (fig. 4.2a) and in soft tissue window (fig. 4.2b).

The bone-window (W = 1400 to 4000 HU, L = 150-400 HU) is indicated for all bone pathology (traumatic, degenerative, tumoral, inflammatory or infectious).

The soft tissue window (W = 150 to 300 HU, L = 10 to 60 HU) is suitable for all ligament, tendon and muscle pathology.

Contrast agent

The contrast agent used in CT is an iodized product. It can be used in different ways.

Intravenous injection

The iodized agent used intravenously increases the contrast of all vascular or highly vascularized structures. It is useful in tumoral, infectious or, to a lesser extent, inflammatory pathology. In standard foot pathology, indications are rare.

Intra-articular injections, CT arthrography (fig. 4.3)

Injection can be done either into the ankle joint, or more rarely into the talocalcaneal joint. This can be done either in the radiography room under scopic control, or directly on the CT table, always under strict asepsis. The main CT arthrography indications are for traumatic ligamentous lesions and cartilage examination.

Injections into tendonous sheaths, CT tenography (fig. 4.4)

CT tenography always follows standard tenography. The main indications [18, 19, 34] are mechanical or inflammatory tenosynovitis and longitudinal splitting of the tendons.

3D CT

Some CT scans, more particularly the latest CT scans called continuous rotation scanning, allow tridimensional image reconstruction. These only concern bone. They are recommended by some authors [1] for particular conditions such as calcaneal fractures.

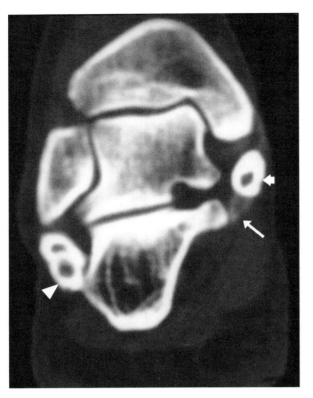

Fig. 4.4. CT tenography of tibialis posterior tendon sheath (⬦), flexor digitorum longus tendon sheath (→) and fibular tendons sheath (▶)

MRI

[2, 5, 6, 9, 10 ,15, 16, 18, 20, 21, 23, 29-31]

As for CT, MRI of the foot is a segmental examination which must be guided by the clinical examination for the best use of the technique. Indeed, as will be shown, the results will be quite different according to the surface to be explored and the pathology sought, the patient's position, the surface coil, the choice of sequences and many acquisition parameters.

Position of the patient

• Unlike CT, it is not necessary to change the foot position during the examination to change the slice plane. Indeed, MRI, as a multiplanar technique, permits slices in all planes. The patient is examined in a supine position, the foot or feet to be explored in neutral position (about 90° between the long axis of the leg and the long axis of the foot). Unlike CT, MRI allows coronal slices of the ankle in the neutral position (without extension).

• Comparative study. As for CT, the comparative study of both feet is often used but less routinely.

• Surface coil. This is essential for a useful examination of the foot. It is a radio-frequency coil located near the scanned structure in order to improve the

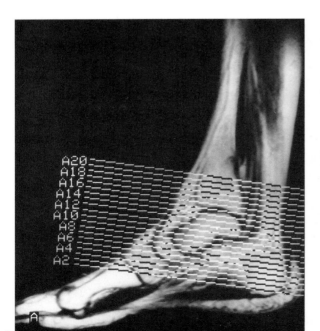

a

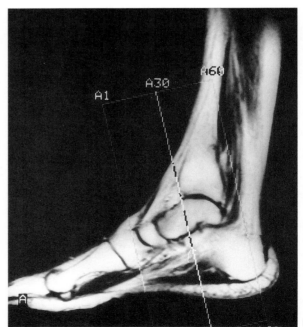

b

Fig. 4.5. Scout view. **a** Axial slice. **b** Coronal slices. Slice planes are slightly angled to be more perpendicular to tendons in the retromalleolar region

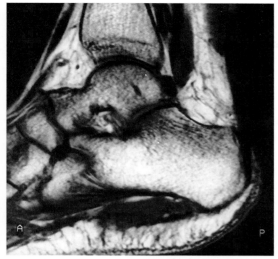

a

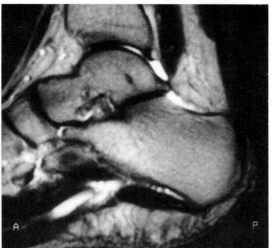

b

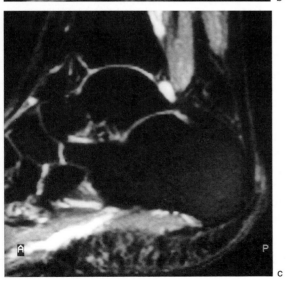

c

Fig. 4.6. Illustration of the main sequences used in MRI. **a** T1-weighted image, **b** T2-weighted image, **c** STIR-weighted image

image quality (increase in the signal-to-noise ratio, S/N). Its size is proportional to the size of the zone to be investigated. The surface coil will be small for unilateral exploration, bigger for bilateral comparative examination. In this case, it is best is to use a head coil.

Slice planes

At least two slice planes will be performed: the axial and sagittal planes are those most commonly used by some authors [29]. We also use many coronal slice planes, but for tendon exploration, we use axial oblique and coronal oblique planes (fig. 4.5) in order to have a more perpendicular position to the long axis of the tendons in the submalleolar regions, favourite sites of tendinous pathologies. The coronal oblique plane proves very valuable in studying the calcaneofibular ligament and talocalcanean joint.

Technical parameters

For MR imaging, the selection of technical parameters is of major importance. For the foot, spatial resolution (clearness and accuracy of images) must be preferred, while keeping a sufficient S/N ratio. With a too low S/N ratio, the slices are less contrasted and "noisy".
• Acquisition field of view (FOV): This must be small, between 10 and 15 cm for a unilateral study and between 18 and 24 cm for a bilateral study.
• Matrix: high resolution matrix: 256 × 256 or even sometimes 512 × 512.
• Slice thickness: thin slices, from 3 to 5 mm routinely. Much thinner slices can be performed (0.5 to 1 mm) by using sequences called "volumic" but to the detriment of other advantages (worse S/N for instance).

Sequences

Contrary to CT, MRI is a multiparameter technique. That is to say that, according to the choice of some technical parameters (repetition time TR, echo-time TE, inversion time TI), the images obtained will be totally different, especially of tissue structure signals. The information obtained from different sequences are different and generally complementary. They are mainly three (fig. 4.6):
• T1-weighted sequence (fig. 4.6 a) gives anatomic images. Fluid is in low signal intensity (black) and fat in high signal intensity (white). For the foot,

tissue contrast is excellent between fat (high signal) and ligaments or tendons (low signal).

• T2-weighted sequence (fig. 4.6b) gives images of lower quality but often supplies more information about pathology, especially for soft tissues (muscles, ligaments, tendons).

Fluid is in high signal; fat has a decreasing signal and appears in low or intermediate signal (gray).

• STIR-weighted sequence (fig. 4.6c), or other fat-suppression techniques. The fat signal is suppressed. These sequences are used in some particular cases, notably for examining bone-marrow pathology and articular cartilage.

Contrast agent

The contrast agent used in MRI is gadolinium (gado-pentetate dimeglumine), intravenously injected. Its influence on the tissue signal is essentially visible on T1-weighted sequences. As for the iodized contrast agent used in CT scan, gadolinium enables us to increase the signal of vessels and highly vascularized tissues. It is also used for tumoral or inflammatory pathology, and for all traumatic muscular, tendinous or ligamentous pathology. Some authors, especially American [4], perform MR arthrography after diluted intra-articular gadolinium injection, although the marketing of gadolinium as an intra-articular contrast material is not yet authorized.

● Normal CT and MR images of the foot and ankle

[6, 17, 19, 22]

CT

All slices presented here have been made with a Siemens Somatom Plus Scanner, with a 2 mm slice thickness. We only deal with soft tissue windows, which are the most difficult to interpret. Indeed, the bone structures are more easily identified. The different types of anatomic structures constituting the foot are the following:

• Bone: the bone-marrow and especially the cortical bone are shown as "white" matter (very high density) in soft tissue windows. In bony windows the trabeculae of the bone-marrow are more accurately visualized.

• Tendons: round or oval structures with regular outlines. Their density is considerable and they appear as "light gray" matter.

• Ligaments: thin, flat structures with regular edges, more or less well visualized over their entire length. Their density is less than that of the tendons and they appear as "gray" matter.

• Muscles: their aspect is generally homogeneous, slightly "punctate". Their density is equal or inferior to that of the ligaments' ("gray" or "dark gray" matter).

• Fat: its density is very low (negative in the Hounsfield scale); it appears black, more or less homogeneous.

• Cartilage: is not directly visualized. Only the articular space is delineated. Cartilage can only be studied by CT arthrography.

MRI

All scans were obtained on a T5 II Philips Gyroscan unit, with a 1.5 mm slice thickness and T1-weighted gradient-echo sequences. T1-weighted sequences are the most anatomic. The various component foot structures are as follows:

• Cortical bone: signal-void (hypointense in all sequences).

• Bone-marrow: hyperintense in T1, hypointense in T2 and signal-void in STIR-weighted images.

• Tendons: hypointense in all sequences.

• Ligaments and aponeuroses: hypointense in all sequences.

• Muscles: intermediate signal (gray) in T1 and STIR, hypointense in T2.

• Fat: hyperintense in T1, intermediate signal or hypointense in T2, signal-void in STIR.

• Cartilage: intermediate signal in T1, generally hypointense in T2 and STIR.

• Fluids (physiologic effusions): hypointense in T1, hyperintense in T2 and STIR.

Abbreviations used in figures of pages 34 to 45

I. Tendons

ct	Calcaneal tendon
edlt	Extensor digitorum longus tendon
ehlt	Extensor hallucis longus tendon
fbt	Fibularis brevis tendon
flt	Fibularis longus tendon
fdlt	Flexor digitorum longus tendon
fhlt	Flexor hallucis longus tendon
tat	Tibialis anterior tendon
tpt	Tibialis posterior tendon

II. Muscles

abd dmm	Abductor digiti minimi muscle
abd hm	Abductor hallucis muscle
add hm	Adductor hallucis muscle
edmbm	Extensor digiti minimi brevis muscle
edbm	Extensor digitorum brevis muscle
edlm	Extensor digitorum longus muscle
ehlm	Extensor hallucis longus muscle
fbm	Fibularis brevis muscle
flm	Fibularis longus muscle
fdmbm	Flexor digiti minimi brevis muscle
fdbm	Flexor digitorum brevis muscle
fdlm	Flexor digitorum longus muscle
fhbm	Flexor hallucis brevis muscle
fhlm	Flexor hallucis longus muscle
qpm	Quadratus plantae muscle
sm	Soleus muscle

III. Ligaments

atfl	Anterior talofibular ligament
attl	Anterior tibiotalar ligament
atifl	Antero-inferior tibiofibular ligament
cfl	Calcaneofibular ligament
dl	Deltoid ligament
dcnl	Dorsal cuboideonavicular ligament
dtnl	Dorsal talonavicular ligament
itcl	Interosseous talocalcaneal ligament
ll	Lateral ligament
ml	Medial ligament
pcacl	Plantar calcaneocuboid ligament
pcanl	Plantar calcaneonavicular ligament
pcunl	Plantar cuneonavicular ligament
ptfl	Posterior talofibular ligament
ptifl	Posterior tibiofibular ligament
pttl	Posterior tibiotalar ligament
tcl	Tibiocalcaneal ligament
tnl	Tibionavicular ligament

IV. Bones

ca	Calcaneus
cub	Cuboid
fi	Fibula
ic	Intermediate cuneiform
lc	Lateral cuneiform
lm	Lateral malleolus
mc	Medial cuneiform
mm	Medial malleolus
M1, M2, M3, M4, M5	Metatarsals
na	Navicular
ta	Talus
ti	Tibia
ptub	Peroneal tubercle

V. Retinacula and aponeurosis

er	Extensor retinaculum
fr	Fibular retinaculum
flr	Flexor retinaculum
pa	Plantar aponeurosis

VI. Vessels and nerves

ata	Anterior tibial artery
atn	Anterior tibial nerve
atv	Anterior tibial vein
dfn	Deep fibular nerve
gsv	Great saphenous vein
lpa	Lateral plantar artery
lpn	Lateral plantar nerve
lpv	Lateral plantar vein
lsv	Lesser saphenous vein
mpa	Medial plantar artery
mpn	Medial plantar nerve
mpv	Medial plantar vein
pta	Posterior tibial artery
ptv	Posterior tibial vein
sn	Saphenous nerve
sfn	Superficial fibular nerve
sun	Sural nerve
tn	Tibial nerve

Legends for figures of pages 34 to 38

Figs. 4.7-4.13. CT. Axial slices presented from above downward

Figs. 4.14-4.20. CT. Coronal slices presented from the most posterior to the most anterior

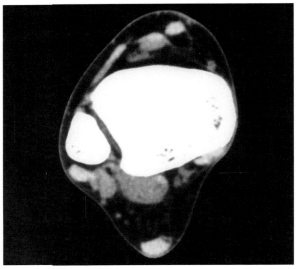

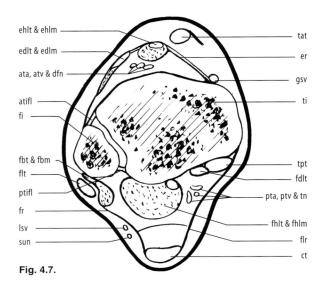

Fig. 4.7.

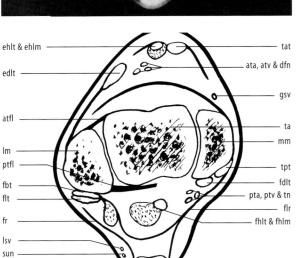

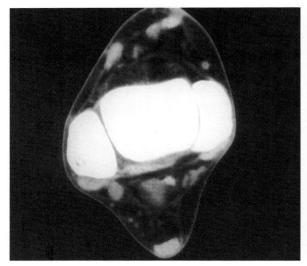

Fig. 4.8.

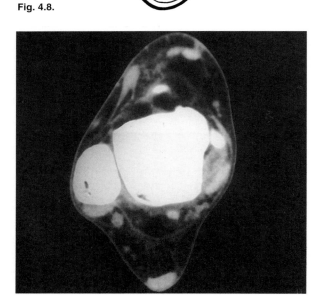

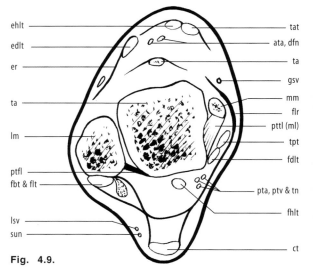

Fig. 4.9.

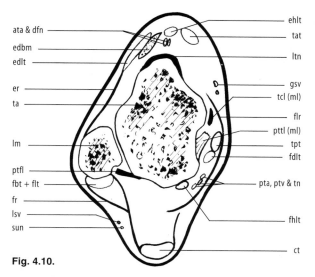

ata & dfn
edbm
edlt
er
ta
lm
ptfl
fbt + flt
fr
lsv
sun

ehlt
tat
ltn
gsv
tcl (ml)
flr
pttl (ml)
tpt
fdlt
pta, ptv & tn
fhlt
ct

Fig. 4.10.

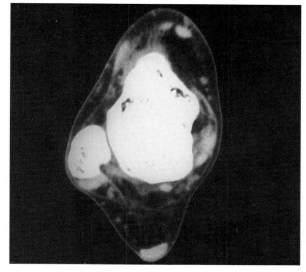

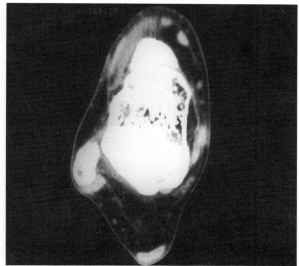

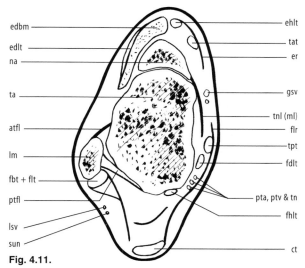

edbm
edlt
na
ta
atfl
lm
fbt + flt
ptfl
lsv
sun

ehlt
tat
er
gsv
tnl (ml)
flr
tpt
fdlt
pta, ptv & tn
fhlt
ct

Fig. 4.11.

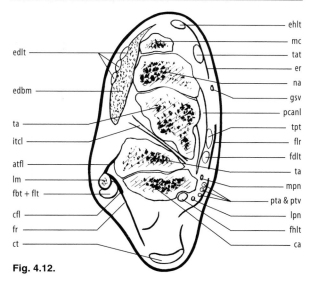

edlt
edbm
ta
itcl
atfl
lm
fbt + flt
cfl
fr
ct

ehlt
mc
tat
er
na
gsv
pcanl
tpt
flr
fdlt
ta
mpn
pta & ptv
lpn
fhlt
ca

Fig. 4.12.

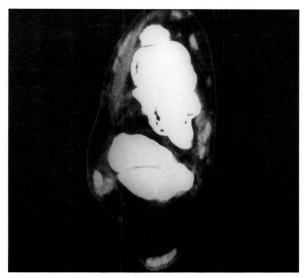

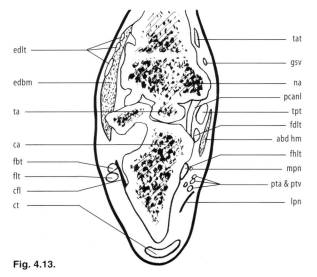

edlt
edbm
ta
ca
fbt
flt
cfl
ct

tat
gsv
na
pcanl
tpt
fdlt
abd hm
fhlt
mpn
pta & ptv
lpn

Fig. 4.13.

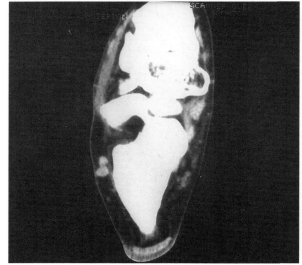

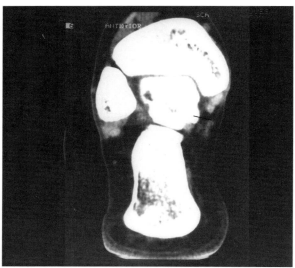

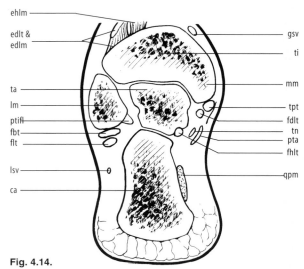

ehlm
edlt &
edlm
ta
lm
ptifl
fbt
flt
lsv
ca

gsv
ti
mm
tpt
fdlt
tn
pta
fhlt
qpm

Fig. 4.14.

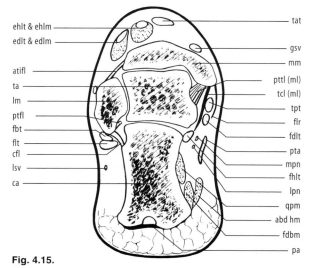

ehlt & ehlm
edlt & edlm
atifl
ta
lm
ptfl
fbt
flt
cfl
lsv
ca

tat
gsv
mm
pttl (ml)
tcl (ml)
tpt
flr
fdlt
pta
mpn
fhlt
lpn
qpm
abd hm
fdbm
pa

Fig. 4.15.

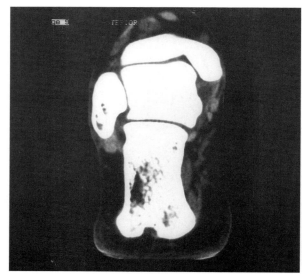

ehlt & ehlm		tat
edlt & edlm		
dfn		gsv
ata		mm
ta		pttl (ml)
lm		tcl (ml)
		tpt
ptfl		fdlt
fbt		flr
cfl		mpa & mpn
flt		fhlt
sun		lpa & lpn
fr		qpm
ca		abd hm
		fdbm
		abd dmm
		pa

Fig. 4.16.

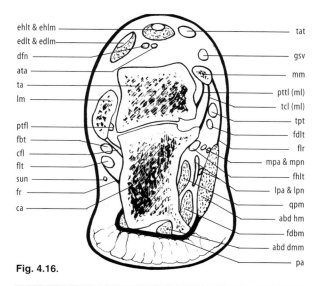

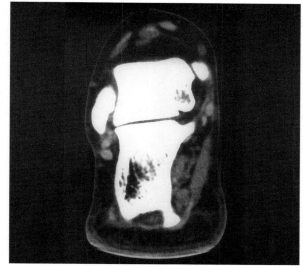

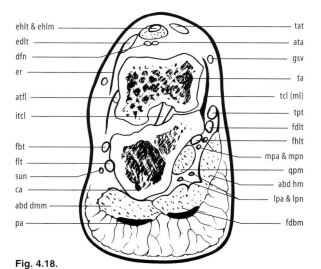

ehlt & ehlm		tat
edlt & edlm		
dfn		gsv
ata		tcl (ml)
ta		flr
atfl		tpt
		itcl
ca		fdlt
fbt		fhlt
flt		mpa & mpn
		qpm
		lpa & lpn
		abd hm
abd dmm		fdbm
		pa

Fig. 4.17.

ehlt & ehlm		tat
edlt		ata
dfn		gsv
er		ta
atfl		tcl (ml)
itcl		tpt
		fdlt
		fhlt
fbt		mpa & mpn
flt		qpm
sun		abd hm
ca		lpa & lpn
abd dmm		
pa		fdbm

Fig. 4.18.

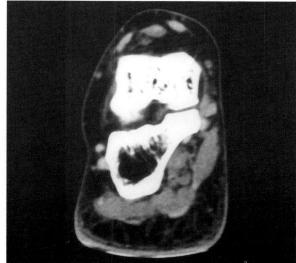

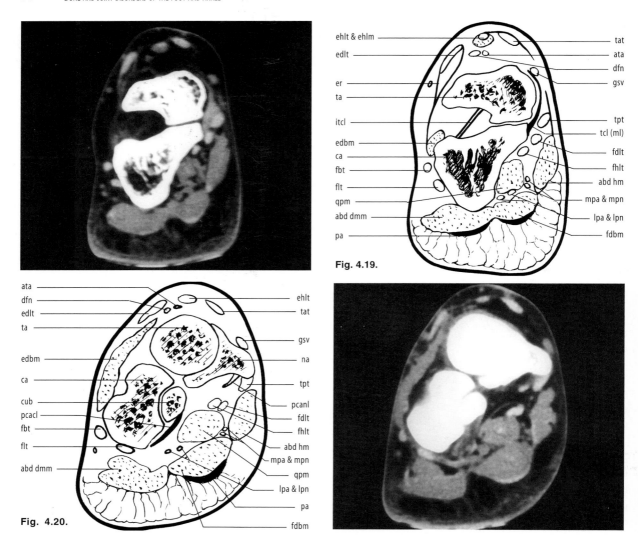

Fig. 4.19.

Fig. 4.20.

Legends for figures of pages 39 to 45

Figs. 4.21-4.27. MRI. Axial T1-weighted slices, presented from above downward
Figs. 4.28-4.34. MRI. Coronal T1-weighted slices, presented from the most posterior to the most anterior
Figs. 4.35-4.41. MRI. Sagittal T1-weighted slices, from the medial malleolus to the lateral malleolus

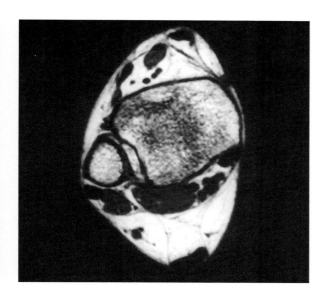

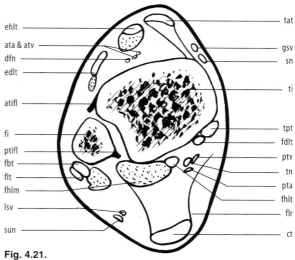

ehlt — tat
ata & atv — gsv
dfn — sn
edlt — ti
atifl
fi — tpt
ptifl — fdlt
fbt — ptv
flt — tn
fhlm — pta
lsv — fhlt
sun — flr
— ct

Fig. 4.21.

ata & atv — gsv
edlt — sn
dfn — mm
er — ta
atifl — tpt
lm — fdlt
— ptv
ptifl — tn
fbt — pta
flt — fhlt
lsv — fhlm
sun — ct

Fig. 4.22.

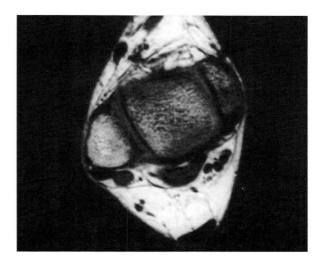

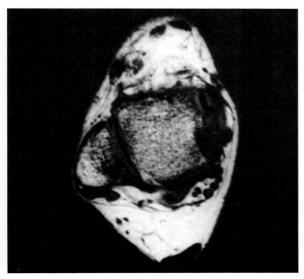

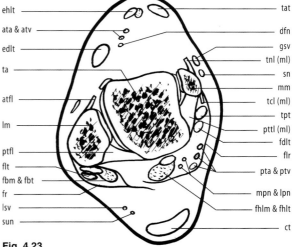

ehlt — tat
ata & atv — dfn
edlt — gsv
ta — tnl (ml)
— sn
atfl — mm
lm — tcl (ml)
— tpt
ptfl — pttl (ml)
flt — fdlt
fbm & fbt — flr
fr — pta & ptv
lsv — mpn & lpn
sun — fhlm & fhlt
— ct

Fig. 4.23.

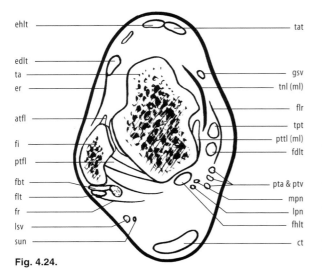

Fig. 4.24.

ehlt — tat
edlt
ta — gsv
er — tnl (ml)
atfl — flr
fi — tpt
ptfl — pttl (ml)
fbt — fdlt
flt — pta & ptv
fr — mpn
lsv — lpn
sun — fhlt
— ct

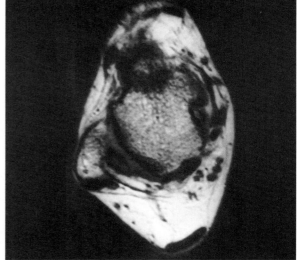

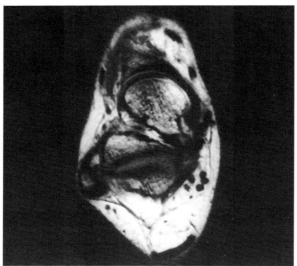

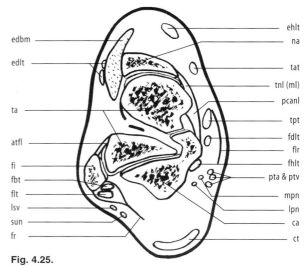

Fig. 4.25.

edbm — ehlt
edlt — na
— tat
ta — tnl (ml)
atfl — pcanl
fi — tpt
fbt — fdlt
flt — flr
lsv — fhlt
sun — pta & ptv
fr — mpn
— lpn
— ca
— ct

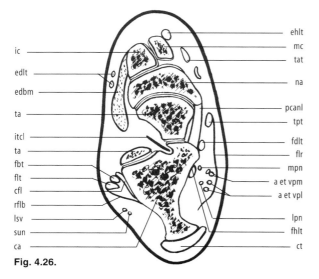

Fig. 4.26.

ic — ehlt
— mc
edlt — tat
edbm — na
ta — pcanl
itcl — tpt
ta — fdlt
fbt — flr
flt — mpn
cfl — a et vpm
rflb — a et vpl
lsv — lpn
sun — fhlt
ca — ct

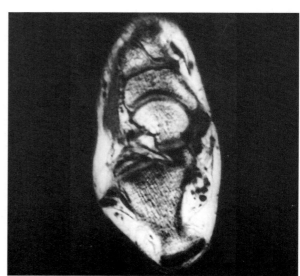

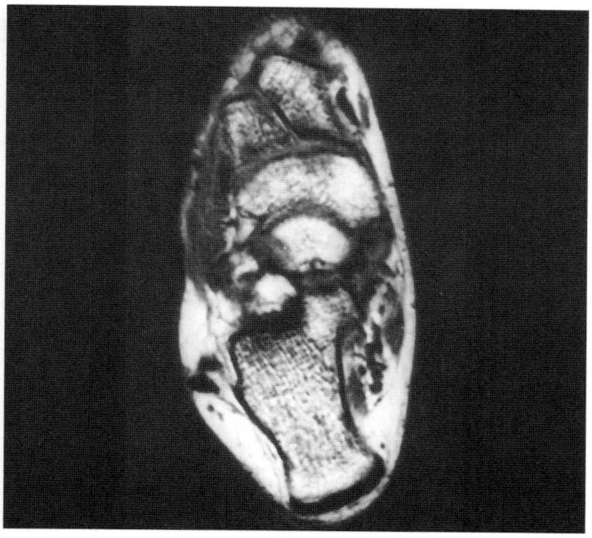

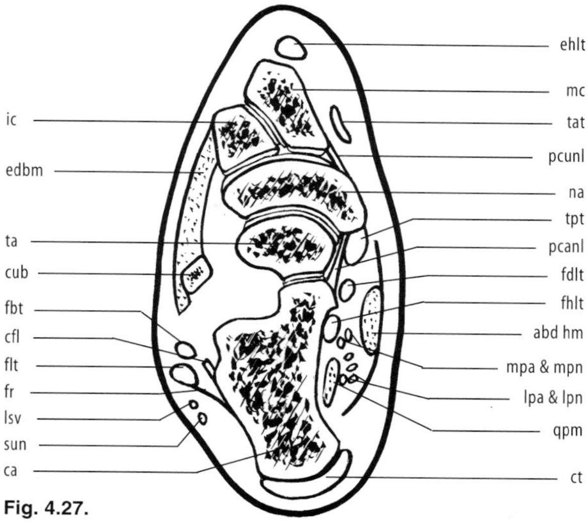
ehlt
mc
ic
tat
pcunl
edbm
na
tpt
ta
pcanl
cub
fdlt
fbt
fhlt
cfl
abd hm
flt
mpa & mpn
fr
lpa & lpn
lsv
qpm
sun
ca
ct

Fig. 4.27.

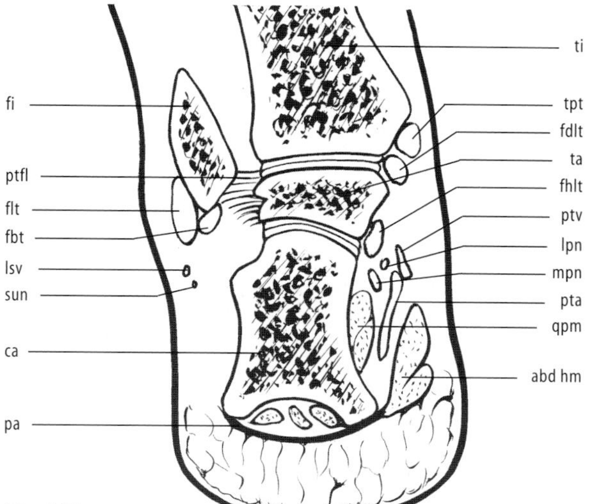
ti
fi
tpt
fdlt
ptfl
ta
fhlt
flt
ptv
fbt
lpn
lsv
mpn
sun
pta
qpm
ca
abd hm
pa

Fig. 4.28.

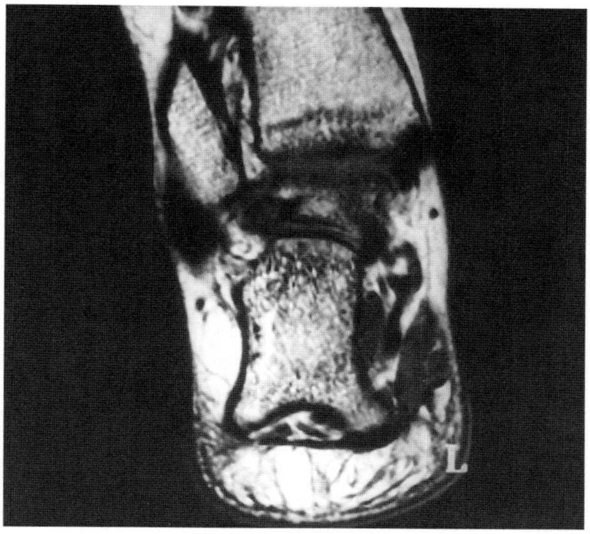

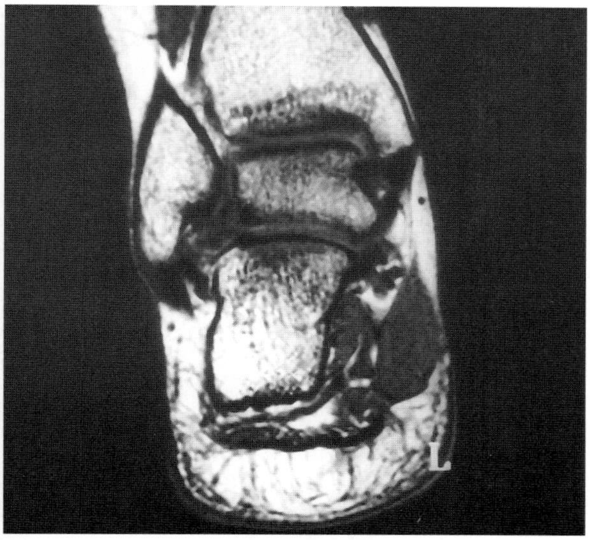

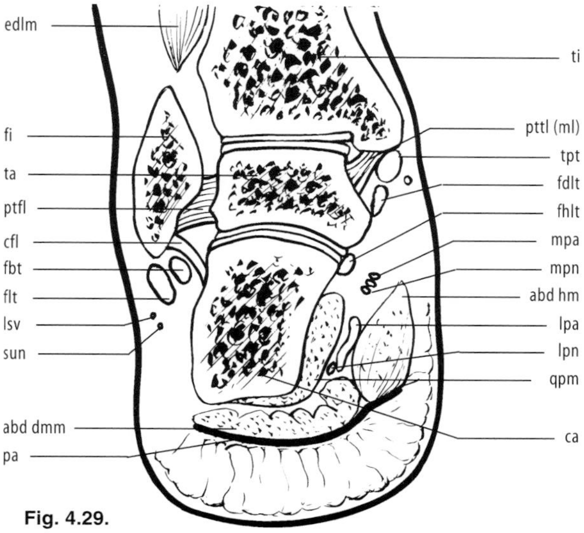
edlm
ti
fi
pttl (ml)
tpt
ta
fdlt
ptfl
fhlt
cfl
mpa
fbt
mpn
flt
abd hm
lsv
lpa
sun
lpn
qpm
abd dmm
ca
pa

Fig. 4.29.

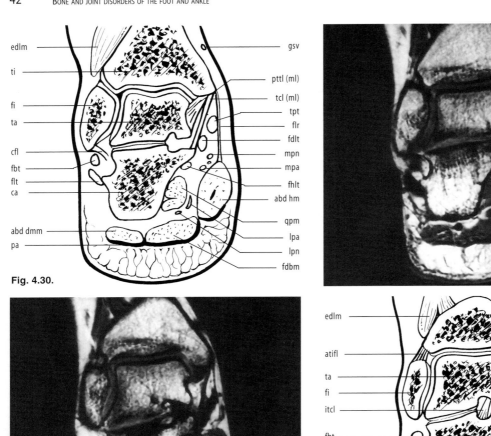

Fig. 4.30.

edlm
ti
fi
ta
cfl
fbt
flt
ca
abd dmm
pa

gsv
pttl (ml)
tcl (ml)
tpt
flr
fdlt
mpn
mpa
fhlt
abd hm
qpm
lpa
lpn
fdbm

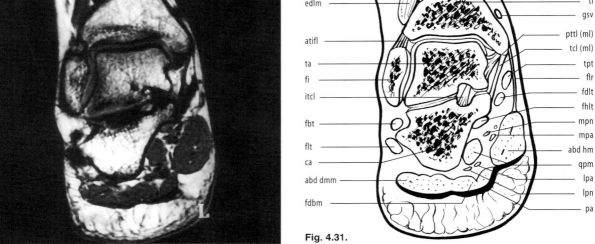

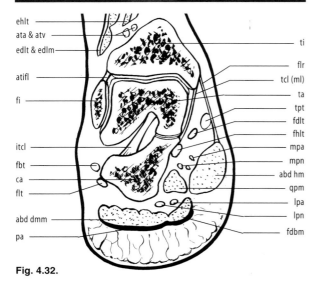

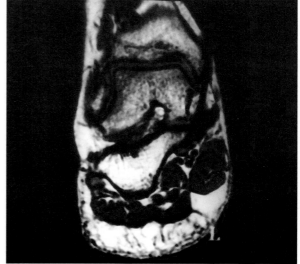

Fig. 4.31.

edlm
atifl
ta
fi
itcl
fbt
flt
ca
abd dmm
fdbm

ti
gsv
pttl (ml)
tcl (ml)
tpt
flr
fdlt
fhlt
mpn
mpa
abd hm
qpm
lpa
lpn
pa

Fig. 4.32.

ehlt
ata & atv
edlt & edlm
atifl
fi
itcl
fbt
ca
flt
abd dmm
pa

ti
flr
tcl (ml)
ta
tpt
fdlt
fhlt
mpa
mpn
abd hm
qpm
lpa
lpn
fdbm

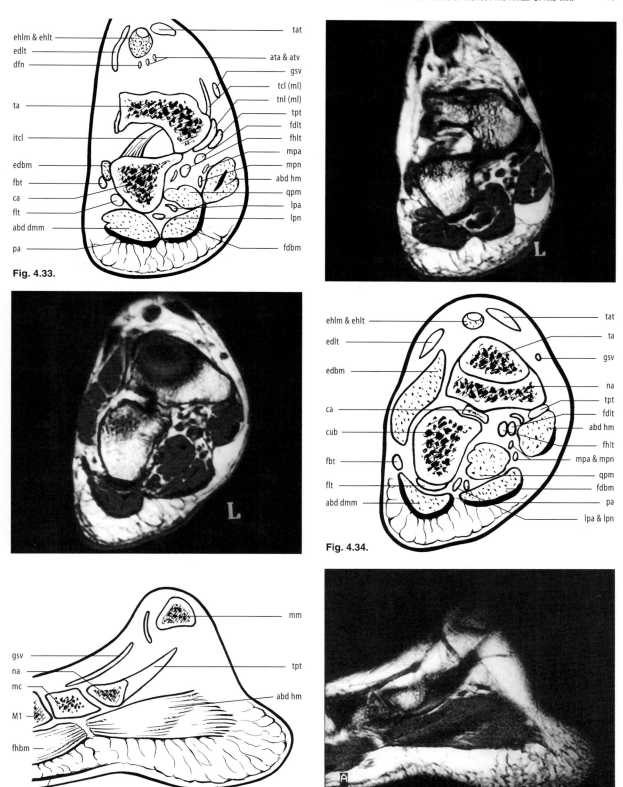

ehlm & ehlt
edlt
dfn
ta
itcl
edbm
fbt
ca
flt
abd dmm
pa

tat
ata & atv
gsv
tcl (ml)
tnl (ml)
tpt
fdlt
fhlt
mpa
mpn
abd hm
qpm
lpa
lpn
fdbm

Fig. 4.33.

ehlm & ehlt
edlt
edbm
ca
cub
fbt
flt
abd dmm

tat
ta
gsv
na
tpt
fdlt
abd hm
fhlt
mpa & mpn
qpm
fdbm
pa
lpa & lpn

Fig. 4.34.

gsv
na
mc
M1
fhbm
pa

mm
tpt
abd hm

Fig. 4.35.

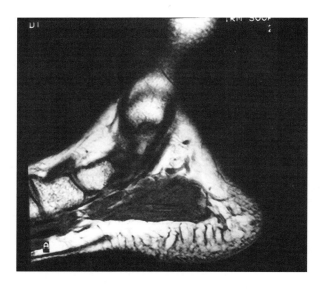

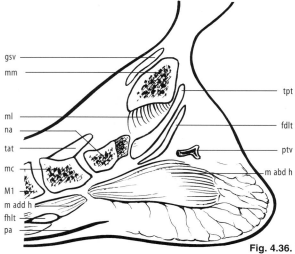

Fig. 4.36.

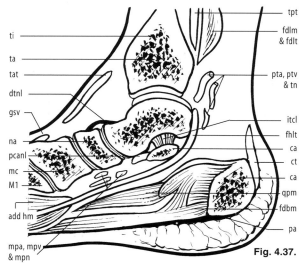

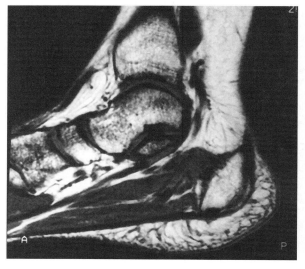

Fig. 4.37.

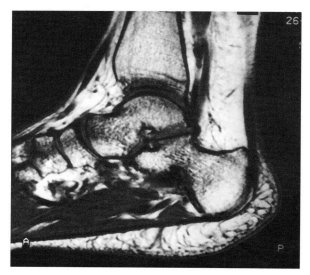

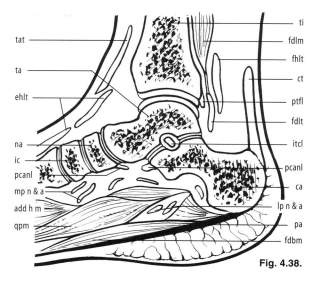

Fig. 4.38.

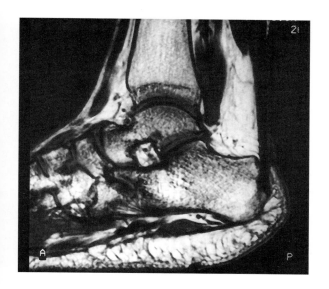

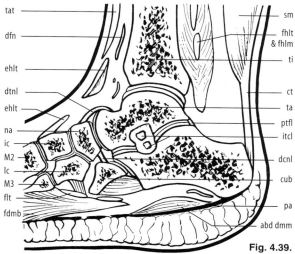

tat — — sm
dfn — — fhlt & fhlm
ehlt — — ti
dtnl — — ct
ehlt — — ta
na — — ptfl
ic — — itcl
M2 — — dcnl
lc — — cub
M3 — — pa
flt — — abd dmm
fdmb

Fig. 4.39.

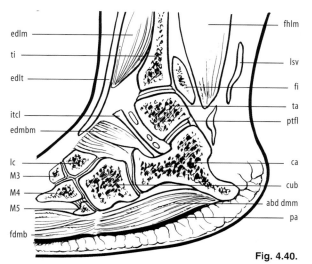

edlm — — fhlm
ti — — lsv
edlt — — fi
itcl — — ta
edmbm — — ptfl
lc — — ca
M3 — — cub
M4 — — abd dmm
M5 — — pa
fdmb

Fig. 4.40.

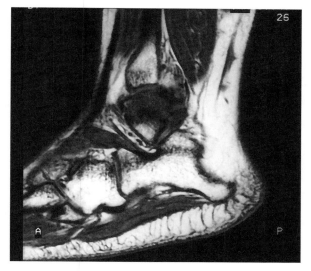

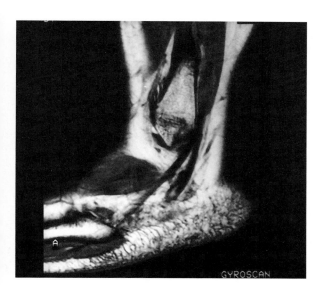

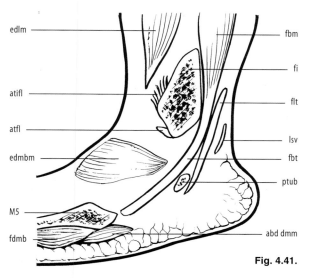

edlm — — fbm
atifl — — fi
atfl — — flt
edmbm — — lsv
M5 — — fbt
fdmb — — ptub
— abd dmm

Fig. 4.41.

● Advantages and disadvantages of both techniques

CT

Advantages

• Excellent spatial resolution, with possible slice thickness of 1 mm or less;
• easy comparative study, without spatial resolution impairment;
• easy interpretation for the clinician, because of the uniparametric technique, with no parameters other than a gray matter scale;
• patient immobility less important than in MRI;
• no contraindications;
• excellent study of the bone structure and cortex, identification of loose bodies;
• excellent study of the cartilage (CT arthrography);
• cheaper technique.

Disadvantages

• Contrast resolution highly inferior to MRI, (especially troublesome for the soft tissues);
• coronal installation sometimes difficult, even impossible, especially in traumatology;
• sagittal slices difficult to perform
• radiation exposure;
• uniparametric technique.

MRI

Advantages

• Excellent contrast resolution, especially in T1-weighted sequence, where spontaneous contrast is maximal between ligaments and tendons (hypointense) and fat (hyperintense);
• multiplanar capabilities: slices are possible in all planes. Great value of the sagittal foot slices;
• longitudinal study of tendons, thanks to the sagittal slices (in CT the tendons are always axially "cut"). Major value for the achilles tendon for instance;
• multiparametric technique: as mentioned, the use of different sequences is of great diagnostic help;
• useful +++ in acute traumatology, for the soft tissues (ligaments, tendons, muscles); thanks to the multiplicity of sequences and the use of gadolinium, edema and inflammatory reaction are not a disad-

vantage (as for CT), but on the contrary, an advantage;
• excellent study of the bone-marrow and its pathology;
• no radiation exposure.

Disadvantages

• Spatial resolution still inferior to CT;
• the comparative study is made to the detriment of spatial resolution;
• the multiparametric aspect makes interpretation more difficult for the clinician: difficulties in identifying the different sequences, signal modification of normal and pathologic structures according to the sequence used;
• poor analysis of cortical and bony fragments. Limited value in detecting loose bodies, or studying bony displacements in traumatology;
• cartilage analysis inferior to CT arthrography;
• strict immobility is required during the examination;
• contraindications: pace-maker, some neurosurgical vascular clips, some artificial heart valves, some intravascular filters, intraocular metallic loose body.

● CT and MRI performances related to the pathology

In this section, the value of CT and MRI is studied for each pathology. The CT and MRI presentations are summed up both by the text and illustrations of the pathology.

Table 4.1 summarizes the value of CT and MRI on a subjective scale from 0 to +++ according to the explored structure and the pathology under investigation.

Bone pathology

Fractures

In traumatic injuries of bone, CT is much more useful than MRI. It is nearly always essential in fractures of the calcaneus (fig. 4.42), the talus or the mediotarsus (figs. 4.43 & 4.44). Indeed, a much more precise analysis is possible compared with conven-

Table 4.1. Contribution of MRI and CT according to pathology

Pathology	CT	MRI
Cortical fracture	+++	+
Osteochondral injuries (talar dome)	+++ (CT arthro)	++
Bone bruise	+	+++
Osteonecrosis (talus)	++	+++
Algodystrophy	+	+++
Osteitis and osteomyelitis	++	+++
Loose bodies	+++ (CT or CT arthro)	+
Synostosis	+++	+
Bone tumor	+++ (characterization)	+++ (extension)
Arthritis	+++ (late check-up)	+++ (early diagnosis)
Arthrosis	+++	++
Soft tissue tumor	+	+++
Tenosynovitis	+	+++ (except stenosing tenosynovitis)
Tendinitis, tendon degeneration	+	+++
Tendon rupture	++	+++
Longitudinal splitting (tibialis posterior tendon & fibularis brevis tendon)	+ (CT)	+++
Dislocation (fibular tendons, tibialis posterior tendon)	+++	+++
Achilles tendon	+	+++
Collateral ligaments	++ (CT arthro)	++
Interosseous talocalcaneal ligament	++	++
Plantar aponeurosis	+	+++
Synovial pathology	++ (CT arthro)	+++
Morton's neuroma	++	+++
Bursitis	+	+++
Accessory muscles	++	+++
Posterior ankle impingement	+++	++

tional radiographs, where the different bony elements are superimposed.

The CT enables us to evaluate the number of fracture lines, their direction and their articular or nonarticular nature. It clearly identifies bony displacements. In the chronic stage, after consolidation, CT and MRI are both useful. CT visualizes malunion and evaluates articular congruence. Both techniques analyse the soft tissue lesions (ligaments, tendons) (fig. 4.45); MRI accurately determines the degree of articular damage and reveals any bone-marrow edema (fig. 4.46).

Occult fractures, microfractures, stress fractures

CT is highly superior to MRI in identifying small bony fragments and detecting stress fractures or occult fractures.

Fig. 4.47 depicts one of the favourite sites of stress fractures of the foot, ie., the navicular bone, with the

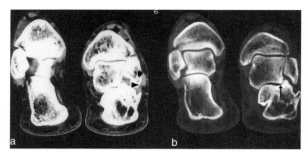

Fig. 4.42. CT: bone window, comminuted calcaneal fracture. *Left*: inverted Y-shaped fracture with extension of fracture lines into articular facet of talocalcanean joint and inferior cortex of calcaneus. *Right* (more anterior slice): comminuted fracture at level of sinus tarsi

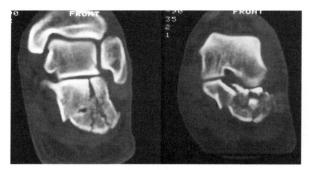

Fig. 4.45. CT: coronal slices. **a** Incarceration of fibularis brevis tendon between calcaneus and lateral malleolus (►). Luxation of fibularis longus tendon (◆). **b** Sequel of old calcaneal fracture with recess (→)

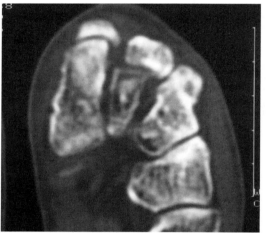

Fig. 4.43. CT: axial slice. Bone window. Lateral subluxation of tarsometatarsal joint, well shown on this slice at level of first and second rays

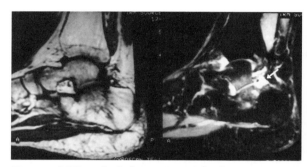

Fig. 4.46. MRI: sagittal slices. **a** T1-weighted image. **b** STIR-weighted image. Damage to talocalcanean joint after **thalamic** fracture. Bone-marrow edema extends on both sides of joint. Effusion in talocalcanean joint (→)

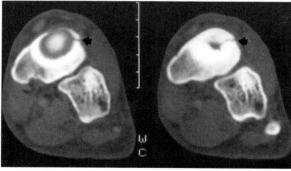

Fig. 4.47. CT: coronal slice. Bone window. Stress fracture (◆) of the navicular bone

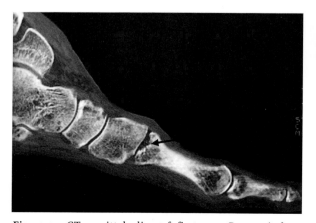

Fig. 4.44. CT: sagittal slice of first ray, Bone window. Osteochondral fracture of base of first metatarsal (→)

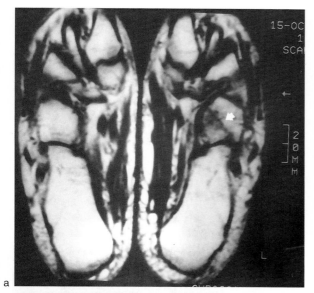

a

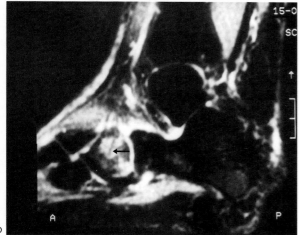

b

Fig. 4.48. MRI: occult fracture of left cuboid. The fracture line is well shown in T₁-weighted image (➡) (a). The STIR sequence (b) shows major bone-marrow edema, with increased signal (→)

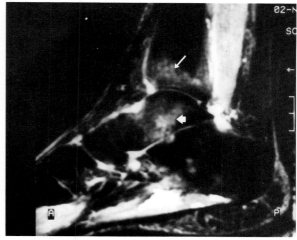

Fig. 4.49. MRI: STIR-weighted image, sagittal slice.Stress response (old patient, hyperparathyroidism). Nonuniform, poorly-defined bone-marrow edema (➡,→) with strikingly increased signal in STIR sequence

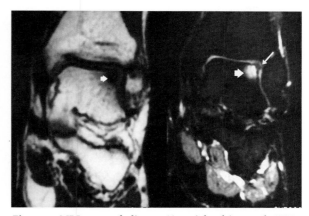

Fig. 4.50. MRI: coronal slices. **a** T₁-weighted image. **b** STIR-weighted image. Osteochondral injury of talar **dome**. The area of subchondral damage is hypointense on T₁-weighted image and hyperintense in STIR-weighted image (➡). The articular cartilage is irregular (→)

"split target" sign described by Morvan [19]. In MRI, fracture lines are often more difficult to identify; they are generally seen as serpiginous lines of low signal intensity, well shown in T₁-weighted images (fig. 4.48). MRI is nevertheless much more sensitive than CT for the diagnosis of these microfractures, because it displays a very good indirect sign, i.e., a more or less diffuse edema of the bone-marrow, appearing hypointense in T₁-weighted images and hyperintense in STIR-weighted images. STIR sequence or other fat-suppressing sequences are the most efficient in detec-

tion of this bone-marrow edema, allowing us to suspect stress reactions (fig. 4.49), which are not diagnosed on CT.

Osteochondral injuries of the talar dome

MRI is the most precise technique for the early detection of osteochondritis dissecans. At a more advanced stage, CT will best determine the position of the sequestrum. For osteochondral fractures, MRI remains the most sensitive technique; notably, it

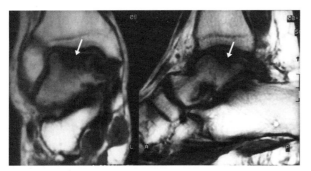

Fig. 4.51. MRI. **a** Coronal T1-weighted image. **b** Sagittal T1-weighted image after intravenous injection of gadolinium. Osteonecrosis of talar **dome**. Necrosed zone (→) remains hypointense after IV injection of gadolinium

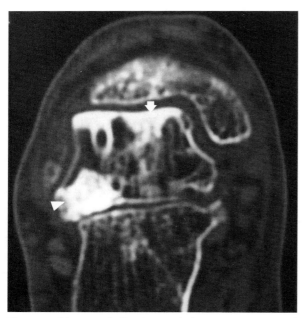

Fig. 4.52. CT: coronal slice. Bone window. Osteonecrosis of talus. Necrotic zone appears as osteosclerotic areas (▶, ►)

enables the identification of a bone bruise (fig. 4.50) which CT cannot visualize at the early stage. In cases of cortical fracture, CT shows the fractures lines and the possible displacement better.

In all cases, CT arthrography still remains the best technique for the evaluation of cartilage injuries (see fig. 4.3).

Osteonecrosis

MRI diagnoses osteonecrosis at a much earlier stage than CT, demonstrating a well-defined low signal intensity line demarcating the margin of the necrotic segment (fig. 4.51). At an early stage, the necrotic segment exhibits signal characteristics similar to those of normal bone-marrow. Later, the necrotic segment demonstrates decreased signal intensity in both T1- and T2-weighted sequences. In CT (fig. 4.52), more or less osteosclerotic zones associated with osseous collapse may be observed.

Algodystrophy

MRI is far superior to CT and combines great sensitivity (even compared with bone scan) with high specificity; it points out a striking area of signal abnormality of the bone-marrow: decreased signal intensity in T1-weighted sequence, increased signal in T2- and STIR-weighted sequences, with enhancement after IV injection of gadolinium.

Loose bodies

CT is the best technique to detect these, even when of extrinsic origin. CT arthrography proves their articular or nonarticular location. MRI is much less effective.

Synostosis and synchondrosis

Detection is possible with either CT or MRI, but CT is always essential to assess the complete aspects of a synostosis and its morphologic consequences on the different bony parts. Both slice planes (coronal and axial) are necessary and complementary. Sagittal slices (or sagittal reconstructions) will complete the examination if surgery is contemplated.

Osteitis, osteomyelitis, arthritis

MRI allows an early diagnosis, but the picture is not specific to the acute or subacute stage, and diagnosis will only be established by numerous clinical and paraclinical features. At a more advanced stage, CT will show more specific signs, notably in arthritis. For chronic osteomyelitis, MRI precisely locates the infected area and is a guide to possible surgery [35]. CT can supplement MRI in detecting a sequestrum in the infected area.

Bone tumors

For benign tumors, diagnosis is established from conventional radiographs and may possibly be confirmed by CT.

For malignant tumors, CT will only be necessary if conventional radiographs cannot give a precise diagnosis. MRI usually remains essential before surgery to accurately determine the locoregional extent (intramedullary and extraosseous extension). MRI examination is superior to CT for determining the soft tissue extension of malignant bone tumors. Bone tumors are best identified in T1-weighted and STIR-weighted images. Most lesions exhibit low signal intensity in T1-weighted images and extension into the soft tissues is best evaluated in T2-weighted or STIR-weighted images.

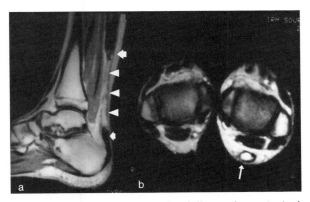

Fig. 4.53. MRI: old rupture of left achilles tendon. a Sagittal T1-weighted image slice: rupture gap exceeds 6 cm (▶) and both tendon ends are well shown (◆). b Axial T2-weighted image slice: achilles tendon is normal on the right. On the left, "empty sheath" aspect in fluid hypersignal (→)

Soft tissue pathology

Calcaneal tendon (Achilles tendon)

CT is not relevant. Ultrasonography (US) is in competition with MRI.

Acute and chronic tendinitis

Both techniques are equally effective. Advantages of MRI compared with US are better spatial resolution, and the possibility of a complete study of the tendon in its entire length. Indeed, as the field of view of the ultrasound probe is limited, complete examination of the tendon can only be performed by a succession of segmental studies. Nevertheless, US is a less expensive technique. In MRI, tendinitis generally combines widening of the tendon contour and moderate intratendinous signal alteration (only visible in T1 or proton density-weighted images, but not in T2-weighted images). Sometimes, especially in chronic tendinitis, there are only morphologic changes.

Rupture

Here again, US and MRI performances are nearly equivalent. In the acute phase, MRI is more accurate. It discriminates better between the tendinous discontinuity and the locoregional inflammatory reaction. The tear size and the tendinous retraction are better identified. The MRI appearance (fig. 4.53) is one of complete tendinous discontinuity with a gap of high signal in T2 sequence and an enhance-

ment of the gap after intravenous injection of gadolinium. Generally, for all tendinous pathology, the T2 sequence with two echos and the T2 fat-suppressed sequence are the most valuable. The T1 sequence is less valuable since edema and inflammatory reactions appear in hyposignal (increase in water content) among the tendons, also spontaneously in hyposignal. For acute ruptures, gadolinium (IV) is useful, especially with T1 fat-suppressed sequence.

For monitoring operated achilles tendons, post-surgical modifications make ultrasound interpretation much more difficult and here MRI is the best technique.

Other tendons

The pathology of other ankle tendons includes tenosynovitis, tendinopathies, rupture, longitudinal splits and dislocations. They mainly affect the tibialis posterior and fibular tendons.

Tenosynovitis

CT perfectly shows major tenosynovitis as a hypodense, well-delimited zone surrounding the tendon in several successive slices. Moderate tenosynovitis may not be shown by CT because of its low tissue resolution and this may lead to the wrong diagnosis of a tendinopathy (apparent increase in tendon size). Tenography followed by CT tenography is much more effective: tenography images show the inflammatory and "spiculated" aspect of the sheath and

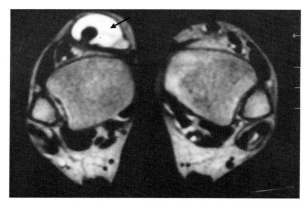

Fig. 4.54. MRI: sagittal T2-weighted image slice. Teno-synovitis of tibialis anterior tendon. Major effusion (→) distending tendon sheath

especially detect stenosing tenosynovitis if this is not diagnosed by other techniques. CT tenography allows evaluation of the tendon state in its sheath and reveals any longitudinal splits.

MRI is reliable for detecting tenosynovitis, even in moderate cases. The T2 sequence shows a hyper-intense fluid in the sheath, surrounding a tendon in hyposignal (fig. 4.54). The T1 sequence with intravenous gadolinium injection distinguishes inflammatory tenosynovitis (enhancement after injection), from mechanical tenosynovitis (no enhancement).

Tendinopathies
(tendinitis, tendon degeneration):

In CT as in MRI, these appear as a more or less marked increase in tendon size. As mentioned, the low tissue resolution of CT may create problems of differential diagnosis from tenosynovitis. On the contrary, MRI is very reliable [29]. Slight intratendinous signal alteration may be present, essentially in short TR sequences.

Ruptures

For accurate diagnosis of ruptures in young patients, both techniques are effective; but in the very early stage MRI is superior to CT, which allows better differentiation of the tendinous gap from associated edema and blood (thanks to T1 sequences with intravenous gadolinium injection. In CT, in the rupture area the tendon is replaced by a hypodense material (fluid). In MRI, tendinous discontinuity appears hyperintense in T2 sequence and is enhanced after intravenous gadolinium injection (in

T1 sequence). Sagittal slices permit better definition of the extent of rupture by showing the proximal and distal extremities of the tendon.

For degenerative ruptures in chronic tendinitis, the Rosenberg staging [29] in three types is generally used (cf. chapter 24). Thus, MRI is ideally suited for diagnosis of partial tears of types I and II.

Longitudinal splits

These lesions mainly involve the tibialis posterior and fibularis (peroneus) brevis tendons. They are not identified in CT but are well visualized in CT tenography. MRI is an appropriate technique, without the invasive nature of CT tenography. The four stages described by Sobel [32, 33] can be easily found [36].

Subluxation and dislocation

Excellent performance for both CT as MRI (fig. 4.55). In transitory dislocation, CT has the theoretic advantage of making slices with dynamic positioning of the ankle, reproducing the dislocation.

Ligamentous lesions

Collateral ligaments
(medial and especially lateral)

In the acute stage, when the diagnosis of the sprain is clinically evident, slice imaging is not necessary and conventional radiographs are sufficient.

In the chronic stage, with chronic ankle instability, or when the diagnosis is uncertain, MRI can define the lesions and exclude other pathologies (especially tendinous pathologies). CT is not very accurate, showing only a ligamentous thickening, which does not allow the establishment of ligamentous rupture. CT tenography (after ankle joint arthrography) is only valuable when it is positive, ie., when it demonstrates passage of contrast through the ligament. For the calcaneofibular ligament, rupture can be assessed when there is opacification of the fibular tendons sheath [3, 8] (fig. 4.56). On the contrary, opacification of the flexor tendons sheaths has no pathologic value [19]. MRI performance is variously assessed depending on the authors [4, 6, 21, 31] and has still to be confirmed. As in CT, MRI can show a ligamentous thickening which does not allow distinction between a simple acute sprain and an old rupture with fibrous cicatrization; but it can also show (especially in T2 sequence and in T1 sequence with intravenous gado-

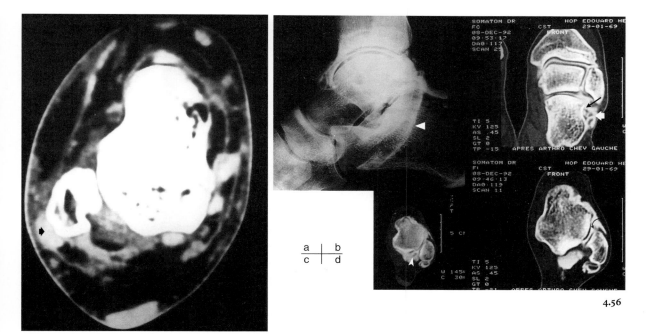

Fig. 4.55. CT: axial slice. Soft tissue window. Antero-lateral subluxation of fibular tendons (➡)

Fig. 4.56. Arthrography and CT arthrography. Rupture of anterior talofibular ligament (atfl), posterior talofibular ligament (ptfl) and calcaneofibular ligament (cfl). **a** Ankle joint arthrography. Contrast enters sheath of fibular tendons (➤) = rupture of the cfl. **b** CT arthrography, coronal slice. Indirect sign (contrast in fibular tendons sheath) (➡) and direct sign (ligament discontinuity) (⟶) of rupture of the cfl. **c, d** CT arthrography, axial slices: rupture of the atfl (⌒) and ptfl (➤)

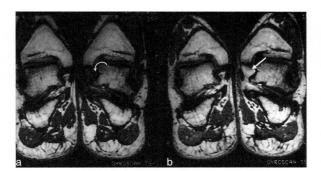

Fig. 4.57. MRI: coronal T1-weighted slice image before (**a**) and after (**b**) IV gadolinium injection. Rupture of medial collateral ligament. The posterior tibiotalar ligament is replaced by edemato-inflammatory hypointense material in T1-weighted image (⌒), intensively enhanced after IV gadolinium injection (⟶)

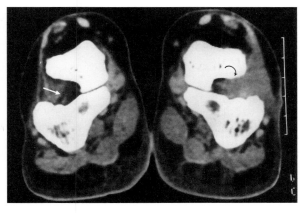

Fig. 4.58. CT: soft tissue window, comparative study, lesion of interosseous talocalcanean ligament. *Right:* normal aspect (⟶). *Left:* filling of sinus tarsi with edemato-inflammatory material (⌒); ligament is no longer visualized

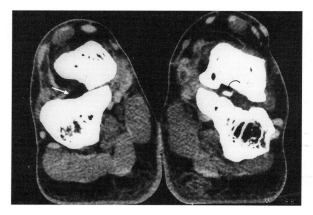

Fig. 4.59. CT: soft tissue window, old rupture of interosseous talocalcanean ligament *Right side: normal aspect*(⟶). *Left side:* fibrous filling of sinus tarsi by osteo-ligamentous avulsion (⌒)

linium injection) true ligamentous discontinuity (with a hyperintense gap) which confirms the rupture (fig. 4.57).

Interosseous talocalcaneal ligament (ITCL)

Its examination is as reliable by CT as by MRI. In both, a serious sprain of the ITCL frequently appears as a disorganization of the soft tissues in the sinus tarsi: the sinus tarsi is diffusely filled with edema and hemorrhage (fig. 4.58); the ligament is thickened and irregular. CT will confirm the rupture in cases of osseous avulsion in the sinus tarsi (fig. 4.59).

Plantar aponeurosis

MRI is undoubtedly the best exploratory technique, by means of sagittal slices. The features revealed are well discriminated [2, 24] and allow the distinction of aponeurositis, myoaponeurositis and ruptures.

Morton's neuroma

Diagnosis is essentially clinical. Nevertheless clinical investigation is not always reliable and imaging is useful before surgery. The best imaging technique is MRI, which can distinguish the Morton's neuroma (hypointense in T1- and T2-weighted images) from intercapito-metatarsal bursitis (hypointense in T1-weighted images and uniformly hyperintense in T2-weighted images).

Accessory muscles

Identical performances: slight superiority of MRI thanks to sagittal slices and better tissue contrast.

Soft tissue tumors

Great superiority of MRI, thanks to numerous slice planes, excellent tissue resolution, and the multiparameter aspect. Most soft tissue tumors are isointense in T1-weighted images, hyperintense in T2-weighted images and enhance after intravenous gadolinium injection. Extensive fibromatosis is an exception and can appear hypointense in T1- and T2-weighted images.

To sum up, CT is to be preferred for traumatic injuries of bone, malformational pathology (synchondrosis), accurate cartilage analysis (talar dome), and for the search for foreign bodies. MRI will be required for tendinous, muscular and aponeurotic disease, for soft tissue tumors and synovial pathology, and for bone-marrow pathology (osteitis, algodystrophy, osteonecrosis; stress fractures, bone bruise). For bone tumors, CT will give better tumoral characterization, whereas MRI offers better determination of locoregional extension. For ligamentous pathology, both MRI and CT arthrography are suitable.

References

1. Allon S M, Mears D C (1991) Three dimensional analysis of calcaneal fractures. In: Deutsch AL, Mink JH, Kerr R (eds) MRI of the foot and ankle. Raven Press, New York, p 254
2. Berkowitz JF, Kier R, Rudicel S (1991) Plantar fasciitis: MR imaging. Radiology 179: 665-668
3. Bleichrodt RP, Kingma LM, Binnendijk B, Klein JP (1989). Radiology 173: 347-349
4. Chandnani VP, harper M, Ficke JR, Gagliardi JA, Rolling L, Christensen KP, Hanser M (1994) Radiology 192: 189-194
5. Conti S, Michelson J, Jahss M, (1992). In: Deutsch A L, Mink J H, Kerr R (eds) MRI of the foot and ankle. Raven Press, New York, p 208
6. Crues JV, Shellock FG (1992). In: Deutsch AL, Mink JH, Kerr R (eds) MRI of the foot and ankle. Raven Press, New York, p 1
7. Devred Ph, Longin-Magnan D, Boorione F, Panuel M, Du Lac P, Girard N, Roumieu G (1989) Étude par tomodensitométrie des fractures du calcanéum. À propos de 30 cas. J Radiol 70: 455-463

8. Dory MA (1986) Arthrography of the ankle joint in chronic instability. Skeletal Radiol 15: 291-294

9. Erickson SJ, Rosengarten JL (1993) MR imaging of the forefoot: normal anatomic findings. AJR 160: 565-571

10. Erickson SJ, Smith JW, Ruiz ME, Fitzgerald SW, Kneeland JB, Johnson JE, Shereff MJ, Carrera GF (1991) MR imaging of the lateral collateral ligament of the ankle. AJR 156: 131-136

11. Guyer BH, Levinsohn EM, Fredrickson BE, Bailey GL, Formikell M (1985) Computed tomography of calcaneal fractures: anatomy, pathology, dosimetry, and clinical relevance. AJR 145: 911-919

12. Hoskins CL, Sartoris DJ, Resnick D (1992) Magnetic resonance imaging of foot neuromas. J Foot Surg 31: 10-16

13. Kabbani YM, Mayer DP (1993) Magnetic resonance imaging of tendon pathology about the foot and ankle. J Am PodiatR Med Assoc 83: 466-468

14. Keyser CK, Gilula LA, Hardy DC, Adler S, Vannier M (1988) Soft-tissue abnormalities of the foot and ankle: CT diagnosis. AJR 150: 845-850

15. Kier R, Dietz MJ, McCarthy M, Rudicel SA (1991) MR imaging of the normal ligaments and tendons of the ankle. J Comput Assist Tomogr 15: 477-482

16. Klein A, Spreitzer AM (1993) MR imaging of the tarsal sinus and canal: normal anatomy, pathologic findings, and features of the sinus tarsi syndrome. Radiology 186: 233-240

17. Möller TB, Reif E (1993) Anatomie IRM des membres. Arnette, Paris

18. Morvan G (1990) L'imagerie nouvelle du pied et de la cheville. Cours de perfectionnement post-univesitaire 6-9 novembre

19. Morvan G, Busson J, Wybier M (1990) Tomodensitométrie du pied et de la cheville. Masson, Paris

20. Noto AM, Cheung Y, Rosenberg ZS, Normal A, Leeds NE (1989) MR imaging of the ankle: normal variants. Radiology 170: 121-124

21. Oloff LM, Sullivan BT, Heard GS, Thornton MC (1992) Magnetic resonance imaging of traumatized ligaments of the ankle. J Am Podiatr Med Assoc 82: 25-32

22. Pomeranz S J (1992) MRI total body atlas, Orthopedic, MRI-EFI publications, Cincinnati,

23. Quinn F, Murray WT, Clark RA, Cochran CF (1987). Radiology 164: 767-770

24. Roger B, Christel P, Poux D, Montalvan B (1991) L'imagerie de l'aponévrose plantaire. In: Pied et cheville. Imagerie et clinique. Sauramps medical, Montpellier, p 159

25. Rosenberg ZS, Feldman F, Singson R, Kane R (1988) Ankle tendons: evaluation with CT. Radiology 166: 221-226

26. Rosenberg ZS, Feldman F, Singson RD (1987) Intra-articular calcaneal fracures: computed tomographic analysis. Skeletal Radiol 16: 105-113

27. Rosenberg ZS, Feldman F, Singson RD, Price GJ (1987) Peroneal tendon injury associated with calcaneal fractures: CT findings. AJR 149: 125-129

28. Rosenberg ZS, Feldman F, Singson RD (1986) Peroneal tendon injuries: CT analysis. Radiology 161: 743-748

29. Rosenberg ZS, Cheung Y, Jahss MH, Noto AM, Normal A, Leeds NE (1988) Rupture of posterior tibial tendon: CT and MR Imaging with surgical correlation. Radiology 169: 229-235

30. Schneck CD, Mesgarzadeh M, Bonakdarpour A, Ross GJ (1992) MR Imaging of the most commonly injured ankle ligaments. Radiology 184: 499-506

31. Schneck CD, Mesgarzadeh M, Bonakdarpour A (1992) MR Imaging of the most commonly injured ankle ligaments. Radiology 184: 507-512

32. Sobel M, Bohne WHO, Markisz JA (1991) Cadaver correlation of peroneal tendon changes with magnetic resonance imaging. Foot Ankle 11: 384-388

33. Sobel M, Geppert MJ, Olson EJ, Bohne WHO, Arnoczky SP (1992) The dynamics of peroneus brevis tendon splits: a proposed mechanism, technique of diagnosis, and classification of injury. Foot Ankle 13: 413-422

34. Solomon MA, Gilula LA, Oloff LM, Oloff J (1986) CT Scanning of the foot and ankle: 2. Clinical applications and review of the literature. AJR 146: 1204-1214

35. Tavernier T, Furhmann M, Boibieux A, Bochu M (1992) Apport de l'IRM dans le diagnostic et le suivi évolutif des ostéites et ostéomyélites. In: L'imagerie ostéo-articulaire post-thérapeutique. Sauramps médical, Montpellier, p 205

36. Tavernier T, Bonnin M, Bouysset M (1997) Syndrome fissuraire du tendon court fibulaire. Mise en évidence et classification en IRM. J Radiol 78: 353-357

Additional references

37. Bonnin M, Tavernier T, Bouysset M (1997) Split lesions of the peroneus brevis tendon in chronic ankle laxity. Am J Sports Med 25: 699-703

38. Breitenseher MJ, Haller J, Kukla C, Gaebler C, Kaider A, Fleischmann D, Helbich T, Trattnig S (1997) MRI of the sinus tarsi in acute ankle sprain injuries. J Comput Assist Tomogr 21: 274-279

39. Breitenseher MJ, Trattnig S, Kukla C, Gaebler C, Kaider A, Baldt MM, Haller J, Imhof H (1997) MRI versus lateral stress radiography in acute lateral ankle ligament injuries. J Comput Assist Tomogr 21: 280-285

40. Khoury NJ, El-Khoury GY, Saltzman CL, Brandser EA (1996) MR imaging of posterior tibial tendon dysfunction. AJR 167: 675-682

41. Khoury NJ, El-Khoury GY, Saltzman CL, Kathol MH (1996) Peroneus longus and brevis tendon tears: MR imaging evaluation. Radiology 200: 833-841

42. Nishimura G, Yamato M, Togawa M (1996) Trabecular trauma of the talus and medial malleolus concurrent with lateral collateral ligamentous injuries of the ankle: evaluation with MR imaging. Skeletal Radiol 25: 49-54

43. Rosenberg ZS, Beltran J, Cheung YY, Colon E, Herraiz F (1997) MR features of longitudinal tears of the peroneus brevis tendon. AJR 168: 141-147

44. Schweitzer ME, Eid ME, Deely D, Wapner K, Hecht P (1997) Using MR imaging to differentiate peroneal splits from other peroneal disorders AJR 168: 129-133

45. Tan RCF, Wilcox DM, Frank L, Shih C, Trudell DJ, Sartoris DJ, Resnick D (1996) MR imaging of articular cartilage in the ankle: comparison of available imaging sequences and methods of measurement in cadavers. Skeletal Radiol 25: 749-755

46. Tjin A, Ton ER, Schweitzer ME, Karasick D (1997) MR imaging of peroneal tendon disorders AJR 168: 135-168

47. Zanetti M, De Simoni C, Wetz HH, Zollinger H, Hodler J (1997) Magnetic resonance imaging of injuries to the ankle joint: can it predict clinical outcome? Skeletal Radiol 26: 82-88

5.

Nuclear medicine in foot pathology

P Chauvot and F Giammarile

Scintigraphy is a non-invasive, functional method of imaging. It provides early information and is highly sensitive. Thus, it can give fundamental diagnostic or prognostic information in various foot disorders [8].

Tracers

The tracers employed are all gamma-emitting and generally bound to a vector. At present, diphosphonates labeled with technetium-99m (99mTc) are the most employed in bone scintigraphy. Because of its short half-life and its exclusive gamma emission, 99mTc irradiation is low (5 mGy for the skeleton) in this kind of examination, thus allowing bone scintigraphy even in children and, if necessary, repeated scans. The examination is highly sensitive but, due to its lack of specificity, the clinical context is of primary importance.

More specific tracers can be employed in order to characterize infection (99mTc or indium-111-labeled autologous leukocytes or IgG), cancer (gallium-67 or thallium-201) or vascularization status (99mTc-labeled microspheres) [18, 21].

Techniques

Usually, scintigraphic procedures require no specific patient preparation and present no risk of allergy. For foot disorders, a bone scintigraphy with 99mTc-diphosphonates is performed in more than 90% of cases. Gamma camera images are obtained about 2.5 hours after the intraveinous injection of the tracer, when the signal-to-noise ratio is optimal. This time may be even longer, in the case of the foot, particularly when a peripheral hypovascularization occurs.

Views can be standard (parallel holes collimator) or "enlarged" (pin-hole collimator), planar, or tomographic in particular cases. For the foot, in particular, centered views performed with a pin-hole collimator better define localized pathologies [11].

Generally, for foot disorders, a three-phase scintigraphy should be performed:
• dynamic phase, during 3 to 5 minutes after injection (gamma camera centered on feet), studies local and regional vascular situations. During the dynamic phase, sequential images at short intervals (1 to 2 seconds) are acquired. Localized or global time/activity diagrams may be constructed;
• early static views at 3 to 5 minutes give information on inflammatory status, in articular or soft tissue disorders;
• delayed images, standard or specific for the study of bone metabolism.

Some authors even perform a fourth phase, 24 hours later, in order to increase the specificity of the examination, especially with infectious problems.

"Normal scintigraphy"

Bone tracer uptake is proportional to blood-flow and to local bone metabolism. In a "healthy" foot, the uptake is uniform in all bony segments. The smallest articular or bony lesion which modifies blood-flow or local bone (osteoblastic) reaction will modify tracer uptake, which is generally increased. This explains the extreme sensitivity and early information provided by the examination.

Image analysis is made in comparision with the opposite side but should be undertaken carefully. In interpreting the images, one must take into account the particular physiology of the foot, its supportive function, the complex pathologies, clinical history, past or current static disturbances and their possible correction, the radiologic appearances, previous surgery or trauma, the skin state, possible walking with crutches and the date of renewed mobility or cessation of the standing position.

Thus, due to the particular physiology of the foot, any factor that can influence the static position may induce scintigraphic abnormalities which are important to characterize. For instance, a calcaneal osteitis that has been evolving for more than a week appears as an increased uptake by the calcaneus and the entire foot because of resulting walking difficulties, and not because of spread of the infectious process. Bone scintigraphy is more specific if done early in a patient without associated orthopedic disorders. Thus, acute osteomyelitis in children is better identified than chronic osteomyelitis in diabetic patients [4, 20].

Indications

Infectious

Bone scintigraphy is frequently asked for, mostly in diabetic patients [9, 10, 16, 19]. Standard three-phase examination should always be performed and can answer most questions.

Scintigraphy with labeled leukocytes may sometimes supplement the usual scan. It necessitates blood sampling, labeling of the white cells in a sterile atmosphere, and reinjection. This examination is thus more complex and costly and should be performed initially only exceptionally.

The traditional three-phase scintigraphy, when carefully done, allows differentiation between cellulitis, arthritis and osteitis. Possible associated arthrosis makes this diagnosis more difficult.

This examination is particularly recommended in the therapeutic follow-up of chronic osteitis, with a reference image at the beginning of treatment.

Roughly, the three phases of the examination should be positive in osteitis, with a delayed uptake by the infected bone segments. The juxta-articular regions are more difficult to evaluate. In isolated arthritis only the first two phases should be positive; the late phase will be positive only subsequently [14]. In cellulitis, the vascular phase shows the soft tissues involved; the early static views will still be weakly positive but the delayed views will be subnormal.

Injuries and stress fractures [1]

When these are suspected, a negative bone scan can unequivocally exclude the diagnosis. The examination is typically performed in three phases, possibly with pin-hole views, lateral views (for calcaneal or trigonal fractures) and particular views when the sesamoids are concerned.

Some images may characterize a clinical context, for instance metatarsal stress fractures [17].

Vascular disorders, necrosis and osteochondritis

In the reflex sympathetic dystrophy syndrome, three-phase examination is imperative [2, 5, 7, 12, 15]. The forms with increased uptake are the most frequent. The "cold" forms (reduced uptake), global or local, are found mainly in children. It is essential to allow for static disturbances and previous trauma. The examination must also look for a diffuse increased uptake in the homolateral limb due to associated osteoporosis.

For frostbite, the use of intra-arterial 99mTc-labeled microspheres is a very demonstrative prognostic test, showing immediately the "excluded" areas. However, it is easier to perform a typical three-phase bone scan for these patients, often in bad general condition. The areas showing no uptake in delayed views, and with increased uptake at the junction with healthy tissue should be amputated [6, 13].

Scintigraphy is of particular value not only for navicular bone necrosis but also for post-traumatic talar necrosis (pin-hole views centered on the talo-crural region).

Neoplastic or degenerative diseases, dysplasia

If a primary tumor is situated in the foot, a three-phase examination centered on the foot and a whole body bone scan should be performed. The examination is particularly important in the case of doubtful lesions. A negative examination can usually identify non-progressive benign lesions.

Specific tracers can be used, such as thallium-201 for osteosarcomas; gallium-67 is not very specific and is not useful for the foot. Iodine-labeled MIBG (in the case of a neuroblastoma or pheochromocytoma), or indium-111-labeled somatostatin have no theoretical value in the foot on its own.

Among benign tumors, osteoid osteoma has a particular place because of the typical clinical findings and its difficult demonstration by conventional imaging. Bone scintigraphy should seek for the lesion both near to and remote from the source of the pain. The focal increased uptake (nidus) is characteristic. Emission tomography (SPECT) can complete the examination in order to better locate the lesion.

In fibrous dysplasia, Paget's disease or metastases, isolated forms in the foot are rare but the initial clinical symptoms may be situated in the foot. A whole-body bone scan will complete the staging. Paget's disease is often recognized by very functional, characteristic images.

In noninfective arthritic spondylitis, bone scintigraphy quantitatively evaluates the sacroiliac uptake [3]. The discovery of periosteal tendinitis or enthesitis (insertional lesions) allows early diagnosis.

Particular orthopedic problems

Bone scan is indicated for possible pseudoarthrosis (rare) but mainly for evaluating the quality of an arthrodesis. In some cases, the conventional bone scan can solve the problem of an uncertain arthrodesis. The views must be programmed according to the problems posed. In arthrodesis, normal uptake is a sign of fusion, whereas increased uptake observed a long time after surgery is a sign of pseudarthrosis. A minor uptake must be interpreted according to the date of surgery. It is reasonable to wait 2 or 3 months; in doubtful cases, the evolution of the images on a second examination performed at least 2 months later may be conclusive.

The uptake by exostoses clarifies their degree of potential development and the more active regions, in particular at their base.

Summary

Radioactive tracers play an important role in the diagnosis and treatment of various foot disorders. Since metabolic abnormalities are detected earlier than anatomic changes, the examination will be positive and informative at the onset of the disorder. However, the examination requires particular attention to the clinical context, a good knowledge of the pathology and optimal quality (good gamma camera, suitable collimators, perfect immobility, optimized acquisition time related to the injected activity and the local uptake), and must be interpreted in relation to the clinical and radiologic data.

Bone scintigraphy is a very sensitive examination (almost 100%), so that a negative scan can exclude osteoarticular pathology. Specificity is less but the above precautions greatly improve this parameter. Sometimes, however, comparison with a "reference" bone scintigraphy can lead to a formal conclusion. For this reason, it is important to perform bone scintigraphy at an early stage of the diagnostic procedure.

References

1. Anderson E G (1990) Fatigue fractures of the foot. Injury 21: 275-278
2. Doury P (1994) Les algodystrophies à forme froide d'emblée. Sem Hôp Paris 33: 1005-1009
3. Doury P, Gaillard J F, Pattin S, Eulry F, Bloch J G (1989) Intérêt de la scintigraphie osseuse dans le diagnostic précoce des spondylarthropathies séronégatives. In: Actualités en physiopathologie et pharmacologie articulaires. Vol 1. Masson, Paris, pp 34-39
4. Elgazzar AH, Abdel-Dayem HM, Clark JD, Maxon HR (1995) Multimodality imaging of osteomyelitis. Eur J Nucl Med 22: 1043-1063
5. Eulry F (1993) Algodystrophies: Étiologie, diagnostic, évolution, traitement. Rev Prat (Paris) 43: 2299-2304
6. Foray J (1991) Gelure grave des extrémités. Chirurgie 117: 550-556
7. Granier Ph, Manicourt DH, Pauwels S, Nagant de Deuxchaisnes Ch, Beckers C (1994) Analyse semi-quantitative des données de la scintigraphie osseuse

en trois temps dans l'algodystrophie des extrémités. Rev Rhum 61: 179-188

8. Karl RD, Hammes CS (1988) Nuclear medicine imaging in podiatric disorders. Clin Podiatr Med Surg, 5: 909-929

9. Keenan AM, Tindel NL, Alavi A (1989) Diagnosis of podal osteomyelitis in diabetic patients using current scintigraphic techniques. Arch Intern Med 149: 2262-2266

10. Larcos G, Brown ML, Sutton RT (1991) Diagnostic of osteomyelitis of the foot in diabetic patients: value of ¹¹¹In-leukocyte scintigraphy. AJR 157: 527-531

11. Mandell GA, Harcke HT, Hugh J, Kumar SJ, Maas KW (1990) Detection of talocalcaneal coalitions by magnification bone scintigraphy. J Nucl Med 31: 1797-1801

12. Manicourt DH (1994) L'exploration scintigraphique dans l'algodystrophie sympathique réflexe. Sem Hop Paris 33: 1023-1042

13. Mehta RC, Wilson MA (1989) Frostbite injury: prediction of tissue viability with triple phase bone scanning. Radiology 170: 511-514

14. Möttönen TT, Hannonen P, Toivanen J, Rekonen A, Oka M (1988) Value of joint scintigraphy in the prediction of erosiveness in early rheumatoid arthritis. Ann Rheum Dis 47: 183-189

15. O'Donoghue JP, Powe JE, Mattar AG, Hurwitz GA, Laurin NR (1993) Three-phase bone scintigraphy. Asymmetric patterns in the upper extremities of asymptomatic normals and reflex sympathetic dystrophy patients. Clin Nucl Med 18: 829-836

16. Oyen WJG, Netten PM, Lemmens JAM, Claessens RAMJ, Lutterman JA, Van der Vliet JA, Goris RJA, Van der Meer JWM, Corstens FHM (1992) Evaluation of infectious diabetic foot complications with indium-111-labeled human nonspecific immunoglobulin G. J Nucl Med 33: 1330-1336

17. Santi M, Sartoris DJ (1991) Diagnostic imaging approach to stress fractures of the foot.J Foot Surg 30 : 85-96

18. Schauwecker DS, Park HM, Burt RW, Mock BH, Wellman HN (1988) Combined bone scintigraphy and indium-111 leukocyte scans in neuropathic foot disease. J Nucl Med 29: 1651-1655

19. Shults DW, Hunter GC, McIntyre KE, Parent FN, Piotrowski JJ, Bernhard VM (1989) Value of radiographs and bone scans in determining the need for therapy in diabetic patients with foot ulcers. Am J Surg 158: 525-530

Additional references

20. Harvey J, Cohen MM (1997) Technetium-99-labeled leukocytes in diagnosing diabetic osteomyelitis in the foot. J Foot Ankle Surg 36: 209-214

21. Nijhof MW, Oyen WJ, van Kampen A, Claessens RA, van der Meer JW, Corstens FH (1997) Evaluation of infections of the locomotor system with indium-111-labeled human IgG scintigraphy. J Nucl Med 38: 1300-1305

6.

Correct use of auxiliary investigations in foot and ankle disorders

M Bouysset, M Bonnin and T Tavernier

Auxiliary investigations seek to confirm the diagnosis. Their employment depends on the simplicity of the procedure and the quality of the information provided. Their cost must be considered as well as the risk undergone by the patient. Sometimes the value of a test comes from comparison with a previous examination.

In current practice

A precise history and an accurate clinical assessment with a basic radiographic study and, if indicated, minimal laboratory evaluation are sufficient for most cases. The clinical features alone very often indicate or strongly suggest the diagnosis.

The history investigates the characteristics of the pain: circumstances of its occurrence, progress since the onset, localization and irradiation, whether mechanical in rhythm (in weight-bearing) or more inflammatory in nature (pain increasing during the night). It is important, also, to search for previous pathologic features, whether localized to the foot or other parts of the body, which sometimes help to establish the diagnosis of the causal disease.

• In some cases the diagnosis seems obvious: the acute painful crisis of the hallux with pain increasing during the night, appearing after a large meal, suggests gout. Metatarsalgia occurring during walking and forcing a female patient to take off her shoe, strongly suggests a Morton's syndrome.

• In other cases the attention of the clinician is attracted by certain features:

- A metatarsalgia or painful heel of rapid or abrupt onset, is not always due to a static metatarsal disorder, a plantar aponeurositis or a calcaneal tendinopathy. The diagnosis of stress fracture must not be overlooked. Any circumstances which may provoke the development of this lesion should be noted and, after clinical assessment, a radiograph and especially a technetium bone scan should be requested at the outset, if there is any doubt.

- The presence of painful heel in a young man suggests a diagnosis of ankylosing spondylitis and invites a search for criteria of this disease.

Clinical assessement

Inspection by itself may provide important information. It will reveal a triangular forefoot deformation, a valgus hindfoot deformation, or a laterally deviated angle of gait. The common static disorders will be verified during the rest of the clinical evaluation; radiography is not always essential. Sometimes the clinician will be alerted by particular features: for instance, the observation of a flat-foot deformity in an adolescent with painful crises and spasms suggests a diagnosis of tarsal synostosis. Sometimes an X-ray, but more often CT, will confirm the diagnosis.

Decreasing dorsiflexion of the first metatarsophalangeal joint may cause lateral metatarsalgia due to walking on the outer side of the foot. X-ray confirms the hallux rigidus.

Bilateral involvement of the metatarsophalangeal and metacarpophalangeal joints with pain, redness, swelling and morning stiffness suggest an inflammatory condition, particularly rheumatoid arthritis. These features indicate radiography and laboratory assessment in a search for this pathology.

The clinical assessment must avoid some major faults.
• In a patient who consults for "ankle pain", when this joint does not seem to be involved on clinical assessment, pain and stiffness of the subtalar joint should direct attention towards a disorder of this joint.
• A so-called talocrural sprain with pain under the medial malleolus, particularly when there is valgus calcaneal deformation, suggests a tendinopathy of the tendon of the tibialis posterior muscle which will be confirmed by pursuing the clinical assessment; sometimes the radiograph shows an accessory tibial ossicle.

When the initial picture is acute with intense pain and a crack followed by total flattening of the medial arch accompanied by other typical clinical features, it is possible to make a diagnosis of rupture of the tibialis posterior tendon. A MRI study is not necessary for the diagnosis; the same applies to recent and typical ruptures of the calcaneal tendon.
• Plantar pain with a rather diffuse burning sensation and little evidence after assessment of the foot is suspicious. It suggests a search for factors predisposing to neuropathy, particularly diabetes or alcoholism. A minimal neurologic assessment may lead to the diagnosis of polyneuritis.

The standard radiologic assessment in weight-bearing confirms and clarifies static disorders of the foot and may give many signs, such as the presence of exostoses and their nature. In some cases, another pathology is noted: Freiberg's disease, Sever's disease, necrosis of a sesamoid bone or a fractured os tibiale. There is rarely a stress fracture line; the radiographic diagnosis is often made later, when bony callus is observed. A bony avulsion secondary to a previously overlooked talocrural sprain is sometimes observed.

The standard laboratory assessment - sedimentation rate, C-reactive protein - requested on the least suspicion sometimes confirms or evaluates an inflammatory lesion. The level of uricemia, in relation to observed predisposing factors in men or after the menopause in women, is easily determined.

When these first investigational stages are negative

Consideration should be given to the following:
• Repetition of the history and physical assessment, with a meticulous review of the pathologic past of the patient in relation to present circumstances: thus, familial cutaneous psoriasis or a record of tenosynovitis of a toe (sausage-like) or finger suggests the diagnosis of psoriatic arthropathy.
• Supplementary radiographic views, e.g., axial view of the sesamoid bones to better observe their structure (presence of fracture or necrosis), oblique or retrotibial view (to look for a tarsal synostosis). In the case of ankle instability after injury, comparative frontal views of both talocrural joints in forced varus will be indicated. Sometimes a tibiotalar diastasis is observed.
• To make, when it is possible, a synovial fluid aspiration with study of the synovial fluid. This laboratory investigation is of great value, particularly when there is an isolated arthritis of the talo-crural joint.
• Further laboratory tests if there is the least doubt, sometimes immediately. The Rose-Waaler and latex tests for rheumatod arthritis and the searching for HLA-B27 antigen in ankylosing spondylitis are aids to diagnosis. In some cases the laboratory findings will suggest contraindications to some forms of treatment and can be used to monitor tolerance of a treatment programme as it proceeds.
• Supplementary assessment of a site other than the foot sometimes helps in diagnosis: radiography of the hands and wrists in rheumatoid arthritis may show bone erosion, radiography of the sacroiliac joints for anklyosing spondylitis.
• Repetition of the basic clinical, radiologic and laboratory examinations at an interval after the first assessment, chiefly in diseases with recurrent acute episodes.

● Auxiliary investigations (table 6.1)

Certain points must stressed about additional investigations:

Bone scintigraphy

The technetium bone scan is very useful when the basic examination gives no guidance (a rare situation in common practice). This procedure may highlight very suggestive localized foci of isotope hyperfixation, particularly suggestive of inflammatory lesions, microcrystalline arthritides or infective arthritis. It may also suggest a diagnosis of bone tumor or a degenerative chondritis with arthrosis. It also permits the diagnosis of algodystrophy at an early stage, when clinically it often resembles an inflammatory foot. It will show up typical early signs of stress fractures while the X-rays are still normal; in other cases it will lead to the diagnosis of spondylarthropathy in cases of mechanical heel pain with hyperfixation at several tendon or ligament attachments.

Often the need for some other additional examination is suggested by the bone scan, which indicates the affected site:
• in some cases with pain in the proximal tarsus or ankle pain, isotope hyperfixation suggests the diagnosis of osteonecrosis, particularly of the talus, which will be confirmed by MRI at an earlier stage and CT at a later stage;
• in cases of diffuse midtarsal pain, hyperfixation at the navicular bone suggests a stress fracture, while the clinical diagnosis remains difficult; here CT is indicated;
• the same problem exists with bone tumors, particularly osteoid osteoma, where CT will pinpoint the diagnosis, to be confirmed by histologic study after removal.
• in septic or microcrystalline arthritides, bone scan and often CT may suggest joint aspiration and examination of the synovial fluid for micro-organisms or micro-crystals of gout or chondrocalcinosis.

The bone scan also allows verification of the soundness of an arthrodesis.

Computed tomography

CT rather concerns cortical bone. Thus, in the case of a patient with a history of trauma, sometimes minimal and old, previously considered as an ankle sprain, the presence of mechanical midtarsal pain suggests CT, at a level defined by the clinical assessment or bone scan, in the search for a fragmented fracture of the tarsus which was not recognized initially.

Arthrography with CT

This better evaluates the cartilage and possible foreign bodies.

Tenography with CT

This seems very useful in some cases, as in the search for tendon ruptures and longitudinal fissures. However it remains an invasive procedure, is difficult to perform properly and a specialist practitioner is often necessary.

MRI

MRI rather concerns soft parts and spongy bone; this more expensive procedure is sometimes essential to confirm a partial rupture of the plantar aponeurosis, or a tendon or ligamentous rupture. The great sensivity of the recent MRI sequences with fat saturation (FAT-SAT) must be stressed in traumatic or inflammatory lesions of spongy bone; in the area observed these last sequences combine technetium bone scan sensitivity and anatomic accuracy.

It must be remembered that pieces of metal near the explored area make the MRI findings uninterpretable because of artefacts. Likewise, a CT view passing through metal presents artefacts which sometimes necessitate the use of tomography. It must be added also that MRI cannot be used in a patient with a pacemaker, with certain artificial cardiac valves, or with metal particles that may be mobilized.

Ultrasonography

Ultrasonography chiefly appears useful for studying the calcaneal tendon; the value of this cheaper procedure depends very much on the experience of the practitioner. Some recent apparatus have a greater accuracy, high-frequency probes (10 MHz).

Table 6.1. Strategy in diagnosis of painful foot and ankle

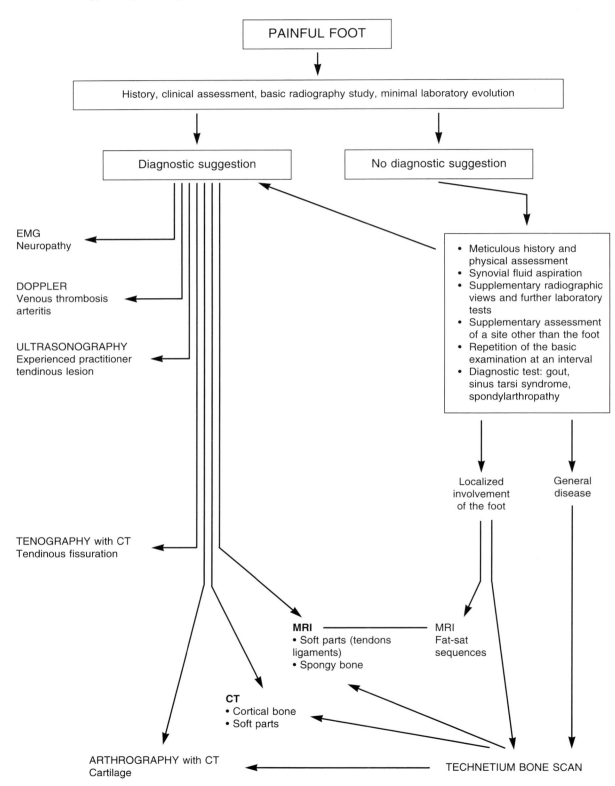

Electromyography (EMG)

This is a procedure whose performance is difficult in the foot and whose value also largely depends on the practitioner. Moreover, it is well-known that some quite obvious clinical conditions do not always present electromyographic features. However, the entrapment neuropathies of the lower extremities or some systemic neuropathies localized to the foot are sometimes difficult to assess initially and then EMG is indicated if in doubt.

Other procedures

Procedures unrelated to bone and joint diseases may be useful for etiologic research. When there is a painful ankle and hindfoot with localized swelling, the doppler technique, a noninvasive procedure, may be used to detect localized venous thrombosis. Arterial doppler may also be employed if the pain seems to be due to arteritis in the lower limb.

Biopsy-arthroscopy of the ankle

The biopsy of a swelling observed on CT or MRI allows histologic confirmation of the diagnosis. Sometimes ankle arthroscopy is used, a procedure which is at the borderline between investigation and operation.

● The procedure varies with every diagnostic possibility

Table 6.2 cites some cases but cannot be exhaustive about such a varied subject. The case of the sinus tarsi syndrome may be stressed because treatment itself may be a diagnostic test (by corticosteroid injection into the sinus). Often, bone scan is the indicated procedure. The absence of isotopic hyperfixation leads one to ask, in terms of the context, for procedures like CT which can suggest certain lesions like foreign bodies, or MRI in the search for ligamentous or tendinous lesions difficult to detect by clinical or radiologic evaluation. It may be very diffi-

Table 6.2. Some examples of diseases sometimes difficult to diagnose at their onset and methods for their better definition

midtarsal arthrosis	bone scan - CT
stress fracture	bone scan - X-ray - (MRI)
algodystrophy	bone scan
polyneuritis	clinical assessment - EMG
entrapment syndromes	clinical assessment - EMG - MRI
sinus tarsi syndrome	clinical assessment - corticosteroid injection - (MRI)
degenerative tendinopathy of the tibialis posterior tendon	clinical assessment - MRI
tumor	X-ray - bone scan - CT
tarsal synostosis	clinical assessment - X-ray - CT

culty to detect some conditions at their onset: degeneration of the tendon of the tibialis posterior muscle, midtarsal arthrosis, or some neuropathies for long localized to the foot whose diagnosis is only made later. Other diagnoses may be suggested, particularly an arteriopathy, disease at a higher level (knee), fibrositis, etc. Mention of these etiologies underlines how important a role the whole pathologic context plays in obscure situations.

● Conclusion

In the foot the analysis of functional symptoms, clinical assessment bilateral and comparative, standard X-rays, and sometimes some simple laboratory tests are often suggestive of the diagnosis in everyday practice. A minimal knowledge of foot pathology, but also of general pathology, makes the investigation easier and contributes to a better interpretation of the results of the above-mentioned investigations. When other additional examination procedures appear necessary, they depend on the pathologic context. Whatever the circumstances, the clinical evaluation must come first in the etiologic search and the practitioner should not use supplementary examinations to conceal his ignorance.

7.

The neuropathic foot

A Bardot, AB Ward and G Curvale

Pathophysiology

Neurological

The foot is essentially adapted for plantargrade bipedal standing and for locomotion. Through its precise and complex biomechanics, it has developed phylogenetically from a part of a posterior limb to a part of an inferior limb. It can only function normally under control of an intact nervous system. There are two major nerve pathways which, through their network, regulate all aspects of the foot's function: first, centripetal afferent pathways supplying the brain and spinal cord with indispensable conscious and subconscious information; second, centrifugal efferent motor pathways providing the working foot with the necessary energy (both in quantity and distribution) for an adequate "kinetic" function which immediately adapts to the specific requirements for each of the foot's tasks, and which must be biomechanically harmonious with the overlying kinetic chains.

The problems affecting the sensory pathways are essentially twofold: first, trophic conditions, among which the most important manifestations are plantar ulcers and neuropathic arthropathy resulting from a loss of sensation. The plantar soft tissues are able to resist considerable mechanical pressure and shear forces but their integrity is dependent on normal nociceptive inputs to allow for a reaction to remove the effects of these forces. Plantar anesthesia is therefore serious. The same is also true for deep sensory loss, notably in capsulo-ligamentous

dysfunction which can lead to neuropathic arthropathy as classically seen in tabes dorsalis. Second, from conditions affecting balance and the postural control of the foot during standing and walking which results in an "ataxic foot" when proprioception is lost or is abnormal.

Conditions of the foot caused by motor-pathway disorders reflect the very diverse anomalies of muscular performance. These can be anomalies due to weakened or excessive muscular contractions. Spatial anomalies from imbalance of synergistic forces lead to architectural and postural disorders within the foot and temporal anomalies caused by inopportune muscular contraction or relaxation.

In order to simplify the description of the various disorders in the foot caused by sensory and motor neurologic impairments, it is useful to consider two major categories separately: those of the central nervous system (CNS) and those of the peripheral nervous system (PNS). CNS disorders arise from the brain and spinal cord lesions and, according to conventional terminology, coexist with the motor units and dorsal root cells that are still intact. PNS disorders are those affecting the anterior horn cells, spinal nerve roots, plexuses and trunks. In clinical podiatric practice the former are characterized by intact distal structures which are capable of functioning, but sensory feedback and voluntary and involuntary motor control are impaired. The muscles can be weak or overactive, but they are not denervated and the distal sensory pathways are intact. Possible eventual amyotrophy results from disuse and trophic problems are rather uncommon in conscious patients. In PNS disorders, however, partial or total denervation of muscles is the norm. Sensory problems are noted which range from simple paresthesiae to total anesthesia. Trophic lesions are frequently found but the integrity of the CNS provides for an awareness of the problems and the possibility to compensate for the motor deficiency to the extent that the preserved regions permit. One of the features of these two expressions of neurologic pathology concerns clinical assessment and auxiliary examinations. There is no point in using clinical analytic muscular assessment for CNS disorders, as denervation is not present and analysis is impossible. As for the use of electromyography (EMG) in this situation, it can only reveal the intensity and chronology of muscular contraction as the lines will be electrologically normal. On the other hand, clinical analytic muscular assessment (muscle testing) and EMG are indispensable aids in PNS disorders. These two sorts of disorders as specified are responsible for the majority of causes of the "neuropathic foot" that respond to relatively straightforward clinical presentations [15]: in CNS pathology, one can observe pyramidal, extrapyramidal, cerebellar and ataxic signs. Peripheral neurologic anomalies are found in the other category. However, these clinical expressions do not cover all aspects and the clinician can encounter less typical pictures corresponding to ailments that overlap the two major functional divisions. These include dystonic feet and lesions of the spinal cord at the interneuronal level such as in amyotrophic lateral sclerosis (Charcot's disease) or hereditary spinocerebellar degeneration.

Biomechanical

Anomalies are considered in a three-dimensional analysis of the different points in the gait cycle in relation to the joints of the other segments of the lower limb. Deficits due to neurologic disorders are usually dynamic and only present themselves during standing and walking. They can eventually become fixed to create deformity depending on the patient's age and the duration, cause and extent of the problem.

Kinetics

The analysis of imbalance in the neuropathic foot assumes a knowledge of fundamental biomechanics as discussed above. It is important to emphasize the interdependence of the talocrural and midtarsal joints given the fact that the talus has no tendinous insertions, and no muscle acts alone on the talocrural joint. All the muscles acting on the ankle do so on both joint complexes. Each muscular group couple (for example invertors and evertors) functions normally in a harmonious balanced fashion for mobility and load stability. Muscular imbalance may appear in neurologic conditions due to underactivity (more commonly in peripheral nerve lesions) or overactivity (more often in central pathology).

Muscle imbalance in the sagittal plane:

Dorsiflexor muscle weakness

This is primarily apparent during the swing phase of the gait cycle. During this phase, foot-drop requires compensation to ensure toe clearance, either through lower limb shortening by increased hip and knee flexion (steppage gait), or through hip abduction and circumduction. Partial weakness (for example of the tibialis anterior) can be compensated by an increased activity of other dorsiflexor muscles (e.g. extensor digitorum longus).

Plantarflexor muscle weakness

This does not alter the swing phase of the gait cycle but becomes disabling during single foot weight-bearing. If dorsiflexion of the ankle is not restricted by secondary calf muscle shortening, body weight forces cause forward movement of the tibia, resulting in knee flexion and subsequent increased work for the quadriceps muscle. If the latter is impaired as well, the knee will give way in flexion. Weakness of the posterior calf muscles (gastrocnemius and soleus) is not compensated for by action of the other plantar flexors (tibialis posterior, flexor hallucis, flexor digitorum, and fibular muscles). In addition, their respective actions can make transverse imbalance additionally apparent. The small muscles of the foot are often impaired. This weakness appears as clawing of the toes, revealing the predominance of the long flexors and extensors of the toes over the short muscles.

Plantarflexor muscle hypertonia or spasticity

This is rarely expressed by equinus alone. In effect, with the exception of the fibular muscles, all the flexors also have a supinator action. Spasticity of the flexor muscles leads to a reducible even an irreducible equinus due to calf-muscle contracture. This can cause the foot to have a dysfunction during the swing phase. There are also consequences for weight-bearing in the stance phase: transmitting an overload onto the forefoot and relative lengthening of the lower limb. The latter occurs if the heel cannot achieve contact with the ground and if there is no proximal skeletal shortening. Irreducible equinus foot causes either a compensatory flexion of the knee, conditions permitting, or a secondary knee recurvatum deformity which will evolve until the equinus deformity is corrected.

Muscle imbalance in the frontal plane

Spasticity in muscles causing plantar flexion and inversion of the foot (as seen in hemiplegic adults) is characterized during the swing phase by an equinovarus posture resulting from a spastic "pseudo foot-drop". This posture of the foot is due not only to dorsiflexor and evertor weakness, but also and mainly to prevalent contraction of the flexor and invertor muscles. During stance, persistent foot inversion results in external instability. Isolated tibialis posterior muscle weakness can be responsible for a developing weight-bearing flat-foot through sagging of the medial arch. The relative deficiency of the supinator muscles results in a valgus foot. Isolated weakness of the fibular muscles can cause ankle inversion instability, while relative deficiency of the anterolateral compartment muscles simply causes a varus foot. Monopodal upright stability, either static or during walking, is disturbed by disturbance of transverse muscular balance. Functional anomalies of the "metatarsal balance platform" usually lead to excessive cutaneous pressure under the first or fifth metatarsal heads.

Muscle imbalance in the horizontal plane

Hypertonicity or predominance of the tibialis posterior muscle leads to a certain degree of forefoot adduction in the horizontal plane. Vertical obliquity in front of and within Henke's axis in the midtarsal joint, which is really a 45-degree hinge between the foot and the leg, explains how each varus/supination action of the weight-bearing foot leads to external rotation of the adjacent lower leg segment and vice versa. A hip internal rotation deficit at the end of the

step cycle can thus decompensate the lateral instability of a weight-bearing ankle.

Deformities of the neuropathic foot [68]

Neuromuscular imbalance tends to lead to fixed deformities. These are linked to muscular shortening and articular and periarticular fibrosis eventually occurs. This is particularly obvious in children by the effect of growth on the morphology of osteocartilaginous structures.

Hindfoot deformities

In the sagittal plane, equinus deformities are more frequent and are defined by an incomplete and reducible horizontalization of the calcaneus as a consequence of calf plantarflexor predominance over the dorsiflexors, particularly when there has been no weight bearing on the forefoot for some time as in prolonged bedrest. The calcaneocavus deformity, on the other hand, is an excessive verticalization of this bone and appears to be most often associated with a paralysed plantar flexor with normal or near normal dorsiflexors.

In the frontal plane, schematically, valgus is a consequence of relative supinator weakness whereas varus is due to relative pronator weakness. In fact, varus is most often associated with equinus or pes cavus. However, one can observe a valgus high-arched foot in poliomyelitis.

Midfoot deformities

High-arched insteps are common in the neuropathic foot. Associated with hindfoot equinus, they increase the slope between the hind- and forefoot and compromise heel weight-bearing.

Flat feet are usually associated with hindfoot valgus but can also be the consequence of equinus (ie, equinus caused by plantarflexor muscle shortening which is compensated by secondary laxity of the midfoot in dorsiflexion and eversion).

Forefoot deformities

Excess load under the metatarsal heads is a result of acquired hind- and midfoot deformity which is often aggravated by clawed toes. It is incapacitating to a greater or lesser degree depending on whether it is shared equally by the five metatarsals or is concentrated on the lateral side (varus foot) or medial side (valgus foot).

Equinus and calcaneocavus foot

These two terms must be defined according to the biomechanical results. While calcaneal equinus refers to an excessive horizontalization of this bone, the expressions "equinus foot" or "equinism of the foot" refer to a foot which, when loaded under a vertical tibia, applies more load on the forefoot than on the heel. Biomechanically, this has the effect of the ground tending to push the tibia backwards. Inversely, calcaneocavus refers to the verticalization of the calcaneus and to a foot which, under a vertical tibia, applies more load on the heel than on the forefoot. This has the biomechanical effect of the ground tending to push the tibia forwards. In the neuropathic foot, this terminology based on biomechanics permits the practitioner to evaluate the respective effects of these foot deformities in the sagittal plane, those of the knee and those of the hip on the stability or the instability of standing and on the therapeutic, surgical, or orthotic results that are applied.

Clawed toes

The short intrinsic muscles, metatarsophalangeal flexors and interphalangeal extensors (interossei, lumbricals and flexor hallucis brevis) play a major biomechanical role in the neurological foot. In peripheral neurologic impairment, their normal function contributes to the stability of the weight-bearing knee if the quadriceps muscle is weak and if the foot plantar flexors are not totally paralyzed, or even if they are mildly shortened (for example, as a consequence of poliomyelitis). In return, their deficit in relation to the long plantar and dorsiflexors of the toes in central or peripheral neurologic disturbance gives rise to clawed toes that are often disabling. Any disharmony between the long and intrinsic muscles can result in reversible deformities which eventually become fixed and are distinguished as three types [8]. **Type I** clawing associates metatarsophalangeal (MTP) dorsiflexion with proximal and distal interphalangeal plantar flexion (PIP and DIP) and results from a deficit of the intrinsic muscles but preservation of long muscle action. **Type II** associates MTP and DIP dorsiflexion with PIP plantar flexion. Thus, flexor digitorum brevis predominates over the flexor longus during standing. **Type III** associates plantar flexion of the three joints rolling the toe under the forefoot. This type is always of neurologic origin and most frequently occurs after severe diffuse cerebral injury.

A general guide to the examination

Examination of the neurologic foot is part of the overall assessment of the disabled individual and implies a number of other work-ups: general medical, neurologic, orthopedic, trophic and functional. An outline can be adapted to account for the most complex situations with a structured, systematic and methodical examination. The extent of the examination depends on the neurological diagnosis and the degree of severity of the condition. A supportive neurologic or neuro-orthopedic opinion can be requested and in very complex cases combined consultation with rheumatologists, rehabilitationists, neuro- and orthopedic surgeons in order to make a comprehensive assessment of these patients.

Past history and etiologic enquiry at the first consultation

The first contact with the patient should attempt to gain as much as possible of the relevant history and to assess the patient's cognitive and intellectual status. It is necessary to define the patient's complaints (pain and disability, which are often different from what is suggested in the clinical examination), needs and lifestyle. Past history taken from former files, the patient and his or her family is all recorded. It is important to arrive at a neurologic diagnosis, if this has not already been made, and to evaluate the progression of the disease process as each will have a direct effect on the choice of treatment strategy. Observation permits an overall appreciation of the patient's functional abilities (whether standing is possible or not, whether walking is possible with or without a stick/crutch, with or without shoes, whether dressing/undressing is possible and if the patient can perform transfers). More particularly, it comprises a study of walking gait, if possible [43], with or without aid, with and then without shoes, analyzing in particular the stance and swing phases of both legs as well as the stability of one or both legs. Deformities, posture, visible difficulties with tone and stability, cutaneous lesions can all be noted immediately. An examination of the footwear is also of great value.

General assessment

The following parameters are taken into account: age, weight and general condition (which is often impaired), mental and cognitive state, possible infection, domestic situation and occupational activity.

Neurologic examination

Neurologic examination is the norm but with the notion of assessment with a view to therapeutic intervention.

Peripheral nerve pathology

Motor assessment

There are two important examinations: muscular function analysis and electromyography. Manual **analytic muscle testing**, assessing the force of voluntary contraction muscle by muscle can only be roughed out at the time of the consultation. It is best performed by a specialist and permits the site and degree of muscular weakness to be precisely determined [33, 38, 41, 67]. It should be systematic and preferably complete in order to avoid neglecting muscle weakness outside of the lower leg or foot. It can therefore, at times, clarify or correct the neurologic diagnosis. Mapping out the deficit provides useful diagnostic information on the level of damaged motor units [29, 65]. It can evaluate the evolution of a deficit, give precise information for rehabilitation and, with the EMG, propose the eventual indications for possible tendon transfers. **EMG** [18, 52, 54, 70] principally focuses on segmental deficits as highlighted by manual analytic muscle testing and defines the extent of denervation, identifies the site and measures the size of the lesion. In certain cases, evoked potentials [71] and nerve and muscle biopsy can provide further diagnostic and prognostic information. Sensory assessment: mapping out sensory, proprioceptive and superficial loss is noted and quantified [26, 48, 69]. Both sensory and motor conduction studies are often useful to specify the site of the lesion.

CNS pathology

Motor assessment

This evaluates tone, reflexes and control of voluntary movement. Methodical examination looks for and notes the obvious signs of pyramidal, extrapyramidal and cerebral problems. Increased muscular tone is clinically assessed with care and skill (progressive slow mobilization of joints can distinguish the difference between straightforward increased tone and muscle shortening). If necessary, spasticity assessment is established [5, 32, 40].

Sensory assessment

This evaluates not only cutaneous sensation but also proprioceptive and perceptual loss.

Orthopedic examination

This looks at anomalies of static and dynamic alignment, not only of the foot and ankle but also of the whole weight-bearing lower limb from the front, the side and in the horizontal plane in order to note the transmission of forces. Joint assessment measures the range of movement, whether excessive or restricted, and attempts to determine an anatomic cause of possible stiffness (bony, capsular ligamentous or muscular). Weight-bearing anomalies are often present with plantar hyperkeratoses and can be evaluated by podoscopic studies. Precise and comprehensive imaging further supports clinical findings.

Trophic and vascular assessment

The association of neurologic problems with vascular anomalies (including lymphatic) alters the prognosis and complicates treatment. Neuropathy in diabetics frequently aggravates the consequences of arteriolar lesions [31] Trophic problems are the classical complication of an anesthetic sole [56], with the development of infected ulcers from which sinuses to deeper tissues can extend into joints, the most common being the metatarsophalangeal joints.

Functional assessment

This is essential for a basis of treatment. It must take into account the cognitive conditions, comprehension and wishes of the patient and can require consultation with the family and/or entourage. Functional problems are analysed in stance and swing phases of gait with stance problems (imbalance, instability, propulsion deficits, pain) being more disabling than swing problems. In the swing phase, foot-drop must be considered, especially if it causes falls. Assessment involves both limbs. Foot disorders must be situated among other possible disabilities due to the neurologic impairment [4]. It is also important to identify, among the troubles cited by the patient or his entourage, those which must be treated and those which must be maintained. Certain anomalies can be exploited to benefit a patient. This is for instance the case in certain equinus problems in poliomyelitis patients, which need to be preserved to stabilize the knee or to compensate for limb-length inequality. Certain spastic patients only stand because of their spasticity. In this context, a therapeutic trial of tibial nerve block using alcohol can be useful [66]. This functional assessment can only be fully relevant with the knowledge gained from simultaneous kinetic and other analyses (neurologic, therapeutic) of the problems by a multidisciplinary team.

● Therapeutic measures

Medication

Apart from analgesics, which are sometimes required in the neuropathic foot, the main drugs indicated are antispasmodic agents which are in four categories [25]: dantrolene sodium, the only antispasmodic with a peripheral effect; benzodiazepines, which work through an indirect GABA-mimetic effect; baclofen, which acts at a pre-synaptic level in the CNS; tizanidine, which preferentially acts on the polysynaptic pathways. The foot, as part of a wider clinical picture, is nevertheless sometimes the most affected part of a spastic lower limb. Antispasmodic drugs used in combination with rehabilitation can often provide satisfactory results in moderately severe spasticity. In severe cases, however, they may be somewhat disappointing since the high doses that are required will cause generalized disabling weakness and frequent side-effects.

Physical medicine

Rehabilitation [51]

Apart from when symptoms are exclusively sensory or trophic, re-education is an integral part of a ther-apeutic program. A co-ordinated process is integrated to include the interventions of physiotherapists and subsequently occupational therapists, medication, orthoses, electrotherapy, neurolysis and neurological and orthopedic surgery.

Physiotherapy

Physiotherapy is carried out over the entire lower limb rather then localized to the neurologically impaired foot, taking into account the following goals: prevention, maintenance, functional restoration and finally rehabilitation. Physiotherapeutic prevention is applied to foreseeable functional deformities through articular and muscular testing, manipulation, mobilization, postural retraining and, if necessary, positioning by orthoses. Maintenance physiotherapy preserves the range of joint movement, orthopedic condition, muscular health and general fitness through massage and an active analytic and complete rehabilitation. Rehabilitation for functional restoration consists, when possible, in exploiting through appropriate muscular activity, the progressive improvement of neurologic weakness - translated into reinnervation in peripheral neuropathies and neuronal plasticity in certain central lesions. Physiotherapy also intervenes in the field of rehabilitation (together with occupational therapy) to teach the patient all of the palliative resources that could improve performance for comfort, the quality of life and coping with any residual deficiencies.

In PNS lesions, physiotherapy must first and foremost carry out analytic re-education, muscle by muscle, based on data obtained from manual muscle testing. It is individually tailored and evolves according to the results of a periodic checkup. Multijoint maneuvers are only secondary and in a complementary fashion except for Kabat's method [37] which is sometimes useful from the start but must not overshadow analytic re-education.

Analytic re-education is impossible in CNS pathology. Physiotherapy calls for multi-joint methods based on proprioceptive neuromuscular techniques and on motor reprogramming, e.g. the methods of Kabat, Bobath and Brunnstrom [39]. Physiotherapy can be enhanced through the use of electrotherapy in the form of functional electrical stimulation, especially in the hemiplegic or the patient with cerebral palsy [3].

Electrotherapy
[13, 14, 53, 57, 79]

This is useful in two situations: either to achieve maintenance of muscular trophic fitness in denervated muscles, or in upper motor neuron pathology. The effect of electrical stimulation on partially or totally denervated fibers during the treatment of denervated muscles has been the subject of a number of studies concerning the various types of electrical currents used in order to avoid possible harmful effects and to identify the minimal requirements for effective therapeutic action. Electrical stimulation is employed in two ways in CNS pathology: as an additional resource in the treatment of spasticity with results that are quite limited and as a form of functional electric stimulation (FES) during hemiplegic gait retraining.

Orthoses and special shoes

Preventive orthoses

Static orthoses, which position the foot to withstand a tendency to cause deformity through muscle shortening, are applied during rest, as at night. They are used continuously throughout the night in the initial phase of a peripheral neuropathy. The most commonly used is an anti-equinus ankle-foot orthosis or cast. The design and adaptation of this orthosis take into account frequent associated deforming valgus or varus tendencies. Conversely, posterior calf-muscle paralysis causing calcaneocavus deformity increasing with growth in children, as in poliomyelitis and spina bifida, can be treated by an anterior brace or cast. Thermoplastics offer a suitable choice of available materials. The principle of the orthosis is to place the shortened structure (-muscular or capsulo-ligamentous) under as reliable and effective a tension as tolerable. When the deforming tendency is associated with anesthesia, great care must be taken to ensure that a pressure sore does not form to further aggravate the problem.

Functional orthoses

Their role during standing and walking is essentially palliative but is also partially preventive as in the case, for example, of certain corrective plantar orthoses in static reducible problems or in protective plantar orthoses where there is plantar anesthesia. Orthoses can be designed to protect against excessive load on the metatarsal heads, the 5th metatarsal styloid and the heel. The material can be covered by a thin layer of silicone polymer and such coverings are now increasingly available commercially. They provide good cutaneous protection but at the cost of other problems related to perspiration. The other plantar orthoses are purely palliative for comfort. Their goal is to adapt and correct, if possible, the static imbalance in the foot induced by muscular inequality. The other palliative orthoses for walking most often extend from the leg to the foot [44, 50]. The most frequent orthoses are those designed to compensate for foot-drop and stabilize weight-bearing. There are essentially two types: either a posterior ankle-foot orthosis made from one piece of thermoplastic material and fitted into a standard shoe or a leg iron fixed into the medial or lateral part of the shoe heel. The latter is heavier and less esthetic but is biomechanically more efficient. The choice depends on the severity of the problem and patient acceptance of the latter. Biomechanical factors include the extent of muscular power in the leg, imbalance, the ensuing deformities, the patient's weight and his or her lifestyle. In certain cases, the foot is part of a neurologically impaired lower limb requiring extension of the ankle-foot orthosis to include the knee. Orthotic mechanisms for the knee and ankle are thus interdependent.

Surgical shoes

Corrective or palliative shoes are prescribed when they appear to be preferable to the combination of an orthosis and a normal shoe or when the foot cannot accommodate a standard shoe.

Factors common to the various bracing methods

Certain useful and important characteristics are worthy of note in the application of an orthosis or a shoe. An orthosis or a surgical shoe must be regularly reviewed for inspection and adjustment. In neurologic impairment where there is poor quadriceps control, altering the thickness of the sole to adjust the height of the forefoot or heel allows for better locking of the knee. As a corollary, an overweighed heel destabilizes a similarly affected knee. Prescription of an orthosis or surgical shoe is often an alternative to surgery.

Neuroablative procedures

Chemical neurolysis or blockade [6, 24]

Troublesome spasticity which is usually found in the territory of the posterior tibial nerve, can be temporarily controlled by chemical blockade at a motor point or in a nerve. Local injection acts on interacting gamma fiber conduction and the principle of the therapeutic action is to partially reduce the reflex arc response while at the same time preserving voluntary muscle activity. There are two primary agents in common usage: ethyl alcohol and phenol. Motor point injections are best indicated for patients who have a relatively small number of muscles to be treated, whereas chemical neurolysis of the tibial nerve trunk is better indicated for more widespread spasticity of the posterior calf. The duration of effect ranges from a few weeks to at least 2-3 months and is somewhat reduced following motor point blockade compared with nerve trunk blockage. However, the latter can be associated with troublesome painful dysesthesia which fortunately rarely persists. Chemical neurolysis is a valuable adjunct to overcome exacerbations of spasticity and is also a useful therapeutic test to predict the effect of surgical neurolysis. It is also worth mentioning at this point the use of a new treatment by botulinum toxin A injections into the center of a spastic muscle [72, 73, 74]. This substance, which acts by blocking the release of acetyl choline at motor points, has many advantages that include painless injections and the possibility of repeated use. However, its high cost and relative lack of experience in its use in large spastic muscles make it a therapy that is not completely mastered for this indication. However, experience in this technique is growing all the time and in Britain and the USA it is actually preferred to phenol blockade [72, 74, 77, 78].

Neuroablative surgical procedures

In practice, these are neurotomies. Progress in microsurgery and in peroperative neurostimulation techniques [46] over the last 20 years has allowed for the development of partial surgical denervation for patients with intractable spasticity or resistance to medication. Sectorial posterior rhizotomy [58] or microsurgical drezotomy [64] (DREZ: dorsal root entry zone) mainly addresses spasticity affecting a whole limb. Selective fascicular neurotomy is indicated for a spastic foot [46, 59], dividing the individual fascicles of the gastrocnemius, soleus and tibialis posterior muscles. This further brings surgeons and rehabilitationists together for neuroablative treatment of the spastic equinovarus foot when noninvasive treatment is ineffective and the foot deformity is reducible.

Orthopedic surgery

Its goals are multiple, associated or isolated, depending on the case: to relieve pain or treat a plantar ulcer by better distribution of plantar forces, improve stability in the weight-bearing foot or knee, or improve the swing phase of gait. It can also avoid or overcome the need for an orthosis or surgical shoe. The surgical means are multiple: tendon surgery, osteotomy, arthrorisis and arthrodesis. Tendon surgery involves lengthening and transfers. Calcaneal tendon (Achilles tendon) lengthening has both advantages and disadvantages [27]. It is a simple operation which treats equinus effectively when there are good talocrural joint conditions and when the talus is not deformed. It reduces tension on muscle fibers in the posterior calf muscles and provides fusimotor relaxation that reduces spasticity. Nevertheless, it also has the effect of permanently shortening the muscle fibers of the posterior calf muscles and their antagonist dorsiflexors of the foot, thus reducing plantarflexor power, if not its force [9]. It modifies the architecture of the foot. However, it is necessary to preserve some equinus and not overcome it totally for fear of losing the ability of the patient to stand freely on the limb. Excessive lengthening can destabilize the weight-bearing knee as a consequence. For tendon transfers, it is advisable during the work-up to take the following neurophysiologic fact into account [42, 49]: in peripheral neuropathy, the muscle whose distal tendon insertion is displaced should be able to contract in a timely and desirable fashion both in postural activities and during gait, following the establishment of easily and newly acquired synaptic circuits (e.g. the tibialis posterior muscle whose tendon is transferred to the tibialis anterior to treat a foot-drop acts opportunely as a dorsiflexor during the swing phase of gait, the exact opposite of its design function). On the other hand, in a central lesion after transferring this muscle, its mechanical effect will be modified but it will continue to contract, more or less powerfully, at the same time as the agonist muscles to which it belongs. Supramalleolar tibiofibular and calcaneal osteotomies aim to alter the weight-bearing area of the foot to improve stability. Metatarsal osteotomies are performed to reduce the excessive weight-bearing load for the treatment of pain or plantar ulcers. Arthrorises are surgically-obtained juxta-articular bony abutments, one of the oldest of which is the anterior talocrural abutment. Tarsectomies, which encompass bone and joint resection and arthrodesis, improve weight-bearing stability and load distribution in the foot. Most current authors usually avoid resorting to quadruple arthrodesis which fuses the talocrural articulation together with the subtalar and midtarsal joints. Triple arthrodesis is the most currently used procedure for the neuropathic foot which requires surgical stabilization [7, 20].

Clinical forms and principles of treatment

The foot in peripheral nerve impairments, called the "peripheral neuropathic foot", presents with functional symptoms and objective signs which are more dependent on the muscular weakness and any subsequent sensory loss than on the nature of the neurological deficit. This is why the principles of treatment depend on accurate analysis of motor and sensory signs. The choice of treatment does not specifically take the etiology into account except in children where it can have an influence on morphologic evolution. Therapeutic principles are dictated by the peripheral problems, taking the biomechanical conditions of the overlying lower limb, the patient's lifestyle and his or her wishes into account. For these reasons, after reviewing the various etiologies, the principles of the treatment of the peripheral neuropathic foot will be considered according to the anatomo-clinical picture that defines the problems to be treated. The foot in upper motor neuron lesions, called the "central neuropathic foot", presents to the clinician in a form that is clearly dependent on the etiology. The same applies to the foot in neurodegenerative conditions: the "neurodegenerative foot". For the latter two categories, the principles of treatment will be considered according to the etiology.

The peripheral neuropathic foot

The symptomatology can be purely motor, predominantly motor, sensori-motor, or purely sensory.

Clinical pictures

Pure motor or sensori-motor

The motor deficit is of a flaccid type with muscle wasting and is confirmed by EMG. Alpha motor neuron impairment can be found at the anterior horn cell (in poliomyelitis), the nerve roots (L5, S1, S2) of the sacral plexus and in the sciatic nerve or its subsequent divisions. The site of the lesion can be ascertained through clinical examination and muscle testing which can be confirmed by EMG, with sensory loss being confirmed by nerve conduction studies [29, 52, 65]. The diagnosis of poliomyelitis is usually already known. Non-traumatic radicular impairments, except for those of inflammatory and usually regressive polyradiculitis, have an intradural cause (meningioma, epidermoid cyst, or tumor) or an extradural cause (herniated disk, primary, or more often, metastatic tumor). Neuro-radiologic imaging contributes to making the diagnosis. Either the foot alone is involved, depending on the nature and the size of the problem, or it is part of a clinical picture along with associated sphincter problems. Taking this example, one can distinguish the foot in lumbo-sacral dysraphism of variable severity [17], from the patient with a meningomyelocele operated at birth to one with spina bifida occulta which is perhaps only revealed by an isolated muscle weakness in the foot. The deficit of the foot owing to sacral plexus lesions is usually well known and may be due to trauma, radiotherapy, or to a tumor. Among the polyneuropathies, those principally affecting the foot are due to alcohol (causing a foot drop, painful anesthesia and sometimes ataxia), the Charcot-Marie-Tooth syndrome (although it is a peripheral neuropathy, it will be considered under hereditary neurodegenerative conditions) and leprosy (large nerves, particularly well recognized by impairment of the common fibular nerve). Finally, lesions of the sciatic nerve and its divisions usually have a cause with a clear cut diagnosis: trauma, tumors (local more often than of the nerves themselves [55, 60]), ischemia, compartment and tunnel syndromes. It goes without saying that treatment for the foot in these conditions must be directed at the etiologic cause if possible, as well as addressing the local effects on the foot.

Predominantly sensory symptoms

The peripheral neuropathic foot with sensory manifestations can generally be classified in one of two large groups: hereditary degenerative polyneuropathies and distal localized compressive neuropathies, as in tunnel syndromes. There is no specific treatment for the former which includes Déjérine-Sottas syndrome, Thévenard's disease and congenital sensory neuropathies [15]. Although Déjérine-Sottas syndrome is a sensory motor neuropathy, it is predominantly sensory and distal. It is slowly progressive and enlarged nerves are easily found. Clinically, it has a sensory picture with an ataxic element and sometimes presents searing pain. Pupillary abnormalities occur, such as Argyll-Robertson pupil. Thévenard's disease is characterized by a progressive distal neurotrophic syndrome with autosomal dominant transmission which starts indolently with plantar ulcers and vasomotor problems (excessive sweating, bounding pulse, etc.) and more or less early development of neuro-arthropathies. Congenital sensory neuropathies are marked by congenital loss of pain sensation with areflexia and neurotrophic problems of variable severity. There can occasionally be major vegetative problems such as in Riley-Day disease. Whatever the underlying cause, severe trophic lesions within an insensitive limb produce soft tissue problems (plantar ulcers) [47] or arthropathies [30] and do not benefit from improvement or stabilization other than owing to prolonged unloading of the affected foot. This can only be achieved at the cost of a weight-bearing orthosis [63], a typical pendular gait with crutches in unilateral lesions, or life in a wheelchair in bilateral lesions. In very long-standing lesions, an amputation may need to be considered if walking without excessive risk from an insensitive stump is to be allowed. Tunnel syndromes, discussed elsewhere in this book, have a predominantly sensory symptomatology as they affect more distal nerves. Some present with sensori-motor features (tarsal tunnel syndrome), but compression of the superficial fibular nerve, the sural nerve and the interdigital nerves (Morton's syndrome) produces essentially sensory symptoms. Depending on the case, these syndromes are relieved by conservative treatment (infiltrations) or simple surgery by decompression or neurotomy.

Principles of treatment

The main treatments will be discussed here in terms of functional deficits and clinical types. The final choice of treatment is determined by the etiology and the clinical context.

Flail foot

This is a completely paralysed foot without any articular stiffness or muscular tone. All of the muscles that control it are denervated. It is observed in three circumstances:
- Severe poliomyelitis, nearly always occurring in children. This flaccid monoplegia is due to major generalized atrophy - both skeletal and longitudinal - of the lower limb, with normal sensation. In this situation, there is a need for major orthotic intervention since effective surgical indications for such a foot are rare.
- Sciatic neurotmesis. This is either due to trauma or tumor and is particularly serious because of the subsequent anesthesia of the foot accompanying the paralysis. In this lesion, two therapeutic options are available: either a surgical shoe with a high and rigid leg iron with protective in soles or a double arthrodesis with Lambrinudi's effect [7, 20], which allows for normal footwear and a protective plantar orthosis.
- Complete flaccid paraplegia due to a lesion of the conus or cauda equina resulting from trauma, tumor or a meningomyelocele: the clinical picture and the therapeutic possibilities are the same as above but with additional sphincter problems. Given the bilateral extent of the disabilities, life in a wheelchair may be indicated.

Foot drop. Equinus foot

Paralysis of the dorsiflexors causing a foot-drop may be accompanied by a shortening of the plantarflexors, notably of the gastrocnemius and soleus muscles, i.e. an equinus effect. The most frequent causes of this are poliomyelitis and common fibular nerve lesions. In the absence of an associated equinus, an ankle-foot orthosis fitted with a normal shoe is indicated. Surgery is possible for those who do not wish this option. Function can be improved by transfer of an intact muscle from the posterior compartment of the leg. The tibialis posterior is more effective than the flexor digitorum longus and is transferred through the interosseous membrane into the tendon of the tibialis anterior [16]. However, this sacrifices horizontal and frontal stability of the ankle and should be accompanied by a triple arthrodesis of the foot. It must be remembered that the transferred muscle must be at least 4/5 on the MRC scale* and must produce a normal EMG trace. When there is associated equinus, lengthening of the calcaneal tendon is nearly always required to allow dorsiflexion of the foot, whether orthotic or surgical treatment is carried out. Calcaneal tendon lengthening contributes to destabilization of the knee which is particularly regrettable when quadriceps muscle is weak.

Paralytic valgus foot (poliomyelitis, L5 palsy, certain types of spina bifida)

This is the result of a supinator muscle deficit, more particularly of the tibialis posterior muscle and is better tolerated than the varus foot. Midtarsal joint disease can produce pain and often leads to an associated equinus, thereby further aggravating the situation. If a plantar orthosis with a surgical shoe fails to provide a satisfactory outcome, surgery may be justified in the form of a triple arthrodesis, together with calcaneal tendon lengthening if it has a valgus equinus action.

Paralytic varus foot

This is due to a deficiency of the pronator muscles, essentially the long and short fibular (peroneal) and the common extensor of the toes. In peripheral neuropathies, its cause may be poliomyelitis, spina bifida, a common fibular nerve lesion, or Charcot-Marie-Tooth disease. It is disabling due to the lateral instability and pain it causes, especially the pain from excessive load on the 5th metatarsal along with the usual hyperkeratosis. In its early stages, the varus deformity is reversible before becoming fixed and it is possible to make do with a surgical shoe or with an orthosis within a normal shoe but this could mean an earlier need for tendon surgery to restore balance through a partial or total lateral transfer of the tibialis anterior tendon [11, 49]. One can rarely fit a surgical shoe on a fixed irreversible varus deformity and surgery is almost always required in the form of triple arthrodesis and a lateral or superolateral tarsectomy if it is a cavo-varus foot. An associated

severe calcaneo-varus may simultaneously require a lateral calcaneal osteotomy (Dwyer's operation) [23]. A varus-equinus association, giving an equinovarus foot, may require equinus treatment during the same operation, either by lengthening the calcaneal tendon or by dorsal basal tarsectomy. There are many available surgical options and the surgeon relies on the deforming elements within the foot, clinical muscle testing and the relationship with the rest of the paralysed limb.

Paralytic calcaneocavus foot

Posterior calf muscle paralysis is infinitely more disabling than an equinus foot because of the need to sustain a permanent and steady contraction of the ipsilateral quadriceps muscle in order to ensure locking of the weight-bearing knee. This is seen in poliomyelitis, in spina bifida and in posterior tibial nerve lesions. In the latter two, plantar anesthesia is usually an accompanying aggravating factor and a usually normal quadriceps muscle acts in compensation: these patients stand on a continually flexed knee because of tibial obliquity in the sagittal plane. In poliomyelitis, a paralysed quadriceps muscle is a strong aggravating factor on the calcaneocavus foot, but intact plantar sensation limits the problem to biomechanical disturbance. Treatment of the poliomyelitic calcaneocavus foot depends on the functional benefit of the quadriceps muscle and the severity of the deformity. It may be necessary to operate on the deformity itself if the forefoot is irreversible high in position in order to accommodate the shoes. Surgery is also justified if it allows for stabilization of the weight-bearing knee and avoids the need for a brace. In fact, surgical treatment of the poliomyelitic calcaneocavus foot is extremely difficult and very often disappointing [21]. Tendon transfers appear to have been abandoned. Triple resection, described by Crenshaw, performed on the transverse tarsal articulation and on the subtalar joint is a laborious procedure and does not provide convincing results. Arthrorisis using Putti's anterior tibiotarsal abutment, vertically embedding a bone graft in the head and neck of the talus, is a simpler and more certain technique (fig. 7.1). Supramalleolar osteotomy with cuneiform and posterior base resection can be the last resort of value. The biomechanical principles upon which one bases the choice of surgical technique can be expressed as follows: either achieve weight-bearing on the forefoot or an advanced position of the tibial shaft on the foot (i.e.

---

* This refers to the muscle power grading of the British Medical Research Council

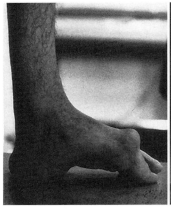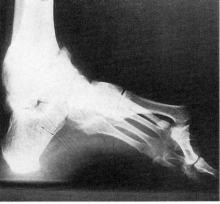

Fig. 7.1. Poliomyelitic calcaneo-cavus foot. The vertical position of the weight-bearing tibia results from a torque made up of ground-reaction of the great toe and Putti's anterior tibio-tarsal abutment

a retroposition of the calcaneus under the tibia). The decision not to operate or the failure of surgery when a locked weight-bearing knee is impossible requires a major knee-ankle-foot orthosis with a surgical shoe. The calcaneocavus foot in spina bifida or in posterior tibial nerve denervation, due to associated trophic problems, essentially requires a surgical shoe with a long leg iron equipped with suitable interior protection in order to reduce the risk of pressure sores or plantar ulcers.

Pes cavus

Two elements characterize pes cavus or arched foot: angle closure at the summit of the arch of the foot and minimal foot contact with the ground. A specific chapter in this book is related to the general problems of the cavus foot. Neurologically induced pes cavus is observed in peripheral neuropathies and in hereditary degenerative diseases. In the former, morphogenetic mechanisms of the deformity result from an imbalance between the forces of the preserved digital long extensors and flexors on the one hand and the weakness or complete denervation of the interossei muscles on the other. This imbalance results from two potential neurologic lesions: either an advanced stage of an untreated tarsal tunnel syndrome or more frequently the situation seen in certain forms of cauda equina syndrome and in spina bifida. This imbalance produces type I toe clawing [8], which in itself provokes verticalization of the metatarsals. The latter, accompanied by atrophy of nearly all the intrinsic muscles, causes excessive load on the metatarsal heads and thus hyperkeratosis. Plantar anesthesia usually completes the clinical picture, giving rise to potential ulcers. In

the right context, it can be helpful to perform surgery which will be described in the section on the neurodegenerative foot. When there is total anesthesia, however, the prognosis must be very guarded.

The neurodegenerative foot

Two neurodegenerative conditions will be addressed here because of their frequency: pure peripheral neuropathy (Charcot-Marie-Tooth disease) and spino-cerebellar degeneration (Friedreich's ataxia).

Clinical features

Charcot-Marie-Tooth disease

This disease is a hereditary sensori-motor neuropathy characterized by a very slowly progressive distal neurogenic amyotrophy. It usually starts in childhood or adolescence with weakness of the anterolateral compartment of the leg, producing foot drop or repetitive ankle strains [12, 15, 34]. Later, intrinsic hand muscle and then calf muscle wasting become apparent. Muscular weakness starts in the intrinsic muscles of the foot and continues in the fibular muscles, tibialis anterior and the digital extensors. However, Barry [12], quoting Fenton, noted a relatively prolonged preservation of fibularis longus and tibialis posterior activity which corresponds well with the morphogenesis of the observed deformities. In Charcot-Marie-Tooth disease, the foot is narrow, arched, in varus and adducted with type I clawed toes and with lost ankle dorsiflexion. These problems give rise to the characteristic pain, which is due to the compressed soft tissue covering bony prominences.

Friedreich's ataxia [15]

This disease has a more complex clinical picture and a more ominous course. It is characterized by the association of a cerebellar syndrome, a pyramidal syndrome and a posterior root syndrome, kyphoscoliosis and arched feet. It has a progressive course with commonly associated cardiac features and leads to death. The pes cavus of these two conditions (Charcot-Marie-Tooth and Friedreich's ataxia) results in a morphologic mechanism comparable to that described above (see Pes cavus above).

Principles of treatment

There is no specific therapy for either of these two disorders [15]. Charcot-Marie-Tooth disease only gradually causes major impotence and does not shorten life. Surgical correction of the affected foot is relatively commonly indicated in situations where plantar orthoses have been inadequate [12]. Stabilising tendon surgery which could theoretically be indicated in children and adolescents, does not appear to be justified in progressive disease. It is more logical to wait for bone maturation before proceeding with triple arthrodesis for a painful pes cavo-varus. This usually involves three-plane tarsectomy [7, 20] and possibly calcaneal osteotomy. During the course of surgery, correction of forefoot supination often creates an excessive cavus of the first metatarsal which may require an osteotomy to correct it. Clawed toes are indications for tendon surgery or proximal interphalangeal joint resection/arthrodesis. In the case of Friedreich's ataxia, reasonable surgical indications are rare because of the more rapidly progressive nature of the disease, but painful clawed toes and metatarsalgia may exceptionally be treated by simple surgical procedures. It is better to reduce pain as much as possible by prescribing adapted plantar orthoses. If those are not sufficient for patients who still have appreciable locomotion, tendon surgery for clawed toes is preferable to other procedures such as metatarsal osteotomy. In Charcot-Marie-Tooth disease as in Friedreich's ataxia, clawed toe surgery consists in restoring active plantarflexion in the MTP joints by transfer of the long flexor muscle tendon into each of the five toes on the first phalanx [8]. The restoration of active metatarsophalangeal flexion relieves meta-

tarsalgia and toe pain at the price of a short immobilization with indoor walking possible the day after surgery. In Friedreich's ataxia, it should be noted that despite the sometimes insistent demands of patients or families, one should lean toward simple surgical palliation permitting a rapid return to walking.

The central neuropathic foot

Clinical features and treatment

In upper motor neuron syndromes, disabling symptomatology in the foot is only a part of the whole clinical picture. Progression may be slow or rapid and other more disabling problems may be evident. This is typically observed in Parkinson's disease, syringomyelia, various myelopathies, multiple sclerosis, amyotrophic lateral sclerosis and pure progressive spinal muscular atrophies. Notable among the latter is Stark-Kaeser's scapulo-fibular syndrome [15, 28], which starts with calf and dorsiflexor wasting and for which a stabilising orthosis can be employed. Three conditions require further attention because of their involvement of the foot in the overall symptomatology: paraplegia, cerebral palsy and cerebral lesions.

The paraplegic foot

• Flaccid paraplegia: destruction of the lumbo-sacral cord and conus gives rise to a lower motor neuron paraplegia. The effects on the feet are the same as in the chapter on peripheral nerve lesions. If standing is possible despite the deficit then assisted walking and correction of any subsequent deformities by simple tenotomies can be justified in order to fit footwear.

• Spastic paraplegia: whatever the clinical picture, treatment is based on whether or not standing is possible and desirable. If the paraplegic person can only live and get around in a wheelchair, then treatment may be beneficial for two types of foot problem: disabling spasticity and deformities, which make the wearing of footwear impossible. Disabling spasticity is rarely confined to the feet and then may benefit from repeated chemical nerve blockade. A variety of treatments has been outlined above to attempt to relieve major spasticity, which usually involves the whole of the lower limb. Deformities making footwear impossible for non-ambulatory

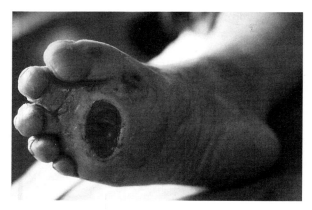

Fig. 7.2. Ulcer on the sole of the forefoot in a paraplegic patient, due to total plantar anesthesia in association with equinus

paraplegics can justify the use of tenotomies to restore a better morphologic aspect and above all, allow a flat foot in order to prevent pressure sores (fig. 7.2). But certain complete or incomplete spastic paraplegics can stand and even move around, either due to useful spasticity or to orthoses. Spasticity treatment must therefore be cautious and clearly defined in these patients. Foot deformities (equinovarus foot is the most common) prevent the use of comfortable footwear and can generate pressure sores by abnormal weight-bearing. Surgical correction should only be indicated after multidisciplinary consideration. If this treatment is an option, then tendon procedures are preferable to osteoarticular surgery as they avoid the need for a 10-12-week period of immobilization following arthrodesis or tarsectomy.

Cerebral palsy foot

Flaccid for the first few months of life, the foot in cerebral palsy invariably becomes increasingly spastic and unstable in the sagittal plane due to the predominance of calf muscle tone. This spastic imbalanced muscular hypertonicity is not confined to the foot and affects the whole of the lower limb [35]. The most common neurologic problems arise from pyramidal impairment which is bilateral in spastic diplegia (Little's disease) and unilateral in infantile (cerebral) hemiplegia. The other deficit arises from extrapyramidal impairment, giving rise to athetosis more commonly than to chorea. In extrapyramidal complaints, equinus is more rarely observed and is less fixed than in pyramidal impair-

ment. Equinus therefore causes most of the problems in the feet of the cerebral palsy child and will, as the child learns to walk, determine the morphology of the foot in terms of balance or imbalance of muscle tonicity controlling inversion/eversion. This equinus is due to posterior calf muscle hypertonicity which during development will be further aggravated by progressive shortening of this muscle. The osteoarticular structure is only rarely normal in the ambulant cerebral palsy child in terms of morphology as a consequence of excessive biomechanical stresses on the weight-bearing forefoot under the constraints of equinus. It is usually deforming, sometimes in equinovarus, but more often in equinovalgus. Because of the difficulties and dubiousness of such surgery and its outcome, doctors are conservative in their recommendations for surgical intervention. Multidisciplinary consultation is preferable and should discuss the indication for surgery and the technique with the surgeon. Physiotherapy and discontinuous static orthoses should be employed to prevent the early development of equinus even before the child learns to walk [41, 62]. In addition, some authors describe the use of Perlstein's splint [45] in the recumbent or seated child. This has been designed for adaptation in surgical shoes, then fitted to moulded soft leather booties. From the time the child is erect in the assisted standing position which should ideally be at 8-10 months to allow for normal structural development of the hip and certainly from the moment walking starts, the feet must rely on weight-bearing structures which will eventually result in equinus. The plantar orthoses should be suitably fitted to preserve correct osteoarticular architecture during walking in sufficiently but not excessively supporting shoes and neither in varus nor in valgus. Strict follow-up of these children during their growth is aimed at slowing the development of or correcting any evolving deformity. The range of available treatments is large. Tibial nerve or calf muscle motor point blockade, corrective plaster casts, static orthoses and surgery. Selective fascicular tibial neurotomy is uncommon in the cerebral palsy child [1]. Orthopedic surgery provides a choice between gastrocnemius aponeurotomy and calcaneal tendon lengthening, depending on the most significantly shortened muscle. Whatever procedure is chosen, it is important that equinus correction be incomplete since an over-zealous approach can impair standing by worsening the flexed position of the weight-bearing knee [27, 36]. Resorting to tendon transfers in the foot of the cerebral palsy patient is less common because postoperative function in upper motor neuron lesions is difficult to predict and is thus inadvisable. Whatever procedure is chosen, any immobilization thereafter is always quite prolonged in these children (not less that three weeks, for example, following tendon lengthening) and is followed by a loss of locomotor skills for which a long recuperation is required. From the age of 13 or 14 and in the ambulant cerebral palsy adult, calcaneal tendon lengthening must be considered as excessively risky. Triple arthrodesis with a possible tarsectomy is possible when valgus or varus deformity causes pain which is insufficiently controlled by suitably adapted therapeutic footwear.

The foot in adult cerebral lesions

As there is a wide variety of conditions, this section will concentrate on the feet of patients after prolonged coma (e.g. following traumatic brain injury) and on the hemiplegic foot.

Despite physiotherapy and preventive correct positioning, lower limb orthopedic deformities of the three main joint levels are quite frequent in patients coming out of a coma and require a surgical strategy, which is irrelevant here. When the foot is the only or the last remaining obstacle preventing standing or walking, surgery can be considered. The choice is between neuro-ablative surgery [46] if non-deforming spasticity is the predominant problem and orthopedic procedures which can be supplementary to the first [10]. The great diversity of problems encountered does not permit a detailed description of surgical intervention for each.

The hemiplegic foot (fig. 7.3)

With the exception of a few variants, motor disorders of the hemiplegic foot due to hemispheric lesions (vascular, tumoral, traumatic) are relatively constant in the great majority of cases. However, Dimitrijevic was able to describe six different lower limb muscular attitudes during the swing phase [22]. The two most common are worthy of description here: the spastic equinovarus foot and clawing of the toes. The former is now much better controlled thanks to the combined efforts of better re-educative methods, notably physiotherapy, supplemented if necessary by antispasmodic medication. When noninvasive methods are insufficient, a complemen-

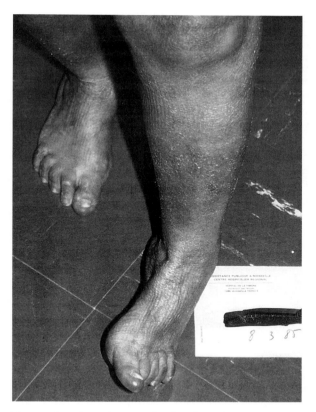

Fig. 7.3. Spastic equinovarus foot in a hemiplegic patient

tary therapeutic approach is possible depending on the result of the clinical assessment. When there is hypertonicity and spasticity without constant muscle shortening, the initial course is to perform a posterior tibial nerve or calf muscle motor point block which can be repeated once. If this therapeutic trial is positive but the clinical effect is not total or sufficiently long-lasting, a selective fascicular neurotomy is possible on the motor branches chosen after clinical and neurophysiologic testing of the gastrocnemius, soleus and tibialis posterior muscles [46, 59]. If muscle shortening is confirmed on clinical examination, orthopedic surgery is worth considering in terms of calcaneal tendon lengthening [19] which may be sufficient although this is rare. It is also usually necessary to treat the dynamic varus problem by a tendon or osteo-articular procedure depending on the patient's individual requirements. Corrective varus tendinous restabilization is performed by giving the tibialis anterior muscle a valgus action, either by transferring its tendon, carrying out an external bifurcation of its tendon

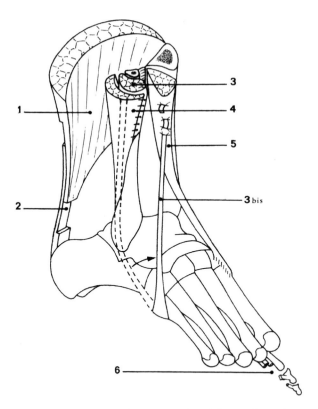

Fig. 7.4. Palliative tendon surgery in adult spastic equinovarus foot [9]. *1* soleus; *2* heel-cord lengthening; *3* peroneus brevis; *3 bis* its tendon, separated from the muscle bulk, sutured to the tibialis anterior tendon; *4* peroneus longus; *5* tibialis anterior; *6* tenotomy of toe-flexors (Courtesy of: Bardot A (1991) Orthopedic surgical corrections of spastic disorders. In: Sindou M, Abbott R, Keravel Y (eds) Neurosurgery for spasticity. Springer-Verlag, Heidelberg)

painful, it can be treated by long flexor muscle partial selective denervation [46], which is at least partially irreversible. However, simple tenotomy of each toe long flexor is a simpler procedure for both types, in which fixed clawing should additionally be treated by proximal interphalangeal joint capsulotomy. Experience shows that calcaneal tendon lengthening in the hemiplegic foot always results in the appearance or worsening of toe clawing and, for this reason, it is sensible to carry out systematic digital flexor tenotomies whenever calcaneal tendon lengthening is undertaken in hemiplegic patients [9].

[11], or by retrograde transfer on the tendon of the fibularis brevis muscle [9] (fig. 7.4). Varus correction by osteoarticular surgery is obtained by triple arthrodesis, which inevitably requires calcaneal tendon lengthening and a minimum of 10 weeks in plaster. Tendon surgery is thus preferable in older and less active patients. However, a successful outcome is dependent on the tibialis anterior muscle's contracting with sufficient force during the ambulatory swing phase. Triple arthrodesis is useful either in young patients with weak or dysfunctional tibialis anterior muscles, for which Lambrinudi's technique is indicated, or in a particularly active young person. Toe clawing in the hemiplegic foot is always type I and is either tonic or fixed. Tonic toe clawing is intermittent and reversible and appears only during standing or walking [2]. When it is

References

1. Abbott R (1991) Indications for surgery to treat children with spasticity due to cerebral palsy. In: Sindou M, Abbott R, Keravel Y (eds) Neurosurgery for spasticity. Springer-Verlag, Heidelberg, pp 215-217

2. Alajouanine Th, Castaigne P, Held JP, et al (1968) Flexion tonique des orteils au cours de la marche chez l'hémiplégique. Essai d'analyse séméiologique; possibilités thérapeutiques. Rev Neurol (Paris) 118: 343-354

3. André JM, Brugerolle B, Beis JM, Chellig L (1993) La stimulation électrique neuromotrice dans le traitement de la spasticité. Ann Readaptation Med Phys 36: 329-335

4. d'Angeli-Chevassut M (1994) Analyse de la marche de l'hémiplégique adulte. Thèse de Médecine, Montpellier

5. Ashworth B (1964) Preliminary trial of carisoprodol in multiple sclerosis. Practitioner 192: 540-542

6. Awad EA, Dykstra D (1990) Treatment of spasticity by neurolysis. In: Kottke FJ, Lehmann JF (eds) Krusen's Handbook of Physical Medicine and Rehabilitation. W.B. Saunders, Philadelphia, pp 1154-1161

7. Bardot A, Dobbels E, Martin G, Olivares JP (1984) Les arthrodèses du tarse postérieur dans les pieds neurologiques. In: Claustre J, Simon L (eds) Pied neurologique, trophique, et vasculaire. Masson, Paris, pp 165-171

8. Bardot A, Delarque A, Curvale G, Groulier P (1989) Orteils en griffe de cause neurologique. In: Bardot A, Pelissier J (eds) Neuro-orthopédie des membres inférieurs chez l'adulte, Masson, Paris, pp 221-227

9. Bardot A, Delarque A, Curvale G, Peragut JC (1991) Orthopedic surgical corrections of spastic disorders. In: Sindou M, Abbott R, Keravel Y (eds) Neurosurgery for spasticity. Springer-verlag, Heidelberg, pp 201-208

10. Bardot A, Viton JM, Pellas F, Curvale G, Delarque A (1993) La place de la chirurgie orthopédique dans le traitement de la spasticité. Ann Réadaptation Med Phys 36: 373-376

11. Barouk LS, Richer L, Deliac M, Laurent F (1989) La chirurgie du membre inférieur de l'hémiplégie séquelle de traumatisme crânien. In: Bardot A, Pelissier J (eds) Neuro-orthopédie des membres inférieurs chez l'adulte. Masson, Paris, pp 104-110

12. Barry LD, Fluellen J (1991) Charcot-Marie-Tooth disease. Podiatric and systemic considerations. J Am Podiatr Med Assoc 81: 490-494

13. Basford JR Jr (1990) Electrical therapy. In: Kottke FJ, Lehmann JF (eds) Krusen's Handbook of Physical Medicine and Rehabilitation. W.B. Saunders, Philadelphia, pp 375-401

14. de Bisschop G, Dumoulin J, Aaron C (1989) Électro-thérapie appliquée en kinésithérapie et rééducation, en rhumatologie et médecine du sport. Coll. Monographies de Bois-Larris. 2e édn. Masson, Paris, pp 21-29 & 82-83

15. Cambier J, Masson M, Dehen H (1994) Neurologie. Masson, Paris

16. Carayon A, Bourrel P, Bourges M, et al (1967) Dual transfer of the posterior tibial and flexor digitorum longus tendons for drop-foot. J Bone Joint Surg 49A: 144-148

17. Carroll NC (1987) Assessment and management of the lower extremity in myelodysplasia. Orthop Clin North Am 18: 709-724

18. Chantraine A, Onkelinx A (1971) Électromyographie et traitement dans les lésions traumatiques du nerf scia-tique. Ann Med Phys 14: 43-49

19. Chantraine A, Taillard W (1989) Allongement du tendon d'Achille chez le traumatisé crânien spastique. In: Bardot A, Pelissier J (eds) Neuroorthopédie des membres inférieurs chez l'adulte. Masson, Paris, pp 98-103

20. Crenshaw AH (1966) Stabilisation des articulations du pied et de la cheville. In: Crenshaw AH (ed) Traité de chirurgie orthopédique de la clinique Campbell. Maloine, Paris, pp 1471-1480

21. Crenshaw AH (1966) Pied bot talus. In: Crenshaw AH (ed) Traité de chirurgie orthopédique de la clinique Campbell. Maloine, Paris, pp 1516-1530

22. Dimitrijevie MR, Faganel J, Sherwood AM, McKay WB (1981) Activation of paralyzed leg flexors and exten-sors during gait in patients after stroke. Scand J Rehabil Med 13: 109-115

23. Dwyer FC (1959) Osteotomy of the calcaneum for pes cavus. J Bone Joint Surg 41B: 80

24. Enjalbert M, Viel E, Toulemonde M, et al (1993) Neurolyse chimique à l'alcool (alcoolisation) et spasticité de l'hémiplégique. Ann Réadaptation Méd Phys 36: 337-342

25. Eyssette M, Boisson D (1993) Les médicaments anti-spastiques: actualités. Ann Réadaptation Méd Phys 36: 343-348

26. Frykman GK, Waylett J (1981) Rehabilitation of peripheral nerve injuries. Orthop Clin North Am 12: 361-379

27. Gaines RW, Ford TB (1984) A systematic approach to the amount of Achilles tendon lengthening in cerebral palsy. J Pediatr Orthop 4: 448-451

28. Gamstorp J, Sarnat HB (1984) Progressive spinal muscular atrophies. Raven Press, New York

29. de Godebout J, Ster J, Thaury MN, Avon-Nicolas C (1984) Bilan clinique lors des paralysies "sciatiques". In: Claustre J, Simon L (eds) Pied neurologique, trophique, et vasculaire. Masson, Paris, pp 121-130

30. Gougeon J, Seignon B (1978) Ostéoarthropathies nerveuses. Encycl Med Chir, Paris, Appareil Loco-moteur, 14285 A 10: 4

31. Haas LB (1993) Chronic complications of diabetes mellitus. Nurs Clin North Am 28: 71-85

32. Held JP, Pierrot-Deseilligny E (1969) Rééducation motrice des affections neurologiques. Baillere, Paris

33. Herlant M, Voisin P, Vanvelcenaher J, et al (1993) Bilans musculaires. Editions techniques. Encycl Med Chir, Paris, Kinésithérapie-Rééducation Fonc-tionnelle, 26-010-A-10, 48 p

34. Holmes JR, Hansen ST (1993) Foot and ankle manifes-tations of Charcot-Marie-Tooth disease. Foot Ankle 14: 476-486

35. Jones ET, Knapp DR (1987) Assessment and manage-ment of the lower extremity in cerebral palsy. Orthop Clin North Am 18: 725-738

36. Joseph B (1992) A modification of the Cincinnati approach for obtaining adequate lengthening of the tendo achillis in the presence of severe equinus defor-mity. J Pediatr Orthop 12: 403

37. Kabat N (1961) Proprioceptive facilitation in thera-peutic exercise. In: Licht S (ed) Therapeutic exercise, 2nd edn. Elisabeth Licht, Newhaven-Connecticut

38. Kendall HO, Wadsworth GE (1974) Les muscles, 2e edn. Maloine, Paris

39. Kottke FJ (1990) Therapeutic exercise to develop neuromuscular coordination. In: Kottke FJ, Lehmann JF (eds) Krusen's Handbook of Physical Medicine and Rehabilitation. W.B. Saunders, Philadelphia, pp 452-479

40. Kurtzke JF (1965) Further notes on disability evalua-tion in multiple sclerosis with scale modifications. Neurology 15: 654-666

41. Lacote M, Stevenin P, Chevalier AM, et al (1982) Évaluation clinique de la fonction musculaire. Maloine, Paris

42. Le Cœur P (1973) Axiomatique des transplantations musculaires. In: Orthopédie-Traumatologie, Confé-rences d'enseignement 1971. L'Expansion scientifique française, Paris, pp 207-226

43. Lehmann JF, de Lateur BJ (1990) Gait analysis: diag-nostic and management. In: Kottke FJ, Lehmann JF (eds) Krusen's Handbook of Physical Medicine and Rehabilitation. W.B. Saunders, Philadelphia, pp 108-125

44. Lehmann JF, de Lateur BJ (1990) Lower extremity orthotics. In: Kottke FJ, Lehmann JF (eds) Krusen's Handbook of Physical Medicine and Rehabilitation. W.B. Saunders, Philadelphia, pp 602-646

45. Lombard M (1981) Infirmité motrice cérébrale. In: Grossiord A, Held JP (eds) Médecine de Réédu-cation. Flammarion Médecine Sciences, Paris, pp 350-363

46. Mertens P, Sindou M (1991) Selective peripheral neurotomies for the treatment of spasticity. In: Sindou M, Abbott R, Keravel Y (eds) Neurosurgery for spasticity. Springer-Verlag , New-York, pp 119-132

47. Meynadier J, Vidal C, Guillot B, Alirezai M (1984) Conduite pratique devant un mal perforant plantaire. In: Claustre J, Simon L (eds) Pied neurologique, trophique, et vasculaire. Masson, Paris, pp 188-192

48. Omer GE Jr (1981) Physical diagnosis of peripheral nerve injuries. Orthop Clin North Am 12: 207-228

49. Orst G, Vidal J, Boisard JL (1984) Les transpositions tendineuses dans le pied neurologique. In: Claustre J, Simon L. Pied neurologique, trophique, et vasculaire. Masson, Paris, pp 159-164

50. Paquin JM, André JM (1980) L'appareillage des paralysies du sciatique et de ses branches. In: Simon L (ed) La sciatique et le nerf sciatique. Masson, Paris, pp 258-265

51. Pease WS, Johnson EW. Rehabilitation management of diseases of the motor unit. In: Kottke FJ, Lehmann JF (eds) Krusen's Handbook of Physical Medicine and Rehabilitation. W.B. Saunders, Philadelphia, pp 754-764

52. Pelissier J, Georgesco M, Cadilhac J (1981) Place de l'électromyographie dans le bilan du pied. In: Claustre J, Simon L (eds) Pied normal et méthodes d'explorations du pied. Masson, Paris, pp 135-146

53. Pelissier J, Roques CF (1992) Electrostimulation des nerfs et des muscles. Masson, Paris

54. Peterson GW, Will D (1988) Newer electrodiagnostic techniques in peripheral nerve injuries. Orthop Clin North Am 19: 13-25

55. Petit E, Paquis P, Brocq O, et al (1991) Compression du nerf sciatique poplité externe par un kyste synovial extraneural. À propos d'un cas exploré par échographie et tomodensitométrie. Ann Réadapation Méd Phys 34: 155-159

56. Planchon B, Mussini JM, Freland JC, et al (1984) Les neuroacropathies. In: Claustre J, Simon L (eds) Pied neurologique, trophique, et vasculaire. Masson Paris, pp 181-192

57. Pouget J (1992) Electrostimulation neuromusculaire: bases expérimentales. In: Pélissier J Roques CF (eds) Électrostimulation des nerfs et des muscles, Masson, Paris, pp 20-24

58. Privat JM, Benezech J, Frerebean Ph, Gros C (1976) Sectorial posterior rhizotomy; a new technique of surgical treatment of spasticity. Acta Neurochir 34: 181-195

59. Privat JM, Privat C (1993) Place des neurotomies fasciculaires sélectives des membres inférieurs dans la chirurgie fonctionnelle de la spasticité. Ann Réadaptation Méd Phys, 36: 349-358

60. Radek A, et al (1992) Gelatinous cyst of the common peroneal nerve. Neurol Neurochir Pol 26: 743-747

61. Rattey TE, et al (1993) Recurrence after Achilles tendon lengthening in cerebral palsy. J Pediatr Orthop 13: 184-187

62. Ricks NR, et al (1993) Effects of inhibitory casts and orthoses on bony alignment of foot and ankle during weight-bearing in children with spasticity. Dev Med Child Neurol 35: 11-16

63. Saltzman CL, et al (1992) The patellar-tendon bearing brace as treatment for neurotrophic arthropathy: a dynamic force monitoring study. Foot Ankle 13: 14-21

64. Sindou M, Jeanmonod D, Mertens P (1989) Microsurgical drezotomy for the treatment of spasticity and pain in the lower limbs. Neurosurgery 24: 655-670

65. Sunderland S (1978) Nerves and nerve injuries, 2nd edn. Churchill-Livingstone, Edinburg

66. Tardieu G, Hariga J (1964) Traitement des raideurs musculaires d'origine cérébrale par l'alcool dilué (résultat de 500 injections). Arch Fr Pediatr 21: 25-41

67. Tobis JS, Hong CZ (1990) Muscle testing. In: Kottke FJ, Lehmann JF (eds) Krusen's Handbook of Physical Medicine and Rehabilitation. W.B. Saunders, Philadelphia, pp 33-60

68. Vogler HW (1990) Complex deformations: paralytic and non-paralytic. In: Levy LA, Hetherington VJ (eds). Principles and practice of Podiatric Medicine. Churchill Livingstone, Edinburgh, pp 953-966

69. Waylett-Rendall J (1988) Sensibility evaluation and rehabilitation. Orthop Clin North Am 19: 43-56

70. Wiechers DO, Johnson EW (1990) Electrodiagnosis. In: Kottke FJ, Lehmann JF (eds) Krusen's Handbook of Physical Medicine and Rehabilitation. W.B. Saunders, Philadelphia, pp 72-107

71. Ziegler D, et al (1993) Tibial nerve somatosensory evoked potentials at various stages of peripheral neuropathy in insulin dependant diabetic patients. J Neurol Neurosurg Psychiatry 56 (1): 58-64

Additional references

72. Dunne JW, Heye N, Dunne SL (1995) Treatment of chronic limb spasticity with botulinum toxin A. J Neurol Neurosurg Psychiatry 58: 232-235

73. Hesse S, et al (1994) Botulinum toxin treatment for lower limb extensor spasticity in chronic hemiparetic patients. J Neurol Neurosurg Psychiatry 57: 1321-1324

74. Koko C, Ward AB (1997) The management of spasticity. Br J Hosp Med 58: 400-405

75. Koman LA, et al (1993) Management of cerebral palsy with botulinum-A toxin: preliminary investigation. J Pediatr Orthop 13: 489-495

76. Konstanzer A, Ceballos-Baumann AO, Dressnandt J, Conrad B (1993) Local injection treatment with botulinum toxin A in severe arm and leg spasticity. Nervenarzt. 64: 517-523

77. Pierson SH, Katz DI, Tarsy D (1996) Botulinum toxin A in the treatment of spasticity: functional implications and patient selection. Arch Phys Med Rehabil 77: 717-721

78. Roques CF (1997) Pratique de l'électrothérapie. Springer, Paris

79. Young RR (1994) Spasticity: a review. Neurology 44: S12-S20

8.

Septic arthritis of the foot and ankle

F Gaillard and G Rémy

Septic arthritis of the foot is a type of medico-surgical emergency where rapidity in diagnosis and treatment is essential to limit functional and sometimes fatal damage, and where microbiologic diagnosis is essential and imperative. While it shares the general characteristics of all forms of septic arthritis [18, 19], it also has several features specific to its site and diagnosis, and related to its course and prognosis.

Frequency

It represents about 10% of septic arthritis cases. Among 1080 patients with 1152 septic foci, 127 cases of septic arthritis were found in the foot, including 42 located in the talocrural joint, 49 in the tarsus, 39 in the metatarsophalangeal joints, and 3 in the toes [6, 7].

Diagnosis

The diagnosis is generally made when faced with [19]:
• an infectious state with a rapid onset followed by 2 or 3 days with fever,
• local signs with a red, hot, swollen joint, impossible to move, and sometimes signs of extension (tenosynovitis, lymphangitis, swollen nodes). Incapacity is often severe.

The diagnosis is simple in a context of septicemia, with multiple arthritides and positive blood cultures. It is often more difficult when the affection is monarticular.

Aspiration is easy when there is a fluid collection, or when there is a talocrural arthritis: the synovial fluid is turbid or purulent, hypercellular (often more than 25,000 polymorphonuclear leukocytes/mm³). Bacteria are isolated by direct examination in half the cases [19] or by culture.

Other examinations may or may not be useful: complete blood count with hyperleukocytosis, elevation of the erythocyte sedimentation rate, and of C-reactive protein. Radiographic findings are always delayed, negative at the beginning but later showing demineralization, joint narrowing and erosions [6]. Bone scintigraphy shows marked and early hyperfixation, which is very useful in giving the exact localization in difficult cases. Some techniques (bone scintigraphy with gallium or with labeled polymorphonuclear leukocytes) are used only in particular cases: subacute arthritis, previous arthropathy). Ultrasound and CT can show an abscess or a soft tissue swelling, a guide to aspiration.

Lastly, MRI proves to be an efficient method to evaluate inflammatory involvement of soft parts and bones [9].

Bacteriologic diagnosis

This depends on isolation of the bacteria from multiple samples:
• joint aspiration with irrigation and reaspiration of synovial fluid,
• systematic blood cultures, repeated after synovial aspiration,
• bacteriologic examination of the urine, or of any cutaneous septic foci,

• in case of failure, surgical biopsy of synovial tissue is essential, which also allows histologic study.

The bacteriologic study must include direct examination, culture, a thorough antibiogram, with study of the effectiveness of combined antibiotics in vitro for organisms of low sensitivity (*Staphylococcus aureus, Pseudomonas aeruginosa*). The laboratory must keep the bacteria for possible studies of combined treatments in difficult cases. The organism usually found is S. aureus (after surgery, arthroscopy, septic metastases, aspiration). Sometimes it can be a *Haemophilus influenzae* (in young children)[14], *Neisseria gonorrheae* (in young females), a streptococcus or pneumococcus. Other bacteria may be found, e.g., *Pasteurella multocida* (after bites), or Gram-negative or fungal organisms (candida, aspergillus).

It is always necessary to find the origin of the septic arthritis: direct inoculation (wound, invasive joint procedures), or hematogenous spread from extra-articular infective foci, such as endocarditis, where a septic arthritis of the foot can be inaugural or co-existent [1]. The patient's history and current state of health (diabetes mellitus, hepatic or renal disease, neoplastic disease, AIDS, corticotherapy) are also important [17].

Several factors explain the particular features of foot lesions

The anatomy

• There are communications between the synovial cavities of the different joints, with a common synovial lining for the midtarsus [17], and sometimes communications between joints and peritendinous synovial sheaths;

• this complexity favours rapid spread to other joints or bones, which explains the frequency of septic osteoarthritis;

• joints and skin are close together in the foot;

• given a rapidly developing swelling, it is difficult to exactly localize the infected joint;

• the multiplicity of joint spaces sets a problem for radiographic diagnosis [6];

• synovial fluid aspiration is more difficult in the foot, except for the ankle joint, and surgical biopsy is more frequently done when no organisms have been found.

The origin

It is very often an adjacent focus:

• frequent wounds after nail care, cutaneous wounds and punctures after podiatric care, plantar warts, rubbing by shoes (friction, bursitis) or callosities secondary to static disorders;

• plantar ulcers (diabetics);

• postoperative infections, benign or serious;

• trauma: postoperative infections are generally localized to the forefoot [10]. Sometimes, after a recent trauma, skin breakdown appears with only moderate infectious signs because of spontaneous drainage even though there is major radiologic destruction. In an old wound, the diagnosis can be more difficult;

• a hematogenous origin is rare in comparison with other causes of septic arthritis [10]: it appears only in the ankle joint, and posterior subtalar joints, often with dramatic signs such as fever and disability;

• a septic arthritis of the foot is rare after corticosteroid intra-articular injection, because such injections are less common that at the shoulder or knee. However, it is possible even with careful asepsis. The symptoms appear 2 or 3 days after an intra-articular injection and become more intense. It must be differentiated from the inflammatory reaction to microcrystalline deposits, which is early and brief. The bacterium is often isolated (7/10), generally *S. aureus*;

• in tropical countries, a sinus from a filarial abscess (dracunculosis) often becomes septic, (often *S. aureus*) [4].

The history

This includes particularly:

• Diabetes mellitus, with a high sensitivity to infections, often with plantar ulcers. Septic spread with osteomyelitis is frequent.

• Plantar ulcers of other types due to alcoholism, neuropathy, malnutrition, poor hygiene and bad foot-wear.

• Vascular diseases: firstly, because the trophic changes can lead to septic foci, and secondly in therapy, because poor vascularization restricts the antibiotic penetration.

• Rheumatoid arthritis: there is an increased incidence of septic arthritis in patients with rheumatoid arthritis [10, 12, 19]; 24 patients with 3 cases in the foot for Dubost [12], with *S. aureus in* all 3; *S. aureus* was found in 19/22 cases by Morris [20]. There are many reasons: hypersensitivity to infection due to impaired phagocytosis and bacteriolysis, increased by corticosteroid and immunosuppressive therapies; preexisting joint lesion favoring bacterial colonization; cutaneous port of entry from an infected rheumatoid lymph node which is infected or discharging; local corticosteroid injection.

The diagnosis is difficult because the septic signs are often mistaken for a rheumatoid flare, sometimes treated by an increase of non-steroidal antiinflammatory drugs or by local steroid injection. The clinical features are often deceptive (subacute onset, irregular fever) and explain a delayed diagnosis (more than a week in half the cases). A sudden increase of local articular signs may indicate a septic etiology (fig. 8.1). The white cell count in the synovial fluid, when a sample is available, gives the diagnosis with isolation of the organisms. *S. aureus* is more frequent in the foot than at other sites [20]. The prognosis is severe, with a fatal risk in 16% of cases of monarticular septic arthritis [12]. For prevention, it is important to treat all cutaneous wounds of the foot by any necessary conservative measures. Some quite benign lesions can lead to septic dissemination to joints having a highly vascular synovial lining (hip, knee) or to joints with protheses.

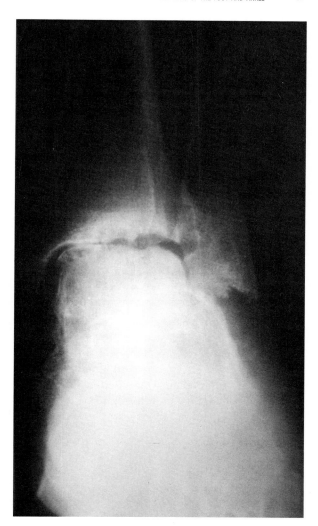

Fig. 8.1. Septic arthritis of the ankle in a patient with a previous rheumatoid arthritis (courtesy of Pierre Cance)

The infected joint

• The ankle joint: a hematogenous origin is possible [8]. The local signs are often marked, with much inflammation, and pain, especially at night, and infectious symptoms. Synovial fluid aspiration is easy.

• The midfoot: an iatrogenic origin is uncommon. Pain is at first only on movement and then becomes constant, with acute inflammation and generalized edema. The exact location is uncertain, and comparative X-ray films and bone scintigraphy are often needed. Sometimes it is possible to aspirate when there is a remittent swelling; a joint puncture is better under TV scopy or CT, followed by reaspiration of the anesthetic agent and by three blood cultures. MRI is also of great value for localization of the lesions. If the result is negative, a surgical biopsy is necessary for diagnosis, and constitutes the first stage of treatment, with excision of the septic tissues [17].

Particular diagnostic problems in septic arthritis of the foot

• Microcrystalline arthritis (gout, chondrocalcinosis and other crystal-forming arthropathies or tendinopathies): the previous history, laboratory findings, the isolation of crystals and sometimes the X-rays confirm the diagnosis [18].

• The first onset of inflammatory rheumatism, especially in its monarticular forms. Rheumatoid arthritis can begin by affecting an metatarso-phalangeal joint or the ankle. It is more frequent with a reactive arthritis, where a foot lesion is inaugural in 6% of cases, and isolated in 7.6%. It is necessary to look for other articular, tendinous or extra-articular features (skin, nails, eyes, urethra, sausage toe), and to check the family history [12].

• When a septic arthritis is suspected, there is no room for doubt: any suspicion must lead to joint aspiration or biopsy, because the functional risk is high with late diagnosis and treatment.

● Treatment

This is determined by the bacteriologic and other findings, and must be instituted very rapidly, using antibiotics, drainage, immobilization and rehabilitation. Preliminary tests (renal and hepatic function, temperature, inflammatory tests: sedimentation rate, CRP principally) allow monitoring of treatment and its tolerance [14, 15, 18].

Antibiotics

A combination of two bactericidal antibiotics is routine and essential [18]. The drugs are selected on the basis of the identification of the bacteria and the antibiogram (table 8.1), and their articular and bony penetration (table 8.2) [8, 15, 18]. It is necessary to use a combination which gives a high concentration of synergic antibiotics in the synovial lining. In the case of early treatment, the lesion is well vascularized and all antibiotics can reach the area easily

The only exception, allowing monotherapy, is the isolation of a Streptococcus A or *Neisseria gonorrheae* [18];

The intravenous route is obligatory during at least 15 days. Then oral administration must be continued for 6 to 10 weeks, at least 8 weeks in the case of an associated bone lesion;

Surveillance is based on the existence, or not, of an associated septicemia or multiple lesions, or the history, on any initial delay in treatment, and on the response to the initial treatment. It is important to take into account all the isolated organisms.

Immobilization

Relief from weight-bearing is essential for 4 to 8 weeks. Immobilization with a plaster or resin cast is useful as long as inflammatory signs are present.

Active muscle contractions are soon possible under a plaster cast, and rehabilitation is carried out, first passive and then active. Early mobilization of non-immobilized neighbouring joints is important, as is, antithrombotic treatment.

Drainage

The aspiration used in diagnosis is also a therapeutic measure, which can be repeated every 48 hours for the ankle joint, as long as there is a joint effusion [15]. The synovial fluid must be studied: persistance of a hyperleukocytosis and of the micro-organism after a week indicates the failure of the treatment, which must be changed. Its efficiency is marked by the return of a low cell-count in the fluid. The results of repeated joint aspirations are better than those of arthroscopic drainage [2].

Particular problems

• Persistence of signs of general infection, clinical as well as laboratory, or in the synovial fluid at the end of the first week of treatment makes it necessary to review the antibiogram, the doses used and their synergy (hence the importance of preserving the identified organism), the absence of any interfering treatment and the quality of the vascularization. Surgical advice is necessary for possible arthroscopic irrigation (of the talo-crural joint) [18] or synovectomy;

• The lack of bacterial isolation leads to a synovial biopsy and then to histologic and bacteriologic examination of the tissue. It is necessary to look for any unusual organisms: KLB, listeria, brucella, candida. The treatment must be adjusted to the organism presumed to be present, on the basis of the: history, port of entry, and any previous hospitalization (multiresistant *S. aureus*, *Pseudomonas aeruginosa*) or not (*S. aureus*, streptococcus);

• Isolation of unusual bacteria or of an organism generally of lowgrade pathogenicity: it is necessary to collect all the available evidence, such as the positivity of different samplings and the presence of

Table 8.1. Antibiotherapy related to bacteria in adults

Bacteria	Initial treatment	Other treatment	Secondary treatment
Staphylococcus aureus, methicillin-susceptible Staphylococcus, coagulase-negative, methicillin-susceptible	Penicillin M + aminoglycoside or Cefazolin + aminoglycoside or Penicillin M + rifampicin	Fluoroquinolone + rifampicin or Lincosamide or Pristinamycin + Rifampicin	idem
Staphylococcus aureus, multiresistant *Staphylococcus*, coagulase-negative, methicillin-resistant	Vancomycin + fucidic acid	Cefotaxime + Fosfomycin or Lincosamide + Phosphomycin/rifampicin	Pristinamycin + rifampicin or Fucidic acid
Enterococcus	Amoxicillin + aminoglycoside	Vancomycine + aminoglycoside	Amoxicillin
Streptococcus sp *S. pneumomiae*	Amoxicillin	Lincosamide or 3rd generation cephalosporin	Lincosamide or Amoxicillin
Cocci Gram –	Amoxicillin	3rd generation cephalosporin	
Gram – (except Pseudomonas)	3rd generation cephalosporin + Aminoglycoside 3rd generation cephalosporin + Fluoroquinolone	Fluoroquinolone + Phosphomycin	Fluoroquinolone
Pseudomonas aeruginosa	Ceftazidime + aminoglycoside or Ceftazidime + fluoroquinolone	Ceftazimide + phosphomycin or Imipenem + phosphomycin or Imipenem + fluoroquinolone	Ciprofloxacin
Anaerobic	Clindamycin	Imipenem or Cephamycin or Imidazol (except Propionibacterium)	Clindamycin or Imidazol (except Propionibacterium

Table 8.2. Bony penetration of antibiotics

Good	Medium	Poor
Fluoroquinolone Rifampicin Fucidic acid Phosphomycin Lincosamide	Betalactamin Glycopeptide Cotrimoxazole Phenicol	Aminoglycoside

adjuvant factors (drug addiction, AIDS, prosthesis, steroid injections);

• In the case of a chronic septic arthritis, it is justifiable to await the microbacteriologic findings to give the most appropriate treatment, which may be very long, sometimes a year.

The criteria for stopping the treatment

There are no formal criteria of healing, except the test of time [18]. They include the disappearance of the clinical signs and evidence of the inflammatory syndrome (CRP) and the absence of scintigraphic hyperfixation, sometimes delayed. If a synovial effusion persists, it must be aseptic and without leukocytoses. The customary rule of at least 3 months' treatment is justified in most cases.

● Course and prognosis

They depend mainly on the rapidity and efficiency of treatment. Sixty to 70% of cases of septic arthritis heal without sequelae [14], but the mortality remains as high as 10%, often due to particular circumstances (late diagnosis, non-identification of the organism or its resistance to treatment, general weakening factors).

An ankle lesion is the most serious, with the possibility of a fatal outcome. The functional prognosis remains poor and there is a mediocre local tolerance, with frequent stiffness of varying extent and a common evolution to osteoarthrosis.

The course of midfoot septic arthritis leads to fusion of the damaged surfaces. The consequences for walking are slight, with good conservation of foot movement, if the adjacent joints stay mobile. It is very important to avoid defective positioning of the hindfoot during immobilization. Rehabilitation, as soon as the painful phase has passed, must limit edema by massage, and manually conserve joint movement (ankle joint, calcaneonavicular joint, forefoot).

Sometimes a Sudeck's atrophy of the foot may complicate the course of a septic arthritis, posing problems of diagnosis with reappearance of infective phenomena [10].

Finally, septic arthritides of the foot and ankle are severe conditions and need urgent treatment. Suspicion of their existence must immediately lead to studies to trace the organism. Treatment must be considered to be an emergency, with close collaboration between the rheumatologist, the specialist in infections, and the surgeon. All therapeutic delay increases the mortality risk and aggravates the functional prognosis, always guarded for these weight-bearing joints.

References

1. Bontoux D, Lambert de Cursay G (1994) Manifestations rhumatismales des endocardites. Encycl Med Chir, Appareil locomoteur, 14-202-A-10
2. Broy B, Schmid F (1986) A comparison of medical drainage (needle aspiration) and surgical drainage (arthrotomy or arthroscopy) in the initial treatment of infected joints. Clin Rheum Dis 12: 501-522
3. Calmels C, Eulry F, Lechevalier D, Dubost J, Ristori J, Sauvezie B, Bussière J (1993) L'atteinte du pied dans les arthrites réactionnelles. Rev Rhum 60: 324-329
4. Carly P (1990) Manifestations articulaires des parasitoses. Concours médical 112: 2447-2752
5. Christol D, Vu Thien H (1991) Pasteurelloses humaines d'inoculation. Concours médical 113: 2511-2513
6. David-Chaussé J (1983) Arthrites infectieuses du pied. Le point de vue du médecin. In: Claustre J, Simon L (eds) Le pied en pratique rhumathologique. Masson, Paris, pp 128-133
7. David-Chaussé J, Dehais J, Boyer M, Darde M, Imbert Y (1981) Les infections articulaires chez l'adulte. Atteintes périphériques et vertébrales à germes banals et à bacilles tuberculeux. Rev Rhum Mal Osteoartic 48: 69-76
8. Dellamonica P (1993) Les infections ostéo-articulaires. Concours médical 115: 3515-3519.
9. Deutsch AL, Mink JH, Kerr R (1992) MRI of the foot and ankle. Raven Press, New York, pp 199-222
10. Dossa J, Picard L (1983) Arthrites infectieuses du pied. Le point de vue du chirurgien. In: Claustre J, Simon L (eds) Le pied en pratique rhumathologique. Masson, Paris, pp 132-136
11. Doury P, Meyer R, Eulry F, Pattin S, Kuntz J, Asch L (1986) Algodystrophies du pied secondaires à des arthrites septiques. À propos de quatre observations. Médecine et chirurgie du pied 8: 125-128.
12. Dubost J, Fis I, Soubrier M, Lopitaux R, Ristori J, Bussière J, Sauvezie B (1994) Les arthrites septiques au cours de la polyarthrite rhumatoïde. Rev Rhum 61: 153-165
13. Goldenberg D, Reed J (1985) Bacterial arthritis. N Engl J Med 312: 764-771.
14. Joseph W (1990) Infections. In: Levy LA, Hetherington VJ (eds) Principles and practices of podiatric medicine. Churchill Livingstone, New York, pp 275-313
15. Legrand E, Le Dantec P, Arvieux C, Guggenbulh P, Meadeb J, Chales G (1992) Conduite à tenir devant une arthrite septique à germe banal de l'adulte. Synoviale 10: 10-16
16. Lemaire V (1991) Les arthrites à pyogènes non gonococciques de l' adulte. Concours médical 113: 3336-3339
17. Pansart E, Segard F, Enjalbert M, Claustre J, Dossa J (1989) Arthrites septiques du médio-pied. In: Claustre J, Simon L (eds). Le médio-pied. Masson, Paris, pp 209-214
18. Pilly E (1994) Infections ostéo-articulaires. In: 2M2 (ed). Maladies Infectieuses. 173-181
19. Siame J (10-1988) Arthrites à pyogènes de l' adulte. Encycl Med Chir Paris, Appareil locomoteur, 1418O A10, 1-6
20. Wu KK (1990) Diagnosis and treatment of foot ulcers. In: Wu KK (ed) Foot orthoses: Principles and Clinical Applications. Williams & Wilkins, Baltimore, pp 227-292.

9.
The diabetic foot

P Vexiau, D Acker and A Belmouhoub

Introduction

Current therapeutic measures have greatly decreased the risks of death directly linked to diabetes, though the increase in life expectancy and the aging of this population have caused a significant increase in the frequency of complications which may give rise to morbidity and mortality. Lower limb lesions, particularly of the foot, are costly from both the human and economic standpoints [1, 70]. All types of diabetes, insulin-dependent or not, are prone to these complications. Prevention through supervision of the feet and education of the patients is therefore a major issue [1, 30].

Epidemiology

Generalities

The prevalence of diabetes is established with difficulty because it is so often latent and unrecognized (almost 50% of cases). Moreover, these unrecognized cases evolve insidiously and favor the appearance of complications. Type I diabetes, i.e., insulin-dependent, has a prevalence rate of 0.25% within the general population. The prevalence of type II diabetes, i.e., non-insulin-dependent, is much less known. In the USA in 1992, the frequency of type II was assessed to be 3.1% of known cases; the rate of unknown cases was estimated at 1.8% [40, 71].

Complications

The increase in the diabetic's duration of life is accompanied by a serious increase in complications, particularly cardiovascular, which are currently the main causes of morbidity and mortality [46, 63]. These complications are responsible for coronary lesions, lesions of the great cervical vessels and especially degeneration of the lower limb arteries. Arteritis is particularly frequent and precocious in diabetic patients [26]: 4.5 times more frequent than in the general population. It is also more severe because it is associated with neuropathy. Other circumstances linked to diabetes such as poor socio-economic conditions also play an important part; the incidence of arteriopathy in the underprivileged population is twice as high as in the general population [22].

Cardiovascular complications are also linked to other common factors among diabetics (hyperlipidemia, arterial hypertension, etc.). This shows their multifactorial nature and the need to treat not only the diabetes, but also lipid dysfunction, arterial hypertension and smoking, which increase the risk of complications.

The frequency of neuropathy depends on the examinations performed to establish a diagnosis.

EMG measurements of dysfunction of nervous conduction are almost routine. This neuropathy plays a major role in the appearance of complications in the diabetic foot [86].

The role of other pathologies associated with diabetes which provoke the appearance of complications in the lower limbs must not be underestimated. Diabetic retinopathy is the leading cause of non-traumatic blindness before the age of 65 in developed countries. Cataracts are the second ocular complication among diabetics. These ocular lesions contribute significantly to the non-detection of foot involvement, particularly among the aged [19].

Trophic risks in diabetics

Twenty per cent of all hospital admissions for diabetes are a result of complications in the foot [33]. In 91.8% of cases, amputation is due to gangrenous lesions, necrosis or ulceration. Furthermore, 33% of diabetic patients who have undergone an amputation in one lower limb will have a surgical operation on the other limb within the 5 years following the first operation. In the same period, the mortality rate in this population is about 50 to 75%. The risk of gangrene among diabetics is 17 times higher than in the non-diabetic population, and 10 times higher after the age of 65. Yet 50 to 70% of these amputations have a minor cause which is certainly curable by early and simple treatment. In numerous cases, these lesions could have been avoided by adequate education in the patient [48].

In 1992, in the USA, the annual average cost for care per known diabetic, was estimated at $11,157 compared with $2,604 for non-diabetics. These amounts estimate the direct costs alone, and not the indirect costs linked to diabetes (sick-leave, invalidity, disability). Hence in 1992, the expenses linked to diabetes represented 11.9% of total expenses for health care. This emphasizes the public health problem that diabetes and its complications represent: it is included among the seven most costly diseases in the developed countries [70, 71]. Lastly, and above all, one must acknowledge that the treatment costs of a diabetic patient without any complications is not very different from those of a non-diabetic patient. The small proportion of diabetic patients is expensive for the welfare state, on account of their complications, notably in the lower limbs [81].

Physiopathology

Arteriopathy

Macroangiopathy is extremely frequent, more especially as other risk factors exist. Although distal lesions are more classical among diabetics, proximal lesions also occur, and are all the more important as it is possible to treat them surgically [52, 77].

Microangiopathy, specific to diabetes, affects the small and capillary vessels, and is particularly linked to the associated neuropathy. This peculiarity leads to the opening of vascular (arterio-venous) shunts, responsible for diversion of the circulation at the site of the microcirculation. The result is that the peripheral pulses are easily palpated or even obviously pulsatile, whereas signs of distal ischemia exist. This phenomenon was considered to justify the surgical sympathectomies that are no longer performed today.

The investigation of arteriopathy is particularly important, as it is almost constantly associated with neuropathy. An accurate lesional survey is essential to establish the therapeutic indications. The investigation of an arteritis of the lower limbs must record the arteritis, specify the topography of the lesions and assess the severity of the ischemia [38, 39, 52]. This arteriopathy is increasingly accessible to surgical procedures in more distal sites.

Neuropathy

Neuropathy plays a major role in the appearance of lower limb lesions [6, 7, 28]. Its origin is essentially metabolic, through accumulation of sorbitol in the nerves, responsible for edema and for axonal destruction [86]. Polyneuritis of the lower limbs is the commonest complication, accompanied by a reduction of sensitivity and loss of the achilles and patellar reflexes. On the one hand, this neuropathy plays a major role in functional anomalies of the foot circulation (shunts) [74]; on the other, it impairs sensation particularly thermo-algesic. If there are lesions, the neuropathy hides the pain, which is normally an alarm symptom [5, 7, 76]. This shows the importance of primary prevention of complications through the education of patients to search routinely for lesions of the feet [65, 77].

Infections

Infections of the feet are multiple among diabetics. Superficial skin infections, particularly mycosis, must be distinguished from bacterial complications such as super-infection or even cellulitis, leading to deep infections with a major general risk.

Mycoses

Mycoses of feet are frequent and dominated by dermatophytes. Yeasts and, more rarely molds, may be observed. Uncontrolled diabetes can encourage their development and rapid extension. Onychomycotic dystrophy, responsible for trophic and infectious complications, is largely linked to the biomechanical characters of the foot and the toes in the shoe.

Intertrigo and onychomycosis are common [3]. Intertrigo arises as a small desquamation which develops a fissure in the depth of the interdigital spaces, particularly the fourth. Pruritus is variable. It can spread to the dorsal aspect or sole of the foot, to its lateral edges and up to the ankle. The skin involvement has different aspects: simple desquamation, hyperkeratosis, vesiculo-bullous or pustulous lesions (to be distinguished from a dyshydrosis or psoriasis). An interdigital soft corn, sometimes over-infected, must be excluded. The fungus can settle in the nails. The mode of penetration determines the major clinical forms [91]:

• **Disto-lateral involvement under the nail** with major ungual callosities (the fungus penetrates under the nail in the horny layer of the hypony-chium and nail-bed; the invasion spreads proximally and may lead to secondary onycholysis); and a form with primary onycholysis (as when the nail becomes detached by overlapping of the second toe over the lateral part of the first toe nail).

• **Proximal subungual lesions** arise in two forms: in the first, the infection begins at the deep side of the subungual fold, and in the second, there is onyxis which is frequently due to candida.

• **Superficial leukonychia**, white opaque spots with clear limits due to *Trichophyton rubrum*, is often interdigital.

• **Onychomycotic dystrophy** may be primary, corresponding to a candida granuloma (involvement of all the tissues of the nail accompanied by severe inflammatory reaction leading to pseudoclubbing). Total onychomycotic dystrophy may also be secon-

dary. Aggravated subungual lesions evolve towards complete involvement of the nail.

Complications are the result of staphylococcal superinfections (cellulitis, spreading deeply towards the articulations and synovial sheaths), streptococci (erysipelas), Proteus, *Escherichia coli*, viral infections (mosaic verruca over interdigital intertrigo), or finally of a spinocellular epithelioma as may occur in any chronic lesion.

It is noteworthy that not every onychopathy is necessarily mycotic; digital dystrophy mechanisms very often cause static and dynamic disturbances that influence the shape and character of the nail through the physical force they exert.

Any abnormal and unexplained aspect of the nail should arouse suspicion of a tumoral lesion, hence the importance of biopsy.

Bacterial infections

Perforating plantar lesions are usually superinfected. A local purulent inflammation with signs of lymphangitis is evidence of this infection. Its gravity is variable, ranging from localized infection to possible necrosing fasciitis or lymphangitis in the sheaths and tendons. Infections are mostly caused by aerobic agents, Gram-positive cocci, particularly Staphylococcus aureus or streptococci. Gram-negative organisms are also frequent; *Escherichia coli*, Klebsiella and Proteus [36, 42, 50, 51]. Anaerobic bacteria are classical but rare; they may be responsible for severe extensive lesions such as gas gangrene [87].

● Clinical examination

Clinical examination is carried out in different ways depending on circumstances: simple examination, in the primary or secondary prevention of acute complications, in subacute circumstances, or more urgently in the presence of signs of ischemia or infection.

Clinical examination of the foot

Clinical examination of the diabetic foot is no different from that of the non-diabetic foot. Some issues are more specific and related to trophic risks. In the majority of cases, clinical examination alone provides the indications for treatment and its nature. First, one must assess the existence and severity of a neuropathy or an arteriopathy, on which therapeutic tactics and follow-up depend.

Examination begins as soon as the patient walks in. The type of gait is recorded. Is the patient functionally independent or does he/she require assistance? Is he/she accompanied? Does he/she take off shoes and clothes alone, and how? The condition of the shoe and its quality of upkeep, the state of the socks and their cleanliness, are noted.

Estimation of the functional symptomatology (intermittent limp, decubitus pain, trophic lesions), auscultation and palpation of arteries, skin color and the time of return of color after pressure establish the diagnosis of arteritis and inform us about its severity. The presence of a murmur and absence of pulses suggest the level of the lesions.

The diabetic foot may be ischemic or neuropathic, though both types of disorder are variably associated [86]. It is important in treatment to distinguish an ischemic from a neuropathic origin. The ischemic foot typically presents aching lesions, absence of peripheral pulses, distal lesions, especially at the toes, and absence of hyperkeratosis. The neuropathic foot is not really painful, with presence of pulses, lesions at pressure points, hyperkeratosis at points of support and friction, and increased blood-flow.

The examination must search for deformities of the foot, particularly pes cavus, interosseous muscle atrophy, and arthropathy with destruction of the osseous structure which ultimately evolves towards a Charcot foot [16, 72] (fig. 9.1). Localized hyperkeratosis, particularly opposite the metatarsal heads, sesamoid bones, interphalangeal joints and toe pads, and the tuberosity of the fifth metatarsal express the points of mechanical overloading and the weak points where the risk of trophic plantar lesions is maximal [7, 8, 9, 10, 20] (fig. 9.2). The underside of the heel is often the center of a fissured hyperkeratosis. Xerosis and cutaneous dryness weaken the dermo-epidermal barrier.

The condition of the sole is assessed by inspection and palpation. Any purplish-blue staining, all the more so if surrounded by an inflammatory halo, every subkeratotic hematoma [5, 7, 76] and every case of cellulitis is a therapeutic emergency.

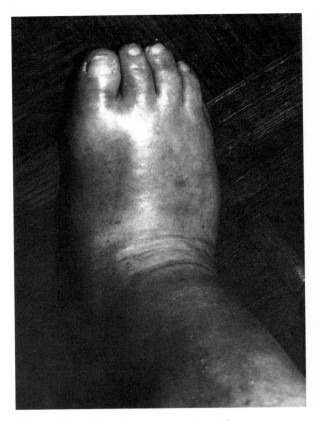

Fig. 9.1. Charcot foot due to neuro-arthropathy

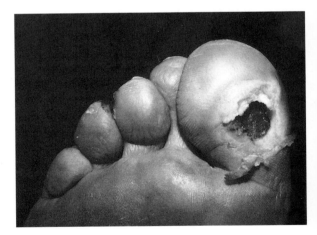

Fig. 9.2. Plantar perforating lesion

The study of superficial and deep sensation is essential. Study by needle, or tuning-fork, which explores deep vibratory sensation but also more superficial sensation (receptors in the deep dermis), is coarse. A fine analysis performed with a flexible nylon filament, allows a much more sensitive study of risk zones [5, 12]. Testing the patellar and achilles tendon reflexes completes the examination.

The interdigital spaces are examined, possibly after cleansing. Nail dystrophies, usually complicated by mycoses, are assessed for their mechanical consequences.

Rigidity of the metatarsophalangeal articulations and clawing of the toes seriously impair uniformity of load distribution over the forefoot. Risk zones are located at the forefoot and heel. Passive dorsiflexion reveals the axis of the talo-naviculo-cuneiform medial column and the presence of a short calcaneal tendon syndrome, especially in cases of neuro-arthropathy, with risk of flattening of the midfoot. The head of the talus, the navicular bone and even the medial cuneiform bone may be in contact with the ground and cause a lesion by localized overloading [22, 31].

Investigation continues with a semi-dynamic study by putting the patient in a monopodal standing position and making him/her walk on the spot. This will assess the biomechanical characters of the foot and display any deviations and the movements of different bony segments, which leads to a reasoned choice of the different types of orthoses. Walking barefoot and wearing shoes is studied. Examination of the footprint allows measurement of the points of maximum pressure, sometimes studied by means of computers though their reliability is still disputed [8, 14, 15, 82].

Lastly, the wear of all parts of the shoe shank is noted. Examination helps to define the trophic risk, which increases with age, neuropathy, arteriopathy, dynamic and static disorders, poor hygiene and footwear, poor social and economic conditions and poor control of glycemia, whether the patient is under insulin or not.

General examination

Examination of the diabetic foot must form part of a more general assessment, including:
• a complete cardiovascular review, searching for a vascular murmur, particularly in the neck, measurement of blood pressure, etc.;
• the ophthalmologic examination is particularly important. It seeks the minimal eye-foot distance, assesses if the patient is able to see his/her sole, completed by the measurement of visual acuity; this examination is fundamental in estimating the degree of independence in foot monitoring and therefore in the prevention of lesions of the foot [19];
• search for infectious signs, but fever and hyperleukocytosis are erratic [37, 61]. It is a major issue in treatment to assess the severity of the infection and of its extension in the soft parts towards the bones. The presence of more general infectious signs, particularly of septicemia, is a grave feature.

● Auxiliary examinations

X-rays without preparation

Radiographs without preparation may suggest a calcified aortic aneurysm or visualize other vascular

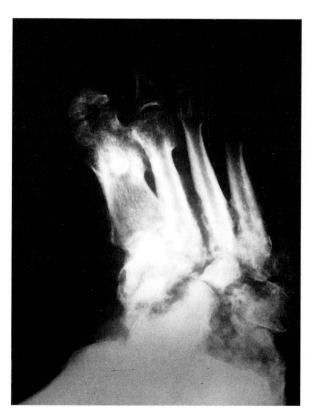

Fig. 9.3. Radiograph of neuro-arthropathic foot with osteolysis. Fragmentation and dislocation of the anterior tarsus, healing arthritis of first and second metatarsophalangeal joints, and of interphalangeal joint of hallux with ankylosis, amputation 2/3 of fifth metatarsal

calcifications, especially medial calcinosis, which is important if surgical operation is being considered. Radiographs also show any osseous demineralization or, at a later stage, bone destruction with arthropathy (fig. 9.3), also the presence of osteitis or arthrosis in trophic disorders. The absence of cortical involvement excludes an osteomyelitis, but cortical destruction does not necessarily confirm the existence of bone infection. It is sometimes quite difficult to distinguish osteitis or arthrotic lesions from neuropathic lesions with osteoathropathy, which is accompanied by severe osteoporosis [44, 61]. Differential diagnosis is all the more important because both types of lesions often coexist.

Vascular examination

Measurement of systolic pressure at the ankle

A doppler apparatus is used to measure the systolic pressure at the ankle, so as to confirm an arteritis, evaluate its severity and follow its course. However, medial calcinosis is frequent in diabetics and can make the arteries incompressible.

Real-time coupled doppler/ultrasound

Ultrasound detects stenosis and occlusion; when coupled to a doppler it helps to evaluate its hemodynamic significance at rest and during effort.

Transcutaneous measurement of oxygen partial pressure (TcPO$_2$)

The apparatus measures transcutaneous oxygen flow. In addition to its simplicity and high reproducibility, this method has a major advantage: it measures a parameter that concerns the skin and its nutrient blood-flow exclusively. The TcPO$_2$ of the dorsal part of the foot can be linked to the pressure measured by the same device in the skin of the thorax below the clavicle. This relation defines the index of regional perfusion [27]. The minimum value of TcPO$_2$, below which it is unrealistic to expect the healing of trophic lesions, is about 30 mmHg. Unlike the systolic pressure measured at the ankle, the TcPO$_2$ is useful in cases of medial calcinosis. When a trophic plantar lesion exists, the responsibility of the peripheral neuropathy is certain, but an underlying

arteritis may jeopardize healing of the wound. A systolic pressure in the hallux above 50 mmHg excludes a causal associated macro-angiopathy, and a TcPO$_2$ above 30 mmHg near the trophic lesion is favorable to healing under medical care [64, 89].

Arteriography

Arteriography remains indispensable whenever a revascularization surgical procedure is contemplated, or an endoluminal angioplasty. Digitilized angiography minimizes the use of iodized contrast. Nevertheless, this test is a source of risk in vascular problems in diabetics, who often present renal deficiency. Possible aggravation of this deficiency during the examination requires strict monitoring [4].

Good management of the radiologic examination is therefore essential since the major cause of acute renal failure is successive examinations with iodine injections, as in arteriography of the lower limbs followed by aortic assessment before operating on a carotid stenosis. Furthermore, treatment with biguanides must be discontinued 48 h beforehand, because of the risks of lactic acidosis.

Additional examinations searching for infective lesions

A bacteriologic swab, with antibiogram, must be made. Swabs must be inserted as deeply as possible to get rid of contamination by superficial saprophytic organisms [51, 73, 87]. Estimating the spread of infection and particularly the existence or not of a bony lesion, is a major issue but is sometimes hard to establish.

Scintigraphy using Tc-99 m [44] or scintigraphy with labeled polynuclears [44, 61] can help to detect the presence of infected bone when significant cutaneous inflammatory signs are absent. However, even if inflammatory signs exist, diffuse isotope fixation will not establish or invalidate osseous involvement. However, if there is a mild superficial inflammatory lesion, scintigraphy can determine whether pathologic fixation exists or not in the bones [29, 54, 85]. MRI may specify the extent of destructive osseous lesions which give rise to osteomyelitis. It also aids the search for spread of the infection by showing necrotic exudate which suggests the extension of an abscess.

Treatment

Preventive treatment

Education

Education is of major importance in teaching patients how to detect, and above all prevent, lesions of the foot [23, 77]. The global amputation rate over the same population at the cantonal hospital of Geneva decreased by half between 1970 and 1978 after an education program was set up. Moreover, for the same surgical team, the level and frequency of amputations were modified by an earlier diagnosis. Thus, among uneducated patients who underwent an amputation, 67% had an amputation halfway down the leg and only 33% an amputation of a toe, whereas these rates were 14% and 86% respectively in the educated population. A ratio of 1:11 was noted for the amputees, depending on whether they were properly educated beforehand or not. In the same way, the average duration of hospital stay decreased from 10 days to 1 day per year [1].

Hygiene

Attention and care of the feet by the diabetic may prevent several trophic complications. Simple preventive measures are the basis of foot care. At each examination, one must ensure that the patient and his/her close relations understand these measures and confirm their application [22]. The practitioner must not forget to repeat this, however banal and tedious it may seem in every day life.

Ten measures are essential [12]

• Daily examination of the feet, in detail, especially between the toes. Any cutaneous or nail modification is suspicious: color, shape, size, consistence. If visual acuity or functional performance is insufficient, one of the patient's close relations must be trained to carry out these measures.
• Foot cleansing with tap-water using a glove with simple or very fatty soap. Foot baths make the cutaneous barrier more fragile; running water (shower) is better than stagnant water; rinsing is important and so is drying, especially between the toes with a special towel;
• Hydration and lubrication of the skin, which is often very dry, must be done every day, morning and evening, except between the toes; never use corn applications, never scratch or pumice, never rasp the skin. The more supple the skin becomes, the more it resists attack.
• Nail cutting with nail-clippers cleaned with bleach after use; never cut too short or bevel the edges, which can be filed with a disposable nail-file. Always clean with an antiseptic solution after cutting. If bad eye sight or functional handicap makes cutting impossible for the patient himself, a trained person among close relations or a chiropodist may perform it. Thickened dirty nails or nails with onychomycotic dystrophies are ground with special scrapers rather than cut [21].
• Hyperkeratoses are cleaned without causing any bleeding, leaving a thin layer of the hyperkeratosis rather than damage the skin. Cleansing with an antiseptic after this operation is also necessary, and should be performed by an experienced professional who knows the risks [21, 90].
• Immediate treatment of any wound with a strong antiseptic (not alcohol) after cleansing and copious irrigation with tap-water; the wound is covered by a thin compress (sterile unit-bag), fixed by a hypoallergenic film without tension or strong adhesion and over a large cutaneous area. Then medical advice should be rapidly sought.
• Tetanus immunization is verified.
• Heat and cold are feared, as in the case of a patient who warms himself directly from a heat source: radiator, hot-water bottle, electric blanket, or near the fire.
• Shoes must be carefully chosen. Walking barefoot, at home or on the beach, is forbidden to patients who have a neuropathy or an arteriopathy. Every day, the patient must verify manually the absence of foreign bodies inside his shoes; it is better to wear two pairs of shoes alternately. Stockings and socks should not have a tight band in their upper part; the distal part must end mesh to mesh and must not include a terminal knot. The choice is not limited to cotton but can include cotton mixed with other fibers. The weave must be soft to the touch.
• Any hesitation or doubt calls for medical consultation even if, knowing that pain or its absence is not an index of severity, this consultation may prove to be negative.

Treatment

Neuropathy and arteriopathy are characteristic of the vulnerability of the diabetic foot and provoke it. Trophic complications can and must be avoided. Everything must be done to eliminate and prevent:
• any external aggression (poor local care and

hygiene, inadequate shoes, mechanical and thermal shocks and trauma);

• any endogenous aggression (overloading by stato-dynamic disorders, aggravation due to dryness and thinness of the skin and/or atrophy of the plantar pad).

It is a fact that every prolonged local stress leads ineluctably, if nothing is done, to amputation, and to trophic and functional disasters with all their economic, social and personal costs [60].

Treatment of lesions

Local care is given during the usual consultation. Each hyperkeratotic, non-homogeneous, hematic area, surrounded by an inflammatory halo, even if minimal, must be checked for ulceration, an accumulation of pus or an underlying sinus.

In the case of a lesion of arterial origin, which is frequently very painful, careful cleansing should be limited to the necrosed and sclerotic tissue if there is an underlying granulation and the appearance of bleeding. Preliminary application of local anesthetics will suppress or reduce the pain.

In the case of a neuropathic ulceration, it is necessary to practice a broad excision, removing the hyperkeratotic areas and the sclerotic tissue in the search for a bleeding substrate on curettage. The cleansing is more mechanical than chemical. The wound must bleed. The absence of pain in neuropathy facilitates care, which must be renewed at each consultation. It does not usually require an anesthetic. Minimal asepsis is adequate (instruments, gloves, sterile area, apron) An osteo-articular lesion calls for curettage of the bone and ablation of sequestra. No wonder product exists to promote healing and the first step is to eliminate overload or friction, de-stressing the wound by bed-rest, orthoses, prostheses, plaster or resin cast immobilization, care with shoes and socks, special custom-made shoes [11, 59, 62].

Preferred antiseptics and antibiotics are iodized polyvidone, iodoform gauge, chlorhexidine, hexomidine and rifamycin. These are more particularly indicated for staphylococcal infections [47]. Their application must be discontinued before their toxicity limits the granulation process; one must then use sterile isotonic saline [47, 49]. The mechanical action of irrigation with an enema syringe or even with shower water is beneficial for this purpose.

Many locally applied agents are used to promote healing: powder, liquid, ointment, hydro-colloids, natural products such as sugar or honey. Local applications of insulin are inappropriate. Hydro-colloidal dressings are difficult to use over arterial lesions; compresses with lipids or soaked in sterile isotonic saline are better. Aqueous eosin at 2% [41, 88] dries out the involved area before regrowth of skin. Treatment by growth factors has not yet been shown to be efficient [45, 55, 78].

Surgery [34]

There is little indication for amputations at levels between transmetatarsal procedures and those located at the lower third of the leg. Even transmetatarsal amputations, when they are too high, as well as amputations at the tarsometatarsal or midtarsal joints or involving the calcaneus or talus, lead to an appreciable risk of necrosis due to the tissue and cutaneous stripping involved. These amputations are subject to biomechanical disorders accompanied with varus deformation and calcaneal verticalization, which are often impossible to correct because of neuro-arthropathic bony fragility or the arteriopathic factor. The special appliances required are dangerous because of mechanical exposure of the stump.

A transmetatarsal amputee can wear standard shoes. The appliance for an amputation through the upper third of the leg has less trophic risk to the stump and its periphery and restoration of weight-bearing is faster.

The amputation of a toe creates a gap which is difficult to control with a prosthesis, which cannot keep the adjacent rays straight without risk of injury. Amputation of a whole ray with the corresponding metatarsal seems to lessen this risk, while hallux amputation leads to major biomechanical disorders; in both cases, architectural transformations modify the level of ground contact stress on the adjacent rays. This risk must be well evaluated and if required one must improve the distribution of pressure by using a plantar orthosis. When there is an indication for amputation of several toes on the same side, amputation of the remaining toes may be considered in order to simplify the appliance and improve function. Amputation is decided with due regard to local vascularization and/or osteitis, but must also take into account that the subsequent appliance should incur minimal trophic risk to the stump and give the best functional outcome [34, 35, 56].

Corrective surgery of the forefoot is limited, and contraindicated when arteriopathy is associated with a macro- or microangiopathy, because of problems in healing.

Ingrowing nails must be systematically treated early on. They are responsible for too many amputations. The surgical treatment of a hallux valgus or a disorder of other rays does not pose problems differing from those in non-diabetics.

Plantar orthoses

These are similar to those discussed in chapter 32. They are most useful in cases with a neuro-arteriopathic context. The shoes must leave enough room for the orthoses to provide their relieving effects without reducing shoe space, which leads to rubbing of the toes against the distal part of the shoe. One must be strict in the choice of a model and not hesitate to prescribe a special appliance or a custom-made shoe for foot disorders. The orthosis must palliate a structural fault which gives rise to a localized plantar overloading, usually opposite a metatarsal head, the sesasmoids, toe extremities or heel. When this is not relieved, a callosity usually develops and acts like a foreign body, and there is underlying bleeding. This favors infection and its spread to deeper tissues down to the osteo-articular level. A plantar orthosis must eliminate the subkeratotic hematoma by reducing ground contact and shear forces. Therefore, they are made of foam; cork and hard materials are forbidden. The common orthoses include supports behind the metatarsal heads, or under the medial arch and behind the sesamoid area, heel lifts of different densities, layers of various materials, and thermo-formed and shaped orthoses allowing appropriate distribution of the body-weight. These are reviewed after a very short period of use, and at the beginning the orthosis must be considered as temporary. This temporary wear and its macroscopic results suggest possible modifications of the orthoses. Very localized areas, where noxious pressure may damage the tissues, soon leave their mark on the orthosis, so that it is easy to redistribute the loads in a better way.

The persistence of a subkeratotic hematoma leads to modification of the orthosis. An abrupt anterior edge in too rigid a material behind the head of the metatarsal can produce a traumatism which must be detected promptly. Therefore, strict and frequent inspection of the feet of a patient wearing an orthosis is essential and the patient and his/her close relations should be taught the critical signs of a possible lesion.

Toe orthoses

As for any appliance for a diabetic foot their adjustment must be perfect so as not to traumatize the areas where they take their support, especially at the bottom of the interdigital spaces under the toes. Indeed they represent foreign bodies. At the beginning supervision of their adjustment is frequent. They cannot be corrective because they could be too aggressive towards the skin. They essentially limit dorsal and toe-pulp loads in the case of clawing of the toes (pad corns and interphalangeal dorsal corns). The protection of the bunion of a first or fifth metatarsal head (hallux valgus, quintus varus) is more often an indication for a special or custom-made shoe. They are really stop-gaps, pending the construction of a plantar orthosis in an adapted shoe. They can be used in the case of a clean ulceration which does not involve the joints or when there is no surgical indication. They must not fill the empty space left by amputation of a toe because, in a neuro-arteriopathic context, friction against the adjacent toes or the stump is too risky.

Shoes

Shoes for diabetics must be discussed and criticized on the evidence at the time of consultation. All the shoes are brought including sports shoes, work shoes and slippers. In trying to efficiently prevent trophic lesions, it is insufficient to ask only for a leather of sufficient width; characterization must be very precise [15, 83].

General criteria of choice

The upper part of the shoe is made of supple leather. The part covering the toes and forefoot is plain, without laces or pinking, particularly in front. Shoes should be bought in the late afternoon to allow for any static edema. The sole of the shoe is in rather thick leather or rubber depending on individual tolerance (hyperhidrosis, mycosis, skin sensitivity). One must run one's hand inside the front of the shoe to detect any sewing or backstitching which may injure the toes and the extreme metatarsal heads. The toe-cap must be as soft as possible.

The shoe must not be too easily twisted or folded. Resistance to these tests is evidence of the quality of the shank. There should not be too great a difference between the suppleness of the upper with insufficiency of the counter and the stiffness of the sole. Support of the tarsus is essential. The insoles of shoes, which come into contact with the sole of the foot, must be of high quality without any roughness. The posterior counter must not be too rigid or have sewing which irritates the calcaneal tuberosity.

Therefore, one does not only talk about shoes in general but gives precise advice from the model worn. Shoes are to be considered as actual orthoses and inspected at clinical examination time. This forms part of the care of the diabetic foot in the prevention of trophic lesions [13, 18, 66, 75, 83, 84].

Specialized shoes

Mass-production shoes may be harmful, for various reasons: excessive size of the foot, presence of dress-ings or orthoses with characteristics due to local conditions, presence of neuropathy and/or arteriop-athy. In these cases, specialized shoes, therapeutic mass-produced shoes and custom-made shoes for foot disorders may be useful.

The ideal shoe for a given condition of the foot does not exist; the choice is always made with respect to the pathology encountered, the functional aspects and the avoidance of abnormal friction.

Various types of mass-produced therapeutic shoes

These are made in series for feet which need support, something which ordinary shoes cannot ensure. They are designed to accommodate, plantar orthoses if necessary:
• shoes for total relief of the forefoot, used for the immediate results of surgery for deformities of the forefoot, have the support at the heel or at the ante-rior part of the tarsus;
• shoes with total aperture have a large available volume and are very adaptable but support the foot less. The fasteners are made of velcro;
• thermo-molded shoes are made of a material which can be adapted to deformities of the forefoot by heating and manipulation;
• slippers and shoes with an open and adjustable end, or without pattens covering the toes;
• shoes for total unloading of the heel;
• shoes with a medial edge.

Custom-made shoes for foot disorders

Their prescription is detailed and reflects the clinical elements to be taken care of. Factors to be defined include the shape, the nature of the leather, upper and fasteners, compensations, orthoses, the orthoses-prostheses for amputations, along with their physico-chemical characteristics, the padding and the sole. They should be supplied as soon as indicated. Their perfect construction is sometimes difficult because of the vulnerability of the foot; once again, it is essential to obtain accurate adjustment of the shoe: absence of cork in the insoles, a sufficient degree of freedom for the toes and lateral metatarsal heads, and a wide and ultra-supple anterior com-partment.

Finally, special shoes for diabetic feet are an orthotic tool for the prevention and treatment of trophic lesions. They are medically prescribed with precise indications according to the condition of the foot; their adjustment is subject to strict surveillance.

The role of rehabilitation

Rehabilitation cannot develop or restore lost vascu-larization. It allows better muscular adaptation to effort and combats stiffening of the joints. Particular attention is given to metatarsophalangeal joint func-tion, giving priority to passive maneuvers; the poste-rior muscles and tendons must be stretched and the transverse stability of the foot and ankle is main-tained by neuromuscular reprogramming exercises.

Treatment of mycosis

The fungal infection is usually dermatophytic, rarely by yeasts or molds. Dermatophytic contamination is by cross-infection and involves prophylactic meas-ures (shoes, socks, communal facilities where one walks bare-foot, hygiene, heat and moisture). Intertrigo and onychomycosis involves also prophy-lactic measures.

General drugs are used, classical ones (griseo-fulvin, ketoconazole) or more recent ones (flucona-zole, itraconazole, terbinafine).

Treatment of diabetes

Diabetes control is a fundamental element in the supervening of complications. There is a direct rela-tion between the glycemic level and the development of complications in both primary and secondary prevention [79]. The proper control of diabetes is therefore essential in limiting the risk of both micro-angiopathic and macroangiopathic complications. In the case of acute lesions, whether arterial or neuro-pathic, in particular when an infectious factor exists, perfect metabolic control becomes imperative. This usually requires resort to insulin: multi-injections (3 or 4 per day) for insulin-dependent diabetics but also often for non-insulin-dependent patients, at least temporarily, possibly by means of a subcuta-neous insulin pump with continuous flow, rarely by intravenous administration.

Antibiotherapy

Antibiotics play a significant role in the treatment of infected lesions, but their efficiency depends on their specificity towards the responsible organisms, on good diffusion into the infected tissues, and finally on the attainment of good control of the glycemia. Their use depends on the type of lesion. With a superficial lesion or intertrigo, the organism usually responsible is the staphylococcus aureus. Preventive systemic treatment with long-term antibiotics is not advisable, because of the evolution of resistant strains and the absence of evidence of its efficiency [2, 12, 43, 68, 80].

Anticoagulant treatment

The indications for anticoagulant treatment in diabetics do not differ from those in non-diabetic patients suffering from arteritis. Preventive treat-ment of phlebitis by low molecular weight heparin is essential in immobilized patients, in non-weight-bearing, and of course when any kind of cast is used.

Treatment of neuropathy

No specific treatment for neuropathy exists to date. Inhibitors of aldose-reductase (inhibiting sorbitol synthesis, involved in the physiopathology of diabetic neuropathy), are efficient in animals, but this has not been confirmed in humans. The treat-ment of neuropathy is therefore based on control of the diabetes and the eradication of the aggravating factors [79]. Other possible factors responsible for neuropathy must be sought and treated because neuropathy is usually multifactorial. Therefore one must exclude alcoholic or drug-induced neuropa-thies, which aggravate the diabetic neuropathy. If there is a lesion (plantar perforating lesion), relief from weight-bearing by rest, or by a de-stressing appliance (plaster or resin cast), or by an orthosis, is the main treatment to avoid microtrauma [11, 32, 62].

Treatment of arteriopathy

The treatment is medical or surgical. The medical treatment of diabetes is little different from that of non-diabetic arteritis. It requires classical arterial vasodilators. The advent of new molecules which are similar to prostacyclins such as Ilomedine may modify the therapeutic indications, though these molecules are difficult to handle.

Fighting the pains in decubitus is a major problem to allow the patient to sleep with his/her feet in bed, even with the aid of strong antalgics.

Recent work has cast doubt on the view that arteritis in diabetics is not usually amenable to surgery. When surgery is technically possible for a diabetic revascularization, functional results do not differ from those of revascularization operations on nondiabetics [67]. Therefore, therapeutic indications are usually difficult to decide in diabetic patients with arteritis, especially in case of trophic lesions of the foot, whose pathogenesis is multifactorial. The use of noninvasive modern techniques of studying vascular function allows a more rapid and reliable selection of patients to be treated medically, revascularized or amputated. Treatments of arteritis, whether more or less classical, are not very different in diabetics from those applied in nondiabetics; the indications mostly depend on the site of the arterial disease and on monitoring of the lesions [38, 39, 53, 69].

Treatment of other risk factors

The treatment of other risk factors is as important as the treatment of the diabetes itself in the prevention of complications.

Smoking is a major risk factor for foot complica-tions in diabetics; investigations show that nico-tinism is twice as common in patients suffering from arteritis as in other patients [88].

The treatment of arterial hypertension, which plays a significant role in microangiopathy, is funda-mental. Arterial hypertension has been recently defined by WHO among diabetics as values exceeding 140 mmHg for the systolic pressure and 85 mmHg for the diastolic pressure [57].

Disorders of lipid metabolism must also be treated thoroughly because of their influence on microangiopathy. Finally, a real risk factor in com-plications because of its mechanical effects on the feet is obesity, which is present among 80% of non-insulin-dependent diabetics and must be treated [17, 21].

The treatment of retinopathy is fundamental, because proper supervision and laser treatment can prevent the onset of blindness. The second ophthal-mologic complication, cataract, is important because of its effect on visual acuity, especially in diabetics over 60, who are the most exposed to complications in the feet [19].

Conclusion

Several complications of diabetes are originally provoked by mistakes in hygiene, wearing of unsuit-able shoes, absence of supervision and failure to prevent static troubles linked to neuropathy and arteriopathy. Aged and isolated patients usually present a very high risk. By promoting access to health care, these patients can quickly benefit from specialized treatment, which is essential to improve primary and secondary prevention. The "Saint Vincent declaration", a European consensus on the management, care and treatment of diabetics, also called "the rights and duties of the patient and the doctor" has stated as its object: "a reduction by at least half of the number of amputations of lower limbs because of diabetic gangrene" [25]. The objec-tive of the USA health department is a 40% reduc-tion in amputations of the lower limbs in diabetics by the year 2000 [24].

References

1. Assal JPh, Albeanu A, Peter-Riesch B, Vaucher J (1993) The cost of training a diabetic patient. Effects on prevention of amputation. Diab Metab 19: 491-495
2. Bamberger DM, Daus GP, Gerding DN (1987) Osteomyelitis in the feet of diabetic patients. Long-term results, prognostic factors and the role of anti-microbial and surgical therapy. Am J Med. 83: 653-660
3. Baran R, Dawber RPR (1990) Guide médico-chirur-gical des onychopathies. Arnette, Paris
4. Billström A, Hietala SO, Lithner, et al (1989) Nephrotoxicity of contrast media in patients with diabetes mellitus. Acta Radiol 30: 509-515
5. Birke JA, Sims DS (1986) Plantar sensory threshold in the ulcerative foot. Lepr Rev. 57: 261-267
6. Boulton AJM (1988) The diabetic foot. Med Clin North Am 72: 1513-1530
7. Boulton AJM (1990) The diabetic foot of neuropathic aetiology. Diabetic Med 7: 852-856
8. Boulton AJM, Hardisty CA, Betts RP, et al (1983) Dynamic foot pressure and other studies as diagnostic and management aids in diabetic neuropathy. Diabetes care 6: 26-33
9. Boulton AJM, Kubrusly D, Bowker JH, et al (1986) Impaired vibratory perception and diabetic foot ulceration. Diabetic Med 3: 335-7
10. Brand PW (1988) Repetitive stress in the development of diabetic foot ulcers. In: Levin ME, O'Neal LW (eds) The diabetic foot, 4th edn. Mosby, S. Louis, pp 83-90
11. Burden AC, Jones GR, Jones R, Blandford RL (1983) Use of the "Scotchcast boot" in treating diabetic foot ulcers. Br Med J 286: 1555-1557
12. Caputo GM, Cavanagh PR, Ulbrecht JS, Gibbons GW, Karchmer AW (1994) Assessment and management of foot disease in patients with diabetes. N Engl J Med 331: 854-60
13. Cavanagh PR, Hewitt FG Jr, Perry JE (1992) In-shoe plantar pressure measurement: a review. Foot Ankle 294: 185-94
14. Cavanagh PR, Ulbrecht JS (1991) Biomechanics of the diabetic foot: a quantitative approach to the assess-ment of neuropathy, deformity, and plantar pressure. In: Iahss MH (ed) Disorders of the foot and ankle: medical and surgical management, 2nd edn. Vol. 2. WB Saunders, Philadelphia, pp 1864-1907
15. Cavanagh PR, Ulbrecht JS (1993) Biomechanics of the foot in diabetes mellitus. In: Levin ME, O'Neal LW, Bowker JH (eds) The diabetic foot, 5th edn. Mosby-Year Book, St Louis, pp 199-232
16. Cavanagh PR, Young MJ, Adams JE, Vickers KL, Boulton AJM (1994) Radiographic abnormalities in the feet of patients with diabetic neuropathy. Diabetes Care 17: 201-209
17. Coleman WC, Brand PW, Birke JA (1984) The total contact cast: a therapy for plantar ulceration on insen-sitive feet. J Am Podiatr Assoc 74: 548-552
18. Coleman WC (1993) Footwear in a management program for injury prevention. In: Levin ME, O'Neal LW, Bowker JH (eds) The diabetic foot. 5th edn. Mosby-Year Book, St. Louis, pp 531-547
19. Crausaz F, Clavel S, Liniger C, et al (1988) Additional factors associated with planter ulcers in diabetic neuropathy. Diabetic Med. 5: 771-775
20. Ctercteko GC, Dhanendran M, Hunon WC, Le Quesne LP (1981) Vertical forces acting on the feet of diabetic patients with neuropathic ulceration. Br J Surg 68: 608-614
21. Davidson JK, Alogna M, Goldsmith M, Borden J (1981) Assessment of program effectiveness at Grady Memorial Hospital, Atlanta. In: Steiner G, Lawrence PA (eds) Educating diabetic patients. Springer, New York, pp 329-348
22. Delbrige L, Appleberg M, Reeve TS (1983) Factors associated wiith developement of foot lesions in the diabetic. Surgery 1: 78-82

23. Delbridge, Perry P, Marr S, et al (1988) Limited joint mobility in the diabetic foot: relationship to neuropathic ulceration. Diabetic Med 5: 333-337

24. Department of Health and Human Services. Healthy People 2000: national health promotion and disease prevention objectives. Washington. D.C.: Government Printing Office (1991): 73-117. [DHHS publication no. 91502 1 3.]

25. Diabetes care and research in Europe: the Saint Vincent Declaration (1990) Diabetic Med 7: 360.

26. Diabetes Drafting Group (1985) Prevalence of small vessel and large vessel disease in diabetes from 14 centers. The WHO multinational study of vascular disease in diabetics. Diabetologia 28: 615-40

27. Editorial (1984) Transcutaneous oxygen measurement in skin ischaemia. Lancet 2: 329

28. Edmonds ME (1987) Expenence in a multidisciplinary diabetic foot clinic. In: Connor H, Boulton AJM, Ward JD (eds) The foot in diabetes: proceedings of the First National Conference on the Diabetic Foot. Malvem, England. May 1986, John Wiley, Chichester, England, pp 121-134

29. Eymontt MJ, Alavi A, Dalinka MK, Clayton Kyle G (1981) Bone scintigraphy in diabetic osteoarthropathy. Radiology140: 475-457

30. Falkenberg M (1990) Metabolic control and amputations among diabetics in primary health care - a population-based intensified programme governed by patient education. Scand J Prim Health Care 8: 25-29

31. Fernando DJ, Masson EA, Veves A, Boulton AJM (1991) Limited joint mobility: relationship to abnormal foot pressures and diabetic foot ulceration. Diabetes Care 14: 8-12

32. Frykberg RG (1984) Podiatric problems in diabetes. In : Kozak GP, Hoar CS Jr, Rowbotham JL, Wheelock FC Jr, Gibbons GW, Campbell D (eds) Management of diabetic foot problems: Joslin Clinic and New England Deaconess Hospital. WB Saunders, Philadelphia, pp 45-67

33. Fylling CP (1992) Wound healing: an update. Comprehensive wound management for prevention of amputation. Diabetes Spectrum 5: 358-3549

34. Gibbons GW (1987) The diabetic foot: amputations and drainage of infection. J Vasc Surg 5: 791-793

35. Gibbons GW (1991) Toe and foot amputations. In: Ernst SB, Stanley JC (eds) Current therapy in vascular surgery, 2nd edn. BC Decker, Philadelphia, pp 694-696

36. Gibbons GW (1992) Diabetic foot sepsis. Semin Vasc Surg 5: 244-248

37. Gibbons GW (1984) Eliopoulos GM. Infection of the diabetic foot. In: Kozak GP, Hoar CS Jr, Rowbotham JL, Wheelock FC Jr, Gibbons GW, Campbell D (eds) Management of diabetic foot problems: Joslin Clinic and New England Deaconess Hospital. WB Saunders, Philadelphia, pp 97-102

38. Gibbons GW, Marcaccio EJ Jr, Burgess AM, et al (1993) Improved quality of diabetic foot care. 1984 vs 1990: reduced length of stay and costs. Insufficient reimbursement. Arch Surg 128: 576-581

39. Gupta SK, Veith FJ (1990) Inadequacy of diagnosis related group [DRG] reimbursements for limb salvage lower extremity arterial reconstructions. J Vasc Surg 11: 348-357

40. Harris MJ, Hadden WC, Knowler WC, Bennett PH (1987) Prevalence of diabetes and impaired glucose tolerance and plasma glucose levels in US population aged 20-74 yr. Diabetes 36: 523-534

41. Hutchinson JI, McGuchn M (1990) Occlusive dressings: a microbiologic and clinical review. Am J Infect Control 18: 257-268

42. Jones EW, Edwards R, Finch R, et al (1984) A microbiologic study of diabetic foot lesions. Diabetic Med 2: 213-215

43. Joseph WS, Axler DA (1990) Microbiology and antimicrobial therapy of diabetic foot infections. Clin Podiatr Med Surg 7: 467-481

44. Keenan AM, Tindel NL, Alavi A (1989) Diagnosis of pedal osteomyelitis in diabetic patients using current scintigraphic techniques. Arch Intern Med 149: 2262-2266

45. Knighton DR, Fiegel VD (1993) Growth factors and repair of diabetic wounds. In: Levin ME. O'Neai LW, Bowker JH (eds) The diabetic foot, 5th edn. Mosby-Year Book, St Louis, pp 247-257

46. Krolewsky AS, Kosinski EJ, Varram JH, et al (1987) Magnitude and determinant of coronary artery disease in IDDM. Am J Cardiol. 59: 750-755

47. Kucan JO, Robson MC, Heggers JP, Ko F (1981) Comparison of silver suifadiazine. povidone-iodine and physiologic saline in the treatment of chronic pressure ulcers. J Am Geriatr Soc 29: 232-235

48. Levin ME, O'Neal LW (1983) The diabetic foot, 3rd edn, Vols 11 & 12. CV Mosby, S. Louis, pp 1-55

49. Lineaweaver W, Howard R, Soucy D, et al (1985) Topical antimicrobial toxicity. Arch Surg. 120: 267-270

50. Lipsky BA, Pecoraro RE, Ahroni JH (1990) Foot ulceration and infections in elderly diabetics. Clin Geriatr Med 6: 747-769

51. Lipsky BA, Pecoraro RE, Wheat Ll (1990) The diabetic foot: soft tissue and bone infection. Infect Dis Clin North Am 4: 409-432

52. LoGerfo FW, Coffman JD (1984) Vascular and microvascular disease of the foot in diabetes: implications for foot care. N Engl J Med 311: 1615-1619

53. LoGerfo FW. Gibbons GW, Pomposelli FB Jr, et al (1992) Trends in the care of the diabetic foot: expanded role of arterial reconstruction. Arch Surg 127: 617-621

54. Maurer AH, Millmond SH, Knight LC, et al (1986) Infection in diabetic osteoarthropathy. Use of indium-labeled leukocytes for diagnosis. Radiology 161: 221-225

55. McGrath MH (1990) Peptide growth factors and wound healing. Clin Plast Surg 17: 421-432

56. McIntyre KE Jr, Bailey SA, Maione JM, Goldstone J (1984) Guillotine amputation in the treatment of non salvageable lower-extremity infections. Arch Surg 119: 450-453

57. Members of the Working Group on Hypertension and Diabetes (1987) Statement on hypertension and diabetes. Diabetes Care 10: 764-776

58. Most R, Sinnock P (1983) The epidemiology of lower extremity amputations in diabetic individuals. Diabetes Care. 6: 87-91

59. Mueller MJ, Diamond JE, Sinacore DR, et al (1989) Total contact casting in treatment of diabetic plantar ulcers: controlled clinical trial. Diabetes Care 12: 384-388

60. Myerson MS, Papa J, Eaton K, Wilson K (1992) The total-contact cast for management of neuropathic plantar ulceration ol the foot. J Bone Joint Surg Am 74: 261-269

61. Newman LG, Waller J, Palestro CJ, et al (1991) Unsuspected osteomyelitis in diabetic foot ulcers: diagnosis and monitoring by leukocyte scanning with indium-111 oxyquinoline. JAMA 266: 1246-1251

62. Novick A, Birke JA, Graham SL, Koziatek E (1991) Effect of a walking splint and total contact casts on plantar forces. J Prosthet Orthop 3: 168-178

63. O'Brien JAD, Corral RJM (1988) Epidemiology of diabetes and its complications. N Engl J Med 318: 1619-1620

64. Oh PJT, Provan JL, Ameli FM (1987) the predictability of the success of arterial reconstruction by means of transcutaneous oxygen tension measurements. J Vasc Surg 5: 356-362

65. Pecoraro RE, Reiber GE, Burgess EM (1990) Pathways to diabetic limb amputation: basis for prevention. Diabetes Care 13: 513-521

66. Perry JE, Ulbrecht JS, Cavanagh PR. Non-therapeutic footwear can play a role in reducing plantar pressurre in the diabetic foot. J Bone Joint Surg [Am] (in press)

67. Pomposelli FB Jr, Jepsen SJ, Gibbons GW, et al (1990) Efficacy of the dorsal pedal bypass for limb salvage in diabetic patients: short-term observations. J Vasc Surg 11: 715-752

68. Peterson LR, Lissack LM, Canter K, et al (1989) Therapy of lower extremity infections with ciprofloxacin in patients with diabetes mellitus, peripheral vascular disease or both. Am J Med 86: 801-808

69. Pomposelli FB Jr, Jepsen SJ, Gibbons GW, et al (1991) A Flexible approach to infrapopliteal vein grafts in patients with diabetes mellitus. Arch Surg 126: 724-729

70. Reiber GE (1992) Diabetic foot care: financial implications and practice guidelines. Diabetes Care 15:Suppl 1: 29-31

71. Rubin RJ, Altman WM, Mendelson DN (1994) Health care expenditures for people with diabetes mellitus, 1992. J Clin Endocrinol Metab 78: 809A-809

72. Sammarco GJ (1991) Diabetic arthropathy. In: Sammarco GJ (ed) The foot in diabetes. Lea & Febiger, Philadelphia, pp 153-172

73. Sapico FL, Wine JL, Canawati HN, Montgomene JZ, Bessman AN (1984) The infected foot of the diabetic patient: quantitative microbiology and analysis of clinical features. Rev Infect Dis 6 Suppl l: S171-S176

74. Sinha S, Munichoodappa CS, Kozak GP (1972) Neuroarthropathy [charcot joints] in diabetes mellitus. Medicine 51: 191-210

75. Soulier SM (1986) The use of running shoes in the prevention of plantar diabetic ulcers. J Am Podiatr Med Assoc 76: 395-400

76. Sosenko JM, Kato M, Soto R, Bild DE (1990) Comparison of quantitative sensory-threshold measures for their association with foot ulceration in diabetic patients. Diabetes Care 13: 1057-1061

77. Spencer F, Ronald S, Graner J (1985) The incidence of foot pathology in a diabetic population. J Am Podiatr Assoc 11: 590-592

78. Steed D, Goslen JB, Holloway GA, Malone JM, Bunt TJ, Webster MW (1992) Randomized prospective double-blind tnal in healing chronic diabetic foot ulcers: CT- 102 activated platelet supernatant. topicai versus placebo. Diabetes Care 15: 1598-1604

79. The Diabetes Control And Complications Trial Research Group (1993) The effect of intensive treatment of diabetes on the development and progression of long-term complications in insulindependent diabetes mellitus. N Engl J Med 329: 977-986

80. Tillo TH, Giunni JM, Habershaw GM, Chizan JS, Rowbotham JL (1990) Review of metatarsal osteotomies for the treatment of neuropathic ulcerations. J Am Podiatr Med Assoc 80: 211-217

81. Triomphe A, Flori YA, Costagliola D, Eschwege E (1988) Le coût du diabète en France. Rev Méd Assurance Maladie 3: 7-11

82. Ulbrecht JS, Norbtis A, Cavanagh PR (1994) Plantar pressure and plantar ulceration in the neuropathic diabetic foot. In: Kominsky SJ (ed) The diabetic foot. Vol.1. Mosby-Year Book, Chicago, pp 29-45

83. Ulbrecht JS, Perry JE, Hewitt FG Jr, Cavanagh PR (1994) Controversies in footwear for the diabetic foot at risk. In: Kominsky SJ (ed) The diabetic foot. Vol.1. Mosby-Year Book, Chicago pp 441-453.

84. Veves A, Masson EA, Fernando DJS, Boulton AJM (1989) Use of experimental padded hosiery to reduce abnormal foot pressures in diabetic neuropathy. Diabetes Care 12: 653-635

85. Visser JH, Jacobs AM, Oloff L, Drago JJ (1984) The use of differential scintigraphy in the clinical diagnosis of osseous and soft tissue changes affecting the diabetic foot. J Foot Surg 23: 74-85

86. Ward JD (1982) The Diabetic Leg. Diabetologia. 22: 141-147

87. Wheat Ll, Allen SD, Henry M, et al (1986) Diabetic foot infections: bacteriologic analysis. Arch Intern Med 146: 1935-1940

88. Witkowski JA, Parish LC (1992) Rational approach to wound care. Int J Dermatol 31: 27-28

89. Wyss CR, Matsen FA, Simmons CW, Burgess EM (1984) Transcutaneous oxygen tension measurements on limbs of diabetic and nondiabetic patients with peripheral vascular disease. Surgery 95: 339-346

90. Young MJ, Cavanagh PR, Thomas G. Johnson MM, Murray H, Boulton AJM (1992) The effect of callus removal on dynamic plantar foot pressures in diabetic patients. Diabetic Med 9: 55-57

91. Zaias N (1992) Clinical manifestations of onychomycosis. Clin Exp Dermatol 17 (suppl 1): 6-7

10.

Metabolic arthropathies of the foot

R Westhovens, Th Conrozier and J Dequeker

Different inflammatory and degenerative articular disorders are grouped under the heading of metabolic arthropathies. These arthropathies result from a generalized or a local metabolic abnormality. In this review we shall not discuss the articular problems due to diabetes, which are reviewed in Chapter 9.

Metabolic arthropathies pose an important diagnostic challenge for the clinician. They include not only those diseases that typically affect the foot, such as gout, but also are a great number of disorders which are characterized by extra-articular manifestations, and where the foot involvement is part of but not the hallmark of the metabolic abnormalities.

Gout

Gout is the most frequent crystal arthropathy, and has the most typical clinical presentation of all the inflammatory arthropathies. The first classical description is attributed to Hippocrates and was refined by Sydenham in 1683. Van Leeuwenhoek, in 1679, was the first to detect the typical crystals in a tophus. Gout is the commonest inflammatory arthropathy in men over 40, but is not exclusively limited to the male sex; the male/female ratio has changed from 20:1 to 2.7:1 in recent decades [23, 31].

Even though the plasma concentration of uric acid is the most important determinant of gouty arthritis, the epidemiology of gout must be differentiated from that of hyperuricemia as such [4]. Risk factors for developing hyperuricemia and gout are: male sex, familial predisposition, obesity, alcohol consumption, lead exposure, use of diuretics, high blood pressure and renal dysfunction.

In more than half the cases of gouty arthritis the first attack is located at the first metatarsophalangeal joint. Other joints frequently affected are the ankle (11%) and the midfoot (8%). In 90% of patients, the initial attack remains monarticular, though oligo- and polyarticular presentations may occur in the course of the disease [10, 15, 29]. The characteristic acute crisis may be preceded by local prodromes such as discomfort in the involved joint, or by extra-articular manifestations such as fatigue and insomnia. Excessive food intake or starvation, intake of diuretics and anti-uricemic drugs, and local trauma can initiate the attack. In addition, generalized disease (infection), overwork, and surgery are known to provoke acute attacks. Within a few hours after the onset of the attack the inflammation reaches its peak. This characteristic presentation is one of the diagnostic criteria defined by the American College of Rheumatology (ACR). There is often excruciating pain and the patient cannot bear any pressure on the affected joint. Typically, the swelling is reddish-blue and often extends beyond the joint. The pain is worse at night, quietening down by morning, and lasting up to 4 to 10 days. Within a few days, symptoms will disappear without sequelae, excepting for desquamation of the skin overlying the affected joint. The arthritic episodes may become less severe later in the course of the disease [3, 28].

Not all patients present with typical attacks. More insidious cases may be encountered: chronic arthropathies, pseudo-septic presentations, atypical localizations (tendinitis of the calcaneal tendon, heel pain, etc.). In chronic tophaceous gout degenerative lesions caused by uric acid deposits or tophi may develop, as well as destructive arthritis. The development of chronic gout depends on the level of the plasma uric acid concentration, and is rarely seen in the first years of the disease. After a minimum of 10 years with gout a typical tophus may be formed and presents as a painless nodule with a yellowish-white content. When located in the environment of a joint, tophi may cause serious morbidity. The tophi form typical cavitary erosions, often at some distance from the articular margin, in those joints that are a regular site of acute attacks (fig. 10.1). In addition, tophi may cause skin ulcers or form tendon nodules, which may be prominent in the calcaneal tendon. Inflammatory episodes are less pronounced in patients with chronic gouty arthropathy.

Acute gouty arthritis has to be differentiated from septic arthritis, spondylarthropathies, and other crystal arthropathies such as chondrocalcinosis or hydroxyapatite crystal disease. If the acute attack is located at midfoot level, a stress fracture may be difficult to exclude. Chronic gouty arthropathy is sometimes difficult to differentiate from psoriatic arthropathy, rheumatoid arthritis or neurogenic arthropathy. Associated morbidity factors such as obesity, high blood pressure, diabetes, hyperlipidemia and vascular problems should be sought in gouty patients [12, 16, 18, 30]. An inverse relationship is noted between rheumatoid arthritis and gout [22] as well as lupus [11] and gout.

In most cases, diagnosis can be made on the clinical characteristics, and confirmed by synovial fluid analysis. The synovial fluid has inflammatory features (5,000 to 100,000 leukocytes with up to 90% of polymorphonuclear cells). One must remember that hyperuricemia is not synonymous with gout, and a transient decrease in uricemia may even occur during an acute attack of gouty arthritis. The single diagnostic test is the identification of intracellular needle-shaped urate crystals, with typical birefringence, in the synovial fluid [19]. The sedimentation rate is increased, usually to between 20 and 50 mm/h, but may peak to 100 mm/h at the time of an acute crisis. Plasma concentrations of uric acid should be retested after the acute attack and will usually exceed 70 mg/l.

Early in the disease, X-rays will show only soft tissue swelling at the time of an acute attack [21]. Definite articular involvement with bony erosions is seen only after some years, often preceded by an

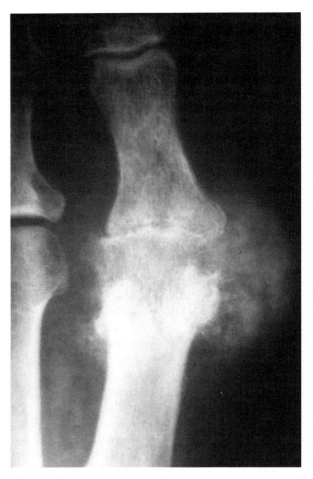

Fig. 10.1. Gouty arthropathy of the 1st metatarsophalangeal joint

increased density of the extra-articular soft tissues, due to periarticular tophi which may calcify or ossify. Bony erosions may occur in or adjacent to the joint, or may even be located at some distance from the joint. They are generally asymmetric and associated with soft tissue swelling. Erosions usually have a cavitary aspect, typically located in the first metatarsal head, with a so-called "punched-out" appearance. Periarticular osteoporosis is rare and joint-space narrowing is a late sign. Secondary degenerative changes with calcification of juxta-articular location or in the bone may be seen. Typical of late chronic gouty arthropathy is secondary degenerative disease of the midfoot, seen in lateral X-rays of the foot.

Treatment of gouty arthritis has not changed for 20 years. The acute attack usually responds to nonsteroidal agents or colchicine, with rest and avoidance of predisposing factors such as intake of diuretic drugs. Prevention is the key measure. Normalization of plasma uric acid can be attained with an appropriate diet and increased alkaline fluid intake, in addition to an inhibitor of uric acid synthesis or a uricosuric drug, but only if the urinary concentrations of uric acid and renal function permit.

Hydroxyapatite crystal arthropathy

Deposits of hydroxyapatite crystals in and around joints can present in different ways: as an acute or more chronic periarthritis, an acute synovitis, but also as an arthrosis or destructive arthropathy in the elderly [7, 8]. Frequently these deposits remain asymptomatic. One seldom sees foot problems in this disease [1, 5], the ankle being affected only occasionally in contrast to the frequent shoulder involvement.

The diagnosis should be considered in an acute painful attack of "pseudo-gout", when the X-rays show periarticular calcification of ligaments and tendons (perimalleolar region, calcaneal tendon, plantar region). Metatarsophalangeal and interphalangeal calcification may be seen at the toes. Sometimes these calcifications disappear after an acute attack of arthritis or tendinitis. The diagnosis is made on the clinical and radiologic findings. Absence of periarticular calcification at the symptomatic joint should lead to an X-ray examination of other joints, particularly the shoulders, hands and hips.

As there is no specific plasma marker, laboratory diagnosis is based on the detection of hydroxyapatite crystals in the synovial fluid. This may be extremely difficult, especially in the small joints of the foot. Moreover, identification of these crystals can only be made by electron microscopy examination [6]. Frequently, hydroxyapatite crystals are composed of a mixture of different phospho-calcium salts, and typically an association with calcium pyrophosphate crystals is found. In most cases, hydroxyapatite crystal arthropathy is idiopathic. The occurrence of hydroxyapatite deposits is well-known in connective tissue disorders such as dermatomyositis and scleroderma. They may also be found in patients with renal insufficiency on chronic haemodialysis, where an increased calcium-phosphorus product is found in the plasma [13].

Chondrocalcinosis (Calcium pyrophosphate deposition disease - CPPD)

This form of crystal arthropathy is associated with intra-articular deposits of calcium pyrophosphate dihydrate crystals. Chrondrocalcinosis can present as acute attacks of painful monosynovitis of short duration, reminiscent of acute gouty attacks, and these attacks are referred to as "pseudogout". Often, CPPD mimics a chronic arthropathy, which differs from classical polyarthrosis by its more severe character and by its occurrence in joints usually spared from arthrosis (e.g., wrists). In exceptional cases, it may present as a chronic polyarthritis mimicking rheumatoid arthritis. Calcium pyrophosphate deposits are often seen in asymptomatic persons [9, 17], especially in the elderly. The female/male ratio is estimated at between 2 and 7/1. An isolated symptomatic foot is rather exceptional. In contrast to gout, involvement of the first toe is extremely rare. Ankle involvement may be destructive. Calcium pyrophosphate deposits can also be seen at the calcaneal tendon and the plantar fascia.

Diagnosis of CPPD is based on the X-ray finding of linear calcifications of cartilage and fibrocartilage. Confirmation may be obtained by synovial fluid analysis, using a polarization microscope on a fresh substrate. If CPPD is present, hyperparathyroidism, hemochromatosis, or hyperthyroidism should be excluded. However, 80% of cases are idiopathic. The treatment of acute attacks is similar to that of acute gout. Because specific prophylactic measures are not possible, treatment of chronic CPPD arthropathy is identical to that of chronic primary arthrosis.

Other crystal arthropathies

Oxalate crystals may be found in the joints of patients with chronic renal failure [20]. In addition, oxalate crystals may complicate renal failure in rheumatoid arthritis with amyloidosis [26]. The knees and hands are especially involved, but the feet or ankles may also be affected. Definite diagnosis is based on crystal identification in the synovial fluid or synovial biopsy.

Hyperlipidemia

Many studies suggest an association between abnormalities of lipid metabolism and painful articular manifestations. However, the exact prevalence of lipid-associated arthropathies is difficult to estimate, because of difficulties in diagnosis and problems of classification in lipid disorders. It is well-known that familial hypercholesterolemia and mixed hyperlipidemia are associated with intratendinous xanthomata, calcaneal tendinitis or transient aching of the calcaneal tendons. Oligoarthritides have been reported to be associated with hyperlipidemia. However, whether intra-articular cholesterol crystals can cause arthritis is debatable. In 60% of cases, rheumatologic symptoms precede the diagnosis of hyperlipidemia. In 63%, the treatment of the lipid disorder improves or even cures the articular symptoms [25].

Hemochromatosis and Wilson's disease

Hemochromatosis is a hereditary disorder that presents with iron deposits in different organ systems. Secondary hemochromatosis is seldom complicated by arthropathy. The severity of the disease is variable. Hepatic iron storage is usually the key presentation, although degenerative arthropathy can cause serious morbidity [24]. The arthropathy is not influenced by venesection [27]. A destructive arthropathy, usually at the ankle, may be the presenting feature. Most of the arthropathies in hemochromatosis are mild. An association with chondrocalcinosis has been reported, presenting as acute attacks of pseudogout.

Wilson's disease is a rare autosomal recessive disorder characterized by copper deposits in the liver and brain. Articular lesions may develop after 10-15 years of the disease [2]. In radiographs of the ankle, the articular surface may be blurred and irregularly sclerosed. In addition, sclerosis of the subchondral bone, para-articular calcifications, or erosions at the epiphysis may be seen. In rare cases chondrocalcinosis may be encountered. The metatarsophalangeal and interphalangeal joints exhibit cavities and para-articular lacunae in association with a local or regional osteoporosis.

Thyroid acropachy

Thyroid acropachy may present some years after the initial diagnosis of hyperthyroidism. Thyroid acropachy consists of exophthalmia associated with painless swelling of the soft tissues, especially in the fingers and toes, clubbing of the digits and pretibial myxedema [14]. Asymmetric periostitis, more pronounced than the periostitis of other arthropathies, may be seen in the X-rays.

Acromegaly

Acromegaly is caused by growth hormone overproduction, most frequently due to a tumor of the hypophysis. The soft tissues thicken, especially at the heel, and this may be an important diagnostic sign. Enlargement of the feet is also typical, but is often less prominent than enlargement of the hands and face.

Hereditary storage disorders

Hereditary storage disorders, such as Gaucher's disease and mucopolysaccharidosis (Hurler, Morquio, Sanfilippo), but also ochronosis, are only occasionally symptomatic in the feet.

References

1. Amor B, Cherot A, Delbarre F (1977) Le rhumatisme à hydroxyapatite (la maladie des calcifications tendineuses multiples). I. Étude clinique. Rev Rhum 44: 301-308

2. Boudin G, Pepin B, Hubault A, Goldstein B, Lidy C (1977) Les arthropathies de la maladie de Wilson. Ann Méd Int Paris 128: 853-856

3. Campbell SM (1988) Gout: how presentation, diagnosis and treatment differ in the elderly. Geriatrics 43: 71-77

4. Campion EW, Glynn RJ, Delabry LO (1987) Asymptomatic hyperuricemia. Am J Med 82: 421-426

5. Cherot A (1976) Le rhumatisme à hydroxyapatite. Thèse Médecine, Paris, p 140

6. Dieppe PA (1979) Crystal deposition and the soft tissues. Clin Rheum Dis 5: 807-822

7. Dieppe PA, Doherty M, Macfarlane DG et al (1984) Apatite associated destructive arthropathy. Br J Rheumatol 23: 84-91

8. Dieppe PA, Huskisson EC, Crocker P, Willoughby DA (1976) Apatite deposition disease: a new arthropathy. Lancet 1: 266-269

9. Doherty M, Dieppe PA (1988) Clinical aspects of calcium pyrophosphate dihydrate crystal deposition. Rheum Dis Clin North Am 14: 395-414

10. Emmerson BT (1983) Hyperuricemia and gout in clinical practice. ADIS Health Science Press, Sydney

11. Greenfield SI, Forg JS, Barth WF (1985) Systemic lupus erythematosus and gout. Semin Arthritis Rheum 14: 176-179

12. Herman JB, Goldbourt Cl (1982) Uric acid and diabetes: observations in a population study. Lancet 2: 240-241

13. Hoffman GS, Schumacher HR, Paul H, et al (1982) Calcium oxalate microcrystalline associated arthritis in end-stage renal failure. Ann Intern Med 97: 36-42

14. Kinsella RA, Black DK (1968) Thyroid acropachy. Med Clin North Am 52: 393

15. Lawry GV, Pan PT, Bluestone R (1988) Polyarticular versus monoarticular gout, a prospective comparative analysis of clinical features. Medicine (Baltimore) 67: 335-343

16. Matsubara R, Matsuzawa J, Jiao S, Takama T, Kubo M, Tarui S (1989) Relationship between hypertriglyceridemia and uric acid production in primary gout. Metabolism 38: 698-701

17. McCarty DJ (1976) Calcium pyrophosphate dihydrate crystal deposition disease 1975. Arthritis Rheum 19 (suppl): 275-286

18. Messerli FH, Frohlich ED, Dreslinski GR, Suarez DH, Aristimuno GG (1980) Serum uric acid in essential hypertension: an indication of renal vascular involvement. Ann Intern Med 93: 817-821

19. Phelps P, Steele AD, McCartey DJ (1968) Compensated polarized light microscopy: Identification of crystals in synovial fluids from gout and pseudogout. JAMA 203: 508-512

20. Reginato AJ, Kurnik BRC (1989) Calcium oxalate and other crystals associated with kidney diseases and arthritis. Semin Arthritis Rheum 18: 198-224

21. Resnick D, Niwayama G (1988) Gouty arthritis. In: Diagnosis of bone and joint disorders, 2nd edn. WB Saunders Company, Philadelphia, pp 1619-1671

22. Rizzoli AJ, Trujeque L, Bankhurst AD (1981) The coexistence of gout and rheumatoid arthritis. J Rheumatol 8: 989-992

23. Roubenoff R (1990) Gout and hyperuricemia. Rheum Dis Clin North Am 16: 539-550

24. Schumacher HR (1964) Hemochromatosis and arthritis. Arthritis Rheum 7: 41-50

25. Schumacher HR, Michael R (1989) Recurrent tendinitis and Achilles tendon nodule with positively birefringent crystals in a patient with hyper-lipoproteinemia. J Rheumatol 16: 1387-1389

26. Schumacher HR, Reginato AJ, Pullman S (1987) Synovial oxalate deposition complicating rheumatoid arthritis with amyloidosis and renal failure. J Rheumatol 14: 361-366

27. Schumacher HR, Straka PC, Krikker MA, Dudley A (1988) The arthropathy of hemochromatosis. Ann NY Acad Sci 526: 224-233

28. Ter Borg EJ, Rasker JJ (1987) Gout in the elderly, a separate entity? Ann Rheum Dis 46: 72-76

29. Wijngaarden JB, Kelley WH (1976) Gout and hyperuricemia. Grune and Stratton, New York

30. Yamashita S, Matsuzawa Y, Tokunaga K, Fujioka S, Tarui S (1986) Studies on the impaired metabolism of uric acid in obese subjects: marked reduction of renal urate excretion and its improvement by a low caloric diet. Int J Obesity 10: 255-264

31. Yu TF (1977) Some unusual features of gouty artritis in females. Semin Arthritis Rheum 6: 247-255

11.

The rheumatoid foot

M Bouysset

General remarks

The incidence of rheumatoid arthritis in the general population is 0.3 to 1.5%. This progressive disease affects 3 times as many women as men and occurs at any age, but especially between 40 and 60 years; initially, it may remain localized to the foot and ankle for a long time. During its progress, the foot is affected in 90% or more of cases [1, 16, 54, 67, 72]. Despite therapeutic progress, rheumatoid arthritis often remains a serious disorder with severe morbidity [3, 62]. Disability related to the foot in rheumatoid arthritis has not been objectively assessed but the frequency of foot surgery enables us to give an estimate: it occurs in approximately 20 to 30% of cases [61, 69]. This high incidence is an argument for optimal management of the foot in rheumatoid arthritis.

Pathomechanics

Biomechanical factors account for the main deformities of the rheumatoid foot; the great variety of factors involved is evidenced by the numerous atypical forms. It is impossible to summarize the pathophysiology of the foot in rheumatoid arthritis in a few lines but the following schema may be suggested.

Inflammatory synovitis predominates and is the initial factor. It leads to weakening of the structures which support the foot: joint capsules, ligaments, tendons and certain muscles. Some authors make a comparison with the hyperlaxity of Ehler-Danlos disease [42, 63].

At a later stage there is osteoarticular destruction with subsequent dislocation (or, in certain cases, ankylosis). In some lesions, the healing process with postinflammatory contracture plays a part in causing deformities [2, 55, 68].

In this weakened setting mechanical stresses, which are common, appear as factors predisposing to deformity. These are anatomic or functional factors of congenital or acquired origin. They are situated not only in the feet (morphotype of the forefoot, more or less marked pronation of the hindfoot), but also at the hips and knees (genu valgum, fixed flexion of the knee) [2, 55, 68].

Other factors promote and aggravate the deformities: the footwear may either stress the foot or fail to support it (wearing of slippers or worn-out shoes). Weight-bearing is particularly harmful during inflammatory crises.

The causes cited increase muscular imbalance: between the flexor and extensor muscles, and between the abductor and adductor muscles. Not only are the intrinsic muscles affected (lumbricals, interossei, extensor digitorum brevis) but also the extrinsic muscles, whose eccentric action gives rise to deformity [1, 55, 68, 76]. Ordinary movements, and particularly intense activity, accentuate the imbalance of forces. Thus, inflammatory rheumatism makes certain deformations appear, or worsens them when previously these deformities had been prevented by healthy supporting structures. The mechanism of deformation, if understood, enables us to better envisage treatment programs.

Hindfoot deformities

Pes planovalgus is the commonest deformity of the rheumatoid hindfoot. Its causes are varied and complex. Even the minimal calcaneal valgus, which is present beforehand and which is usual in the general population, is a predisposing factor in the great majority of cases. The inflammatory disease impairs the structures which stabilize the talo-calcaneo-navicular joint and the valgus deformity appears as a result of lesions of the supporting soft tissues [42, 68, 71, 72]. Other causes exist but are often more difficult to distinguish (see below).
• Several disease sites promote this tendency: the tarsus and especially the medial articular chain of the foot; the talonavicular and subtalar joints, which are more subject to mechanical stress, are the most frequently affected [11, 21, 72]. Tillmann emphasizes the role of tarsometatarsal arthritis which is also frequently observed by Resnick [56, 68]. The increased susceptibility to torque accentuates the tendency to valgus deformity (or sometimes varus, if there was prior varus) [1, 32, 61, 63, 65, 68, 72, 76]. On the whole, the flat-foot is initially flexible, and then becomes rigid. This secondary rigidity of the deformity is due to the consequences of tarsal arthritis [69, 71, 72]. Some authors state that the rigid flat-foot is caused by spasm of the fibular muscles, which may be provoked by any cause of stiffening or ankylosis of the tarsus. The principal muscle concerned is the fibularis brevis [2]. The two deforming processes - weakening of the supporting structures of the foot and spasm of the fibular muscles - can combine to lead to pes planovalgus [71].
• The importance of retromalleolar tenosynovitis in the development of pes planovalgus is generally undervalued [8, 15, 25, 45, 72]. The tendon of the tibialis posterior muscle is of primary importance as it plays a major role in maintaining the dynamic stability of the foot. All lesions of this tendon, simple stretching of inflammatory origin or even rupture, may explain the flattening of the midfoot and the valgus deviation of the hindfoot. Loss of function of the fibular tendons does not have such repercussions on the structure of the foot. The tendons of other muscles can be affected, in particular those of flexor hallucis longus and flexor digitorum longus

muscles [4, 15, 26, 42, 60, 68]. The respective roles of tenosynovitis and arthritis in the appearance of pes planovalgus are debatable [15, 26, 39, 60].

Ankle arthritis appears later [11, 40, 68, 72]. The lateral talocrural narrowing, which is found more frequently, promotes valgus deformation [68, 72] or may itself be caused by preexisting calcaneal valgus.
• Other factors may be involved in the appearance of pes planovalgus: abnormal gait and/or antalgic positions. Arthritis of the first metatarsophalangeal joint prevents the patient from standing on this painful joint and causes supination of the forefoot. If, after the inflammatory crisis, the forefoot resumes its initial position, the compensatory deformation of the hindfoot into pronation, relative to the forefoot, may remain fixed and thus cause planovalgus [68, 72]. This clinical sequence may explain the varus of the forefoot observed by Vavahnen [68, 71] and corresponds to Hohmann's description of "pes postice pronatus, antice supinatus" [68].

Deformities of the other joints of the lower limb also play a part: a varus knee may sometimes give rise to a valgus hindfoot. If there is a calcaneal valgus and then a valgus knee develops, the latter worsens the valgus hindfoot, though it may sometimes bring about a varus hindfoot [68]. Likewise, a large angle of gait while walking stresses the mid-hindfoot and favors the tendency of the hindfoot to pronate. Numerous other factors may be involved in the development of valgus foot [2, 68].

The frequency of **cavus foot** varies according to the authors: 4% for Potter [55], higher for others [16]. Among other causes, sclero-inflammatory contracture of the soft parts may be responsible [2, 16]. It can be in a valgus or varus position. An initial hindfoot varus seems to ensure relative protection from the development of hindfoot deformities.

Stiffness in flexion of the hip or knee may make the pathology of the foot more pronounced and provoke functional imbalance; abnormal gait or an antalgic position can have the same effect. Thus, contracture of the triceps surae muscle following fixed flexion of the hip or knee causes plantarflexion and inversion of the foot with dorsiflexion of the proximal phalanges and plantarflexion of the distal phalanges [2, 23]. Persistence of this position may lead to secondary cavus deformity (modern knee and hip replacements have certainly reduced the frequency of these conditions). Direct inflammatory involvement of the plantar aponeurosis can have the same result [2]. For some authors, cavus foot is due to spasm of the fibularis longus muscle, which causes a valgus cavus foot with heightening of the longitudinal arch, forefoot abduction and calcaneal valgus [2].

Forefoot deformities

Forefoot and hindfoot deformities, whether of mechanical or inflammatory origin are interrelated, with each influencing the other [5, 12, 13, 68, 70].

Hallux valgus and metatarsus varus of the first ray are examples of deformities of both mechanical and inflammatory origin [68]. Hallux valgus is logically correlated with other deformities and articular lesions of the forefoot and mid-hindfoot, but the relation between flattening of the arch and metatarsus varus of the first ray is direct; above all, it does not depend on the duration of the disease [12]. Habitual mechanical causes of hallux valgus are metatarsus varus of the first ray, deviation into pronation of the hallux by the tendon of the abductor hallucis muscle, adduction of the hallux by the long flexor and extensor muscles; but an inflammatory component worsens the consequences of the mechanical stresses. The latter favor the appearance of hallux valgus and are diverse:
• prior static disorders, particularly the common marked valgus of the hindfoot [43, 55];
• inadequate footwear and abnormal weight-bearing, especially during an inflammatory period, increased by obesity, over-exertion, too heavy bed covers and any external constraint on the foot;
• certain torsional or flexion abnormalities of the lower limb in the foot (forefoot varus, equinus hindfoot) or in the hips and knees [2];
• gait abnormalities which may or may not be secondary to the preceding causes;
• other general conditions with a weakening effect (articular laxity) [43].

When there is inflammation, the reciprocal influences between the forefoot and hindfoot are exacerbated. Rheumatoid hallux valgus can cause a hindfoot deformity which will then augment the hallux valgus; the reverse order of events may also occur [4, 12, 22, 42, 68].

Other lesions can arise in the development of rheumatoid hallux valgus [68]. Tarsometatarsal arthritis can play a part in splaying of the forefoot; the tendon of the abductor hallucis muscle, which is inserted between two inflammatory sites (superficial

bursitis and deep articular synovitis), can be damaged and weakened; lateral displacement of the extensor hallucis longus tendon is also involved more in rheumatoid arthritis (as with the other extensors), due to synovitis of the first metatarsophalangeal joint.

Sometimes the first ray is unaffected. There is often a favorable morphotype of the forefoot with an intact metatarsophalangeal joint in patients who wear adequate footwear [1, 76]. This respect of the first ray is often the case in male patients [73], stressing the fact that certain deforming factors are more frequent in women (narrow shoes, postmenopausal flat-foot).

Splaying of the forefoot increases in frequency with the duration of the disease [12]. The periarticular edema and intermetatarsal bursitis displace the metatarsal heads [1, 25]. The extra mobility of the first and fifth metatarsals particularly favors their deviation and therefore their role in spreading of the metatarsal bones [35]. Tarsometatarsal arthritis certainly arises in this process [68], and also stretching of the intermetatarsal ligaments [2]. The influence of these different lesions is combined and determines the appearance of the deformity [63, 68].

Deformities of the toes

• **Deformation of the lesser toes** depends on mechanical factors (fig. 11.1): the flattening of the medial arch and spreading of the forefoot increase the tension of the short flexor tendons, which passively flex the proximal interphalangeal joints. The proximal phalanx is not subject to the action of the flexor muscles and the balancing action of the interosseous and lumbrical muscles is lacking, so that the extensor muscles exert a great force on the proximal phalanges [22, 23, 68].

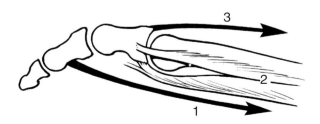

Fig. 11.1. Clawed toes and tendency to subluxation of the proximal phalanges (toes 2, 3, 4). *1* short flexor tendons; *2* interosseus and lumbrical muscles; *3* extensor tendons

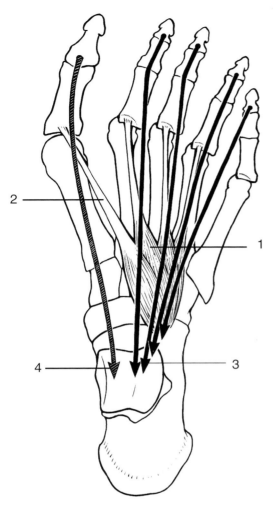

Fig. 11.2. Lateral deviation of toes 2, 3, 4. *1* extensor digitorum brevis muscle; *2* extensor hallucis brevis tendon; *3* extensor digitorum longus tendon; *4* extensor hallucis longus tendon (from K. Tillmann)

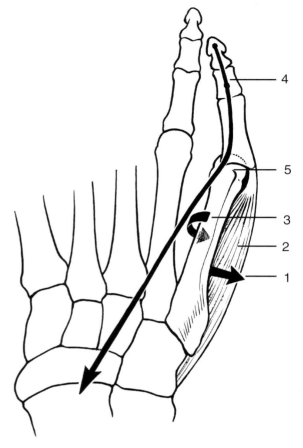

Fig. 11.3. Specifics of the fifth toe. *1* Abduction of the fifth metatarsal; *2* stretched abductor digiti minimi tendon; *3* pronation of fifth metatarsal bone; *4* insertion of the long extensor tendon of fifth toe becomes medial; *5* the fifth metatarsal head displaces outwards because there is a lateral displacement of the tendon of the flexor digitorum longus to the fifth toe (from K. Tillmann)

In rheumatoid arthritis, the tendency to deformity worsens as the muscular involvement particularly affects the interosseous and lumbrical muscles. These muscles are active in 40% of the gait cycle [46] and their reduced efficiency, of inflammatory origin, becomes evident during this cycle. At the end of stance, the metatarsal heads tend to be placed under the proximal phalanges [2, 68, 76]. The other articular support structures (capsules, ligaments) are also weakened and subluxation of the first phalanx is accentuated. The cartilaginous and bony destruction worsens the deformity and healing with secondary fibrosis can make it become fixed [1, 68].

Other causes also play a part in this dorsal subluxation of the proximal phalanx, with flexion of the interphalangeal joint: tenosynovitis of the flexor [2] or extensor muscles [68]; inflammatory lesions of the plantar aponeurosis which is situated between the deep articular pannus and the more superficial plantar bursitis [68]; and inflammation of the tarso-metatarsal joints. At a late stage interdigital displacement of the flexor tendons also plays a part [68].

• **The lateral deviation of the toes** is largely due to the role of the extensor digitorum brevis muscle (fig. 11.2). Flattening of the medial arch and abduction of the forefoot deviate the axis of traction of this muscle outwards and upwards; lateral deviation of the toes occurs in this way. On the other hand, the varus of the first metatarsal increases the tension of the extensor hallucis brevis tendon and favors valgus deformation of the hallux in addition to the other causes of hallux valgus. The metatarsophalangeal joint capsules are weakened early on by the inflammation, facilitating this process, which also affects the long extensor tendons of the toes [1, 68, 76]; it has been suggested that the deviated hallux may displace the lateral toes [1, 38, 76].

• **The fifth toe** is not subject to the action of the extensor digitorum brevis muscle but (like the hallux), is particularly subject to footwear constraints. Other influences exist [68] (fig. 11.3): inflammation of the tarsometatarsal joints accentuates the abduction of the fifth metatarsal, stretching the tendon of the abductor digiti minimi muscle; the fifth toe can then deviate into adduction. Moreover, the flattening of the anterior arch favors pronation of the fifth metatarsal and in consequence the insertion of the long extensor tendon of the fifth toe becomes medial and the pull of this tendon takes a medial direction. Finally, lateral displacement of the tendon of the flexor digitorum longus to the fifth toe displaces the fifth metatarsal head outwards, just as the first is displaced inwards.

• **The congenital morphotype of the forefoot** influences the deformities. Viladot distinguishes two types of rheumatoid forefoot [76]:

- **the triangular forefoot**, caused by combined hallux valgus and varus of the fifth toe. This deformity, which Morton called the atonic foot, is characterized by the weakened intrinsic musculature of the first and fifth rays and shortness of the first metatarsal, with consequent spreading of the metatarsal bones. This results in a predominance of the extrinsic musculature: the long flexor and extensor tendons of the first and fifth rays deviate outwards the first and the fifth metatarsals and the corresponding toes inwards, resulting in the typical triangular forefoot deformity;

- **the forefoot with lateral deviation of the toes** is characterized by a long first metatarsal and a predominating intrinsic musculature. The reflex contracture of the tendons of the abductor hallucis and flexor hallucis brevis muscles due to inflammatory involvement deviates this hallux into valgus. This favors the lateral deviation of the median toes. The extensor digitorum brevis, as we have seen, accentuates this deviation except at the fifth toe, which is unaffected by the deviation [76].

These deformities often occur with a long hallux, which, as it is subject to more mechanical strain, becomes deformed more easily. A short hallux is less sensitive to the pressure of the shoe and becomes deformed less frequently [76]. Needless to say, these rules do not apply uniformly. Other factors influence the deformities as we have already seen and account for the numerous atypical forms where they are not correlated with any particular metatarsal or digital morphotype.

Clinical features

At the onset

In the great majority of cases, the first signs are an inflammatory and symmetric involvement of the metatarsophalangeal joints [16, 25, 40] which is often also present at the metacarpophalangeal joints. These two localisations dominate the pathology of rheumatoid arthritis at the onset, even if their relative frequency varies [25, 32, 49, 67]. Radioclinical involvement of the forefoot may be the inaugural manifestation of rheumatoid arthritis in 10 to 25 % of cases [1, 16, 21, 54, 56, 61, 64]. The initial symptoms are sometimes asymmetric [49, 64].

Clinically, the lateral metatarsophalangeal joints are those most affected in the initial stage [25]. Braun particularly emphasizes the prime localisation at the fifth metatarsal head; this is a lesion which must be searched for clinically as it is not always painful spontaneously [16]. First metatarsophalangeal joint involvement appears less frequently. Nevertheless, some patients who have generalized rheumatoid arthritis, and who have undergone a recent operation for hallux valgus, suggest that the pain was caused by the arthritis and not of mechanical origin [25].

The examination shows swelling of the metatarsophalangeal region with edema on the dorsal side of the forefoot and global widening of the forefoot. This inflammatory involvement may be detected early on by pain on lateral compression of the metatarsal bones, which is not painful in a normal foot [25]. Selective pressure between the thumb and index on each metatarsophalangeal joint highlights those most affected and the radiologic detection of early bony erosion may confirm the examination [16, 25]. At its maximum, when the forefoot is enlarged by the periarticular edema, the toes are separated ("daylight sign") [25].

Radiography at this early stage of the disease is often characteristic enough to permit the detection of other signs which are not specific at this time [16, 49]. Regional demineralisation is frequent at the inflamed joints and is initially juxta-articular [16, 32, 49]. Edema of the soft tissues with articular synovitis, effusion and periarticular edema can be detected at the metatarsophalangeal joints [49]. A slight enlargement of the metatarsophalangeal space is rarely observed [49]. Radiographic evidence of cysts is common at this stage [16] but metatarsal bony erosion predominates in the initial radiographic findings. In the forefoot, it precedes joint narrowing [17, 64].

Being the first sign whose observation is uniformly interpreted on the radiograph, erosion is sometimes the prime feature of inflammatory rheumatism [16]. The earliest signs of erosion correspond to the bony areas at the sides of the joint, which are not covered by articular cartilage. These erosions are normally detected on the medial side of the metatarsal heads, apart from the fifth, where the initial erosion is normally found on the lateral side [32, 49]. Generally speaking, erosion of the interphalangeal joints seems to occur later, apart from the interphalangeal joint of the hallux which is affected more often and earlier. Though bony erosion often precedes the clinical onset of the disease or occurs soon afterwards [16, 17, 49, 67], it sometimes appears only after six months or more [49]. Nevertheless, the importance of early radiographic signs in rheumatoid arthritis makes Thould and Simon conclude that, in a patient observed over a year who has no radiographic signs in the feet or hands, we must have doubts about the diagnosis [67]. The joint narrowing is always uniform and is difficult to assess in standard views of the metatarsophalangeal joints.

Other manifestations at the initial phase of foot involvement are possible: involvement of a single metatarsophalangeal joint [77]; tarsitis [25, 29, 58] or retromalleolar tenosynovitis [7, 25]; pain, swelling or widening of the intermetatarsal spaces; the second and third are the most cited but sometimes the fourth. The initial diagnosis is often Morton's metatarsalgia [6, 50, 53] but sometimes the symptoms are those of an ordinary bursitis without neurologic compression [24, 50, 59].

The symptoms of inflammatory rheumatism advance at different joints. If it were not the case before, the lesions become bilateral and symmetric and then in the majority of cases the clinical course, generally progressing with acute inflammatory episodes, is the same with some small variants; the edema of the soft parts, synovitis and articular effusion appear more clearly; the phase of advanced destruction and deformation develops progressively.

The established state

Generally speaking, the clinical manifestations predominate clearly over either the forefoot or hindfoot but rarely at both sites at the same time, except for cases of severe and very progressive diseases [4, 25]. The physical examination specifies the possible reversible character of any deformity.

At the **forefoot**, there is typically deformation with a triangular-shaped forefoot and lateral deviation of the toes 1, 2, 3, 4 [76]. Hallux valgus, the most frequent deformity of the rheumatoid forefoot, appears or is accentuated if it existed before [63, 72] (fig. 11.4). The first metatarsal bone presents a major varus deformation. The incidence of hallux valgus increases with the duration of the disease [12, 63, 72]. In men, the deformity occurs especially in cases of advanced inflammatory lesions of the first metatarsophalangeal joint [73]. The bony hypertrophy which is characteristic of non-rheumatoid hallux valgus is uncommon [41].

The spreading of the forefoot occurs at the same time as the deviation of the first ray and is accompanied by a plantar depression of the metatarsal heads. It also affects the fifth ray and may even start there [72].

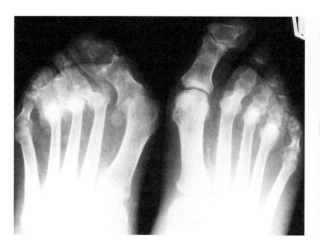

Fig. 11.4. Rheumatoid forefoot: hallux valgus deformation, lateral deviation of toes, and medial deviation of fifth toe

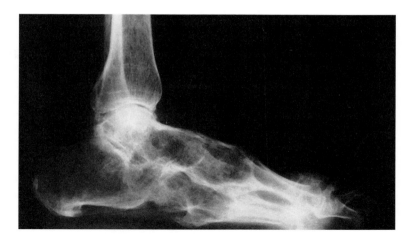

Fig. 11.5. Global spontaneous ankylosis of the tarsus

Clawed toes and subluxation of the metatarsophalangeal joints complete this clinical picture. Deformation of the metatarsophalangeal joints - 2, 3, 4 and 5 - increases in frequency with disease duration [63] and after ten years almost all patients seem to be affected [72]. All types of toe deformities can be variously associated (clawed toes, hammer-toes, swan-neck). The deformity, which is initially flexible, rapidly becomes fixed [72]. The metatarsophalangeal joints become partially subluxed and the toes lose their role in walking, which accounts for the formation of corns, callosities and sometimes bursitis. Malalignment of the metatarsophalangeal joints is typical at a later stage, with lateral deviation of toes 1, 2, 3 and 4 and quintus varus, thus defining the triangular forefoot deformity [1, 16, 68, 76]. Classically, the deviation of the toes decreases from the first toe to the fourth.

Apart from this clinical form of triangular forefoot - the commonest - there are numerous variants of rheumatoid forefoot deformities [16, 76]. First, there is the forefoot with outward deviation of all the toes; this deviation decreases from the hallux to the fifth toe, which may remain centered. Next come numerous atypical forms which include: rare monarticular forms [76, 77] affecting a single metatarsophalangeal joint (in the great majority of cases at the onset of the disease); forms where the hallux remains centered with outward deviation of the other toes; anarchic deformities which defy description [16]; tibial deviation of the toes is more characteristic of rheumatoid arthritis according to Dixon [25].

The hallux may present other lesions such as hallux rigidus: its frequency is variable. Usually there is absent or reduced dorsiflexion of the first metatarsophalangeal joint secondary to fibrous (or, much more rarely, bony) ankylosis [41, 63, 68, 72]. Other deformities of the hallux seem even rarer (hallux flexus, hallux malleus) [41].

Mid-hindfoot involvement is quite frequent [11, 29, 55, 71, 74] and almost always associated with metatarsophalangeal involvement [56, 74]. The lesions, which are less characteristic than those of the forefoot, appear more asymmetrically [64, 66, 71, 72]. In the majority of cases, midtarsal pain is described by the patient as ankle pain. When there is subtalar involvement, walking on uneven ground is painful.

A weight-bearing and non-weight-bearing examination considers the lower limb in its entirety and observes walking. It studies the passive movements of each joint. Active movements against resistance are useful to determine the integrity of the tendons. With this clinical assessment it is possible to detect symptoms early, which allows, the timely institution of medical treatment more adapted to mid-hindfoot involvement. When there is midtarsal involvement, the dorsum of the midtarsus is warm to palpation, and pronation and supination are painful; localized redness is rarer.

Subtalar involvement often presents with swelling behind the medial and lateral malleoli; at the latter site there is a palpable swelling which must also be searched for at the lateral orifice of the sinus tarsi or at the calcano-cuboid joint. Midtarsal and subtalar movements are studied, with particular attention to the presence of subtalar laxity and calcaneal valgus [52]; the deformities of the hindfoot must be assessed in weight-bearing and this clinical assessment will indicate whether a tarsal ankylosis appears to be in an acceptable position from the functional viewpoint (fig. 11.5).

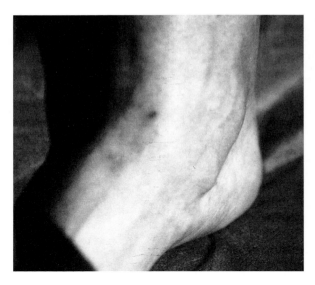

Fig. 11.6. Tenosynovitis of the tibialis posterior tendon

The ankle itself is often spared until a late stage of the disease [11, 25, 40, 72]. The examination may identify an increase in local warmth or anterior joint swelling. However, the detection of an effusion or a proliferative synovitis generally proves difficult due to inflammatory involvement of the neighboring soft parts. Finally, a decrease in talocrural movements may be noted; dorsiflexion is limited in a quarter of the cases [63].

In addition to articular involvement, **tendinous lesions** must be systematically studied and any swelling in the course of the tendons noted. The tibialis posterior tendon which maintains the medial longitudinal arch, has a particular importance. Previous degenerative chronic tenosynovitis and very often also a rheumatoid tenosynovitis weaken the tendon. Repeated corticosteroid infiltrations also have a harmful role. The examination searches for local edema or a swelling under the medial malleolus (fig. 11.6) [15, 16], but also evaluates the loss or decrease of active inversion against resistance; the tibialis posterior tendon is not palpated during this test if it is completely ruptured [26, 60]. The function of this tendon may also be assessed by examining the heel from the rear in order to check if hindfoot inversion is satisfactory when the patient is on tiptoe. These difficulties in clinical examination may make us underestimate lesions of the tendon, whose rupture generally goes unrecognized in its early stage [15, 26]. Other tenosynovial structures in

the foot may be affected by inflammatory involvement [4, 8, 16, 42, 68, 72]. Their functional repercussions are less evident than those of the tibialis posterior tendon and here again, clinical examination appears difficult in the case of rheumatoid arthritis, chiefly during inflammatory crises. In fibular tenosynovitis, there is a typical swelling of the tendinous tract on the lateral side of the heel, localized tenderness and possible weakening or loss of foot abduction. The possibility of rupture of the calcaneal tendon is reported but it may be uncertain whether this is of mechanical or inflammatory origin or both.

If there is a diffuse swelling of the midfoot, hindfoot and ankle, it becomes difficult to make a distinction between different articular and extra-articular rheumatoid pathologies; moreover, one of these lesions is often predominant [42, 49]. Thus, when there is posteromedial pain, a medial retromalleolar tendinopathy can be surmised, and when there is lateral pain a posterolateral tendinopathy or an impingement syndrome may be suggested, and the possibility of a stress fracture should be remembered. The pains normally have mechanical associations and paresthesiae or dysesthesiae of non-mechanical nature must prompt search for a tarsal tunnel syndrome or a peripheral neuropathy. Again, any weakening of the lower limbs must make us consider extra-articular etiologies such as a cervical myelopathy [42].

Frequently, **the disease evolves towards a pes plano-valgus** which is initially flexible. Sometimes the articular laxity worsens, but normally pronation and supination lessen and the flat-foot becomes rigid; consequently the maximum frequency of flexible flat-foot is in the initial period of foot involvement, this then decreases as a rigid flat-foot increases with prolonged disease. However, some mobile flat-feet which arise during inflammatory crises can be cured by suitable treatment, which leads to a normally shaped, stable foot [72].

Radiography

Radiography defines the osteo-articular destruction clearly and shows the malalignment of the axes (fig. 11.4). In rheumatoid arthritis foot involvement is, exceptionally, monarticular [49] and the radiographic signs generally increase in frequency with disease duration [11, 67, 72].

Standard radiographic views must include lateral and frontal views of the foot and ankle with and without weight-bearing. Other may prove useful: 3/4 obliques, axial sesamoid views [25, 31] or others [42].

Erosive features

• In the forefoot, the most affected metatarsal head is the fifth [13, 16, 67] and the first is the least affected from a radiographic viewpoint [13, 67]. When the disease is chronic, the number of involved metatarsal heads increases (approximately 80% of cases after 10 years of disease duration) and the severity of the lesions become more pronounced. Likewise, advanced radiographic changes go hand-in-hand with more symmetric lesions and a more frequent positive latex test [67]. Radiographic signs of rheumatoid arthritis may be observed even when there is no history of clinical symptoms, (15% of cases for Thould and Simon) [16, 67], but if there has not been any foot pain the number of affected metatarsal heads is minimal [67].

The initial image of erosion increases; progressive destruction of the metatarsal head occurs and often tends to prevail at plantar level under the metatarsal head [32]. In rare cases, complete absorption of one or more metatarsal heads occurs [13, 16, 25, 49]. Both sesamoids, embedded in the articular capsule, may be affected by these lesions [32, 49, 57, 68, 72]; tangential radiography of the forefoot specifies their state, but also spike-erosions of the metatarsal heads, thinning of the fibrofatty cushion, and inversion of the transverse arch [25, 31]. Lastly, as the destructions worsen, generalized and progressive demineralisation of the foot occurs.

Radiography of the forefoot helps to identify the patients who have erosive arthropathy and whose prognosis is poor: in this context, X-rays of the feet and hands every six months during the first two years of the disease can be useful in identifying the patients who risk having severe articular lesions [17]. The tests for HLA DR1 and HLA DR4 also help to identify erosive disease.

• In the hindfoot and midfoot (and ankle), radiographic signs are often delayed [11, 66] and are more asymmetric than those in the forefoot. Swelling of the soft parts due to joint effusion, synovial pannus and periarticular edema is common [42]. Articular space narrowing, sometimes with osteosclerosis, is almost always present; it is the first lesion which can be uniformly interpreted at this level and it is irreversible

[49]. Unlike the forefoot, erosions are not frequent in the midfoot [63, 64] or are of small size [56].

The torque joints, posterior subtalar and talocalcaneo-navicular, are affected earlier and more frequently [11, 71, 72, 74]. Joint involvement increases in frequency with disease duration to reach or exceed 50% of cases after 10 years [11, 58, 71, 72]. All the tarsal joints may be involved with different degrees of severity, exhibiting joint-narrowing with variable bone destruction, sometimes very marked. In rare cases talonavicular subluxation is observed.

Talocrural arthritis occurs later, rarely without tarsal involvement, and may represent 14% of cases after ten years of the disease [11, 16, 21, 25, 56, 64, 68, 72]. The joint narrowing rather concerns the lateral side of the joint. The observation of a tibial cyst is not rare. Complete destruction of the joint or bony ankylosis is possible.

Radiography also shows clearly the malalignment of the axes.

Deformations

The forefoot deformations evolve together (fig. 11.4). On the other hand, hallux valgus, splayed forefoot and marked calcaneal valgus increase in frequency with disease duration. Metatarsus varus of the first ray only is correlated with midfoot lesions, tarsitis and flattening of the medial arch, and is independent of disease duration [12]. This last finding confirms the interrelation between mid-hindfoot and forefoot involvement [5, 40, 68, 70, 71, 72]. The incidence of flat-foot is higher in feet affected by tarsitis and generally, there is a relation between tarsal arthritis, disease duration and flat-foot [11]. Sometimes a true articular dislocation will appear. In other cases bony ankylosis is observed in the tarsus, exceptionally it is global (fig. 11.5). Osteophytosis is noted in certain cases, either prior to inflammatory rheumatism or secondary in late cases of arthritis [17].

Inflammatory involvement can also affect the accessory bones; the structures of the foot are weakened, especially if the os tibiale is concerned, whose involvement is often followed by a pes planovalgus [72]. The trigonal and fibular accessory bones can also be affected [72].

Additional imaging techniques

The X-ray assessment may be supplemented, when necessary, depending on the results of the clinical assessment, by CT, MRI with gadolinium injection, or arthrography with CT [15, 26, 60]. CT displays the bone and joint involvement better. MRI with gadolinium injection detects soft part lesions better chiefly of the tendons (tenosynovitis, rupture) [15] and the degree of synovial proliferation. However, it must be kept in mind that the information supplied by additional imaging, whatever its quality, must not be interpreted without comparison with the clinical findings.

Other rheumatoid features

• **Plantar rheumatoid heel pain** seems to be rare (2-3% of cases) and perhaps no commoner than in the general population; posterior talalgia is less frequent [14, 19, 72]. These heel pains appear more often on clinical examination [30, 74] and are often mechanical in origin [14, 16, 19, 30]. In the rheumatoid foot, as in the general population, there is no relation between talalgia and the presence of a plantar or posterior spur [15], or between talalgia and tarsitis [14, 30].

• **Calcaneal spurs** seem to be more common in rheumatoid arthritis than in the general population [7, 14]. Age and perhaps disease duration play a part in their incidence; the inflammatory involvement certainly causes a modification in a preexisting spur or leads to its development [14, 19]. Typically, an inflammatory exostosis is large and rounded-off; rarely, a periosteal reaction gives it a fluffy appearance [19, 30]. The common mechanical exostosis is often small, well defined and generally sharp-pointed [19]. There are numerous intermediate aspects between these typical forms [14] and these radiographic observations are not characteristic of the rheumatoid process as they are also found in spondylarthropathies [14, 56]. The mechanical tension of the plantar aponeurosis, secondary to midfoot flattening, certainly explains the frequency of the plantar spur in flat-foot [75], but local inflammation also plays a part [14, 19, 72].

Retrocalcaneal bursitis is not painful or only slightly [14, 19, 72] and a local swelling is rarely noted. Bony posterosuperior erosion of the calcaneus appears in 5 to 8% of cases in lateral radiographs [14, 16, 30, 73, 74]. Its evolution is as follows: inflammatory bursitis is the first stage; then the underlying bone has a dimineralized and sometimes cavitary aspect; finally, an erosion appears just above the insertion of the calcaneal tendon. The cortical bone on the upper and posterior part of the calcaneus often remains intact and rarely appears to be burnt out by the rheumatoid process [16, 19]. A subchondral sclerosis may emphasize the bony erosion [16, 19]. Hypertrophic modifications are rarely observed among elderly patients; they give the posterosuperior part of the calcaneus an irregular appearance and can be caused by rubbing of the counter of the shoe against the posterosuperior region of the calcaneus [16, 72]. In the majority of cases, this posterosuperior bursitis heals spontaneously [19, 30]. On radiography, when the thickening of the soft tissues decreases, remineralisation may occur, sometimes giving a surface of roughened appearance [19]. The bony erosion often persists as a witness of burnt-out inflammation [19, 72]. Histologic changes are no different from those noted in the joints in rheumatoid arthritis. This also applies to plantar calcaneitis, which is much rarer (1 to 2% of cases) and which exceptionally erodes the bone to a depth of 1 cm [14, 16, 19, 72]. Rheumatoid calcaneitis increases in frequency with disease duration [14] and almost always appears associated with tarsal arthritis or metatarsophalangeal involvement [56]; it is therefore evidence of an advanced stage of the disease [73].

• The **tarsal tunnel syndrome** can arise at any stage of the disease and in some cases is inaugural [20]. It is very rare in ordinary practice in rheumatoid arthritis [25, 74] but some systematic electromyographic studies show a higher proportion of cases, though often subclinical [33, 44]. Paresthesiae of the toes, often nocturnal, are sometimes accompanied by pain [8, 20, 42]. The electromyogram confirms the diagnosis. Treatment using local infiltration is sometimes effective [20, 44] but when it fails surgery will be indicated. This irritation of the posterior tibial nerve must of course be differentiated from the peripheral neuropathies observed in some advanced and chronic cases of rheumatoid arthritis [25, 44, 74].

• **Nodules and bursitis** between the metatarsal heads are sometimes noted, with certain symptoms reminiscent of Morton's metatarsalgia [6, 24, 47, 50, 53, 72]. The local anatomic configuration explains the symptoms [9, 10]. Pain caused by the nodule or by the bursitis, and widening of the intermetatarsal space and interdigital spaces are sometimes the only features, particularly at the second space [2, 4, 47, 59].

• **Subcutaneous nodules** can appear at the calcaneal tendon [16, 25] or at points of hyperpressure. Due to footwear or to weight-bearing [27, 54]. Their specific treatment must be avoided unless there are local complications (erosions, infection, pain due to hyperpressure) [27].

• **Circulatory abnormalities** may be observed: usually banal disorders of the venous circulation which can lead to ulcers [25, 42, 54, 74]. Foot and ankle edema is frequent, often due to the almost permanent seated position of the patients [25]. Raynaud's syndrome and some signs of vasculitis may be noted, especially in severe cases [25, 42, 54, 74].

• As the disease progresses **atrophy of the soft parts** develops. The thickness of the plantar subcutaneous tissues lessens and cutaneous abnormalities are customary; the skin becomes thin and fragile. The plantar skin, which is subject to hyperpressure, hypertrophies into painful callosities with corns. These can also arise at the toes. Plantar bursitis, which is sometimes very painful, is frequent.

• During the course of the disease **the gait becomes characteristic** with shuffling movements. There is no longer an impact of the heel in walking; the foot is placed flat on the ground with the knee and hip maintained in slight flexion. Elevation of the forefoot is absent and the foot slides forwards. The two stages of swing and stance are short as the gait cycle is shortened. Antalgic abnormalities of gait become common and the patient avoids standing on the painful parts of the foot [25, 48, 54, 76].

• **Stress fractures** seem to be rare [25, 40, 68] and are generally masked by the usual symptoms of rheumatoid arthritis. They must be suspected when there is severe and unexplained pain of sudden onset. Localisation at the lateral malleolus is typical [40, 68]. Hyperpressure due to calcaneal valgus produces painful fibulo-calcaneal contact (impingement syndrome) which may become complicated by a stress fracture of the fibula. In fact, any of the standard sites of such fractures may be affected in these often osteoporotic patients. Deformities of the knee, ankle and subtalar joint are probably predisposing factors [79].

Course

The disease progresses with crises of variable length and intensity. Any articular and tenosynovial structure may be affected. Generally speaking, the fore-foot involvement worsens, then midfoot and hindfoot lesions occur gradually and often insidiously. The symptoms progress and worsen as disease duration increases [11, 12, 25, 63, 72]. At a late stage, the metatarsophalangeal synovitis is less severe but more diffuse [63]; the deformities become fixed by tendinous and muscular contracture. This highlights the importance of early supervision.

Treatment

This aims to preserve the functional capacity of the patient and influence deforming factors. It is a real program which includes different therapeutic means. The contribution made by plantar orthoses and suitable footwear is assessed and the surgical possibilities considered. Everything must be understood by the patients as well as those who carry out the care. We must therefore emphasize the importance of teamwork.

Nonoperative treatment, apart from general drugs

• The nonoperative treatment, apart from general drugs, first uses all **different means of articular protection**; the temporary non-weight-bearing position during an inflammatory crisis remains an indispensable measure and should be recommended untiringly [21, 55]. The lessening of overloading helps to relieve the weakened joints [63]. Devices which immobilize or protect the foot are certainly not used enough; they prevent or delay articular deformation. A support at the bottom of the bed avoids bed-cover pressure and prevents equinus or hallux valgus. Appliances made of thermomodeled material immobilize the joints in a functional position; they are applied in the evening on going to bed and intermittently during the day. For example, a cast maintains the ankle at right angles or corrects a reducible hindfoot valgus. The hallux remains centered by a wedge between the first and second toes [4, 21, 42].

• Concerning **ergotherapy**, the patient needs to be properly trained in order to respect a certain hygiene of life, adapted to each case [4]. By carrying out a complete physical assessment of the patient's daily and professional life, the possible economy of weight-bearing can be evaluated. In the first place, the articular constraints encountered in everyday life must be reduced, e.g., the frequent use of the sitting position in household and professional activities. Standing strains must be reduced by using aids when carrying heavy objects (tea trolleys) and by using appropriate walking aids (sticks). Functional capacity can be greatly improved by the efficient use of such aids [4]. Occupational therapy is used in some centers; it completes the rehabilitation and respects the same cautionary rules [21].

• **Corticosteroid injections** can reduce synovitis when there is no response to medical treatment. They produce rapid improvement and help in the implementation of other treatment. The main sites concerned are the metatarsophalangeal joints, the intermetatarsal bursae and the ankle [21, 63]. Others which are affected more rarely are the midtarsal and posterior subtalar joints or even extra-articular sites such as the tarsal tunnel, tenosynovial sheaths (tibialis posterior, fibularis, flexor hallucis longus), the pre-achillean bursa, a plantar spur or a painful nodule under the heel [21, 25, 63]. Aspiration followed by infiltration is indicated in plantar bursitis [63]. This local corticotherapy must always be carried out very cautiously as the injections promote articular and tendinous deterioration; it carries some of the risks of systemic corticotherapy.

• The **intra-articular injection of radioactive agents** supplements local corticotherapy. The talocrural joint reacts very well to such treatment. The results are even better if the osteo-articular lesion is less advanced. For the metatarsophalangeal joints, erbium-169 seems to be less useful than in the hands. Other sites are rarely so treated [21].

• **Plantar orthoses** can be preventive, corrective or palliative. They should be used early, as soon as there is inflammatory involvement of the foot to provide efficient correction [32, 42, 68]. Their preventive use is justified when there are previous static disorders [55]. Unfortunately, the quality of their therapeutic effect is supported by few objective studies [18, 51] and their prescription only comes with experience. Orthotic treatment can be beneficial after surgery of the forefoot when there is marked calcaneal valgus [65].

• **The footwear for the rheumatoid foot** must be attractive, light and easy to lace; it must also be comfortable, causing no pressure or excessive rubbing [4, 21]. As rheumatoid arthritis is a progressive disease, the shoe must be continually adapted in order to fit the foot which is deformed. In particular, walking conditions are sometimes bettered by small improvements in the heel or sole of the shoe [4]. Numerous forefoot deformities are ascribed to shoe pressure [21, 25]. However, a shoe which is too flexible does not support the foot and gives rise to flattening: slippers which are frequently used indoors, are harmful [21, 72]. The good quality shoe must have a wide forefoot with a thick rigid sole, sometimes rounded off at its anterior and posterior parts to facilitate walking. The sole of the shoe is firm and the heel, not very high (1 to 2 cm). The leather is soft but the calcaneus must be supported by a firm and comfortable counter. When there are talocrural and subtalar lesions, it is better to support these joints [21, 25, 42, 72].

These conditions are sometimes difficult to reconcile and made-to-measure shoes are sometimes an acceptable solution. Depending on their construction and the choice of materials, they can more easily correct a deforming tendency or they can be adapted to fixed deformities [21]. In certain cases, they are molded and give a very satisfactory result if a correct clinical follow-up is carried out [25].

• **Toe orthoses** are small devices which are molded onto one or several toes. They can correct a reversible deformity and slow down its course or even relieve a zone of hyperpressure. Their palliative role proves very useful when there is non-operable fixed clawing. They fill in the gap between the ground and the plantar side of the toes and in this way relieve the metatarsal heads [4, 21, 78].

• **Chiropodal care** makes a valuable contribution and alleviates lesions due to pressure and hyperkeratoses by the excision of corns and nail care. It sometimes abolishes the pain in a forefoot, even a very deformed one [4, 21, 25]. Local hygiene is supplementary in patients who have difficulty in maintaining the hygiene of their feet. The fragile skin cover needs attention by trying to avoid maceration, and by the wearing of cotton socks. Adhesive epidermal protectors relieve the hyperpressure zones [21, 78].

• **Massage, rehabilitation and physical treatment** are contraindicated when there is an acute inflammatory crisis or irreversible deformity. Rehabilitation must be carried out with caution and be related to the stage of the disease. The patient must also be trained to mobilize his joints. Passive mobilisation, if not painful, maintains the remaining range. Manual stretching combats contractures of muscles and ligaments [21].

Therapeutic indications

Invalidity caused by the lower limbs has decreased due to prostheses and foot pathology is comparatively more striking. Often, unfortunately, in the treatment of the rheumatoid foot, the indications remain purely symptomatic: steroid infiltrations or radioactive injections for pain; suitable plantar orthoses for flattening; made-to-measure shoes when there is severe destruction. Finally, if arthritis does not respond to conservative treatment, we resort to arthrodesis. However, therapeutic indications vary widely among different schools of thought; within two similar establishments which treat inflammatory rheumatism, the rate of foot surgery is 20% at Bad Bramstedt in Germany and more than 33% at Heinola in Finland [69].

Some general notions must be stressed as regards treatment:

• In this progressive disease the immediate treatment must not compromise future function. Here are a few examples:

- a plantar orthosis with an empty spot in the middle of the forefoot relieves the inflammatory forefoot but favors deformation into a rigid flattened forefoot which will present its own complications later;

- intra-articular corticosteroid injections permit a spectacular improvement but one wonders, especially if they are repeated, whether they further weaken an already weak joint and accelerate subluxation of the lateral toes;

- one must be cautious about operations limited to the tendons; the fragile development of the supporting structures in this disease is well-known. If one tendon is involved, the others will generally be involved too [15];

- finally, it is risky to do a subtalar arthrodesis to stabilizes the hindfoot and subsequently to modify the axis of the limb by an operation on the knee.

• One must try to control the deforming tendencies in order to keep the foot in acceptable functional condition: malalignment of the axes must be compensated in a vertical plane between the axis of the leg and hindfoot, but also in a horizontal plane between the hindfoot and forefoot (particularly at the first ray) [4, 12, 70].

• Ankle involvement generally occurs later, but its structure and function must be preserved as much as possible. This joint helps the correct progress of the patient's gait and must preserve a good range of movement, especially in dorsiflexion. Ankylosis of the ankle harms the mid-tarsal and subtalar joints. The difficulties increase when the first metatarsophalangeal joint is rigid.

General indications

The patient's contribution and a proper medical follow-up make it easier to implement treatment measures.

The initial treatment remains medical. It is adapted to each case and acts upon the deforming factors: by general and if necessary local anti-inflammatory treatment (steroid or radioactive injections), and by using to the greatest possible extent other local measures which present few secondary risks. In the first place, adequate footwear and appropriate plantar orthoses maintain the foot in a good position. Likewise, relatively non-weight-bearing positions, cast immobilisation and the observation of a suitable hygiene of life are recommended from the onset of inflammatory involvement of the foot. Finally, plantar or toe orthoses, chiropodal care and discerning rehabilitation prove useful aids. All these methods, when properly used, bring relief which enables the practitioner to avoid the use of more aggressive care. They are all the more efficient if they are used early. In this way, improvement in the function of the foot is possible as well as a saving of time, which is useful if surgical operations are scheduled for joints other than those of the foot.

These different types of care can have a preventive aim, particularly when there are static disorders. Plantar orthoses and suitable footwear are sometimes used before inflammatory involvement of the foot has developed, depending on the course of the disease: a support behind the metatarsal heads if there is a flattened forefoot, a support of the midfoot in certain circumstances (marked calcaneus valgus, minimal flat-foot, metatarsus varus of the first ray, or even if there is an increase in the angle of gait which favors hyperpronation and therefore stresses the mid-hindfoot).

Consequently, a systematic clinical examination searches for any involvement which is potentially destructive, especially tarsitis or tenosynovitis of the tendon of the tibialis posterior muscle. In this way, treatment can be prescribed early and in the light of the foreseeable evolution of the disease; when deformities have already appeared, care is essentially palliative in nature.

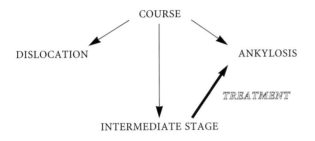

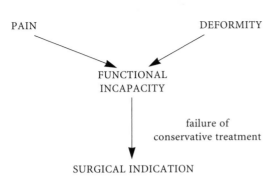

Fig. 11.7. Some feet will dislocate whatever happens, others will develop fibrous or bony ankylosis in good position. The difficulty in treatment is to act for the best in feet at an intermediate stage of the disease

Fig. 11.8. The surgical indications include pain, deformity and functional incapacity and therefore depend on the efficiency of the conservative treatment

This treatment aims to prevent dislocation of the tarsus or its ankylosis in a bad position. To obtain such a result, the causes of the deformity must be controlled as much as possible. Nevertheless, certain feet will dislocate whatever happens, whereas other feet will present fibrous or bony ankylosis. Finally, the best possible solution seems to be the obtaining of a tarsal ankylosis in an acceptable position from a functional point of view [68]; all means which permit this to happen are thus beneficial. In this perspective, the ankle itself must of course retain sufficient mobility. The difficulty in treatment is to act in this way for the feet whose disease state is intermediate (fig. 11.7); the forefoot may be rendered fit for walking by wearing appropriate footwear or by a surgical operation, depending on the stage of the disease.

Surgery is indicated for pain, deformity and functional incapacity and therefore depends on the efficiency of the maintenance treatment [34, 68] (fig. 11.8). It must also take into account the deforming potential of certain situations. In patients whose disease is not very destructive, and who present localized involvement, simple early surgical treatment is sometimes indicated to maintain correct functional conditions of the foot: talonavicular arthrodesis [5, 28] or synovectomy of the tendon of the posterior tibialis muscle. On the contrary, if the arthritis is very destructive, surgery will be more radical at an earlier stage to prevent the dislocation of the tarsus.

Conclusion

The very common involvement of the foot and ankle in rheumatoid arthritis is well-known; generally speaking, forefoot involvement appears earlier and is more obvious, while the tarsal lesion is later, often more insidious and clinically often mistaken for ankle involvement. Repeated corticosteroid infiltrations for tarsitis are not uncommon, but the talocrural joint must spared as much as possible.

When medical treatment fails, forefoot involvement, which is more often and earlier disabling, leads to surgical treatment, generally including arthrodesis of the first metatarsophalangeal joint. Then (or sometimes simultaneously) arthrodesis of the subtalar and midtarsal joints is performed in some cases.

Advanced talocrural disease can lead to the performance of an ankle arthrodesis or to the insertion of a prosthesis.

All these considerations underline the importance of a global overview of the progressive nature of the disease. Consequently, the treatment of foot involvement must be carried out in the context of treatment of the rheumatoid arthritis as a whole.

References

1. Allieu Y, Claustre J, Simon L (1977) Étude anatomo-clinique et genèse des déformations du pied dans la polyarthrite rhumatoïde. In: Le pied inflammatoire. Maloine, Paris, pp 15-33
2. Amico (D') JC (1976) The pathomechanics of adult rheumatoid arthritis affecting the foot. J Am Podiatr Assoc 66: 227-236

3. Amor B, Herson D, Cherot A, Delbarre F (1981) Polyarthrites rhumatoïdes évoluant depuis plus de dix ans (1966-1978). Ann Med Interne (Paris) 132: 168-173

4. Anderson EG (1990) The rheumatoid foot: a sideways look. Ann Rheum Dis 4: 851-857

5. Ascensio G, Bertin R, Megy B, Leonardi C, Combes B (1991) Intrication de l'arrière-pied dans la chirurgie de l'avant-pied rhumatoïde. Médecine et Chirurgie du Pied 7: 185-191

6. Awerbuch MS, Shephard E, Vernon-Roberts B, Morton's metatarsalgia due to intermetatarso-phalangeal bursitis as an early manifestation of rheumatoid arthritis. Clin Orthop 167: 214-221

7. Bassiouni M (1965) Incidence of calcaneal spurs in osteoarthrosis and rheumatoid arthritis and in control patients. Ann Rheum Dis 24: 490-493

8. Blotman F, Claustre J, Allieu Y, Simon L (1977) Ténosynovites et syndromes canalaires du pied rhumatoïde. In: Le pied inflammatoire. Maloine, Paris, p 35

9. Bonnel F, Farenc C, Claustre J, Julian JM, Peruchon E (1989) Étude biométrique et radiographique du pied. Médecine et Chirurgie du Pied 5: 105-111

10. Bossley CJ, Cairney PC (1980) The intermetatarsophalangeal bursa: its significance in Morton's metatarsalgia. J Bone Joint Surg 62B: 184

11. Bouysset M, Bonvoisin B, Lejeune E, Bouvier M (1987) Flattening of the Rheumatoid Foot in Tarsal Arthritis on X-ray. Scand J Rheumatol 16: 127-133

12. Bouysset M, Tebib J, Noel E, Nemoz C, Larbre JP, Bouvier M (1991) Rheumatoid Metatarsus. The Original Evolution of the First Metatarsal. Clin Rheumatol 10: 408-412

13. Bouysset M, Tebib J, Noel E, Nemoz C, Vianney JC, Bouvier M (1991) Le métatarse rhumatoïde: lésions des têtes métatarsiennes, angles M1-P1, M1-M2 et M1-M5. Médecine et Chirurgie du Pied 7: 159-164

14. Bouysset M, Tebib J, Weil E, Noel E, Colson F, Llorca G, Lejeune E, Bouvier M (1989) The rheumatoid heel: its relationship to other disorders in the rheumatoid foot. Clin Rheumatol 8: 208-214

15. Bouysset M, Tavernier T, Tebib J, Noel E, Tillmann K, Bonnin M, Eulry F, Bouvier M (1995) CT and MRI evaluation or tenosynovitis of the rheumatoid hindfoot. Clin Rheumatol 14: 303-307

16. Braun S (1975) Le pied dans les grands rhumatismes inflammatoires chroniques. Rhumatologie 27: 47-56

17. Brook A, Corbett M (1977) Radiographic changes in early rheumatoid disease. Ann Rheum Dis 36: 71-73

18. Budiman-Mak K, Conrad K, Roach J, Moore X, Lertratanakul A, Koch J, Skossy C, Froolich N, Joyce-Clark (1993) Can foot orthoses prevent deformity in rheumatoid arthritis? American College of Rheumatoloy, San Antonio nov. 7-11

19. Bywaters EGL (1953) Heel lesions of rheumatoid arthritis. Ann Rheum Dis 13: 42-50

20. Chatter EH (1970) Tarsal tunnel syndrome in rheumatoid arthritis (letter to the editor). Br Med J (Clin Res) 3: 406

21. Claustre J (1979) Le pied rhumatoïde. Problèmes podologiques pratiques. Rev Rhum 46: 673-678

22. Clayton ML (1960) Surgery of the forefoot in rheumatoid arthritis. Clin Orthop 16:136

23. Clayton ML (1967) Surgical treatment of the rheumatoid foot. In: Giannestras NJ (ed) Foot and disorders. Medical and Surgical Management. Lea and Febiger, Philadelphia

24. Dedrick Dk, Mc Cune J, Smith WS (1990) Rheumatoid arthritis presenting as spreading of the toes. J Bone Joint Surg 72A: 463

25. Dixon A St J (1971) The rheumatoid foot. Mod Trands Rheumatol 2: 158-173

26. Downey DJ, Simkin PA, Mack LA, Richardson ML, Kilcoyne RF, Hansen ST (1988) Tibialis posterior tendon rupture: a cause of rheumatoid flat foot. Arthritis Rheum 31: 441-446

27. Duncan GS (1990) Recurrent rheumatoid nodule of the foot. J Am Podiatr Med Assoc 80, number 10: 552-555

28. Elbaor JE, Thomas WH, Weinfeld MS et al (1976) Talonavicular arthrodesis for rheumatoid arthritis of the hindfoot. Orthop Clin North Am 7: 821

29. Enjalbert M, Claustre J, Herisson C, Simon L (1989) Synovites du médio-tarse révélatrices d'un rhumatisme inflammatoire chronique. In: Claustre J, Simon L (ed). Le médio-pied. Masson, Paris, pp 191-197

30. Gerster JC, Vicher TL, Bennami A, Fallet GH (1977) The painful heel. Ann Rheum Dis 36: 343-348

31. Gheith and Dixon (1973) Tangential X-ray of the forefoot in rheumatoid arthritis. Ann Rheum Dis 32: 92-93

32. Gold RH Basset LW (1982) Radiologic evaluation of the arthritis foot. Foot Ankle 2: 232

33. Grabois M, Puentes J, Lidsky M (1981) Tarsal tunnel syndrome in rheumatoid arthritis. Arch Phys Med Rehabil 62: 401

34. Gracchiolo A III, Kitaoka HB, Pearson S (1988) Treatment of the painful, arthritic hindfoot [abstract]. Orthop Transactions 12: 765

35. Haines RW, Mac Dougall A (1954) The anatomy of hallux valgus. J Bone Joint Surg 36-B: 272

36. Huber-Levernieux C (1993) La rupture du tendon du jambier postérieur. Synoviale 20: 10-17

37. Jakubowski (1959) Early synovectomy in rheumatoid arthritis. Excerpta Medica Foundation: 149-161

38. Jörgensen G (1953) Uber die laterale abduktion der zehen. Zbl Chir 78: 849

39. Kirkham BW, Gibson T (1988) Letter: comment on the article by Downey et al. Arthritis Rheum 31:3

40. Kirkup JR (1974) Ankle and tarsal joints in rheumatoid arthritis. Scand J Rheumatol 3: 50-52

41. Kirkup JR, Vidigal E, Jacob RK (1977) The hallux and rheumatoid arthritis. Acta Orthop Scand 48: 527-544

42. Kitaoka HB (1989) Rheumatoid hindfoot. Orthop Clin North Am 20: 593-604

43. Mac Carthy DJ (1983) Surgical anatomy of the first ray. J Am Podiatr Assoc 73: 244-255

44. Mac Guigan L, Burke D, Fleming A (1983) Tarsal tunnel syndrome and peripheral neuropathy in rheumatoid disease. Ann Rheum Dis 42: 128

45. Mac Master PE (1933) Tendon and muscle ruptures: clinical and experimental studies of the causes and location of subcutaneous ruptures. J Bone Joint Surg 15: 705-722

46. Mann R, Inman VT (1964) Phasic activity of intrinsic muscles of the foot. J Bone Joint Surg 46A: 469

47. Manzi JA, Goldman F (1983) Rheumatoid nodule, an unusual variant. J Am. Podiatr Assoc 73: 205-208

48. Marshall RN, Myers DB, Palmer D (1980) Disturbance of gait due to rheumatoid disease. J Rheumatol 7: 617-623

49. Martel W (1970) Acute and Chronic Arthritis of the foot. Semin Roentgenol 5: 391-406

50. Meachim G, Abberton MJ (1971) Histological findings in Morton's metatarsalgia. J Pathol 103: 209

51. Mereday C, BS, Dolan C, MS, Lusskin MD (1972) Evaluation of the University of California biomechanics laboratory shoe insert in "flexible" pes planus. Clin Orthop 82: 45-58

52. Milgrom C, Giladi M, Simkin A, et al (1985) The normal range of subtalar inversion and eversion in young males as measured by three different techniques. Foot Ankle 6: 143

53. Miller HG, Abadesco L, Heaney J (1983) Morton's neuroma symptoms from a rheumatoid nodule. J Am Podiatr Assoc 73: 311-312

54. Minaker K, Little H (1973) Painful feet in rheumatoid arthritis. CMA Journal 109: 724-730

55. Potter TA, Khus JG (1972) Painful feet. In: Hollander JL (ed) Arthritis and Allied Conditions. Lea and Febiger, Philadelphia

56. Resnick D (1976) Roentgen features of the rheumatoid mid and hindfoot. J Can Assoc Radiol 27: 99-107

57. Resnick D, Niwayama G, Feingold ML (1977) The sesamoid bones of the hands and feet: participators in arthritis. Radiology 123: 57-62

58. Seror P, Claustre J, Kha TD (1983) Les tarsites rhumatoïdes. In: Claustre J, Simon L (eds) Le pied en pratique rhumatologique. Masson, Paris, p 40

59. Serre H, Simon L, Claustre J (1972) Le syndrome douloureux aigu du deuxième espace inter-métatarsien. Rev Rhum 39: 495-503

60. Simkin PA, Downey DJ, Richardson ML (1989) Letter: More on the posterior tibial tendon in rheumatoid arthritis. Arthritis Rheum 32: 8

61. Simon L, Claustre J, Allieu Y (1980) Le pied rhumatoïde. Genèse des déformations. Rev Rhum 47: 117-122

62. Spector TD, Scott Dl (1988) What happens to patients with rheumatoid arthritis? The long-term outcome of treatment. Clin Rheumatol 3: 315-330

63. Spiegel TM, Spiegel JS (1982) Rheumatoid arthritis in the foot and ankle. Diagnosis, pathology and treatment. Foot Ankle 2: 318-324

64. Stiles RG, Resnick D, Sartoris DJ (1988) Radiologic manifestations of arthritides involving the foot. Clin Podiatr Med Surg 5: 1-16

65. Stockley I, Betts Rp, Rowley Di, Getty CJM, Duckworth T (1990) The importance of the valgus hindfoot in forefoot surgery in rheumatoid arthritis. J Bone Joint Surg 72B: 705-708

66. Tenoudji-Cohen M, Perez R, Dessauw Ph, Sany J (1983) Apport de l'exploration radiographique du pied dans les rhumatismes inflammatoires. In: Claustre, Simon (eds) Le pied en pratique rhumatologique. Masson, Paris, p 102

67. Thould AK, Simon G (1966) Assessment of radiological changes in hands and feet in rheumatoid arthritis. Ann Rheum Dis 25: 220

68. Tillmann K (1979) The rheumatoid foot. G Thieme, Stuttgart, pp 44-56

69. Tillmann K (1985) Reconstructive foot surgery. Ann Chir Gynaecol 74: 90-95

70. Tillmann K (1987) The mutual interplay between forefoot and hindfoot affections and deformities in RA. Rheumatoid arthritis surgery of the complex foot. Rheumatology 11: 97-99

71. Vahvanen VAJ (1967) Rheumatoid arthritis in the pantalar joints. Acta Orthop Scand Suppl 107: 1-152

72. Vainio K (1956) The rheumatoid foot. A clinical study wih pathological and roentgenological comments. In: Kallio, Vara (eds) Ann Chir Gynaecol 45 (suppl 1): 1-107

73. Vannimenus PY, Vannimenus-Hayem C, Thevenon A (1987) Étude radiographique du pied rhumatoide et comparaison avec l'atteinte de la main. Médecine et Chirurgie du Pied 3: 197-202

74. Vidigal E, Jacoby RK, Dixon J, Ratliff Ah, Kirkup J (1975) The foot in chronic rheumatoid arthritis. Ann Rheum Dis 34: 292-295

75. Viladot A (1985) Anatomie, physiologie et physiopathologie du système suro-achilléo-calcanéo-plantaire. Médecine et Chirurgie du pied 4: 69-74

76. Viladot A, Viladot R (1983) Biomécanique de l'avant-pied rhumatoïde. In: Claustre J, Simon L (eds). Le pied en pratique rhumatologique. Masson, Paris, p 28

77. Voutey H, Strauss J, Magnet JL (1980) Résultats dans la chirurgie de l'avant-pied rhumatoïde. Rev Rhum 47: 123-125

78. Whitney, Kalan K (1990) Padding and taping therapy. In: Levy LA (ed) Principles and practice of podiatric medicine. Churchill Livingstone, NewYork, pp 709-746

79. Young A, Kinsella P, Boland P (1981) Stress fractures of the lower limb in patients with rheumatoid arthritis. J Bone Joint Surg 63B: 239

Additionnal references

Clayton ML, Leidholt JD, Clark W (1997) Arthroplasty of rheumatoid metatarsophalangeal joints. An outcome study. Clin Orthop 340: 48-57

Cracchiolo A (1997) Rheumatoid arthritis; hindfoot disease. Clin Orthop 340: 58-68

Grifka JK (1997) Shoes and insoles for patients with rheumatoid foot disease. Clin Orthop 340: 18-25

Hamalainen M, Raunio P (1997) Long term follow-up of rheumatoid forefoot surgery. Clin Orthop 340: 34-38

Hoffmann P (1997) An operation for severe grades of contracted or clawed toes. Clin Orthop 340: 4-6

Jahss MH (1992) Foot and ankle pain resulting from rheumatic conditions. Curr Opin Rheumatol 4: 233-240

Jan C, Delagoutte JP, Loeuille D, Blum A, Regent D, Gaucher A (1995) Polyarthrite rhumatoïde et kyste synovial: une localisation inhabituelle. Médecine et Chirurgie du Pied 11: 45-48

Kindsfater K, Wilson MG, Thomas WH (1997) Management of the rheumatoid hindfoot with special reference to talonavicular arthrodesis. Clin Orthop 340: 69-74

Klenerman L (1995) The foot and ankle in rheumatoid arthritis. Br J Rheumatol 34: 443-448

Lapeyre-Gros F (1996) Le chaussage du pied rhumatoïde. Med Chir Pied 12: 196-201

Lauzon C, Carette S, Mathon G (1987) Multiple tendon rupture at unusual sites in rheumatoid arthritis. J Rheumatol 14: 369-371

Loet (Le) X, Vittecoq O, Daragon A (1995) En pratique, peut-on prédire le devenir d'un sujet atteint d'une polyarthrite rhumatoïde, au début? Synoviale 37: 3-5

Mann RA, Schakel ME (1995) Surgical correction of rheumatoid forefoot deformities. Foot Ankle Int 16: 1-6

Masi AT (1983) Articular patterns in the early course of rheumatoid arthritis. Am J Med 75: 16-26

Masterson E, Mulcahy D, McElwain, J, McInerney D (1995) The planovalgus rheumatoid foot - is tibialis posterior tendon rupture a factor? Br J Rheumatol 34: 645-646

Michelson J, Easley M, Wigley FM, Hellmann D (1994) Foot and ankle problems in rheumatoid arthritis. Foot Ankle Int 15: 608-613

Michelson J, Easley M, Wigley FM, Hellmann D (1995) Posterior tibial tendon dysfunction in rheumatoid arthritis. Foot Ankle Int 16: 156-161

Miehlbe W, Gschwend N, Rippstein P, Simmen BR (1997) Compression arthrodesis of the rheumatoid ankle and hindfoot. Clin Orthop 340: 75-86

O'Brien TS, Hart TS, Gould JS (1997) Extraosseous manifestations of rheumatoid arthritis in the foot and ankle. Clin Orthop 340: 26-33

Pisani G (1993) Trattato Di Chirurgia Del Piede (patologia ortopedica) II Edizione, Edizioni Minerva Medica, Torino

Resnick RN, Jahss MH, Choueka J, Kummer F, Hersch JC, Okereke E (1995) Deltoid ligament forces after tibialis posterior tendon ruptures: effect of triple arthrodesis and calcaneal displacement osteotomies. Foot Ankle Int 16: 14-20

Scott DL, Coultom BL, Symmons DPM, Popert Aj (1987) Long-term outcome of treating rheumatoid arthritis: results after 20 years. Lancet 1: 1108-11

Sharp JT, Wilder RR, Hunder Rl (1988) The American Rheumatism Association 1989. Criteria for the classification of rheumatoid arthritis. Arthritis Rheum 31: 315-324

Smyth CJ, Janson RW (1997) Rheumatologic view of the rheumatoid foot. Clin Orthop 340: 7-17

Swanson AB, De Groot Swanson G (1997) Use of grommets for flexible hinge implant arthroplasty of the great toe. Clin Orthop 340: 87-94

Tillmann K (1997) Surgery of the rheumatoid forefoot with special reference to the plantar approach. Clin Orthop 340: 39-47

12.

Surgery of the rheumatoid foot: indications

K Tillmann

General considerations

There is no indication for any surgery as long as conservative treatment has a reasonable chance. Therefore I want to give strong support to the preceding article.

The quality established by our orthopedic shoemakers may be one reason for the low percentage of hindfoot surgery compared to forefoot surgery in our rheumatoid patients. Above all, corrective operative procedures and arthrodeses in the region of the hindfoot can be avoided by a timely institution of protection of shape by very firm and optimally fitting insoles or custom-made shoes. The insoles may be firm but must be comfortable and have to fit snugly (fig. 12.1). One can say that a suitable shoe for a rheumatoid foot has to be hard at the bottom and soft on the top. The use of any soft plantar orthosis - unfortunately still very frequent - is a common and very serious mistake; more harm is done than good. Chosen for a temporary relief of pain, in actual fact it furthers the progress of rheumatoid deformation [35, 39].

When the local and general possibilities of physical and medical treatment are exhausted unsuccessfully, surgery can be considered. In the foot, cosmetic aspects are minor considerations compared to pain and functional disability. We should also beware of treating the X-rays rather than the patients.

Regarding preventive surgery, the patient needs our advice. The indications (and also the differential indications) for reconstructive surgery depend on the demands of the patient.

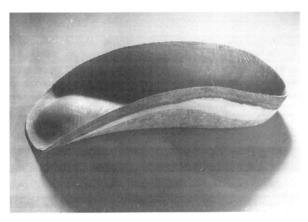

Fig. 12.1. Cork-leather insole, reinforced by laminated thermoplastic acrylate; supporting exactly the transversal and the longitudinal arches, and disloading painfully destroyed metatarsal heads effectively

Technically speaking, there are very few limitations nowadays for an experienced surgeon in the treatment of rheumatoid disabilities. However, if surgery needs to be done, it should be discussed thoroughly, including where should it be carried out and which procedure should be chosen? In this discussion, we should always have in mind the principle of adequacy. Usually the foot is not the only site that needs treatment; in addition to the diseased foot there is also a diseased patient.

Preventive surgery

When the conservative treatment fails, and the joints and tendons are threatened by destruction and

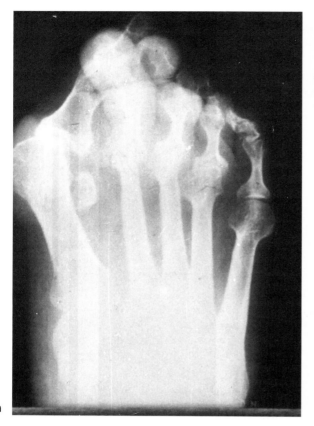
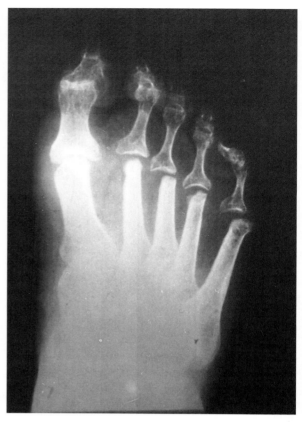

a

Fig. 12.2. Fifty-six year old rheumatoid woman before (**a**) and 3 1/2 years after (**b**) forefoot correction by metatarso-phalangeal arthroplasty

disabling deformities, synovectomy is the treatment of choice. Its benefits are proven by retrospective studies and experience. All earlier attempts to disprove its value [2, 3, 30] have been methodologically unsound and therefore invalid [29, 36, 37, 38].

We practice arthrosynovectomies successfully at the ankle joint [35] and in the tarsal joints, usually in combination with other procedures in this region, but only exceptionally in single metatarsal joints. The latter gave us less satisfactory results than reported in the literature [1, 6].

Tenosynovectomies as an isolated procedure are rarely performed and there are, as far as we know, no reports on results. We have performed very few, mainly in juvenile patients, in particular for the tibialis posterior and also anterior tendons in order to avoid ruptures, which can be followed by sudden loss of the longitudinal arch. Ankle joint synovectomy is nearly always routinely accompanied by tenosynovectomies of the retromalleolar tendons, peroneal and tibial [35].

Reconstructive procedures

Tendon repair

These we have only rarely performed, except for a more or less crude cobbling together of ruptured digital flexor tendons. Mere reconstruction of a spontaneously ruptured tibialis posterior tendon only achieves a temporary lifting of the longitudinal arch; it must be combined with stabilization of lax tarsal joints [5]. Spontaneous rupture of the achilles tendon, occasionally seen in lupus erythematosus disseminatus and "lupoid" cases of rheumatoid arthritis, needs immediate repair, if possible with augmentation by a sound graft (plantaris tendon).

Osteotomy

Distal metatarsal osteotomies without any fixation have been recommended for correction of toe deformities and relief of forefoot pain [17]. The advantage of this undemanding procedure has to be balanced by its less predictable results in comparison with more extensive surgery. We use these operations mainly for burnt-out cases at the 2nd to 4th metatarsals in order to correct toe deformities with a convex transverse plantar arch.

Arthrodesis

Arthrodesis, combined with the correction of deformities, is still the method of choice and it can be ranked as the "gold standard" in cases of severe destruction and deformity of the ankle joint [41]. It is also frequently used for stabilization of severely affected single tarsal joints. Form-correcting triple arthrodesis in case of varus or valgus hindfoot deformity can protect the ankle joint [23, 42, 44] against asymmetric destruction and improve the chances for later endoprosthetic replacement, if necessary.

Arthrodesis is also recommended for excessive deformities of the first MTP joint [4, 43]. The post-operative treatment by plaster immobilization can be demanding for the patient. We feel that this procedure, combined with arthroplasty of the lesser toes, is especially suitable to keep them in good position and to prevent revalgisation.

Corrective procedures for the interphalangeal joints [18] may aim predominantly at ankylosis: bony at the IP joint of the big toe and at least fibrous in the lesser toes [35].

Arthroplasty

The majority of corrective operations on the MTP joints are basically resection procedures. The more demanding they are, the more they approximate to a true arthroplasty. The resection may be performed at the bases of the proximal phalanges [26, 32], or at the metatarsal heads [9, 14, 19, 20, 21, 28, 35]. Due to the main localization of the destruction we prefer resection or reshaping of the metatarsal heads (fig. 12.2) in combination with soft tissue correction. Painful callosities may be excised using a plantar approach

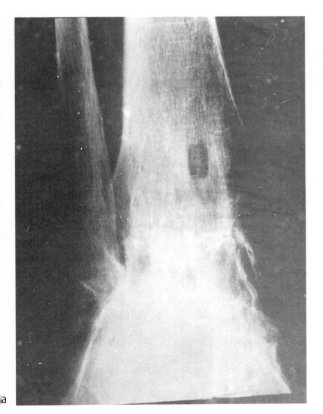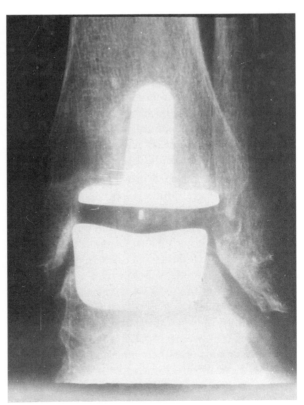

a   b

Fig. 12.3. Sixty-seven years old rheumatoid female patient after ankle surgery: satisfied by an arthrodesis on the right side (**a**), but happy with her uncemented endoprosthesis on the left side (**b**)

(as we do) [35], or they may disappear spontaneously due to the relief from pressure after bone resection.

These surgical corrections of toe and forefoot deformities are generally the most frequently used surgical procedures in the rheumatoid foot: in our hospital about three times more frequent than hindfoot operations. This reflects the disabling effect of forefoot involvement in rheumatoid arthritis.

Endoprosthetic replacement

Alloarthroplasties in the foot still are still controversial. Considering the unfavorable biomechanic effects of ankle joint arthrodesis [13], especially on the gait, it becomes more and more questionable if it is still justified to rank this procedure as the "gold standard" (fig. 12.3). Cemented ankle joint replacements of the St Georg prototype [7] are subjected to a relatively high rate of loosening [25, 27, 31]: about 12% of reoperations in our patients 8 years after implantation on average. The fall-back to an arthrodesis using voluminous bone grafts is problematic.

Newly conceived meniscal endoprotheses, which can be optionally used without cement, seem to be less subject to loosening and promise moreover a lower wear rate of the interposed polyethylene bearings [8, 24]. Our short-term experience seems encouraging [40], but of course the final judgment will need many years of clinical monitoring in order to settle the definitive indications.

The value of endoprosthetic replacement of the metatarsophalangeal joints is even more controversial. Experience worth mentioning exists for the first MTP joint [10, 11, 12, 15, 23, 24]. The failure rate differs considerably from author to author, so that it is very difficult to detect a common pattern. The clinical results are at least better over a considerable follow-up period than the mechanical resistance of the silicone implants mostly used. However, in view of the remarkably good results of nonprosthetic procedures [16], we personally see no real need for artificial implants with their inherent risks. We need and use them in selected cases for salvage procedures after unsuccessful, because inappropriate and inadequate, previous surgery. The origin of these cases is predominantly lack of surgical experience in the special field of arthritis surgery.

Final remarks

We feel that arthritic surgery, and especially its indications in the foot, needs much special training and close cooperation with equally experienced and motivated rheumatologists. The treatment of arthritic patients has to be by permanent teamwork, and surgery in this field can by no means be excluded from this general rule.

References

1. Aho H, Halonen P (1991) Synovectomy of MTP joints in Rheumatoid Arthritis. Acta Orthop Scand 62, suppl. 243: 1
2. Arthritis Foundation Committee on Evaluation of Synovectomy in Rheumatoid Arthritis (1977) Arthritis Rheum 20: 711-765
3. Arthritis and Rheumatism Council and British Orthopaedic Assocation (1976) Controlled trial of synovectomy of the knee and the metacarpophalangeal joints in rheumatoid arthritis. Ann Rheum Dis 35: 437-442
4. Beauchamp CG, Kirby T, Rudge RS, Worthington BS (1984) Fusion of the first metatarsophalangeal joint in forefoot arthroplasty. Clin Orthop 190: 249-253
5. Bouysset M, Tavernier T, Tebib J, Noël E, Tillmann K, Bonnin M, Eulry F, Bouvier M (1995) CT and MRI evaluation of tenosynovitis of the rheumatoid hindfoot. Clin Rheumatol 14: 303-307
6. Brattström H (1973) Synovectomien in den Metatarsophalangeal Gelenken. Orthopäde 2: 81
7. Buchholz HW, Engelbrecht E, Siegel A (1973) Totale Sprunggelenksendoprothese, Modell "St Georg". Chirurgie 44: 241-244
8. Buechel FF, Pappas MJ, Iorio LJ (1988) New Jersey low contact stress total ankle replacement: biomechanical rationale and review of 23 cementless cases. Foot Ankle 8: 279-290
9. Clayton ML (1960) Surgery of the forefoot in rheumatoid arthritis. Clin Orthop 16: 136-140
10. Cracchiolo A III, Weltmer BJ Jr, Lian G, Delseth T, Dorey F (1992) Arthroplasty of the first metatarsophalangeal joint with a double stem silicone implant. J Bone Joint Surg 74-A: 552-563
11. Delagoutte JA (1980) Les endoprothèses dans la chirurgie du pied rhumatoïde. Rev Rhum 47: 135-137
12. Denis A, Debeyre J (1974) L'arthroplastie du gros orteil avec l'implant phalangien en silicone (implant de Swanson). Rev Rhum 41: 251-256
13. Dühr A (1994) Elektronische Messungen von Fussohlendrucken im Abrollverhalten vor und nach Versteifungsoperationen am rheumatischen Rückfuss. Dissertation, Universität Hamburg.
14. Fowler AW (1959) A method of forefoot reconstruction. J Bone Joint Surg 41B: 507-513

15. Granberry WM, Noble PC, Bishop JO, Tuloss HS (1991) Use of a hinge silicon prosthesis for replacement-arthroplasty of the first metatarsalphalangeal joint. J Bone Joint Surg 73A: 1453-1459

16. Hansens Ch, Horstmeyer M, Tillmann K (1987) Mittel und lang fristige Ergebnisse bei kompletter Vorfusskorrektur nach Tillmann bei Patienten mit chronischer Polyarthritis. Acta Rheumatol 12: 222-225

17. Helal B (1975) Metatarsal Osteotomy for Metatarsalgia. J Bone Joint Surg 57B: 187-192

18. Hohmann G (1951) Fuss und Bein: ihre Erkrankungen und deren Behandlung. 5th edn. Bergmann, München

19. Hoffmann P (1911) An operation for severe grades of contracted or clawed toes. Am J Orthop Surg 9: 411-449

20. Hueter C (1881) Klinik der Gelenkkrankheiten, Vol 1. Vogel, Leipzig, p 338

21. Kates A, Kessel L, Kay A (1967) Arthroplasty of the forefoot. J Bone Joint Surg 49B: 552-557

22. Keller Wl (1904) The surgical treatment of bunion and hallux valgus. NY Med J 80: 741-742

23. Kirkup J (1974) Ankle and tarsal joints in Rheumatoid Arthritis. Scand J Rheum 3: 50-52

24. Kofoed H (1990) S.T.A.R. - Prothesis - personnal communication

25. Lachiewicz PF, Hill C, Inglis AE, Ranawat CS (1984) Total ankle replacement in Rheumatoid Arthritis. J Bone Joint Surg 66A: 340-343

26. Lipscomb PR, Benson GM, Sones DA (1972) Resection of proximal phalanges and metatarsal condyles of the forefoot due to rheumatoid arthritis. Clin Orthop 82: 24-31

27. Lord G, Marotte JH (1973) Prothèse totale de cheville. Rev Chir Orthop 59: 139-151

28. Mayo Ch (1908) The surgical treatment of bunions. Ann Surg 48: 300-302

29. Mc Ewen C (1988) Multicenter evaluation of synovectomy in the treatment of rheumatoid arthritis. Reports of results at the end of five years. Rheumatology 15: 765-769

30. Meijers KAE, Valkenburg A, Cats A (1983) A synovectomy trial and the history of early knee synovectomy in rheumatoid arthritis. Rheumatol Int 3: 161-166

31. Sinn W, Tillmann K (1986) Mittelfristige Ergebnisse der TPR Sprunggelenksendoprothese. Akt Rheumatol 11: 231-236

32. Stainsby GD (1992) A modified keller's procedure for the lateral four toes. Unpublished - personnal communication

33. Swanson AB (1972) Implant arthroplasty for the great toe. Clin Orthop 85: 75-81

34. Swanson AB, Lumsden RM, De Groot Swanson G (1979) Silicone implant arthroplasty of the great toe. Review of single stem and flexible hinge implants. Clin Orthop 85: 75-81

35. Tillmann K (1977) The rheumatoid foot. Diagnosis, pathomechanics and treatment. Thieme, Stuttgart

36. Tillmann K (1990) Recent advances in the surgical treatment of rheumatoid arthritis. Clin Orthop 258: 62-72

37. Tillmann K (1990) Value of synovectomy. Revisional surgery in rheumatoid arthritis. Rheumatology 13: 1-13

38. Tillmann K (1991) Die Synovektomie in der Behandlung entzündlich-rheumatischer Krankheiten: historisch oder aktuell? Z Orthop 129: 129-135

39. Tillmann K, Hansens Ch, Hofmann H (1989) Orthopädieschuhtechnische Versorgung rheumatischer Füsse. Med Orth Tech 109:142-146

40. Tillmann K, Straub ML (1993) Early experience with uncemented ankle joint replacements in rheumatoid arthritis [Abstract]. J Bone Joint Surg 75B: 293

41. Uuspää V, Raunio P (1987) Ankle arthrodesis. Rheumatology 11: 104-113

42. Vahvanen V (1967) Rheumatoid arthritis in the pantalar joints. A follow-up study of triple arthrodesis on 292 adult feet. Acta Orthop Scand Suppl 107

43. Vainio K (1955) The rheumatoid foot. A clinical study with pathological and rheumatological comments. Ann Chir Gynaecol Suppl 45: 51

44. Wigren A (1985) Operative treatment with special regard to the hindfoot. Rheumatology 11: 100-103

13.

Foot involvement in spondylarthropathies

F Eulry

The spondylarthropathies are a group of inflamma-tory joint diseases having a strong but inconstant link to the presence of the HLA B27 antigen [3, 5, 49]. They include ankylosing spondylitis; reactive arthritis, of which Reiter's syndrome [41] is the most complete form; psoriatic arthritis; the arthritis of Crohn's disease or ulcerative colitis; and some forms of juvenile chronic arthritis. These arthritides often have a chronic course and may be simultaneous or successive in the same patient [3, 49] exhibiting common articular and extra-articular features. These facts justify the global concept of the spondylar-thropathies. The foot is one of the most important sites of the clinical lesions [3, 20] because its involve-ment is often early and frequent [13], in up to about 75% of cases [11], and because it has three practical characteristics for the physician: it often helps in the diagnosis of spondylarthropathy; it can be related to spondylarthropathy in a given clinical context; it sometimes leads to major problems of prognosis and treatment, because in some cases, the foot involve-ment is the only cause of disability during the evolu-tion of the disease [13].

Both sexes are affected, and the sex ratio is one female/4 or 5 males [34]. Every age group may be affected, including children [38] and old people, in whom a late and misleading onset is possible [24]. However, the disease mainly occurs in the young adult and at the middle period of life. The familial cases are explained by the strong link between spon-dylarthropathies and the HLA B27 antigen [10]. The clinical features may be very different in the involved patients, but foot and ankle localization is a common feature of the disease.

General pathophysiology

Pathology

Spondylarthropathy is a chronic inflammatory rheu-matic disease characterized by an axial and/or a peripheral involvement marked by a double mecha-nism of articular and juxta-articular inflammation. First, a synovitis of the joints is classically present, affecting especially the ankle and foot; a nonspecific, inflammatory cellular infiltration around the vessels of the chorion characterizes this synovitis, with neither hyperplasia of the villi nor fibrinoid necrosis (and hence no pannus). But the spondylarthropa-thies present particularly an inflammation of the entheses (enthesitis) which are the bony attachments [59] of tendons, capsule or ligaments, e.g., vertebral syndesmophytes, sacroiliitis (association of enthe-sitis and synovitis), calcaneal origin of the plantar aponeurosis, or the connections of the nail and distal phalanx in psoriatic arthropathy [31]. Histologic examination reveals that the enthesitis is initially a subchondral aseptic osteitis in the intra-osseous part of the enthesis. This osteitis may induce an inflam-matory periostitis or an aseptic osteomyelitis or a cicatricial hyperostosis, characterized by destruction of the cartilagenous part of the enthesis, followed by ossification [33]. Various stages of the histologic course are observed by light microscopy: granulom-atous tissue, lympho-plasmocytic infiltration, then ankylosing ossifications. Foot enthesitides are local-ized mainly at the inferior side of the calcaneus (at the plantar aponeurosis origin) and/or its posterior aspect (at the calcaneal tendon insertion). Enthesitis is also present on the toes (dactylitis), where the joint synovitis is associated with tenosynovitis. In psoriatic arthropathy, the enthesitis involves the distal interphalangeal joints, where there is almost no synovial tissue, and the nail insertion on the distal phalanx [31].

Pathogenesis

Several factors can favor the onset of spondylarthropathy but none is essential; there are genetic, infectious, and phenotypic factors which may be variously associated.

The frequency of the HLA B27 antigen depends on the clinical type of spondylarthropathy: this antigen is observed in 90% of cases of ankylosing spondylarthritis or reactive arthritis, but in only 30 to 60% [32] of psoriatic arthropathies, where HLA B16 and B17 antigens are also observed, and of other spondylarthropathies (ulcerative colitis, Crohn's disease, some forms of juvenile chronic arthritis).

The infectious factor is of intestinal or genital origin. It is inconstant, more frequent in reactive arthritis than in the other spondylarthropathies, but it can eventually induce an acute arthritic episode of any known or unidentifiable spondylarthropathy. *Chlamydia trachomatis*, and more rarely ureoplasma ureolytica, are the pathogenic agents of genital origin. Campylobacter, Yersinia, Salmonella, Shigella and *Klebsiella pneumoniae* [44] are the most frequent agents of intestinal origin; Shigella and *Klebsiella pneumoniae* have an antigenic resemblance to HLA B27 [26, 61]. The frequency of chronic and latent intestinal infections has been clearly demonstrated in the majority of the spondylarthropathies [47]. The association of one of these pathogenic agents with the Aids virus significantly influences the clinical features and the prognosis in reactive arthritis and other spondylarthropathies [56].

In fact, the patient's past medical history may influence the genesis of the phenotypic features. This is particularly the case for previous articular disease, whether traumatic or not; however, every previous joint injury is considered as a possible factor favoring the subsequent preferential localization of arthritis, even if there had been recovery without

sequelae. This observation has been clearly shown for arthritic lesions in joints previously subjected to moderate or severe trauma [50]. The influence of direct trauma on the onset of spondylarthropathy is highly probable in some rare cases [1] and certain in others [23].

● Diagnostic criteria of spondylarthropathies

Ankylosing spondylitis [63], reactive arthritis [65] and psoriatic arthritis [48, 64] have for a long time been characterized by diagnostic criteria that have sometimes been modified over time. Now the nosology groups these diseases of similar genetic origin under the general term of spondylarthropathies [3, 5, 49], and common diagnostic criteria [4, 17] have been established for the entire group. These criteria (listed in tables 13.1-13.3) seem valid [4].

Table 13.1. Classification criteria of the European Spondylarthropathy Study Group [4, 17]

Inflammatory vertebral pain   OR   synovitis
• asymmetric
• or preferentially involving the lower limbs
AND at least one of the following criteria:
• familial history of spondylarthropathy or uveitis or enterocolopathy
• psoriasis
• inflammatory enterocolopathy
• enthesitis
• radiologic sacroiliitis

Table 13.3. Diagnostic performances of Amor's and European Spondylarthropathy Study Group (ESSG) criteria [4]

Performance	Criteria	
	AMOR	ESSG
Sensitivity (%)	91,94	87,10
Specificity (%)	97,86	96,38
Positive predictive value	73,08	60,34
Negative predictive value	99,48	99,16
Probability ratio	42,96	24,08
Precision	97,50	98,83

Table 13.2. Amor's classification criteria for the spondylarthropathies [4]

A - Clinical signs or history	Points
1 - lumbar or dorsal nocturnal pain and/or morning stiffness	1
2 - asymmetric oligoarthritis	2
3 - gluteal pain	1
or alternate right-left gluteal pain	2
4 - sausage-like toe or finger	2
5 - talalgia or any other lower limb enthesopathy	2
6 - iritis	2
7 - nongonococcal uretritis or cervicitis (at least one month before onset of arthritis)	1
8 - diarrhea (at least one month before onset of arthritis)	1
9 - presence or history of psoriasis, and/or balanitis and/or chronic enterocolopathy	2
B - Radiologic signs	
10 - sacroiliitis (stage $\geq$ 2 when bilateral, or stage $\geq$ 3 when unilateral)	3
C - Genetic background	
11 - presence of HLA B27 antigen and/or family history of ankylosing spondylarthropathy, Reiter's disease, psoriasis, uveitis, or chronic enterocolopathy	2
D - Response to treatment	
12 - pain improvement within 48 hours by NSAIDs and/or immediate relapse (48 h) after NSAIDs with stopping the treatment	2

The diagnosis of spondylarthropathy is certain when the total points are $\geq$ 6

Involvement of the foot joints in the spondylarthropathies

This is characterized by the usual association [13] with generalized articular and nonarticular symptoms elsewhere. Articular features are evocative: inflammatory lumbar pain, bilateral but often alternating buttock pain, anterior and posterior parietal thoracic pain, cervical pain, oligoarthritis of the limbs (nonmigratory and asymmetric), rarely asymmetric polyarthritis, exceptionally monoarthritis; the synovial fluid is of inflammatory type, at least in the acute or subacute phase; it is pluricellular and bacteriologic cultures are sterile. The extra-articular signs involve principally skin and mucosae (recurrent uveitis, balanitis, stomatitis, psoriasis or dermatosis of psoriatic type); the viscera are more rarely affected (heart and lung essentially), generally only after several years of disease duration. Laboratory tests for inflammation are inconstant or moderate, even during acute episodes which are the usual course of spondylarthropathies; however, they are often considerable in recent acute or subacute forms, particularly in reactive arthritis.

Foot involvement is the earliest sign of the disease in about 30% of spondylarthropathies [12, 13]: heel pain (talalgia) in half the cases, involvement of the forefoot in a third of patients. This involvement appears within the first five years of the disease and is the sole feature in 15% of patients, even after 5 years [12]. It concerns mainly the hindfoot and forefoot, and more rarely, the midtarsal joints. Two major clinical features are highly evocative of spondylarthropathy [2, 12]: talalgia and "sausage-like toes". Their diagnostic significance predominates over other articular disorders such as metatarsalgia and the extra-articular symptoms such as skin involvement. All these clinical signs are associated with each other to a variable degree according to the type of spondylarthropathy, and do not play an important part in the precise diagnosis of the clinical type of spondylarthropathy. The radiologic signs [54, 55] include thickening of soft tissues, joint-space narrowing with subchondral erosions, followed by ankylosis and juxta-articular periostitis (periosteal new bone formation).

Hindfoot involvement

Heel pain is a major feature. This calcaneal enthesitis occurs in about 42% of spondylarthropathies [18], and in 40% [11, 28] to 65% [13] of cases of reactive arthritis, mainly during the first six months of their evolution [11], 30% of ankylosing spondylitis, and 77% of psoriatic arthritis [13]. Its initial presence in young people is so important that talalgia of any type, occurring before 40 years of age, must suggest the diagnosis of spondylarthropathy as long as another diagnosis is not proved. Talalgia is often bilateral and it almost never wakes the patient at night: it occurs immediately on getting up, and the pain is especially severe in weight-bearing, then decreases slowly on walking over one to several hours; it is equivalent to the morning joint stiffness of arthritis. The plantar talalgia is localized and rarely diffuse, described by the patients as a very sharp pain in the heel; it is more rarely posterior, and can be accompanied by pain [40] at the calcaneal tendon insertion (local enthesitis) or by a painful retrocalcaneal bursitis [21] produced by a localized inflammation of the soft tissues [53]. Walking and the putting on of shoes, becomes much more difficult. Apart from this rare bursitis, examination elicits the pain by localized pressure on the medial and forepart of the plantar aspect of the heel, or on its posterior and lower part. Talalgia is only disabling at the start of the disease, and tends to completely disappear later, but sometimes becomes chronic and persistent.

For a long time the radiologic posterior calcaneal anomalies are delayed in appearance (lateral or retrotibial view of the calcaneus); they are especially close to the calcaneal tendon or the plantar aponeurosis insertion [28, 40, 46]. These anomalies are clas-

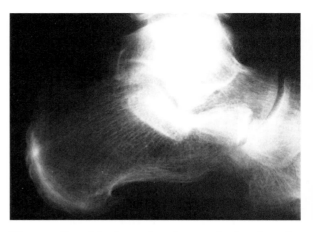

Fig. 13.2. Spondylarthropathy of 19-year's duration; the plantar talalgia has disappeared and the large plantar calcaneal spur is therefore rather regular (stage III) and of a healing nature

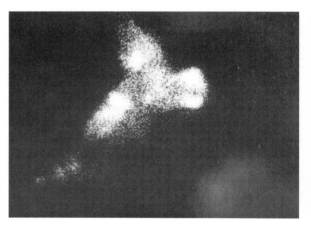

Fig. 13.3. Spondylarthropathy clinically involving talocrural and midtarsal joints and calcaneus (bipolar involvement); 99mTc-methylene diphosphonate bone scan reveals an intense hyperfixation at each clinically active site, especially the calcaneus

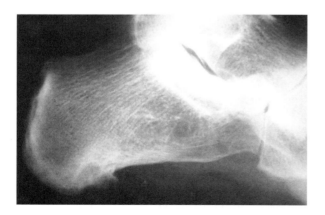

Fig. 13.1. Radiograph of calcaneus in a painful heel spondylarthropathy: posterior and inferior erosion because of a retrocalcaneal bursitis (stage I) and fuzzy, exuberant and irregular calcaneal "false" spur with a persistent interior demineralization (stage II)

sified into three types (figs. 13.1 & 13.2): local isolated erosion (stage I), or erosion associated with a beginning periosteal ossification (stage II), or extensive fluffy periosteal ossification without further erosion, giving an image of a fuzzy, irregular, "false" calcaneal spur (stage III), which is healing, and not painful. At the start of the disease course, careful inspection of the X-rays only detects a small erosion, very localized demineralization, perhaps beginning cortical irregularity. A posterior and upper calcaneal erosion is exceptionally present (fig. 13.1), but at a lower site than in rheumatoid arthritis [46]; when they are present, these posterior calcaneal erosions of spondylarthropathy are generally lower and posterior [53, 55].

At the onset of calcaneal involvement, the X-rays may be normal or difficult to read. In this case, 99m-technetium scintigraphy often shows an intense localized hyperfixation at the painful calcaneal site [11, 28], which is plantar or posterior or both (fig. 13.3). This localized hyperfixation may sometimes be discovered despite the absence of pain or radiologic evidence. [11]. Whole skeleton scintigraphy is of value in order to detect early [22, 27], other clinically quiet sites of enthesitis and/or arthritis (anterior tibial tuberosity, great trochanter, pubis symphysis, sacroiliac joints, sternoclavicular joints). The calcaneal enthesitic pain is characterized by usual complete recovery without functional sequelae, even after a course of many months, or even two or three years in exceptionally resistant forms.

Other hindfoot features

These are not specific. Talocrural arthritis is rarely observed, in about 15% of cases [13], subtalar arthritis in 6% [11]. Clinical symptoms at both these sites are those of an arthropathy of inflammatory nature. Moderate radiologic signs can occur later in the ankle. The subtalar joint is studied better by CT: images of joint-space narrowing, osteosclerosis rather than subchondral demineralization, or periarticular ossifications of enthesitis [57].

Forefoot involvement

This occurs in 20% [27] to 60% [12, 13] of cases of spondylarthropathy, according to its clinical form: 15% [54] to 20% [37] in primary ankylosing spondylitis, about 50% in reactive arthritis [11, 28], and more than 80% in psoriatic arthritis [13, 32]. Forefoot involvement is the first feature in 10 to 30% of cases, unilateral in 65%, and simultaneous with the other early signs in 40%. Its association with talalgia is highly suggestive. It occurs before the age of 50 in 75% of cases [13].

The "**sausage-like toes**" are the other major feature. At examination, the presence of one or several "sausage-like toes" is virtually pathognomonic of the spondylarthropathies (fig. 13.4), occurring in 20% [11] to 50% [13] of patients: the global

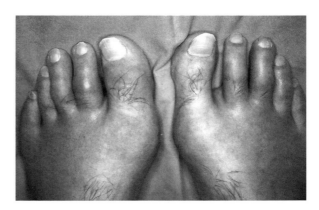

Fig. 13.4. Spondylarthropathy with sausage-like toes; in the left foot the second and third toes are involved and in the right foot the first three toes, especially the hallux, where involvement of the metatarsophalangeal joint is more apparent

inflammatory swelling all along the toes is observed more frequently than on the fingers. The great toe is involved in 30% [11] or 50% [28] of cases with sausage-like toes [28]; it sometimes simulates a gouty attack. The involved toes are initially red in color, later of normal color, but the global swelling can persist for a long time. This involvement corresponds to a plantar and/or dorsal tenosynovitis and not just to a synovitis of the metatarsophalangeal and interphalangeal joints, or to isolated distal enthesitis [31, 32].

Other forefoot symptoms

These are less evocative. Metatarsalgia can be severe, nocturnal and not truly localized. Some of their characteristics, however, can guide the diagnosis to the spondylarthropathies. They are asymmetric in 84% of cases [11]; often they are mild and unrecognized unless the metatarsal heads are palpated to elicit the pain, or a mild swelling is looked for on the dorsal intertendinous spaces of the forefoot; they can accompany the proximal or distal interphalangeal arthritis of toes which sometimes do not present any "sausage-like" aspect. The two first rays are mainly concerned, principally the first [11, 28]. Intermetatarsal bursitis is rare and found mainly in the second intermetatarsal space [13].

The weight of bedclothes, standing or walking, lead to functional complications in the forefoot in every case of sausage-like toe or metatarsalgia:

increasing pain and risk of local deformities followed in some cases, by irreversible ankylosis.

The radiologic anomalies are generally delayed in relation to the beginning of clinical symptoms. No correlation exists between the radiologic and clinical signs. Clear bands of metatarsal demineralization are exceptional, in about 4% of cases [25]; a pseudoalgodystrophic appearance is found in 5% of patients [13]; subchondral geodes, joint-space narrowing, partial or complete joint destruction and, particularly, phalangeal periostitis [6] or joint osteosclerosis are more frequent. As a general rule, the radiologic features of the spondylarthropathies [42], especially in the foot [25], are characterized by no or moderate demineralization and by the preponderance of new bone formation in close proximity to the entheses; this last phenomenon concerns the forefoot as well as the hindfoot.

Other forefoot characteristics of spondylarthropathies are important: possible involvement of the fifth metatarsal head [11], which is more rarely affected than in rheumatoid arthritis [9]; the hallux is the only toe involved in 50% of cases [28]; in the appropriate planar radiographs, the sesamoid bones may also be affected by a very ossified sesamoiditis that is sometimes unassociated with any dactylitis of the hallux [19]; the course can be especially complicated by subsequent inactive deformations and disabling fixed destruction of the toes, which are compressed in the shoes on walking or standing. This last point is essential for the evolution of the spondylarthropathies: forefoot involvement is insidious, recognized late, and can lead to silent forefoot destruction that permanently impairs the local functional prognosis.

Other joint disorders in the foot

These are rare and nonspecific because they can be observed in other inflammatory chronic joint diseases. They include tenosynovitis (15% of cases), especially of the tendon of the tibialis posterior muscle and, more rarely, of the fibular tendons. Involvement of the calcaneal tendon is exceptionally, the first sign of a reactive arthritis [29]. MRI [30] shows an abnormal tendinous signal and the presence of synovial fluid in the peritendinous envelope. It is particularly useful in searching for a clinically mild tendinous rupture.

Midtarsal joint involvement occurs in an average of 17-19% of patients [11, 13, 57] with 5% of clinical symptoms and 16% of radiologic anomalies. This lesion can lead to severe ankylosis of the tarsus [57].

All these disorders are generally moderate, not very inflammatory and not specific. Unlike talalgia and "sausage-like toe", their diagnostic value is very low.

An exceptional mode of onset should be emphasised [24]: it occurs in men of over 50, and is characterized by a very moderate oligoarthritis associated with HLA B27, and particularly with severe deterioration of the general health. The talocrural joint is concerned in 70% of cases and the tarsus and/or toes only in some 20%, but pitting edema of the ankles and feet is constant, initially suggesting the "RS3PE" syndrome [24].

Skin involvement in spondylarthropathies

Although very inconstant, this can be one of the most important clinical features, sometimes integrated into a more general skin disease (fig. 13.5) that extends far beyond the simple spondylarthropathic

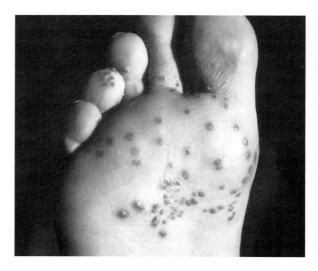

Fig. 13.5. Spondylarthropathy with plantar skin involvement: pustulosis is present in a patient with a known psoriatic arthropathy experiencing a severe acute cutaneous and articular episode suggestive of a recent reactive venereal arthritis, although the patient is HIV-positive [56]

foot localization. The nature of the skin involvement can considerably help in the diagnosis of the clinical form of spondylarthropathy [14]. Four main dermatoses can be associated with a spondylarthropathy: keratoderma palmaris et plantaris; pustulosis palmaris et plantaris; psoriasis and severe acne (fulminans or conglobata). In practice, only the first three dermatoses concern the foot and may have some common clinical and histologic aspects, but some of these are still debatable. The general and localized psoriatic joint disorders of the foot, for example, are sufficiently specific to greatly help in the diagnosis of a spondylarthropathy and in recognizing its psoriatic etiology.

Keratoderma palmaris and plantaris of Vidal-Jacquet

This is one of the features of reactive arthritis in about 10% of cases [11, 28, 41]. It is very similar to the pustular psoriatic lesions and in 20% of cases [14], it is associated with skin lesions of the trunk, scalp, flexures and nails. The palmo-plantar lesions are initially pustular, then keratinoid, and then become true cutaneous horns of nail-head type. They are variable in size (from pin-head to pea), more or less numerous but bulky, and subsequently coalesce. The microscopic examination reveals a spongiform multilocular pustulosis as in pustular psoriasis. From a general point of view, keratoderma palmaris and plantaris is evidence of the gravity of a reactive arthritis [28] because 75% of patients experiencing it have a disease relapse after recovery. In about 75% of these cases, the new attack includes a relapse of keratoderma palmaris et plantaris [11, 15].

Pustulosis palmaris et plantaris

Pustular psoriasis probably remains the most important example and its cutaneous evolution can be isolated, chronic or recurrent [14]. It can be considered either as a chronic pustular psoriasis or as a reactive dermatosis (Andrews' bacterides) induced by a remote infectious focus [14], or sometimes as a specific clinical entity. The sole is covered with an aseptic recurrent pustulosis, often of abrupt onset with recurrences, with negative bacteriologic examinations [51], and with the histologic aspect of possible unilocular pustulosis without a spongiosis

[51]; characteristics those of pustular psoriasis. These lesions are important because of their possible association with an aseptic osteitis and/or arthritis [60] of the spine, or anterior part of the thorax or the limbs, and with a sternoclavicular or manubriosternal hyperostosis, sometimes with sacro-iliitis or peripheral arthritis. This so called "SAPHO": synovitus-acne-putulosis-hyperostosis-osteomyelitis syndrome [8], can sometimes constitute a characteristic spondylarthropathy or a very similar disease picture in which foot joint involvement seems to be rare; the delay between the onsets of the skin and joint disorders may be long as up to 20 years [39].

Psoriasis

This is the most important dermatosis associated with the spondylarthropathies. This specific cause of some spondylarthropathies leads to the definition of psoriatic arthropathy [48, 64], in which the clinical joint manifestations are either solely or predominantly axial or peripheral in type. In these cases, the foot is a very important joint, skin and/or nail target, and is involved in 85% of cases, often at the early stage of the psoriatic arthropathy. The joint involvement generally occurs some years after the onset of the dermatosis, but before in 10% of cases [14]. All clinical forms of psoriasis are possible in cases of psoriatic arthropathy: psoriasis vulgaris is present either as a squamous well-circumscribed erythema of the trunk and/or limbs, or as isolated erythematous papules located between the buttocks, in the umbilicus, behind the ears and on the scalp. Pustular psoriasis with aseptic pustules can be generalized or limited to a palmo-plantar localization, and thus identical to keratoderma or pustulosis palmaris et plantaris. Cutaneous biopsy confirms the diagnosis of each clinical form: parakeratotic hyperkeratosis, acanthosis, absence of the stratum granulosum, presence of polymorphonuclear granulocytes under the stratum corneum, multilocular spongiform pustulosis in case of pustular psoriasis.

Psoriatic nail involvement in the feet and hands is a strong argument for the diagnosis: nail dystrophy (pachyonychia or onycholysis) is more frequent in psoriatic arthritis than in psoriasis vulgaris [14]. The very evocative "Bauer's toe" combines in the same toe a psoriatic dystrophic nail, periungual psoriasis, distal phalangeal enthesitis, and distal interphalangeal arthritis [13]. Onycho-pachydermo-periostitis of the hallux is another specific form [31]. It includes psoriatic onychosis, thickening of the distal soft tissues and radiologic osteoperiostitis of the distal phalanx with phalangeal periostal ossification, and a possible eburnated aspect of the distal phalanx [52], but no lesion of the interphalangeal joint. Other anomalies of the toes are possible: sausage-like toe, pseudogouty aspect of the hallux (the most involved toe) which is the initial lesion in about 12% of cases [31], and sometimes a contracted toe, like a lorgnette, because of phalangeal osteolysis; these last two appearances are suggestive of the diagnosis of psoriatic arthritis.

From a general point of view, the radiologic findings in the forefoot often suggest the psoriasis as the cause of a spondylarthropathy because they explain both the destructive joint involvement and the enthesitis. They are classified in the fingers and toes according to the five criteria of Avila et al [7]:
- erosive arthritis of a distal interphalangeal joint;
- ankylosis of a distal or proximal interphalangeal joint;
- osteolysis of an interphalangeal joint with no joint-space narrowing or even with widening of this space;
- destructive arthritis of the interphalangeal joint of the hallux, with a very large enthesophyte on the base of the distal phalanx, evidence of the association between enthesitis and synovitis;
- very suggestively, resorption of the distal phalangeal tuft.

When the third criterion is followed by the second at the same site, this is almost pathognomonic of psoriatic arthropathy.

It must be emphasised that psoriatic arthropathy is the only spondylarthropathy involving both the distal interphalangeal joint and the distal phalanx, which distinguishes it from rheumatoid arthritis [9, 31, 32, 46].

The clinical features of psoriatic arthropathy of the midfoot and hindfoot are not specific in comparison with other spondylarthropathies, but the radiologic anomalies are evocative enough with images of new bone formation especially seen in lateral X-rays [13]: these show exuberant "onion-skin" periostitis and a "false" calcaneal spur, with buttressing of the posterior part of the calcaneus and sometimes a local superior erosion; a bristly aspect of the upper border of the midtarsal joint is evocative; malleolar periostitis at the ankle is highly specific of psoriatic involvement because no other chronic inflammatory joint disease gives such an image.

Diagnostic difficulties

Two different clinical patterns of foot involvement lead to diagnostic difficulties. In one, involvement of the foot is integrated into a generalized inflammatory joint disease, but its specific characteristics help to identify the spondylarthropathy; in the other, the foot involvement seems isolated, but its nature and/or the investigations, authorize its inclusion in a spondylarthropathy. The use of recent diagnostic criteria [4, 17] has become usual for every individual case because of their highly negative predictive value (> 99%) (table 13.3).

Foot involvement makes the diagnosis of a chronic inflammatory rheumatism easier. A spondylarthropathy can be recognized by the nature of the joint and/or skin involvement: a sausage-like toe and/or a talalgia at whatever stage of an acute, subacute or chronic arthritis (evocative in cases of nonmigratory asymmetric oligoarthritis, less suggestive in cases of polyarthritis or monoarthritis) virtually confirm the diagnosis of spondylarthropathy. It is not necessary for these features to be contemporaneous with the generalized or localized foot joint involvement [4]. On the other hand, the radiologic signs in the hindfoot are fundamental, especially at the calcaneus; great importance has to be attached to a dense periostitis, sometimes extravagant, or to a "false" calcaneal spur in the lateral X-ray; this is irregular, fuzzy, ill-defined and therefore different from the regular spur of mechanical origin observed mainly after the age of 50. The evocative posterior or plantar calcaneal erosions are more difficult to interpret initially, even when associated subsequently with a periosteal osteosclerosis. They have to be distinguished from the rare upper or posterior erosions of the calcaneus which are sometimes observed in rheumatoid arthritis [46]. In this last disease, the distal and symmetric character of the joint involvement aids in the diagnosis, especially in the foot. Confronted with an unclassified polyarthritis, the asymmetric character of the clinical and radiologic features in the forefoot is precisely evocative of spondylarthropathy, especially when the radiologic destruction is associated with ossification, or when there are distal interphalangeal joint lesions evoking a psoriatic etiology.

The suggestive cutaneous features have to be sought in the patient's history, the history of his family, or by examination of his skin: in the history, because a pustulosis may be absent at the time of joint involvement and detected only by detailed questioning about the past medical history; in the family, because the psoriasis may only be present in the members of that family; on the skin, because psoriasis has to be meticulously sought in concealed places (scalp, behind and in the ears, umbilicus, between the buttocks) or at more visible sites (elbows, knees). Lastly, keratoderma palmaris et plantaris directs the diagnosis towards a spondylarthropathy like reactive arthritis [2].

On the whole, the foot involvement is very informative about the possible diagnosis of a spondylarthropathy, even if it is necessary to patiently correlate features which may be spread out over time. An isolated foot involvement can be related to a spondylarthropathy in two situations: it is characterized by local inflammatory manifestations, or it leads to the finding of suggestive features in the patient's history or in the history of his family.

In the former, the general and local inflammatory signs are evocative: swelling of a metatarsophalangeal joint or a sausage-like toe, nocturnal pain; prolonged morning stiffness; talalgia, which is routinely suspicious of a spondylarthropathy when it occurs before 40 years of age; retrocalcaneal bursitis, where aspiration may yield some droplets of synovial fluid of inflammatory character. An increase of the sedimentation rate or of the plasma C-reactive protein provides laboratory evidence of an inflammatory syndrome when the local or remote radiologic and isotopic data are suggestive.

In the latter case, the following past or present features have to be considered when associated with foot involvement: low back pain of inflammatory character, buttock pain, bilateral alternating sciatica, uveitis, psoriasis, chronic colitis, family history of spondylarthropathy, radiologic sacroiliitis, vertebral syndesmophytes, presence of the HLA B27 antigen.

● Problems of prognosis and treatment

These are common to the different types of spondylarthropathies. We refer here only to the problems of the foot disorders, in which local treatment is important and may be associated with general treatment that also influences the prognosis of the foot involvement. It must first be emphasised that the functional prognosis is fundamentally different between hindfoot and forefoot involvement: even when talalgia is apparently severe, recovery is the rule except in a few cases, but forefoot involvement is more sinister because of its insidious course. There is a serious risk of local destruction of the involved foot with later joint ankylosis and/or dislocation [2, 11, 12, 20], largely promoted by inopportune weight-bearing, even in the case of simultaneous general and local treatment.

Practical treatment aims to suppress local inflammation and to prevent deformity, especially in the forefoot, and later this treatment must allow normal walking and avoid the possible complications [12].

The treatment of local inflammation

The basic treatment uses nonsteroidal anti-inflammatory drugs; systemic corticotherapy is used only in some very severe forms with long-lasting crises. More often "second line" anti-inflammatory drugs are prescribed, they are only efficient, if at all, in some peripheral joint disorders of spondylarthropathies like foot involvement. Exceptionally, there is a place for gold salts [12], more reliably sulphasalazine [16, 43] or mesalamine [62], methotrexate [58] and perhaps bromocriptine [36]; etetrinate is effective in the joint and skin disorders of some spondylarthropathies [45], especially with foot involvement.

Fundamental measures have to be locally applied. First, during the acute or subacute phase of the disease, the basic treatment is relief from weight-bearing, either with crutches in the case of unilateral disorders or by bed-rest for bilateral involvement, or when the (exceptionally) affected upper limbs prohibit the use of crutches. The use of local corticosteroid injections is also possible: plantar or retrocalcaneal injection for talalgia, injection of the talocrural or midtarsal joint, injection into the basis of a sausage-like toe, into the metatarsophalangeal joints if necessary, or into an intermetatarsal space. Cortivazole can be chosen, but the intra-articular injection of triamcinolone hexacetonide into the forefoot needs use of the image intensifier to check the precise intra-articular position of the needle before injection.

Spondylarthropathies rarely require intra-articular injections of radioactive isotopes except in some cases of chronic nondestructive inflammatory disorders. Cautious associated physical treatments (wax baths at 35°C, local hydrotherapy) are often useful. Surgery is always contraindicated in case of talalgia with a local exuberant calcaneal periostitis (stage II or III), but the surgical removal of a retrocalcaneal bursitis [21] may be indicated early in the course of an attack.

Prevention of the deformities

This must be immediate and start with relief from weight-bearing (especially by bed rest) in order to protect the forefoot from deformities. A protective cradle placed under the bedclothes prevents aggravation of the forefoot lesions by pressure of the bedclothes against the toes. A splint should be used as early as possible, depending on the degree of pain, to maintain the foot and toes in a nonvicious posture; a light thermoformed material cast directly on the foot, is better than plaster. The patient should be informed about his condition and future prospects at this time.

The cautious and programmed rehabilitation phase starts when the inflammatory disorders have completely or nearly completely disappeared, but it is suspended in the event of a recurrence of pain, or if the local inflammatory disorders reappear. This rehabilitation phase is often prolonged, first in a special center, then at home if necessary. It counteracts the damaging consequences of immobilization, soft tissue contractures and muscular atrophy. When possible, physical treatment and occupational therapy (ergotherapy) are combined.

Physical treatment is given during the non-weight-bearing phase: local drainage-massage of the lower limb, then gentle passive mobilization of the foot joints, especially the metatarsophalangeal joints, then isometric active exercises to prevent contractures of the extrinsic foot muscles. Hydrotherapy helps in physical treatment: localized warm balneotherapy has an anodyne effect and permits active exercises in conditions of partial weightlessness to facilitate cautious active physical treatment and progressive weight-bearing.

Occupational treatment (ergotherapy) uses methods to restore muscular strength and movement; vocational techniques are adapted to the patient's capacity and to the joints which need to be stimulated, particularly in the forefoot.

Obtaining normal walking

Walking can be resumed cautiously in two ways: actual walking rehabilitation and the use of adapted orthoses.

Partial weightlessness in balneotherapy allows progressive resumption of walking in the pool. Functional physical treatment in partial weight-bearing is supplementary: the standing patient moves his foot, stands on tip-toe or on the heel, does antero-posterior foot rolling, and then resumes actual walking by initially leaning on parallel hand-rails.

Plantar orthoses have a triple aim: firstly, to decrease pain in the foot, then to prevent deformity, and finally to correct deformity. In cases of talalgia, an adapted supple heel orthosis is made, which can possibly correct a reducible varus or valgus of the heel; such an orthosis is higher in its posterior part and its height decreases slowly to the midfoot or the metatarsus; a heel orthosis can include a limited excavation placed under the area of painful calcaneal pressure. When an anomaly is present in the forefoot, a supple apparatus is placed under the metatarsal bones to correct and harmoniously distribute the metatarsal load. A toe deformity can be relieved by a silicone orthosis protecting it against the shoe. The shoe itself must be non-aggressive, including a high heel of at least 2 cm, a shank which is wide and supple in front and a thick and supple sole; during the first weeks of recovery, the best shoes seem to be running shoes (trainers).

Treatment of local complications

Two problems have to be considered: first, the rare talalgia resistant to treatment; second, forefoot deformity.

Chronic talalgia can progress for over a year [18] despite a plantar heel orthosis and local corticosteroid injections. At this late stage, the surgical removal of a retrocalcaneal bursitis can be useful [21] but is not enough [12], even when it is exceptionally necessary to operate for Haglund's calcaneal deformity, by removing the posterior-superior angle of the tuberosity [2]. Local anti-inflammatory radiotherapy [2, 12, 20, 35] is sometimes useful in about 2% of cases of resistant talalgia. The technic must be strict: precise focal irradiation with no radiation outside the chosen location, a maximum total dose of about 15 to 20 grays, spread over 3 weekly sessions. Talalgia disappears within 3 to 4 months in 80% of cases [12].

The management of forefoot deformities is more difficult [6, 12]. When there are capsular contractures with stiffening of the metatarsophalangeal joints hindering the last phase of gait, local corticosteroid injections and prolonged cautious physical treatment improve the situation. On the other hand, the rigid flat triangular forefoot with metatarsophalangeal luxations and irreducible toe deformities has a very poor prognosis because of the difficulties of treatment. Initially, foot orthoses, toe orthoplasties and custom-made shoes are adequate. In other rare situations, the irreducible painful deformities require surgical treatment: either treatment of the toe deformities only, or resection of the destroyed 2th to 5th metatarsal heads.

The prognosis of spondylarthropathic foot involvement is generally good when treatment is started early and protects the forefoot.

References

1. Alcalay M, Debiais F, Prieur AM, Azais I, Masson G, Thomas P, Bontoux D (1987) Étude rétrospective du rôle éventuel des traumatismes dans la genèse de la spondylarthrite ankylosante, du syndrome de Fiessinger-Leroy-Reiter et des autres arthrites réactionnelles, des rhumatismes B27 inclassés de l'adulte, et des arthrites chroniques B27 de l'enfant. Rev Rhum 54: 235-241

2. Amor B (1982) Le pied dans le syndrome de Fiessinger-Leroy-Reiter. In: Claustre J, Simon L (eds). Le pied en pratique rhumatologique. Masson, Paris, p 72

3. Amor B (1989) Le concept de spondylarthropathie. Rev Prat (Paris) 17: 1469-1472

4. Amor B, Dougados M, Listrat V, et al (1991) Évaluation des critères des spondylarthropathies d'Amor et de l'European Spondylarthropathy Study Group; une étude transversale de 2228 patients. Ann Med Interne (Paris) 142: 85-89

5. Arnett F (1987) Seronegative spondylarthropathies. Bull Rheum Dis 37: 1-12

6. Aussedat R, Gaunel C, Daum B, Vivard Th, Pourel J (1988) Atteintes de l'avant-pied au cours de la spondylarthrite ankylosante. Annales de Médecine (Nancy) 27: 279-282

7. Avila R, Pugh DG, Slocumb CH, Winkelmann RK (1960) Psoriatic arthritis: a roentgenologic study. Radiology 75: 691-702

8. Benhamou CL, Chamot AM, Kahn MF (1988) Synovitis-acne-pustolosis hyperostosis osteomyelitis syndrome (SAPHO). A new syndrome among the spondylarthropathies? Clin Exp Rheumatol 6: 109-112

9. Braun S (1975) Le pied dans les grands rhumatismes inflammatoires chroniques. Rhumatologie 27: 47-56

10. Calin A, Marder A, Marks S, Burns T (1984) Familial aggregation of Reiter's syndrome and ankylosing spondylitis: a comparative study. J Rheumatol 11: 672-677

11. Calmels C, Eulry F, Lechevalier D, Dubest JJ, Ristori JM, Sauvezie B, Bussiere JL (1993) Involvement of the foot in reactive arthritides. A retrospective study of one hundred five cases. Rev Rhum (Engl edn) 60: 285-290

12. Claustre J, Marcelli Ch (1988) Le pied de la spondylarthrite ankylosante. In: Simon L, Hérisson C (eds) La spondylarthrite ankylosante. Masson, Paris, p 214

13. Claustre J, Miralles D, Simon L (1989) Le pied, miroir des spondylarthropathies. In: Gaucher A, Pourel J, Netter P, Kessler M (eds) Actualités en physiopathologie et pharmacologie articulaires. Les spondylarthropathies. Masson, Paris, p 39

14. Cuny JF, Schmutz JL Terver MN, Weber M, Beurey J (1988) Dermatoses et spondylarthropathies. Annales de Médecine de Nancy 27: 265-268

15. David-Chaussé J, Dehais J, Garnier JP (1975) Rechutes tardives dans dix-sept cas de syndrome de Fiessinger-Leroy-Reiter. Rhumatologie 27: 277-281

16. Dougados M, Boumier P, Amor B (1986) Sulphasalazine in ankylosing spondylitis, adouble bind controlled study. Br Med J 293: 911-914

17. Dougados M, van der linden S, Juhlin R, Huifeldt B, Amor B, Calin A, Cats A, Dijkmans B, Oliveri I, Pasero G, Veys E, Zeidler H. The European Spondylarthropathy Study Group (1991) The European Spondylarthropathy Study Group preliminary criteria for the classification of spondylarthropathy. Arthritis Rheum 34: 1218-1227

18. Dougados M, Contreras L, Maetzel A, Amor B (1992) Les talalgies des spondylarthropathies. Présentation clinique et traitement. Rev Rhum 59: résumé A 12

19. Doury P, Pattin S, Delahaye RP, Metges PJ, Mine J, Casanova G (1979: Sésamoïdite du gros orteil au cours d'un syndrome de Fiessinger-Leroy-Reiter. Rev Rhum 46: 133-134

20. Doury P (1987) Concept de spondylarthropathies séronégatives. Importance du pied. Médecine et Chirurgie du Pied 3: 95-96

21. Doury P, Pattin S, Eulry F (1987) La calcanéite postéro-supérieure par bursite rétro-calcanéene dans le syndrome de Fiessinger-Leroy-Reiter. Medecine et Chirurgie du Pied 3: 203-206

22. Doury P, Granier R, Pattin S, Eulry F, Gaillard JF, Bloch JG (1988) La place de la scintigraphie osseuse dans le diagnostic précoce de la spondylarthrite ankylosante et des autres spondylarthropathies séronégatives. In: Simon L, Hérisson Ch (eds) La spondyl-arthrite ankylosante. Masson, Paris, p 49

23. Doury p (1993) Psoriatic arthritis with physical trauma. J Rheumatol 20: 1629

24. Dubost JJ, Sauvezie B (1989) Late onset peripheral spondylarthropathy. J Rheumatol 16: 1214-1217

25. Durckel J, Sibilla J, Kuntz JL, Bloch JG, Walter JP, Asch L (1989) Spondylarthropathies inflammatoires. Aspects radiographiques particuliers de l'atteinte du pied. In: Gaucher A, Pourel J, Netter P, Kessler M (eds) Actualités en physiopathologie et pharmacologie articulaires. Les spondylarthropathies. Masson, Paris, p 48 26

26. Ebringer A (1992) Ankylosing spondylitis is caused by Klebsiella: evidence from immunologic, microbiologic and serologic studies. Rheum Dis North Am 18: 105-121

27. Esdaile J, Hawkins D, Rosenthall L (1979) Radio-nucleide joint imaging in the seronegative spondylarthropathies. Clin Orthop 12: 46-52

28. Eulry F, Labbe P, Magnin J, Lechevalier D, Doury P (1992) La calcanéite dans 95 arthrites réactionnelles. Rev Rhum 59: résumé A 16

29. Eulry F, Verrière D, Dellestable F, Haguenauer D, Crozes Ph, Lechevalier D, Magnin J (1993) Tendinopathie d'Achille inaugurant un syndrome de Fiessinger-Leroy-Reiter. Médecine et Chirurgie du Pied 4: 224-226

30. Feldman F, Staron RB, Haramati N (1991) Magnetic resonance imaging of the foot and ankle. In: Weissman BN (ed) Imaging of Rheumatic Diseases. Rheum Dis Clin North Am 17: 617-636

31. Fournié B, Viraben R, Durroux R, Lassoued S, Gay R, Fournié A (1989) L'onycho-pachydermo-périostite psoriasique du gros orteil; étude anatomo-clinique et approche physiopathagénique à propos de 4 observations. Rev Rhum 56: 579-582

32. Fournié B, Granel J, Bonnet M, Dromer C, Pagès M, Billey Th, Fournié A (1992) Fréquence des signes évocateurs d'un rhumatisme psoriasique dans l'atteinte radiologique des doigts et des orteils. À propos de 193 cas d'arthropathie psoriasique. Rev Rhum 59: 177-180

33. Fournié B (1993) A broader concept of entheses and the hyperosteosis-osteitis-periostosis (HOP) syndrome. A nosological radioclinical approach to inflammatory spondylarthropathies. Rev Rhum (Engl edn) 60: 399-402

34. Gran JT (1990) Ankylosing spondylitis in women. Semin Arthritis Rheum 19: 303-312

35. Grill V, Smith M, Ahern M, Littlejohn G (1988) Local radiotherapy for pedal manifestations of HLA-B27-related arthropathy. Br J Rheumatol 27: 390-392

36. Guttierez MA, Anaya JM, Cabrera GE, Vindrola O, Espinoza LR (1994) Prolactin, a link between neuroendocrine and immune system. Its role in the pathogenesis of rheumatic diseases. Rev Rhum (Engl ddn) 61: 261-267

37. Hajjaj-Hassouni N, Guedira-Srairi N, Boukhrissi N, Tazi A (1987) Le pied dans la spondylarthrite ankylosante idiopathique. Medecine et Chirurgie du Pied 3: 143-150

38. Jacob JC, Berdon WE, Johnston AD (1982) HLA B27 associated spodyloarthritis and enthesopathy in childhood: clinical, pathologic and radiographic observations in 58 patients. J Pediatr 100: 521-528

39. Kahn MF, Bouvier M, Palazzo E, Tebib JG, Colson F (1991) Sternoclavicular pustulotic osteitis (SAPHO). 20-year interval between skin and bone lesions. J Rheumatol 18: 1104-1108

40. Keat AC, Maini RN, Pegrum GD, Scott JT (1979) The clinical features and HLA associations of reactive arthritis associated with non-gonococcal urethritis. Q J Med 48: 323-342

41. Keat A (1983) Reiter's syndrome and reactive arthritis in perspective. N Engl J Med 309: 1606-1615

42. Kerr R, Resnick D (1985) Radiology of the seronegative spodylarthropathies. Clin Rheum Dis 11: 113-146

43. Kirwan J, Edwards A, Huitfeldt B, Thompson P, Currey H (1993) The course of established ankylosing spondylitis and the effects of sulphasalazine over 3 years. Br J Rheumatol 32: 729-733

44. Leirisalo-Repo M, Turinen U, Stenman S, Helenieus P, Seppalà K (1994) High frequency of silent inflammatory bowel disease in spondylarthropathy. Arthritis Rheum 37: 23-31

45. Louthrenoo W (1993) Successful treatment of severe Reiter's syndrome associated with human immunodeficiency virus infection with etetrinate; report of 2 cases. J Rheumatol 20: 1243-1246

46. Martel W (1970) Acute and chronic arthritis of the foot. Semin Roentgenol 5: 391-406

47. Mielants H, Veys EM, Goemaeres S, Cuveleier C, de Vos M (1993) A prospective study of patients with spondylarthropathy with special reference to HLA-B27 and to gut histology. J Rheumatol 20: 1353-1358

48. Moll JMH, Wright V (1973) Psoriatic arthritis. Semin Arthritis Rheum 3: 55-78

49. Moll JMH, Haslock I, Macrae IF, Wright V (1974) Associations between ankylosing spondylitis, psoriatic arthritis, Reiter's disease, the intestinal arthropathies and Behçet's syndrome. Medicine 53: 343-364

50. Noer HR (1966) An experimental epidemic of Reiter's syndrome. J Am Med Assoc 198: 693-698

51. Prier A, Kaeger AC, Di Crescenzo MC, Canesi MF, Camus JP (1985) Manifestations ostéo-articulaires vertébrales et thoraciques au cours de la pustulose palmo-plantaire. Ann Med Inerne (Paris) 136: 615-619

52. Resnick D, Broderick RW (1977) Bony proliferation of terminal phalanges in psoriasis. The "ivory" phalanx. J Can Assoc Radiol 28: 187

53. Resnick D, Feingold ML, Niwayama G, Georgen TG (1977) Calcaneal abnormalities in articular disorders: rheumatoid arthritis, ankylosing spondylitis, psoriatic arthritis, Reiter's syndrome. Radiology 125: 355-359

54. Resnick D, Niwayama G (1981) Ankylosing spondylitis. In: Resnick D et Niwayama G (eds) Diagnosis of bone and joint disorders. WB Saunders Company, Philadelphia, p 1040

55. Resnick D, Niwayama G (1981) Rheumatoid arthritis and the seronegative spondylo-arthropathies: radiographic and pathologic concepts. In: Resnick D, Niwayama G (eds) Diagnosis of bone and joint disorders. WB Saunders Company, Philadelphia, p 850

56. Reveille JD, Conant M, Duvic M (1990) Human immunodeficiency virus-associated psoriasis, psoriatic arthritis, and Reiter's syndrome: a disease continuum? Arthritis Rheum 33: 1574-1578

57. Roth RD (1986) Tarsal ankylosing in juvenile ankylosing spondylitis. J Am Pediatr Med Assoc 76: 514-518

58. Schnabel A, Gross WL (1994) Low-dose methotrexate in rheumatic diseases; efficacy, side effects, and risk factors for side effects. Semin Arthritis Rheum 23: 310-327

59. Shichikawa K, Tsujimoto M, Mshioka J, Nishibayashi Y, Matsumoto K (1985) Histopathology of early sacroillitis and enthesitis in ankylosing spondylitis. In: Ziff M, Cohen SB (eds) Advances in inflammation research, vol 9. The spondylarthropathies. Raven Press, New York, p 15

60. Sonozaki H, Mitsui H, Miyanaga Y, Okitsu K, Igarashi M, Hayashi Y, Matsuura M, Azuha A, Okai K, Kawashima M (1981) Clinical features of 53 cases with pustolotic arthro-osteitis. Ann Rheum Dis 40: 554-557

61. Stieglitz H, Lipsky P (1993) Association between reactive arthritis and antecedent infection with Shigella flexneri carrying a 2-Md plasmid and encoding an HLA-B27 mimetic epitope. Arthritis Rheum 36: 1387-1391

62. Thomson GTD, McKibbon C, Inman RD (1994) Mesalamine therapy in Reiter's syndrome. J Rheumatol 31: 57-572

63. van der Linden S, Valkenburg HA, Cats A (1984) Evaluation of diagnostic criteria for ankylosing spondylitis. A proposal for modification of the New York criteria. Arthritis Rheum 27: 361-368

64. Veale D, Rogers S, Fitzgerald O (1994) Classification of clinical subsets in psoriatic arthritis. Br J Rheumatol 33: 133-138

65. Wilkens RF, Arnett FC, Bitter T, Calin A, Fisher L, Ford DK, Good AE, Masi AT (1981) Reiter's syndrome: evaluation of preliminary criteria for definite disease. Arthritis Rheum 24: 844-849

14.

Algodystrophies of the foot and ankle

F Eulry

Introduction

Algodystrophy is a primary or secondary disease, due to peripheral vascular disturbances involving local microcirculation and its sympathetic control in a joint region. Every tissue can be involved except cartilage: cutaneous, subcutaneous, tendinous, muscular, aponeurotic, capsular, synovial and bone [7, 46]. Pain and disability of varying degree are the most important diagnostic data. The disease may continue for weeks, months or years but leads to complete recovery; it sometimes has trophic and/or moderate dysfunctional (soft tissue contracture) sequelae; treatment shortens the duration of the disease. The foot involvement was initially described by Südeck [52] as "an acute inflammatory bone atrophy" and is the most frequent localization of algodystrophy of the lower limbs: 122 of 188 localization's in the lower limbs [48], 92 out of 168 cases [7]. The course of foot algodystrophy is often long and leads to difficulties in diagnosis and treatment [5, 7. 19, 41, 48]. The social, occupational and familial consequences are a very important problem for both patients and community [20, 38].

Physiopathology

A local or remote noxious influence acts on one or several joint regions of the foot. This is specific (local or regional traumatism) or nonspecific and generalized (e.g., drug therapy) and may be associated with possible favoring factors [43]. A delayed and abnor-

mally intense sympathetic response appears; it is disproportionate, long-lasting, extensive but reversible and induces local peripheral vascular disturbances of the intermediate channels which connect the terminal arterioles and the venules, including the metarterioles and Surquet's channels which connect the arteriole directly to the venule. Decrease of blood-flow, capillary stasis and dilation, plasmatic edema, secondary hyperplasia of the arteriolar muscularis (a phenomenon specific to algodystrophy [43]), early involvement of the bone and soft tissues of the joint and periarticular region (with subsequent fibrosis) are the most important consequences of this disorder.

The first stage ("hot" or pseudo-inflammatory stage) is characterized by intense and lasting arteriolar constriction and the opening of arteriovenous shunts, vasodilation, capillary hyperpermeability and stasis (edema), leading first to local hyperemia and then to ischemia, anoxia and tissue acidosis. The arteriolar constriction explains neither the capillary dilation nor the plasmatic edema. There are never any inflammatory cells [42] or any laboratory parameters of inflammation [7], and vasoactive-inhibiting drugs (anti-histamines, nonsteroidal anti-inflammatory drugs) are ineffective. Locally, the stasis acts as a tourniquet, inducing a pO_2 and pH decrease and a pCO_2 and K^+ increase. These events enhance the vasodilation and capillary permeability [43]; the area of increased isotope uptake (scintigraphy) extends beyond the bounds of the involved bones. Partial ischemia (second stage: "cold" or ischemic stage) stimulates polymerization of the ground substance, the fibrocysts and fibroblasts inducing subsequent fibrosis. The third stage is one of complete recovery except in a few cases of sequelae (soft tissue contracture). The biomechanical modifications of the tissues induce pain and have a noxious influence on the sympathetic reflex arc, which is auto-stimulated by a vicious circle maintaining the disease. The division of the course of algodystrophy into three successive stages is inconstant because of the possible telescoping or absence or inversion of these stages. Vasoactive crises can induce alternating brief episodes of the hot and cold stages, sometimes even during a single day.

Etiology

Algodystrophy may be encountered in all age groups: children, adolescents, [4, 15, 27, 50], and young adults [19], and not only in adults over the age of 40 [5, 41, 48]. According to the populations studied the disease involves the sexes equally [28] or unequally [19].

Apparently, primary algodystrophies occur in less than 40% of cases [7] and secondary cases are the most frequent. Trauma is the prime cause in cases involving the foot [31, 37], as in 141 of our 199 cases [19]. This trauma may be direct or indirect, loco-regional or remote. It is more often accidental: 93% of cases (fractures, luxations or sprains in 75%; local contusion in 18%), but is surgical in 7% of cases: orthopedic or, more rarely, arterial or visceral surgical procedures [39]. Plaster immobilization and painful rehabilitation or precipitate mobilization are the most frequent provocative and/or promoting factors [19]. Algodystrophy begins either immediately after traumatism or its treatment (77% of cases), or after an average delay of 4 months [19].

Nontraumatic causes are rarer in algodystrophy of the foot [7] and relate primarily to the locomotor apparatus: septic [12], inflammatory [29] or metabolic [7] arthritides [12]; exceptionally, osteoporosis [7] or osteomalacia; metabolic acidosis and renal tubulopathy [33]; diseases of the nervous system [7], e.g., central lesions such as hemiplegia, or peripheral lesions such as sciatic or crural radiculalgia or Morton's disease [17]. Cardiovascular diseases (myocardial infarction), pleuropulmonary disease, endocrine and metabolic diseases (hyperthyroidism, diabetes mellitus), malignant tumors in some cases [6, 14], drug therapy (antituberculous agents, pheno-

barbitals) can all be causal, but more often in the upper limb than in the foot [7, 19].

Particular background-linked favoring factors can be present in secondary or primary cases. Psychiatric disorders like anxiety, depression, hysteria or a context of overprotective parents in childhood disease [15] are found in 35% of patients [19]. Hypertriglyceridemia is classically present in 35% of traumatic and nontraumatic cases [1, 19]; but this is not an etiologic factor but secondary to immobilization at the start of the disease and disappearing after progressive mobilization [21].

Clinical study

The sudden or gradual onset of algodystrophy occurs spontaneously or following an injury. The disease affects the ankle and/or foot, which should always be examined compared with the healthy foot.

Articular features

These concern essentially the talocrural and subtalar joints and the forefoot joints. Pain of various degrees (from discomfort to intolerable pain) limits or prevents weight-bearing and/or walking and can wake the patient during the night. Pain is increased by passive or active mobilization. Stiffness and functional disability are secondary to the pain or to contracture of soft tissues (calcaneal tendon, tendons of the muscles controlling the toes, plantar aponeurosis). These contractures are ominous for the functional prognosis; they are late in most cases but may be precocious or even initiate the evolution of algodystrophy [11, 19]. Joint effusion can be present in the ankle.

Vasomotor disturbances and trophic symptoms

Edema is inconstant, soft or firm, pale or reddish, painful and accompanied by local hyperthermia or more rarely by hypothermia; hypothermia is frequent at the onset of the disease in young patients [15]. Cutaneous hyperesthesia is present in 51% of cases [19] and strongly suggests the diagnosis; it is isolated in some cases [48], particularly in young patients [19]. Permanent sweating, pallor, erythrocyanosis are spontaneously present or induced by dependence of the limb; brief and repeated vaso-motor disturbances are spontaneous or provoked, and are, exceptionally, isolated [19]. Hypotrichosis and local onychopathy are rare but very evocative [46].

Clinical syndromes

These constitute the three standard stages of the disease. The "hot" phase is a pseudo-inflammatory arthropathy that in some cases mimics septic arthritis or thrombotic conditions but without positive laboratory tests. There is edema filling the intertendinous hollows of the forefoot or ankle, erythema, hyperthermia, cutaneous hyperesthesia, intolerance to passive mobilization of the foot joints and exaggerated sweating.

The "cold" phase is of ischemic type (fig. 14.1) with cutaneous hypothermia, hypotrichosis, cutaneous atrophy, pallor, pitting or firm edema, and restriction of joint mobility.

Isolated or predominant contracture of soft tissues is possible (a phase of risk of definitive sequelae which can be precocious) and has a poor functional prognosis due to equinus or contracture of the plantar aponeurosis as in Ledderhose's disease. Sometimes this contracture has a sudden and definitive onset [7].

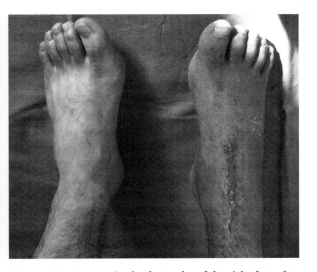

Fig. 14.1. Post-traumatic algodystrophy of the right foot after surgical treatment and plaster immobilization: diffuse edema of ankle and foot filling the intertendinous hollows and cutaneous cyanosis ("cold" or ischemic phase). Compare to opposite side

Complementary investigations

The sedimentation rate and plasma levels of C-reactive protein, fibrin and alpha-2-globulins are strictly normal: there is no laboratory evidence of an inflammatory syndrome. If such anomalies do exist, the diagnosis must be rejected or an inflammatory disease associated with algodystrophy has to be sought as a possible cause of the algodystrophy.

In cases with joint effusion the synovial fluid has no inflammatory characteristics (mechanical type): cells number < 1000 mm³ and there are no pathogens on bacteriologic examination. Synovial biopsy [42] confirms the absence of any inflammatory cells; a vascular hyperemia is observed in the initial stage of the disease and progressive local fibrosis appears later.

Radiologic features

X-rays of normal and involved regions must be compared: ankles (frontal and lateral views), both feet (frontal and lateral views, 3/4 oblique and sesamoid views). They should be repeated as the disease progresses because the clinical signs usually precede the radiologic evidence by several weeks. Radiologic features can be absent during the whole disease duration in about 70% of cases in children, but in less than 20% of cases in adults [15, 19]. The radiologic signs may persist after clinical recovery.

In the involved articular regions osteopenia is predominant in the peri- or juxta-articular area with enhanced subchondral osteolysis. It is uniform or patchy, micro- or macrolacunar, localized or diffuse. In young patients [15] the demineralization may be featured by an appearance of clear bands in the metaphyses [4] of the metatarsals, tibia or fibula (distal extremities) (fig. 14.2), a sign which decreases progressively with aging does not disappear completely after 60. The absolute integrity of the joint-spaces and the total absence of osteosclerosis are the most important radiologic signs throughout the course of the disease. The soft tissues are initially thickened and seem emphasised (hyperemia) by the contrast used in CT (not an indispensable investigation); later, the soft tissues become progressively thinner and insensitive to contrast in CT because of fibrosis.

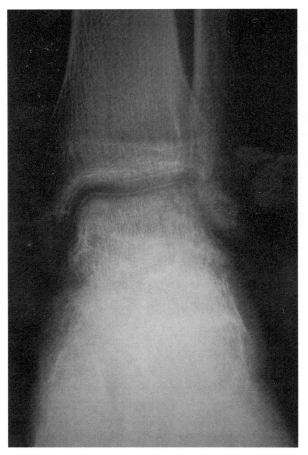

Fig. 14.2. Ankle algodystrophy (frontal X-ray) in a 17-year-old patient: subchondral demineralization delineates the talus very well and the "clear metaphyseal band" enhances the demineralization of the distal tibial extremity

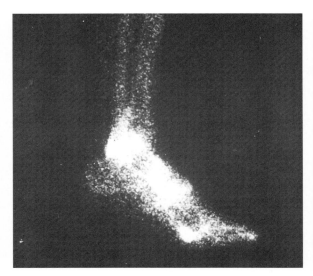

Fig. 14.3. Bone scintigraphy (methylene diphosphonate 99mTc) during an acute episode of foot algodystrophy: diffuse hyperfixation, predominately in the tarsus and the sesamoid bones of the hallux

Magnetic resonance imaging

This is very exceptionally necessary but is positive at a very early stage. It is better known in algodystrophy of the hip [30]. It is characterized by hypersignal (T2) and hyposignal (T1), enhanced by gadolinium in hyperemic forms but not in fibrosis. Distinguishing algodystrophy from avascular osteonecrosis (of the talus for example) can sometimes be difficult [30].

99mTc bone scan

Only rarely is this normal at the early vascular precocious phase or late tissue phase [36]. Loco-regional increased uptake is usual [7] and precedes radiologic signs by many weeks so that bone scintigraphy is of great importance for early diagnosis. Increased regional or loco-regional (fig. 14.3) uptake often involves other joints of the affected limb and persists throughout the disease and sometimes after clinical recovery. In contrast, local hypofixation [16] can be observed in 70% of cases in children [7], but almost never over the age of 40 [19] except in rare cases [47]. The bone scan has good sensitivity: 95% [19] to 100% [32], but very poor specificity of between 66 and 80% [32].

Diagnostic difficulties

The diagnostic difficulties are as numerous as the clinical forms of the disease [7, 19]. The pseudo-inflammatory aspects may suggest septic, inflammatory or microcrystalline arthritis but the absence of laboratory evidence of an inflammatory syndrome helps to rectify the diagnosis. Hot or cold vascular forms sometimes mimic a thrombophlebitis, a diagnosis which must be absolutely excluded at the outset [18], as must an arterial ischemia, exceptionally an acute form [13] but more often chronic with intermittent claudication [7]. Doppler velocimetry or exceptionally arteriography [13] shows no thrombosis but a very narrowed distal arterial system. Locally, migratory forms mimicking recurrent disease [9, 34] have been discovered by bone scintigraphy; a completely recovered episode may seem to recur clinically in the same region of the foot, but bone scintigraphy shows extinction of the initial focal hyperfixation and the appearance of a new focus indicating a new clinical episode. Initially multifocal forms involving the homolateral knee and/or hip are clinically detected in 19% of cases, radiologically in 27% and by scintigraphy in 39% [19]; exceptional extensive forms involving the limbs, vertebral column and thorax lead to consideration of a possible paraneoplastic etiology [6, 14].

Clinical, isotopic and follow-up data facilitate the diagnosis in cases with no radiologic signs throughout the disease, especially in children or young adults [15]. The isotopic hypofixation forms must not be mistakenly interpreted as indicating pathological "hyperfixation" in the opposite sound limb, nor as due to lack of walking on the involved limb (use of crutches); hypofixation forms occur primarily in young people and children (70% of cases) [15], and only exceptionally in adults [47]. All partial forms may involve one ray of the foot (tarso-metatarso-phalangeal ray); patchy forms affect a small part of the bone or a small bone like the cuboid or sesamoids [10], when an intense and very localized hyperfixation is associated later with local demineralization that may subsequently spread to the entire foot [8]. Forms limited to the sesamoids occur in only 2% of foot algodystrophies [19]. These partial or patchy forms may suggest a tumor (osteoid osteoma with nocturnal pain, localized hyperfixation, dramatic effect of aspirin or nonsteroidal anti-inflammatory drugs) or aseptic bone necrosis (talus, sesamoids) characterized by an intense and localized hyperfixation with surrounding demineralization, subsequently associated with patchy osteosclerosis or a stress fracture which is detected by MRI and which may complicate algodystrophy [35, 49].

Algodystrophy in children is characterized by the greater frequency of cold ischemic forms which are directly apparent at the onset of the disease, by hypofixation (70% of cases) and by the virtual absence of radiologic signs (70% of cases) [15]; when present, these radiologic signs often appear as clear metaphyseal bands [4]. In cases of a painful foot of apparently normal clinical aspect [19, 48], hysteria or even malingering may have to be considered even if the foot is cold and painful, and even if there is cutaneous hyperesthesia and no radiologic features; scintigraphy then often corrects this diagnosis by revealing a suggestive hypofixation.

Diagnosis

A group of associated features serves to confirm the diagnosis of algodystrophy: clinical features, laboratory data (no evidence of inflammation), radiologic signs (demineralization but never joint-space narrowing), isotopic data (hyper- or hypofixation), course of the disease (recovery without sequelae or with only moderate sequelae). These diagnostic criteria [7] are useful in difficult cases; the best is complete recovery with no recurrence of disease.

● Clinical course

The disease course is shortened by treatment. Algodystrophy generally recovers, even without treatment but sometimes with sequelae: slow disappearance of pain authorizes progressive weight-bearing and/or use of the involved limb, trophic signs decrease and full joint mobility returns gradually. The duration of foot algodystrophy is about one year in 75% of cases [20], sometimes two years or more. It is significantly longer in post-traumatic forms than in non-traumatic forms [20, 38]. If an accident at work (with insurance compensation) is the cause of post-traumatic disease, the course duration is identical [20], shorter [38] or longer [26] than in cases of other post-traumatic algodystrophies. In the post-traumatic algodystrophies the presence of psychological disorders is accompanied by a significantly longer disease duration than when these are absent [20]. Sequelae are moderate or severe (soft tissue contracture, or localized joint stiffness) and are present in 4.6% [20] to 46% [38] of cases according to two retrospective studies [20, 38]. Painful, intermittent and capricious discomfort, without disability, may persist for months or years [7, 38]. Local clinical recurrence when progressive walking begins may exceptionally be due to stress fracture (because of local bone insufficiency) and not necessarily to locally migratory algodystrophy. In such a case MRI is a good diagnostic procedure during the disease course, showing a (T1) linear hyposignal [35, 49]. These fractures can occur at the same site as a previous episode of algodystrophy cured many years ago [44]. In general, normal life is possible on average 5-6 months after the phase of drug treatment [20].

Treatment

The aim of physical treatment and correct positioning [51] is to combat stasis and pain by non-weight-bearing on the involved limb and bed rest with the distal extremity elevated, postural drainage favoring the venous circulation. Walking has to be limited to the strict minimum and is aided by crutches. Hyperesthesia prohibits any contact with clothes or bedclothes. Passive mobilization is impossible because of the pain and active mobilization must be controlled by the patient himself in order to keep it below the pain threshold. Massage to encourage lymphatic drainage from the involved region, cold or warm hydrotherapy or in alternation at a few minutes' interval can be useful when they are tolerated. The aim of postural casts, if tolerated despite pain, is to prevent the onset of vicious postures. Percutaneous nerve electrostimulation is sometimes useful in children [2].

Systemic drugs against vasomotor disturbances

Calcitonin is given by intramuscular or subcutaneous injection (160 UI/d of porcine calcitonin or the equivalent dose of any other calcitonin) for 15-20 days; longer treatment does not give better results [7]. 60 to 70% of good results are obtained [7, 22, 26] whatever the clinical form and disease duration may be before treatment [20]. Nausea, vomiting and flushes interrupt the treatment in only 8% of cases and are prevented by antiemetic drugs and by giving the calcitonin late in the evening. Allergy to calcitonin is a rare contra-indication.

Beta-blockers are sympatholytic drugs used in dosages giving a heart rate of about 55-60/min. Good results are obtained in 60 to 80% of cases [7, 26]. They are well tolerated in the absence of contraindications.

Griseofulvin is given orally in a daily dose of 50 mg/kg, i.e., some three times greater than in the treatment of mycosis; this daily dosage can induce headache or, exceptionally, a leukopenia which requires interruption of this treatment.

General analgesics

Paracetamol is useful; nonsteroidal anti-inflammatory drugs and corticotherapy are illogical and ineffective, except sometimes for pain. Tricyclic antidepressants and other psychotonic drugs have a very good action on the pain center of the brain; if necessary, they can be combined with anxiolytics and they can be used in children, either alone or associated with other general treatments.

Local and locoregional treatment

Local corticosteroids (intra-articular or intra-canalar) have only an analgesic, vasoactive and anti-fibrotic effect [31, 51].

Regional sympathetic block by reserpine, buflomedil [24] or guanethidine [23], is carried out in special centers: 1 or 2 weekly blocks, 6 at most in ordinary cases [20]. The risk of these blocks (especially with guanethidine) is an increase of pain due to the use of a tourniquet for 20 to 30 min and a possible severe fall of blood-pressure on removal of the tourniquet [23]. The contraindications are arteriopathy, coronaropathy, cardiac rhythm disturbances, venous disorders. Positive results are obtained immediately in 70 to 80% of cases [20, 25] and may be even better six months later [25]. In 17% of cases sympathetic block has to be stopped because of a paradoxical worsening of the algodystrophy or because of intolerance: immediate local pain, transient fall in blood-pressure, severe headache and, exceptionally, prolonged sinus bradycardia, thrombophlebitis or acute reversible ischemia of the treated limb without thrombosis [23].

Intra-arterial injections (femoral artery) of lidocaine and buflomedil may be efficient [20, 40] and are used before regional sympathetic block; their true efficacy is unknown because of the absence of controlled studies.

Management of treatment

Avoidance of weight-bearing and prevention of vicious postures are necessary (protection against bedclothes; postural splints if possible) during the attack phase of treatment (1st-20th day). Calcitonin is chosen first [7, 19], but beta-blockers or griseofulvin are preferred to calcitonin when the clinical form seems to call for caution [20]. A change of drug is often necessary after calcitonin treatment: beta-blockers or griseofulvin in moderate cases or regional sympathetic block in more severe forms [20, 23]. Progressive weight-bearing in the swimming-pool is prescribed by many authors [7, 51] at the end of this phase (21st-60th day).

During the second phase of treatment beta-blockers or griseofulvin are combined for 1 or 2 months with hydrotherapy and self-controlled rehabilitation of the patient without provoking pain by motion. Psychiatric help is often useful, especially for children [15]. The return to a normal family and occupational life is very gradual.

Does a preventive treatment exist?

No possibility exists of preventing the onset of algodystrophy, especially in the field of orthopedic surgery; a controlled study has shown the failure of calcitonin used as preventive treatment [45]. The only possibility is to make the earliest possible diagnosis in an orthopedic context; bone scintigraphy is one of the best means for early detection.

● Conclusion

Foot algodystrophy is a disease of various forms in which diagnosis is difficult, but in which bone scintigraphy is the best additional diagnostic examination. The functional and social prognosis of the disease is uncertain because its average duration is one year. Drug therapy and physical treatment are a powerful combination used to shorten the duration of the disease.

References

1. Amor B, Tallet F, Raichvarg D, Guenee B, de Gery A, Damak A, Kharrat A, Ekindjian OG (1982) Algodystrophie et anomalies métaboliques. Rev Rhum 49: 827-833
2. Ashwal A, Tomasi L, Neumann M, Schneider S (1988) Reflex sympathetic dystrophy syndrome in children. Pediatr Neurol 44: 38-42
3. Bernstein BH, Singsen BH, Kent JJ, Kornreich H, King K, Hicks R, Hanson U (1978) Reflex neurovascular dystrophy in childhood. J Pediatr 93: 211-215
4. Betend B, Lebacq E, Kohler R, David L (1981) Ostéolyse métaphysaire: aspect inhabituel de l'algodystrophie de l'enfant. Arch Fr Pediatr 38: 121-123
5. Bouvier M, Lejeune E, Bocquet B, Richard D (1973) Circonstances d'apparition des algoneurodystrophies (à propos d'une série personnelle de 100 observations). Rhumatologie 25: 27-32
6. Cerf I, Hilliquin P, Blanche P, Renoux M, Menkes CJ (1992) Algodystrophie extensive des membres inférieurs associée à un carcinome bronchique. Rev Rhum 59: 296-297
7. Doury P, Dirheimer Y, Pattin S (1981) Algodystrophy. Diagnosis and therapy of a frequent disease of the locomotor apparatus. Springer Verlag, Berlin
8. Doury P (1982) Les formes atypiques partielles, parcellaires et infraradiologiques des algodystrophies. Rev Rhum 49: 781-786
9. Doury P, Pattin S, Eulry F, Granier R, Gaillard JF, Maurel Ch, Masson Ch (1984) Algodystrophie des pieds localement migratrice. Intérêt de la scintigraphie osseuse. Médecine et Chirurgie du Pied 1: 59-63
10. Doury P, Eulry F, Pattin S (1984) L'algodystrophie des sésamoides du gros orteil. Médecine et Chirurgie du Pied 1: 55-58
11. Doury P, Paffin S, Eulry F (1985) L'atteinte des tendons au cours de l'algodystrophie. Sem Hop Paris, 61: 1627-1632
12. Doury P, Meyer R, Eulry F, Pattin S, Kuntz JL, Asch L (1986) Algodystrophies du pied secondaires à des arthrites septiques. À propos de 4 observations. Médecine et chirurgie du Pied 8: 125-128
13. Doury P, Paffin S, Eulry F, Vasseur Ph, Clément R, Metges PJ, Flageat J, Brunot J (1987) Algodystrophie sévère du pied simulant une artériopathie ischémique. Guérison spectaculaire par bloc régional à la guanéthidine. Ann Med interne (Paris) 138: 45-8
14. Doury P, Wendling D, Pattin S, Eulry F, Delmaire P, Aboukrat P, Rolland Y, Leleoire O (1987) Algodystrophies sévères et tumeurs malignes. À propos de 4 observations. Rev Rhum 54
15. Doury P, Paffin S, Gaillard JF, Eulry F, Paffin C (1988) L'algodystrophie de l'enfant. Ann Pédiatr (Paris) 35: 469-475
16. Doury P, Wendling D, Pattin S, Prost A, Eulry F, Granier R, Sereni D, Gaillard JF, Garrouste O (1988) L'hypofixation isotopique dans les algodystrophies. Sem Hop Paris 64: 1287-1292
17. Eulry F, Pattin S, Doury P (1986) Algodystrophie et maladie de Morton. Médecine et Chirurgie du Pied, 2: 39-41
18. Eulry F, Chazerain P, Magnin J, Demazière A, Clément R, Chanudet X, Pattin S, Doury P (1989) Algodystrophie et thromboses veineuses des membres inférieurs: problèmes diagnostiques (à propos de 5 observations). Rev Rhum 56: 403-407
19. Eulry F, Aczel F, Vasseur P, Pattin S, Vicens JL, Flageat J, Gaillard F, Doury P (1990) L'algodystrophie du Pied. À propos de 199 observations. Rev Rhum 57: 351-356
20. Eulry F, Aczel F, Vasseur Ph, Thomas E, Pattin S, Doury P (1990) Traitement et évolution de l'algodystrophie du pied. Étude rétrospective de 199 observations. Ann Med Interne (Paris) 141: 20-25

21. Eulry F, Chevalier X, Crozes Ph, Chevalier D, Magnin J, Prudat M, Patoz B, Larget-Piet B (1992) Les lipides plasmatiques dans l'algodystrophie: étude à propos de 90 observations. Rev Rhum 59: 721-727

22. Eulry F, Doury P, Lechevalier D, Magnin J, Crozes Ph (1993) Le traitement de l'algodystrophie post-traumatique du pied par la calcitonine injectable. Médecine et Chirurgie du Pied 9: 89-92

23. Eulry F, Lechevalier D, Pats B, Alliaume C, Crozes Ph, Vasseur P, Coutant G, Felten D, Pattin S (1991) Regional intravenous guanethidine blocks in algodystrophy. Clin Rheumatol 10: 377-383

24. Farcot JM, Grasser C, Foucher G, Marin-Braun F, Ehrler S, Demangeat JL, Constantinesco A (1990) Traitements locaux intraveineux des algodystrophies de la main: buflomédil versus guanéthidine, suivi à long terme. Ann Chir Main 9: 296-304

25. Field J, Atkins RM (1993) Effect of guanethidine on the natural history of post-traumatic algodystrophy. Ann Rheum Dis 52: 467-469

26. Friez L, Pere G, Breuillard P, Meignan S (1982) Comparaison du traitement par la griséfuline, les bêtabloquants et la calcitonine dans 55 cas d'algoneurodystrophie post-traumatique. Rev Rhum 49: 857-860

27. Goldsmith DP, Vivino FB, Eichenfield AH, Athreya BH, Heyman S (1989) Nuclear imaging and clinical features of childhood reflex neurovascular dystrophy: comparison with adults. Arthritis Rheum 32: 480-485

28. Gougeon J, Eschard JP, Moreau-Hottin J, Françon J, David-Chaussoe J, Doury P (1982) Les algodystrophies : évolution, formes polyarticulaires, formes à épisodes multiples. Rev Rhum (Paris) 49: 809-814

29. Hannequin JR, Dirheimer Y, Schvingt E, Schmutz G (1986) L'association arthrite-algodystrophie. J Med Strasbourg 17: 549-552

30. Hauzeur JP, Hanquinet S, Genevois PA, Appelboom T, Bentin J, Perlmuter N (1991) Study of magnetic resonance imaging in transient osteoporosis of the hip. J Rheumatol 18: 1211-1217

31. Hérisson Ch, Simon L (1987) Les algodystrophies sympathiques réflexes: une entité. In: Simon L et Hérisson C (eds) Les algodystrophies sympathiques réflexes. Masson, Paris, p 1

32. Holder LE, Cole LA, Myerson MS (1992) Reflex sympathetic dystrophy in the foot: clinical and scintigraphic criteria Radiology 184: 531-535

33. Huaux JP, Malghem J, Maldague B, Devogelaer JP, Esselnckx W, Withofs H, Nagant de Deuxchaisnes (1986) Reflex sympathetic dystrophy syndrome: an unusual mode of presentation of osteomalacia. Arthritis Rheum 29: 918-925

34. Lechevalier D, Crozes Ph, Thomachot B, Magnin J, Doury P, Eulry F (1992) Epiphyseal migration of abnormalities in algodystrophy: the role of bone scintigraphy. J Rheumatol 19: 1486-1487

35. Lechevalier D, Haguenauer D, Dellestable F, Magnin J, Eulry F (1993) Algodystrophie post-traumatique du pied compliquée d'une fracture de l'astragale. Médecine et chirurgie du pied 9: 85-87

36. Mackinnon S, Holder L (1984) The use of three phase radionuelide bone scanning in the diagnosis of reflex sympathetic distrophy. J Hand Surg 9A: 556-563

37. Malkin LH (1990) Reflex sympathetic dystrophy syndrome following trauma to the foot. Orthopedics 13: 851-858

38. May V, Glowinski J (1983) Les séquelles de l'algodystrophie: manifestations cliniques et retentissement socio-professionnel et médico-légal. "R" 13: 355-361

39. Michel Ch, Casillas JM, Giraud JC, Taurand J (1993) Foot algodystrophy following arterial surgery. Rev Rhum (Engl edn) 60: 445-456

40. Queinnec JY, Vilayleck S, Bregeon C, Renier JC (1985) Traitement des algodystrophies du membre inférieur par infiltration intra-artérielle de lidocaïne et buflomédil. Apports de l'angioscintigraphie. Rev Rhum 37: 33-36

41. Ravault PP, Maitrepierre J, Riffat G (1959) Le pied décalcifié douloureux idiopathique (ou ostéoporose algique essentielle du pied). Rev Rhum 26: 393-407

42. Renier JC, Arlet J, Bregeon Ch, Baslem, Seret P (1983) L'articulation dans l'algodystrophie. Le liquide articulaire, la synoviale, le cartilage. Rev Rhum 50: 255-260

43. Renier JC (1992) Les algodystrophies: trois décennies de progrès. Laboratoires Ciba-Geigy, Rueil-Malmaison

44. Renier JC, Baslé M, Masson Ch, Brégeon Ch, Audran M (1993) Regional migratory osteoporosis complicated with stress fractures. Rev Rhum (Engl edn) 60: 383-386

45. Riou C, Daoudi Y, Langlais F, Pawlotsky Y, Cheverry C (1991) L'algodystrophie en milieu chirurgical peut-elle être prévenue par la thyrocalcitonine? Rev Chir Orthop 77: 208-210

46. Schwartzman RJ, McLellan TL (1987) Reflex sympathetic dystrophy. A review. Arch Neurol 44: 555-561

47. Sereni D, Khalifa P, Richard B, Doury P, Cremer GA (1987) Algodystrophie de l'adulte avec hypofixation à la scintigraphie osseuse par le méthylène-diphosphonate de technétium-99m. Rev Rhum 54: 767-769

48. Serre H, Simon L, Claustre J, Sany J (1973) Formes cliniques des algodystrophies sympathiques des membres inférieurs. Rhumatologie 23: 43-54

49. Sibilia J, Javier RM, Durckel J, Krause D, Kuntz JL (1994): Fissure of the navicular bone in a patient with reflex sympathetic dystrophy syndrome: diagnostic value of magnetic resonance imaging. Rev Rhum (Engl edn), 61: 51-53

50. Silbert J, Majd M (1988) Reflex sympathetic dystrophy syndrome in children and adolescents. Report of 18 cases and review of the literature. Am J Dis Child, 142: 1325-1330

51. Simon L, Blotman F, Leroux JL, Claustre J, Azema MT, Brun-Meyer M (1982) Rééducation et algodystrophie. Rev Rhum 49: 861-865

52. Sudeck P (1901) Uber die akute reflektorische Knochenatrophie nach Entzundungen und Verletzungen an der Extremitaten und ihre klinischen Erscheinungen. Fortschr Geb Roentgenstr 5: 277-293

15.

Valgus flat foot and tarsal fusions

Ch Piat and D Goutallier

Definition

The flat foot (pes planus) can be defined as decrease, collapse or inversion of the medial longitudinal arch of the foot. This deformity is sufficient in itself to establish the diagnosis of flat foot, whatever the associated deformities of the forefoot or hindfoot.

The flat foot may be static, that is apparently primary, in origin. More rarely, it follows injury or a rheumatic or neurologic disorder or is the sequel of a congenital deformity. In exceptional instances, it may be related to a hereditary disorder such as Marfan's syndrome, Ehler-Danlos syndrome or the fragile-X syndrome [10] (table 15.1). The deformity appears under the strains of weight-bearing and so the diagnosis of flat foot can only be made when a child has reached walking age. In practice, the term of flat foot cannot be used before the age of three years. Flat foot is a relatively rare disorder which affects only 1 to 3% of the adult population according to the series.

Characteristics

The characteristic of flat foot is collapse of the longitudinal plantar arch. Anatomically, this collapse is reflected by sagittal and frontal malalignment of the talometatarsal axis, generally overlying the talonavicular joint-space. The cuneonavicular or more rarely the cuneometatarsal joint may also be the site

Table 15.1. Secondary valgus flat feet

Neurologic diseases	• Poliomyelitis sequelae • Spastic paralysis • Myopathy	• Spina bifida • Peripheral neuropathy
Traumatic sequelae	• Calcaneal fracture • Bi-malleolar fracture with valgus deformation • Tarsometatarsal fracture dislocation	• Midtarsal sprain • Tarsal dislocation
Rheumatic diseases	• Rheumatoid arthritis • Rupture of the tendon of the tibialis posterior muscle • Midtarsal arthritis	
Congenital diseases	• Talus foot • Convex foot • Surgical hypercorrection of a varus equinus foot	• Tarsal fusions
Other diseases	• Marfan's syndrome • Ehler-Danlos syndrome • Fragile X syndrome	

of malalignment of the medial longitudinal arch. Collapse of the plantar arch is associated with numerous other basic deformities which are always present in the valgus flat foot and which can be interpreted as cause or consequence of this collapse [12, 14, 20, 27, 35]. The following phenomena can be observed:

• hindfoot valgus of more than 10° with calcaneal pronation. The degree of calcaneal deformity is proportional to talometatarsal malalignment. The valgus attitude can be considered as a constant element of the deformity;

• increase in talocalcaneal divergence and forward displacement of the talus in relation to the calcaneus;

• relative lengthening of the medial column, which is increased by backward displacement of the calcaneus and cuboid bone;

• tibiotalar equinus deformity;

• shortening of the lateral column

• forefoot deformity in compensatory supination and abduction which has the effect of increasing the valgus attitude and collapse of the medial arch;

• abnormal bone shape, particularly of the talus, with increased length of the talar neck and increased inclination (normal range 115°-120°) and declination (normal range 150°-160°) (figs. 15.1 & 15.2). The navicular bone is also abnormal in shape, with an elongated and hypertrophic medial part and tuberosity;

• abnormal torsion of the lower limbs, where the main factor is forward displacement of the axis between the two malleoli, the lateral malleolus being brought relatively forward by the downward movement of the talus.

Each of these individual deformities aggravates and increases the flat foot.

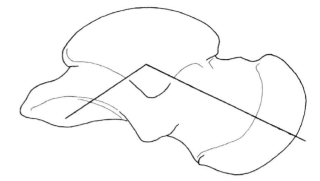

Fig. 15.1. Talus, lateral aspect; angle of inclination

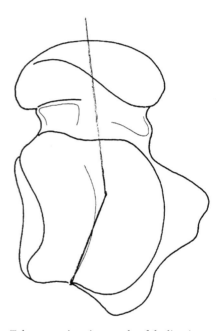

Fig. 15.2. Talus, superior view; angle of declination

● Pathomechanics

In the normal state, in a subject standing on both feet, the medial longitudinal arch is linear even when the muscles are not contracted. The static triangular arrangement described by De Doncker is maintained by the posterior components (talocalcaneal column) and anterior components of the triangle (navicular, cuboid, intermediate and lateral cuneiforms, second and third metatarsals) linked by their joints, capsules and ligaments, while the middle plantar fascia forms the base [12, 14].

Experimental studies of serial sections of plantar support components in cadaveric feet have shown that the main stabilizer is the plantar fascia, followed by the talonavicular and calcaneonavicular ligaments [11, 21]. In the flat foot, collapse of the normal medial longitudinal arch is related to mechanical insufficiency of the capsular and ligamentous components which normally maintain the curve of the arch.

Musculotendinous components also help to support the arch. They play a role in the development of deformity, as shown by the high incidence of bony anomalies of the navicular insertion of the tibialis posterior muscle in flat foot and by the increased activity seen on electromyography of the muscles which accentuate the arch (intrinsic and tibialis posterior muscles). Lastly, a valgus flat foot may develop after rupture of the tendon of the tibialis posterior muscle. Another possibility is lack of tone of the extrinsic muscles which maintain the foot in varus (tibialis posterior and flexor hallucis longus) and increased tone of the evertor muscles fibularis brevis and longus) which abduct the forefoot, lengthen the medial arch, shorten the lateral arch, pronate the calcaneus and bring the lateral malleolus forward. However, the role of the fibularis longus muscle is more debatable as its contraction lowers and gives a vertical angulation to the first metatarsal.

For Meary and Judet [27, 35], the heel valgus is primary and forces the talus, which is no longer supported, to slide progressively downwards, forwards and inwards, increasing talocalcaneal divergence and transmitting mechanical stresses preferentially towards the medial column, which is deformed secondarily. However, some feet have an isolated valgus deformity and do not become flat as long as the capsular, ligamentous and muscular components do not give way.

Forward displacement of the bimalleolar axis by voluntary forced torsion induces valgus angulation of the heel, inward and downward movement of the head of the talus, increased declination of the neck of the talus and abduction of the forefoot by torsion in the opposite direction. Conversely, external rotation of the axis of the leg produces the reverse deformity. Flat foot and increased anteversion of the femur are also frequently associated. However, the primary or secondary role of abnormal torsion in the origin of flat foot cannot be determined with any certainty.

Niederecker [31] has described numerous muscular anomalies in valgus flat foot, such as the presence of a third peroneal muscle which inserts on the shaft of the fifth metatarsal or an abnormally anterior insertion of the tibialis anterior muscle tendon on the first metatarsal, which could be responsible for the deformity.

A shortened calcaneal tendon has also frequently been reported as a possible cause of the deformity, by inducing a horizontal attitude of the calcaneus and pronation which leads to hindfoot valgus and forefoot abduction. Shortness of this tendon is certainly an aggravating factor by limiting talocrural dorsiflexion. Limitation of dorsiflexion of the foot increases the demands on the tibialis ante-rior muscle, aggravating the flat foot by inducing a horizontal and pronated attitude of the calcaneus. Also, the horizontal and valgus angulation of the calcaneus increases the power of the triceps surae muscle by shortening its active moment and has a permanent valgus effect on the calcaneus. In such forms, the calcaneus is more horizontal than would be expected from the degree of flat foot deformity [14].

In the vast majority of cases, flat foot either affects the left foot only or is bilateral but more marked in the left foot. The predominance of the left foot would appear to reflect an asymmetric distribution of forces during weight-bearing [3]. This phenomenon is a reminder that it is weight-bearing and axial constraints which lead to the development of flat foot [22].

Opinions differ as to the influence of footwear. According to accepted opinion, shoes with rigid soles, a high upper and a good shank should be worn to prevent deformity. However, in a recent study of three populations of children who habitually went unshod, wore slippers or sandals, or leather shoes, Rao [34] showed that the incidence of flat foot increased with the rigidity of the footwear.

In many instances there is no obvious cause and in subjects with flat feet, diffuse decreased muscle tone is observed together with joint laxity, genu valgum, dorsal kyphosis and obesity.

In summary, static valgus flat foot appears to be related to the conjunction of ligamentous laxity, neuromuscular anomaly and bone and joint imbalance, of which hindfoot valgus is the main element.

Congenital tarsal fusions are often associated with valgus flat foot. The fusion may be calcaneonavicular, between the calcaneal tuberosity and the posteromedial edge of the navicular bone, or talocalcaneal, between the sustentaculum tali and the medial portion of the talus.

Tarsal fusions consist of a fibrous (synfibrosis), cartilaginous (synchondrosis) or bony bridge (synostosis proper) joining at least two of the tarsal bones. They are frequent, affecting 1 to 2% of the population, but the majority (70%) remain asymptomatic and are perfectly well tolerated, accounting for the small numbers in the series studied [28, 36]. Fifty-three percent of fusions are calcaneonavicular and 37% talocalcaneal. Other sites have been described: talonavicular, calcaneocuboid, cuboidonavicular and cuneonavicular, which are rarely associated with valgus flat foot.

Fusions are located in areas where sesamoid bones and accessory ossicles are found, and it has been suggested that they correspond to abnormal fusion of these ossicles. They may be associated with other congenital malformations in a multiple deformity syndrome. They have been described in the fetus before birth as a result of failure of mesenchymal segmentation, which is generally completed at the eighth week of life in utero. Familial forms of this disorder also exist. Fusions appear to be a hereditary congenital unifactorial malformation with an autosomal-dominant pattern of inheritance with high penetrance. They are bilateral in 50% of cases [28].

Numerous clinical forms of fusion have been reported. However, it is noteworthy that valgus flat foot is associated with calcaneonavicular and talocalcaneal fusions [26, 33].

The presence of a fusion at the center of rotation is revealed by decreased mobility, especially in dorsiflexion of the foot, during which the talus normally moves posteriorly and sagittally and rotates in relation to the calcaneus. When this movement is limited, it is compensated by lengthening of the talonavicular axis, abduction of the calcaneus and increase of the active moment of the fibular muscles [26, 28]. The various elements of the flat foot gradually develop and the earlier stiffness sets in, the more marked the deformity. Fusions become symptomatic when they lead to decreased mobility and valgus deviation of the hindfoot. This generally occurs at adolescence through ossification of the fibrous or cartilaginous bridge which varies according to the type of fusion [18]. In the early stages, the bridge remains fibrous or cartilaginous and allows a certain degree of mobility, accounting for the tolerance of the deformity.

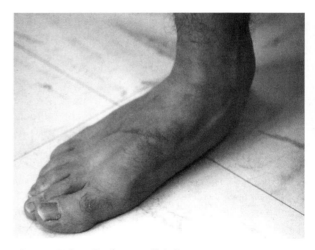

Fig. 15.3. Valgus flat foot: medial view

● Clinical examination

The gait and footwear of the patient and his (or her) foot should be examined in static and dynamic positions. A general examination should then be carried out to search for a possible cause or association with another pathology.

A weight-bearing profile view of the medial aspect of the foot shows collapse of the longitudinal arch (normal range 13-16 mm) (fig. 15.3). The middle part of the medial edge of the foot comes into contact with the ground. The talar head and sometimes the navicular tuberosity can be seen projecting downwards and forwards, forming a double or triple medial malleolus. Sometimes the tibialis anterior muscle can be seen to contract intermittently, resisting plantar collapse.

A dorso-plantar view shows malalignment of the medial tarso-metatarso-phalangeal axis, which is normally rectilinear. This malalignment is revealed by forward abduction in relation to the hindfoot, relative lengthening of the medial edge of the foot, a protruding navicular tuberosity, medial spread of the midfoot and sometimes early signs of hallux valgus. Reduced external rotation of the tibia is revealed by a forward shift of the lateral malleolus.

A posterior view shows decreased height of the hindfoot and above all heel valgus with an angle of more than 10° between the calcaneal tendon and the upper tuberosity (fig. 15.4).

When a fusion is present, limitation of subtalar and mediotarsal mobility may be slight but it increases as the fusion becomes ossified. Any rigidity immediately suggests the presence of a fusion. When the foot is inverted, the fibular muscles may attempt to contract, which also strongly suggests this diagnosis [26]. Tarsal fusion should also be sought if there is lack of response to conservative management or aggravation of flat foot during growth.

After examination of the weight-bearing foot, the correctibility of the deformity can be evaluated passively by letting the foot dangle, which should

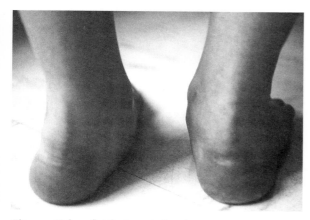

Fig. 15.4. Valgus flat foot: posterior view

totally or partially correct the flat foot and valgus attitude. Correctibility can also be actively assessed by voluntary contraction of the intrinsic, flexor hallucis and tibialis posterior muscles. The valgus flat foot can also be corrected by external rotation of the bimalleolar axis and correction of calcaneal valgus. The flexibility of the various components of the deformity is obviously of prognostic and therapeutic importance, making a satisfactory result of conservative or surgical treatment more likely. Talocrural mobility should also be examined to look for a shortened calcaneal tendon, together with mobility of the subtalar and mediotarsal joints, balance of the forefoot in pronation-supination and excessive joint laxity. The mobility of these joints should be of normal or even more than normal range. If this is not the case, a tarsal fusion may well be present. The foot-progression angle, abnormal rotation and deviations from normal angulation of the lower limbs (genu valgum or more frequently varum) should also be sought. Lastly, a general examination is carried out to search for another etiology, neurologic in particular, or for associated lesions.

● Radiographic investigation

Technique

Radiographic investigation of flat foot includes the standard lateral and dorsoplantar weight-bearing views, preferably of both limbs on the same film,

and a 45-degree oblique view. These three projections confirm the diagnosis of flat foot and evaluate its severity. Other projections can be useful especially if surgical treatment is being considered: non-weight-bearing lateral view, circled anteroposterior view (Meary's projection), lateral view in dorsiflexion then in maximum plantarflexion, then an ascending retrotibial view to look for talocalcaneal fusion, and lastly the specific views described by Harris [19, 22].

This standard radiographic investigation may be completed by CT of the hindfoot, which is particularly useful to look for tarsal fusion or an associated tendon or ligament disorder. MRI is of special value in juxta-articular pathology, particularly of the tendon of the tibialis posterior muscle.

Results

A lateral view makes it possible to measure the talometatarsal axis, look for malalignment, locate it and measure it in degrees (fig. 15.5). Talocalcaneal divergence, normally between 20° and 30°, can also be assessed and measured, together with the angle of the medial arch, the vertical position of the talus and the horizontal position of the calcaneus, decrease in

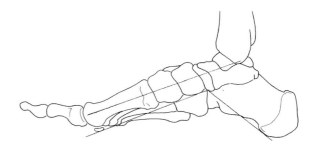

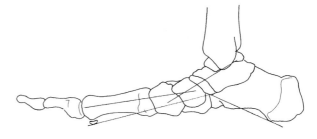

Fig. 15.5. Malalignment of the talar-first metatarsal axis in flat foot

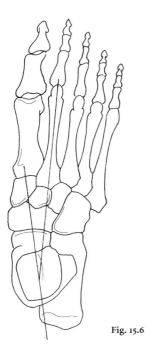

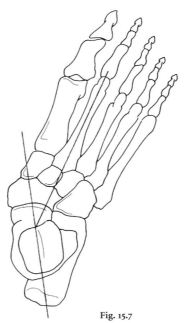

Fig. 15.6

Fig. 15.7

Fig. 15.6. Measurement of abduction of the normal forefoot (angle between the talar and second metatarsal axes)

Fig. 15.7. Measurement of abduction in the flat forefoot (angle between the talar and second metatarsal axes)

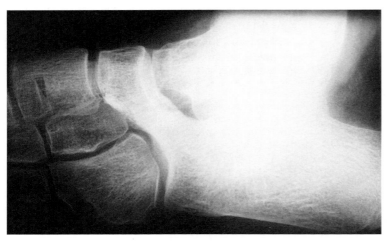

Fig. 15.8. Radiograph: calcaneonavicular fusion

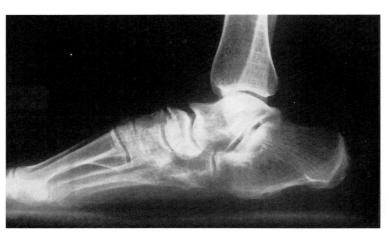

Fig. 15.9. Radiograph: flat foot with talocalcaneal fusion; opposing talonavicular and cuneonavicular bone spur

the slope of the first metatarsal, excessive anteromedial pressure arising secondarily from forefoot supination, superimposition of the navicular and cuboid,
and lastly, indirect visualization of frontal displacement of the bimalleolar mortice by forward shift of
the lateral malleolus. Degenerative arthritic changes
should also be sought, in particular at the talonavicular joint-space.

On the anteroposterior dorsoplantar view, talocalcaneal divergence is measured (normal range 15°
to 25°), and forefoot abduction due to deviation of
the axis of the second metatarsal and the talus
arising in the cuneonavicular, cuneometatarsal and
talonavicular joints (figs. 15.6 & 15.7). Talar declination can be measured and any navicular abnormalities such as an accessory navicular can be seen.

The circled anteroposterior view evaluates the
degree of hindfoot valgus and may sometimes secondarily show signs of subtalar fusion or a fusion
directly opposite the sustentaculum tali.

The 45-degree oblique view reveals any navicular
anomalies, the presence of calcaneonavicular or
more rarely cuboidocalcaneal fusion, and lastly early
osteoarthrosis.

Non-weight-bearing views evaluate the correctibility of each of the above deformities if equivalent
weight-bearing views are available for comparison.

When assessing the severity of deformity, it
should be borne in mind that calcaneal valgus and
forefoot abduction increase malalignment and thus
increase the magnitude of flat foot deformity, at least
as visualized on radiographs. If these two deformities seem marked, it may be useful to obtain
further lateral weight-bearing views after correcting
hindfoot valgus and forefoot abduction by centering
the beam differently.

Tarsal fusions may be revealed directly (fig. 15.8)
or by secondary signs. These are an opposing talonavicular bone spur, still called a talar beak (fig. 15.9),
bar-shaped thickening of the talar neck, widening of
the medial part of the subtalar joint-space whereas
the rest of the joint is narrowed, and hypertrophy of
the calcaneal tuberosity [28, 40]. Secondarily, the
adaptive changes arising from fusion lead to a
domed talus (fig. 15.10) and deformities of the malleolar mortice.

Direct evidence of fusion, a bony bridge or
synotosis, can be visualized on standard radiographs and on the specific projections which have
been clearly described by Harris [19]. If a bony
bridge is present, dorsoplantar anteroposterior

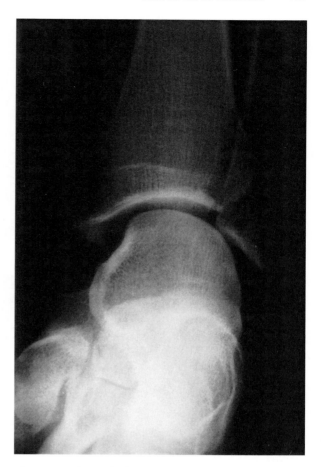

Fig. 15.10. Radiograph: domed talus

views with an oblique beam at 30° and 40° may be
necessary for direct visualization. Talocalcaneal
fusions may begin to ossify from the age of ten
years, calcaneonavicular fusions (fig. 15.8) at the age
of eight, and talonavicular fusions from the age of
three [28] (fig. 15.11). Frontal and especially sagittal
plane CT may also directly or indirectly show the
fusion as a continuous bony bridge, or as a distinct
irregularity with narrowing of part of the joint
surface [18, 40]. Reconstructed images may be easier
to interpret. CT also shows the uninvolved joint
surface.

The diagnosis of fibrous fusions or synchondroses may be suggested by standard radiographs or
by technetium bone scan, which shows focal
increased uptake, and above all by computed tomography which reveals the fibrous bridge and localized irregularities of the joint surface [26, 28] (fig.
15.12).

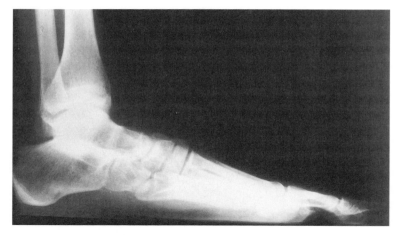

Fig. 15.11. Radiograph: talonavicular (and talocalcaneal) fusion

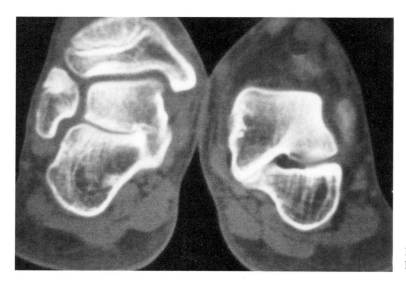

Fig. 15.12. CT scan. Right, talocalcaneal fusion; left, talocalcaneal synchondrosis

● Functional signs

During childhood, the static flat foot remains virtually asymptomatic. The functional complaint comes from parents concerned by the unpleasing appearance of the child's foot and gait, abnormal shoe wear or signs of hyperlaxity, and by the child's tendency to "lack of tone". The flat foot can also be detected by an anomaly of anteversion of the femoral neck, a tendency to walk with the feet turned inwards, genu valgum or a spinal deformity. In practice, during childhood the deformity is characterized by its painlessness.

If the foot is painful, a cause other than static deformity should be sought.

It is during adolescence and adulthood that certain flat feet become symptomatic, essentially through the onset of pain.

Medial pain syndrome

In the adult, this is related to involvement of the tendon of the tibialis posterior muscle, whether tendinopathy, enthesopathy, tenosynovitis or even rupture. This pathology is accompanied by swelling behind and under the medial malleolus, pain on palpation of the body of the tendon or at its insertion on the navicular tuberosity. Pain may also be produced during isometric resisted abduction and on maximal passive stretching. Pure synovitis may be seen, but is more often associated with tendon lesions such as fissures, general or nodular thickening of the tendon, or elongation.

Tendon rupture of the tibialis posterior muscle is highly symptomatic in most cases, with acute pain and sudden severe aggravation of hindfoot valgus and flat foot. Walking on tiptoe is either impossible or can only be achieved by abducting the forefoot and above all by placing the heel in valgus [4, 24, 29, 30]. The adductor muscles are also weakened and mediotarsal mobility increased. All these deformities are either unilateral or clearly asymmetric. Rupture is rarely located at the tendon insertion, but is more often under and behind the medial malleolus. At an early stage, loss of continuity of the tendon can be detected by palpation [4].

Sometimes, rupture is insidious; injury appears minimal or even absent and rupture is revealed secondarily by the asymmetric nature of the flat foot and by swelling behind and below the medial malleolus. The patient has suffered chronic pain or long-standing episodes of tenosynovitis and has already received corticosteroid injections. He or she may have no history of injury, even minor, and the condition is difficult to differentiate from tendinopathy. In such cases, CT with a soft tissue window may show signs indicating rupture. CT with contrast enhanced tenography and MRI, are sometimes more precise but difficult to interpret in long-standing cases.

Medial pain may also be located at the medial edge of the navicular if footwear impinges on the hypertrophic medial edge of this bone or an accessory navicular [22].

In the young subject, the medial pain syndrome presents differently. Pain is chronic, below and in front of the medial malleolus, aggravated by sport which becomes impossible. On examination, there is pain at the navicular insertion of the tendon of the tibialis posterior tendon and on passive eversion. Radiographs suggest "osteochondritis" of the medial tuberosity of the navicular or sesamoiditis of the tendon of the tibialis posterior muscle, and true fractures of the medial tuberosity have been described.

The painful contracted flat foot

In the adolescent, this is revealed by the sudden onset of an acute episode with limping, sharp anterolateral pain and permanent fixed valgus of the hindfoot. On examination, the fibular muscles (fibu-

laris brevis) and the extensor digitorum muscles are contracted. This contraction is permanent, painful and intractable. It is accompanied by stiffness of the center of rotation and fixed forefoot pronation.

In 61% of cases this involvement is associated with tarsal fusion [19, 46]. Even when the fusions are localized at the subtalar and mediotarsal center of rotation, they may be totally asymptomatic and therefore require no treatment [28]. When they ossify, fusions are generally revealed by limitation of mobility and midfoot or posterior tarsal pain produced on walking, on exertion and above all, on mobilization. This pain is alleviated by rest and aggravated by activity, sports in particular. Pain may be elicited by palpation of the fusion and attempts to mobilize the stiffened joint.

Pain of the subtalar and midtarsal center of rotation

This appears progressively due to ligament distension, in particular of the talonavicular ligament, then secondarily by arthrosis of the center of rotation which also originates at this joint. It is revealed by lateral or medial submalleolar pain aggravated on weight-bearing. Osteoarthrosis appears rapidly and is revealed on radiographs by an opposing talonavicular bone spur, exuberant in some cases, and lastly by joint-space narrowing, and occasionally microcavities. Mediotarsal osteoarthrosis is more likely if there is tarsal fusion which should again be sought.

Failure of compensatory mechanisms in the forefoot

The valgus flat foot may be accompanied by anteromedial or median metatarsal pain due to excessive anteromedial pressure or decompensation of a pre-existing rounded forefoot. Claw toe related to progressive insufficiency of the intrinsic muscles is frequent, as is hallux valgus arising from capsular and ligamentous failure, relative lengthening of the medial arch and preferential transmission of mechanical stresses to the medial edge of the foot [25].

Exceptionally, there may be valgus instability of the hindfoot when there is major calcaneal deformity and the malleolar axis has shifted only slightly forward. Callosities may form under the head of the talus in flat foot of long duration.

Evolution of symptoms with age

Childhood is characterized by the painless nature of the deformity, which remains flexible and partially or totally correctible. The parents are concerned because of the unpleasing nature of the deformity, the appearance of the foot when the child walks, and by early wear and deformation of the shoes.

Pain first appears at adolescence, with fatigue, after sports or prolonged standing. This pain is related to a medial navicular syndrome, subtalar ligament stretching, valgus instability or a contracted valgus flat foot. However, the deformity remains flexible. If it does not, a previously unsuspected fusion should be sought.

In the adult, the flat foot is generally well tolerated. Pain reappears after the age of 40 as a medial pain syndrome due to strain of the tendon of the tibialis posterior muscle or the navicular, or to forefoot decompensation with development of hallux valgus or anterior metatarsal pain. The pain is also related to capsular and ligamentous stretching which is permanent once a certain limit has been reached, or which extends to other capsular and ligamentous structures which were previously subjected to little stress. At a later stage, but relatively rarely, mediotarsal osteoarthrosis develops and the deformity gradually becomes fixed, but still painful.

Treatment

The principle of treatment of the static flat foot is to correct the primary deformity, in particular its cardinal elements (medial malalignment, calcaneal valgus, talocalcanear divergence), and to maintain the correction achieved while preserving as much joint motion as possible. In the child and adolescent, bone growth must be safeguarded.

● Conservative treatment

Plantar orthoses

Corrective orthoses

Corrective plantar orthoses are made of a relatively rigid material. A posterior supinator insert with a medial base corrects calcaneal valgus and may be sufficient in itself to correct medial arch collapse and restore normal pressure distribution. The anterior part either has a neutral support behind the metatarsal heads or a corrective support to induce forefoot pronation. This orthosis is suitable for a flexible, reducible foot with a medial arch which is effectively straightened when calcaneal valgus is corrected. It must be inserted in suitable footwear with a sufficiently wide heel and a proper counter. The sole and shoe should be checked for wear.

The orthosis should be replaced once a year and modified according to the evolution of the deformity. Tarsal fusion should be suspected if the foot is refractory to this treatment. Long-term results seem satisfactory but this dogma has been questioned by Wenger [45] in a comparative study of the efficacy of orthoses.

Compensatory orthoses

Here it is no longer a matter of correcting the deformity or one of its elements, but of inserting a padding material which adapts and molds itself to a fixed or partially fixed deformity. The medial arch must be supported by a half-dome and an insert must be designed to correct the deformity and progressive decompensation of the forefoot. The aim is to reduce the pain caused by ligamentous stretching and to obtain even distribution of pressure points.

This type of orthosis is used when compensatory mechanisms fail due to chronic capsular and ligamentous stretching, followed by later degenerative osteoarthritic changes in the flat foot.

Functional rehabilitation

The aim is to strengthen the muscles which act on the arch, increase proprioceptive control of the foot and stretch the contracted muscles. Functional rehabilitation is probably a useful aid in the management of flat foot. Improved tone of the muscles which maintain the curve of the medial arch (intrinsic muscles, fibularis longus) and the encouraging effect of such a rehabilitative program should bring about an improvement, but it is not always easy to put into practice with children.

Tarsal fusions

These may be treated by rest and restriction of painful activities. Manipulation in an attempt to free the fusion should be avoided. On the other hand, rehabilitation as tolerated, plantar orthoses and, if necessary, immobilization in a plaster cast, under anesthesia if the muscles are contracted, are indicated [9, 28].

Surgical treatment

The aim is to restore the medial arch, correct calcaneal valgus, reposition the talus on the calcaneus and preserve whatever mobility is still present in the foot, in order to maintain the correction achieved without over-correcting. Also, the procedure must not in itself be a cause of pain. In the child and adolescent who still have potential for growth, restoration of a normal static position of the hindfoot and normal play of tendons and muscles will correct distribution of muscle strains and loading, recreate the physiologic shape of the foot and, above all, allow growth to continue normally. It is hoped that this will lengthen the lateral column and reduce the relative and the absolute length of the medial arch. A large number of procedures have been proposed. Some involve soft tissues, others involve bone or joints, and mixed procedures are often used which combine osteotomy or a joint insert and tendon transfer.

Soft tissue procedures

These aim to restore the medial capsular and ligamentous plane and attempt to establish better muscular balance by tendon transfer, elongation or stretching The following techniques may be used: transfer of the tendon of the tibialis posterior muscle to the lower aspect of the navicular or medial cuneiform, transfer of the tendon of the tibialis anterior muscle to the navicular bone or the medial cuneiform, inward transfer of the fibularis tertius, elongation of the calcaneal tendon by Green's technique, elongation and varus positioning of the tendon of the fibularis brevis muscle, or tenodesis of the tendon of the tibialis anterior muscle on the tendon of the tibialis posterior muscle. Capsulo-ligamentoplasties are carried out by simple suture or vest-over-pants suture after resection of a medial and plantar-based wedge, or by raising a capsular-periosteal flap on the talonavicular or calcaneonavicular ligaments [5, 38].

Bone and joint procedures

Extra-articular osteotomies to shorten and correct the alignment of the medial arch, usually by resection of a medial and plantar-based wedge, are proposed to restore the curve of the medial arch while reducing forefoot abduction. A single osteotomy may be done at the level of the talometatarsal malalignment or serial osteotomies along the medial column to decrease the height of resection and to keep it extra-articular. This has been proposed for the medial cuneiform, the navicular and even the talar neck. Osteotomy to lengthen the lateral arch is indicated as a supplement to the above procedure. It is generally carried out in the cuboid by interposition of bone from the medial resection [38, 43].

Other procedures have also been proposed to treat anomalies of the talus and calcaneus by correcting calcaneal valgus and pronation, or by restoring normal talocalcaneal divergence. Among these are subtalar insertion of a biologically inert material (silastic silicone sphere, zyrcon, polyethylene) into the sinus tarsi. The aim is to correct calcaneal valgus and, secondarily, to decrease talocalcaneal divergence while avoiding ankylosis of the subtalar joint [1, 41, 43]. These techniques satisfactorily correct heel valgus but have little effect on talocalcaneal malalignment.

Judet's procedure makes use of the same principle by temporary screw fixation of the talus and calcaneus after correction of talocalcaneal divergence and hindfoot valgus. This procedure spares the subtalar and mediotarsal joints and allows normal bone growth after correction. There is a risk of under- or overcorrection if the screw fractures.

Dwyer's osteotomy for calcaneal realignment acts on calcaneal valgus in isolation. It lengthens the posterior tuberosity and gives it a more varus and vertical position. In addition to correcting forefoot pronation, it thus lengthens the lateral arch and has a slightly corrective effect on the collapse of the longitudinal arch of the foot. It has the advantage of being an extra-articular procedure but it would seem to be often insufficient on its own to correct the overall deformity [23].

Partial arthrodesis of the foot makes it possible to immobilize the joint-space which is at the origin of the malalignment, after correction of the valgus attitude, talocalcanear divergence and flat foot. It can be carried out either on the medial column alone in the talonavicular or, more rarely, the cuneonavicular and intercuneiform joint-spaces, or at the level of the center of rotation by immobilizing the medio-tarsal joint alone or the posterior subtalar joint [6]. Posterior subtalar arthrodesis may be intra-articular after the deformity has been corrected by resection of a medial-based wedge, or extra-articular at the sinus tarsi by interposition of a bone graft according to Grice's technique (fig. 15.13).

Lastly, arthrodesis may involve the entire subtalar and mediotarsal center of rotation. It can be carried out in situ, or after the deformities have been corrected by wedge-shaped resection or by sliding and restoration of a normal talocalcaneal divergence. Correction of the overall deformity may reveal forefoot pronation. Before undertaking the procedure, it is necessary to determine the possibilities of preserving forefoot balance after the flat foot has been corrected. This procedure gives even better results if good correction of the flat foot and secondarily of heel valgus have been obtained [42].

Indications

As we have seen, numerous surgical procedures have been proposed to correct the valgus flat foot, but in fact the indications are few, both during growth and during adulthood. It should be borne in mind that flat foot is virtually physiologic in the child under the age of four. In fact, during the growth period talocalcaneal divergence gradually decreases from an average of 30° to 50° at birth to 20° to 30° at the age of six. The incidence of flat foot and valgus heel decreases in a parallel and progressive manner as the bones grow. According to Bedouelle, if the small number of adult flat feet which require treatment is compared with the high incidence of flat feet in the child, it may well be considered that the latter has a favorable prognosis. More precisely, Méary [27] observed that out of 100 flat feet in children aged four, at the end of the growth period 65 had resolved, 30 still had a moderate but above all asymptomatic deformity, and only five still had a marked deformity which was likely to cause problems at a later date. Similarly, Lelièvre found that flat feet persisted in 5% of children and that a third of these feet became painful at adolescence.

In children, surgery is only exceptionally indicated, and should only be performed if the flat foot is severe, can be reduced only slightly or not at all, and above all if the condition progressively worsens in spite of conservative treatment. The following can be considered as predictive factors of gravity: talocrural equinus, talometatarsal malalignment located at the

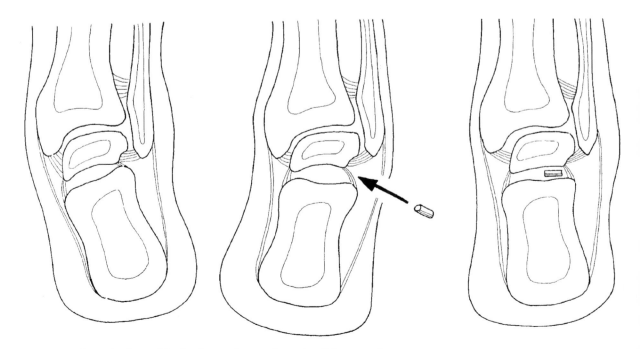

Fig. 15.13. Calcaneal valgus of the flat foot and correction using Grice procedure

talonavicular joint-space, and lastly, the fixed nature of the deformity when spontaneous correction of the valgus attitude does not reduce the flat foot. On the other hand, deformities which are reduced when the foot is relieved of weight-bearing or when the calcaneus is placed in a varus position, or when malalignment is moderate and is located at the cuneonavicular joint-space may be considered as benign.

In feet which show severe signs, talocalcaneal divergence and calcaneal pronation can be corrected by procedures such as Grice's or Judet's technique [35] or by posterior subtalar inserts, often combined with tendon transfer and elongation of the calcaneal tendon if necessary.

If there is no sign of severity, as in the overwhelming majority of cases, the child should be treated non-surgically by a corrective plantar orthosis and a specific rehabilitative program if necessary.

In the asymptomatic adolescent, the choice is open between simple surveillance and plantar orthosis, depending on the severity of the flat foot and above all on the progressive tendency of the deformity. If the flat foot or valgus heel show no gradual spontaneous improvement, use of an orthosis seems appropriate even if long-term results still remain uncertain.

In uncomplicated flat foot, it would seem logical to prescribe a corrective orthosis. While such devices cannot cure the deformity, they appear capable of halting the painful symptoms related to ligamentous stretching and mechanical overload of the components supporting the arch of the foot. In adolescents, rehabilitation is a useful complement.

Surgery may be indicated if the flat foot is serious and refractory to conservative treatment. A combination of a bony procedure and tendon transfer is usually proposed. Grice's technique or subtalar insert are the most common procedures. Used in isolation, they may correct the overall deformity. They are combined with medial capsulorraphy and transfer of the tendons of tibialis anterior and tibialis posterior muscles.

Another possibility is Dwyer's osteotomy to restore the varus position of the calcaneus, either with subtalar insert or in association with tendon transfer. Used alone, this procedure does not appear sufficient to ensure long-lasting correction of flat foot.

At the end of the growth period, such procedures are in general inadequate to ensure good

correction of associated deformities of the midfoot and forefoot, and osteotomy, extra-articular if possible, is often indicated.

If there is a calcaneonavicular fusion and if the center of rotation is still flexible, resection can be proposed before the age of 13. Resection must extend over more than 1 cm and all the adjacent non-ossified cartilage must be excised. Fibrous or muscular interposition using the extensor digitorum brevis muscle is recommended [8, 16, 26, 28, 32, 39]. After the age of 13, resection of the fusion has a poorer prognosis and arthrodesis may be indicated in such cases [16, 42]. In talocalcanear fusion, resection of the bony or bony-cartilaginous bridge can always be attempted if at least one-half of the subtalar joint surface is free, and if there is as yet no osteoarthrotic degeneration of the neighboring joints, in particular the talonavicular joint [40]. To reduce the risk of recurrence, resection must be sufficiently extensive and combined with interposition of the muscle (flexor digitorum brevis). Double arthrodesis is indicated if there is osteoarthrosis of the midfoot or if the fusion involves more than half of the joint surface [27].

If this fails, posterior subtalar arthrodesis can be carried out in isolation unless the center of rotation is markedly stiff, in which case double arthrodesis should be proposed.

In adults, asymptomatic flat foot should not be routinely treated. If the deformity becomes symptomatic, an orthosis should be used to attempt partial correction if the foot is still flexible. If it is not flexible, if the deformity is fixed but without osteoarthrotic degeneration, treatment should include an orthosis to compensate for the deformity, combined with a rehabilitative program to decrease pain and relax the muscles. If this conservative management fails, a surgical procedure may be proposed. Extra-articular osteotomy to realign the joint is indicated. If these osteotomies are to remain extra-articular, relatively little correction is possible. Only moderately flat feet can be treated in this way or in conjunction with a Dwyer osteotomy. In severe flat feet or osteoarthrotic or symptomatic deformity, partial arthrodesis of the center of rotation passing through the arthritic joint can alleviate the pain of arthrosis and correct the main deformities. In longstanding or severely deformed cases, double subtalar and mediotarsal arthrodesis is indicated [17, 42]. The better the correction obtained, the better the result of these procedures, but care must be taken to avoid overcorrection, which is usually less well tolerated than the initial deformity.

Rupture of the tendon of the tibialis posterior muscle can only rarely be repaired by direct suture because of the loss of tendon substance. Repair is carried out by tendon splitting alone, or more often accompanied by transfer of the tendon of the flexor digitorum longus muscle. This procedure generally relieves pain on weight-bearing, but rarely or only partially corrects the valgus deformity and medial arch collapse. Combined partial talonavicular or mediotarsal arthrodesis is proposed either as a complement to the above procedure, or after failure of suture or tendon transfer [4, 17].

● Conclusion

Valgus flat foot is a benign condition which, in the vast majority of cases, gradually resolves as the patient grows. When the deformity does persist at adolescence or adulthood, it is still generally well tolerated. Some severe flat feet are refractory to conservative management and should be treated surgically before major deformity develops. Congenital tarsal fusions are a frequent cause of painful decompensation of the midfoot and forefoot. They are particularly associated with static valgus flat foot and should be sought and detected early, so that appropriate treatment can be instituted.

References

1. Addante JB, Chin MW, Loomis JC, Burleigh W Lucarelli JE (1992) Subtalar joint arthroerisis with SILASTIC silicone sphere: a retrospective study. J Foot Surg 31:47-51
2. Aharonson Z, Arcan M, Steinback TV (1992) Foot-ground pressure pattern of flexible flatfoot in children, with and without correction of calcaneovalgus. Clin Orthop 278: 177-82
3. Azemar G (1985) La gauche et la droite en podologie: considération sur les asymétries fonctionnelles en podologie. Expansion Scientifique Française, Paris, pp 7-10
4. Banks AS, Mc Glamry ED (1987) Tibialis posterior tendon rupture. J Am Podiatr Assoc 77: 170-176
5. Barouk LS (1981) Ostéotomie scaphoïdienne associée à la transposition rétension du jambier postérieur dans les pieds plats valgus. Med Chir Pied 5: 171-176
6. Catanzariti AR (1993) Modified medial column arthrodesis. J Foot Ankle Surg 32: 180-188
7. Chiappara P, Dagnino G, Verrina F, Guzino MT (1992) Le pied plat synostosique douloureux du jeune garçon. Med Chir Pied 8: 25-28
8. Cohen AH, Laughner TE, Pupp GR (1993) Calcaneo-navicular bar resection. A retrospective review. J Am Podiatr Med Assoc 83: 10-17
9. Cowell HR, Elener V (1983) Rigid painful flat foot secondary to tarsal coalition. Clin Orthop 177: 54-60
10. Davids JR, Hagerman RJ, Eilert RE (1990) Orthopaedic aspects of fragile-X syndrome. J Bone Joint Surg 72A: 889-896
11. Deland JT, Arnoczky SP, Thompson FM (1992) Adult acquired flatfoot deformity at the talonavicular joint: reconstruction of the spring ligament in an in vitro model. Foot Ankle 13: 327-332
12. De Doncker E, Kowalski C (1979) Cinesiologie et rééducation du pied. Masson, Paris
13. Funk DA, Cass JR, Johnson KA (1986) Acquired adult flat foot secondary to posterior tibial tendon pathology. J Bone Joint Surg 68A: 95-102
14. Gauthier G (1977) Trouble biomécanique du pied plat. Rev Chir Orthop 63: 736-739
15. Giannestras NJ (1977) Correction chirurgicale du pied plat de l'adolescent. Rev Chir Orthop 63: 766-770
16. Gonzalez P, Kumar S, Jay RM (1990) Calcaneo-navicular coalition treated by resection and interposition of the extensor digitorum brevis muscle. J Bone Joint Surg 72A: 71-77
17. Graves SC, Mann RA, Graves KO (1993) Triple arthrodesis in older adults. Results after long-term follow-up. J Bone Joint Surg 75A: 355-362
18. Gualtieri G, Guastieri I, Gagliardi S (1993) Contracted valgus flat foot caused by tarsal synostosis in the adolescent. Chir Organi Mov 78: 161-165
19. Harris RI (1955) Rigid valgus foot due to talo-calcaneal bridge. J Bone Joint Surg 37A 169-183
20. Henceroth WD, Deyerlew M (1982) The acquired unilateral flat foot in the adult. Some causative factors. Foot Ankle 2: 304-308
21. Huang CK, Kitaoka HB, An KN, Chao EY (1993) Biomechanical evaluation of longitudinal arch stability. Foot Ankle 14: 353-357
22. Isikan UE (1993) The values of talo-navicular angles in patients with pes planus. J Foot Surg 32: 514-516
23. Jacobs AM, Geistler P (1991) Posterior calcaneal osteotomy. Effect, technique, and indications. Clin Podiatr Med Surg 8: 647-657
24. Karasick D, Schweitzer ME (1993) Tear of the posterior tibial tendon causing asymmetric flat foot. Am J Roentgenol 161: 1237-1240
25. Kilmartin TE, Wallace WA (1992) The significance of pes planus in juvenile hallux valgus. Foot Ankle 13: 53-56
26. Kumar S, Jay, Lee MS, Couto JC (1992) Osseous and non osseous coalition of the middle facet of the talo-calcaneal joint. J Bone Joint Surg 74A: 529-535
27. Meary R (1969) Symposium sur le pied plat. Ann Orth de l'Ouest 1: 55-71

28. Mosier K, Pennsylvania H, Asher M (1984) Tarsal coalition and peroneal spastic flat foot. A review. J Bone Joint Surg 66A: 976-984

29. Mueller TJ (1984) Ruptures and lacerations of the tibialis posterior tendon. J Am Podiatr Assoc 74: 109-119

30. Mueller TJ (1991) Acquired flat foot secondary to tibialis posterior dysfuction biomecanical aspect. J Foot Surg 30: 2-11

31. Niederecker K (1959) Der plattfuss. Enke, Stuttgart

32. Olney BW, Asher MA (1987) Excision of symptomatic coalition of the middle facet of the talo-calcaneal joint. J Bone Joint Surg 69A: 539-544

33. Pachuda NM, lasday SD, Jay RM (1990) Tarsal coalition: etiology, diagnosis and treatment. J Foot Surg 29: 474-488

34. Rao UB, Joseph B (1992) The influence of footwear on the prevalence of flat foot. J Bone Joint Surg 74B: 525-527

35. Regnauld B (1986) Le pied. Springer Verlag, Berlin, 189-245

36. Roger A, Meary R (1969) Les synostoses congénitales des os du tarse. Rev Chir Orthop 55: 721-741

37. Rose GK, Welton EA, Marshal T (1985) The diagnosis of flat foot in the child. J Bone Joint Surg 67B: 71-78

38. Salo JM, Viladot A, Garcia-Elias M, Sanchez-Freijo JM, Viladot R (1992) Congenital flat foot: different clinical forms. Acta Orthop Belg 58: 406-410

39. Salomao O, Napoli MM, De Carvalho Junior AE, Fernandes TD, Marques J, Hernandez AJ (1992) Talocalcaneal coalition: diagnosis and surgical management. Foot Ankle 13: 251-256

40. Scranton PE (1987) Treatment of symptomatic talocalcaneal coalition. J Bone Joint Surg 69A: 533-558

41. Smith DK, Gilula LA, Totty WG (1990) Subtalar arthrosis: evaluation with CT. Am J Roentgenol 154: 559-562

42. Tomeno B (1977) La double arthrodèse sous-astragalienne et médio-tarsienne dans le pied plat essentiel après 15 ans. Rev Chir Orthop 63: 761-763

43. Viladot A (1992) Surgical treatment of the child's flat-foot. Clin Orthop 283: 34-38

44. Warren MJ, Jeffree MA, Wilson DJ, MC Lamon JC (1990) Computed tomography in suspected tarsal coalition. Acta Orthop Scand 6: 554-557

45. Wenger DR, Mauldin D, Speck G, Morgan D, Lieber RL (1981) Corrective shoes and inserts as treatment for flexible flat foot in enfants and children. J Bone Joint Surg 71A: 800-810

46. Williamson DM, Torode IP (1992) Cubonavicular coalition: an unusual cause of peroneal spastic flat foot. Aust NZ J Surg 62: 506-507

16.

Pes cavus in the adult

H Mestdagh, C Maynou, E Butin and I Durieu

The sole of the foot, while weight-bearing, is classically compared to an arch, and is in fact a truss consisting of anterior and posterior main rafters, held together by tiebeams [24]. Increasing the slope of the main rafters by shortening the tiebeams elevates the truss and makes it more concave. Thus pes cavus represents an exaggeration of normal plantar concavity, where the anterior and posterior weight-bearing areas of the foot are brought closer together [9].

Pathologic anatomy

There are several types of pes cavus, **depending on the site.**
• The most frequent is anterior pes cavus, characterized by lowering of the forefoot in plantarflexion relative to the hindfoot, which causes an increase in the slope of the forefoot. In total pes cavus this increase involves the whole of the metatarsal range; in medial pes cavus it decreases from the inner to the outer side; the first ray is very vertical whereas the fifth remains horizontal, which causes pronation of the forefoot.
• Posterior pes cavus is characterized by an isolated increase in the vertical slope of the calcaneus.
• Mixed pes cavus includes both deformities.

Tripod foot is rarer; it includes the two deformities already mentioned, but also includes a true transverse anterior arch, i.e., there is a cavus forefoot.

Although dominant, pes cavus is never the only element in a clinical picture which combines several deformities affecting the whole foot.

With Braun [5], three types of pes cavus are distinguished **according to the associated conditions:**
• Classical pes cavus varus, where cavus deformity is usually marked, is accompanied by static varus of the heel in the hindfoot, and in the forefoot by narrowing of the metatarsal range, which is curved transversely and overloaded at either end. Weight-bearing accentuates the varus of the hindfoot, which is transmitted to the forefoot, and the fifth metatarsal head is overloaded. Compensatory pronation of the forefoot shortens, adducts and increases the vertical pitch of the first metatarsal. Therefore, there is overloading of the first metatarsal head. The deformity causes, in addition, clawing of all the toes.
• Pes cavus valgus, where cavus is mild, is accompanied by excessive valgus of the heel in the hindfoot, and in the forefoot by widening of the metatarsal spread, which is flat. Weight-bearing, together with wearing down of the lateral part of the shoes, shows this uncontrolled tendency to be due to a varus deformity whose consequence is overloading of the fourth metatarsal head. If there is insufficiency of the first ray, as in an atavistic foot, the overloading may also affect the third metatarsal head. The characteristics of an atavistic foot are found at the toes: metatarsus primus adductus, hallux valgus, insufficiency of the second ray and quintus varus, all of these anomalies causing the flattened and triangular forefoot.
• Braun described a third variety of pes cavus, with clinical features of a pseudo pes cavus which can be particularly confusing. There is a paradoxically associated widening of the isthmus of the footprint, whose lateral side is made prominent by projection of the fifth metatarsal styloid despite the presence of a cavus, and a varus deformity of the soft parts of the

heel which are crushed outwards, plus overloading of the fifth metatarsal head despite the presence of a calcaneo-valgus deformity.

● Pathophysiology

The pathophysiologic mechanism of pes cavus is variable [2].

Posterior pes cavus is due to triceps surae insufficiency, which causes the inferior posterior center of ossification of the calcaneus to be displaced forwards; ossification of this center produces an increase in the pitch of the calcaneus.

For anterior pes cavus, there are several, sometimes contradictory, pathogenic hypotheses: muscle dysfunction, capsular and ligamentous contracture.

Muscle dysfunction

There are different forms, which have been grouped together by Samilson [32].

Dysfunction of the long plantar flexor muscles

Hyperactivity of the tibialis posterior muscle, because of spastic paralysis or through compensation for triceps surae insufficiency, or because of insufficiency of the anterior muscles, produces flexion and supination of the foot. In the same way, hyperactivity of the peroneus longus muscle, either from spasticity or compensation for insufficiency of the dorsiflexor muscles, causes plantarflexion of the first metatarsal. On the other hand, insufficiency of the triceps surae and peroneus longus muscles forces the foot to follow the flexion of the toes.

Loss of balance between the anterior and posterior muscles

Any muscle deficiency that leaves the tibialis anterior muscle intact produces inversion of the foot. Conversely, deficiency of the tibialis anterior, where the extensor hallucis longus muscle is intact, causes hallux extensus, and the first metatarsal is fixed in plantarflexion [7].

Dysfunction of the intrinsic muscles of the foot

Hyperactivity of the intrinsic muscles, together with a short calcaneal tendon, can cause cavus. On the other hand, insufficiency of the intrinsics produces hyperactivity of the extensor muscles and posterior pressure of the toes on the metatarsal heads, which causes plantarflexion of the forefoot [22].

Capsular and ligamentous contracture

This can occur in certain cases of primary pes cavus, since the truss of the foot is held up by the plantar capsules and ligaments. It is however impossible to tell if the contracture is the result or the cause of the cavus deformity.

During growth, a self-perpetuating vicious circle develops. Tensing of the plantar soft tissues brings the anterior and posterior weight-bearing areas closer together, which causes an increase in the pitches of the metatarsals and calcaneus. The talus on the other hand becomes horizontal. The result is restriction of dorsiflexion and a relative deficiency in the tibialis anterior muscle, the difference between the relaxed and tense positions of this last muscle being reduced. This deficit is compensated by the other dorsal muscles, whose contraction causes extension of the metatarsophalangeal joints. To allow the toe pulp to touch the ground, the flexor muscles of the toes contract, producing clawing of the toes, which is also encouraged by a deficiency of the interosseous muscles. Hicks [16] showed that clawing of the toes accentuates the slope of the metatarsals because there is exaggerated pressure on the metatarsal heads, which in turn increases the tension in the plantar aponeurosis. According to Coleman and Chestnut [8], plantarflexion of the first metatarsal and pronation of the forefoot are the first stage of the process and become irreducible, causing compensatory supination of the hindfoot, which is necessary to stabilize weight-bearing. There are several possible ways in this context for anterior pes cavus to occur. While the cavus is reducible, which is the rule in children and adolescents, stopping this cycle at one point can correct all the deformities. However, in the adult the irreversibility of the lesions requires bone or bone and joint correction.

Etiology

The usual causes of pes cavus fall into four groups of unequal frequency.

• Traumatic causes are rare. The initial trauma may be either local: unrecognized or improperly treated fracture or subluxation of the tarsal bones, scarring from a burn to the sole of the foot or, higher up, destruction of the anterolateral muscle compartment of the leg.

• The causes due to static disorders have also become rare: contracture of the achilleo-calcaneo-plantar system [41] can be due to cast immobilization in an incorrect position, to a Volkmann's syndrome, or sometimes to simple lack of ankle physiotherapy in a bed-ridden patient under the weight of the bed covers.

• Arthritic causes are rare: in rheumatoid arthritis, valgus of the hindfoot is much commoner than varus.

• Neurologic causes are by far the most common. They are classified anatomically from the periphery towards the central structures [42].

Muscular conditions

Myopathies or Duchenne and Becker progressive muscular dystrophies affect the muscles of the anterolateral compartment of the leg selectively, and are accompanied by contracture of the calcaneal tendon and of the triceps surae muscle, leading to walking on tiptoe. Gower's distal myopathy starts by affecting the small distal muscles.

Peripheral neuron diseases

Trunk lesions

These are mainly represented by trauma to the common peroneal nerve.

Polyneuropathies

Acquired polyneuritis of whatever cause (toxic, metabolic, lack of minerals or vitamins, or inflammatory) rarely produces cavus.

Hereditary motor and sensory neuropathy

Charcot-Marie-Tooth's disease causes cavus by atrophy of the distal muscles (fig. 16.1). The progressive interstitial neuritis of Déjérine-Sottas is similar, but also includes noticeable but painless hypertrophy of the peripheral nerve trunks. Roussy-Levy's hereditary areflexic dysplasia has signs of both Charcot-Marie-Tooth's disease and Friedreich's disease. Stark-Kaeser's scapulo-fibular amyotrophy is the result of a neurogenic degenerative process with associated peripheral neuropathy or anterior horn disease, or a myogenic degenerative process similar to myopathy.

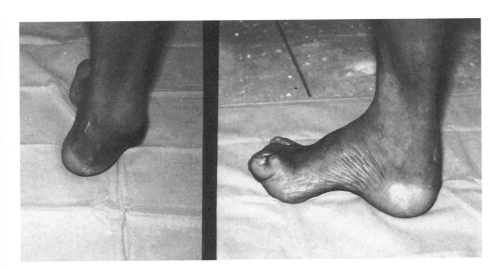

Fig. 16.1. Posterior and medial views of pes cavus due to Charcot-Marie-Tooth's disease

Cauda equina root lesions

Whether they are the result of trauma, tumors or inflammation, they rarely produce cavus, except in the case of complete paralysis of the intrinsic muscles where the toe flexor and extensor muscles are intact. However, in its diverse anatomic forms, spina bifida classically produces a deformity of the foot and pes cavus in particular, sometimes unilateral, with paralysis of the plantarflexor muscles, as a result of sacral nerve root damage (S1-S2).

Anterior horn lesions of the spinal cord

Acute anterior poliomyelitis was historically the main cause, as regards both frequency and orthopedic complications, during the period when this viral infection was still very active. The deficit often affects the plantar and dorsal ankle flexor muscles asymmetrically and produces either posterior pes cavus by triceps surae muscle paralysis, or anterior pes cavus with paralysis of the tibialis anterior muscle. The rare forms of chronic anterior poliomyelitis which begin in the lower limbs and the distal forms of progressive spinal amyotrophy of the adult also have pes cavus.

Hereditary spinocerebellar degenerative diseases

Pes cavus occurs in 75% of cases of Friedreich's disease. In Strumell-Lorrain's familial spasmodic paraplegia, pes cavus is considered as secondary to the pyramidal syndrome, and is unusual in that it disappears on standing because the plantar arch is filled in by movement of the soft tissues. Pierre-Marie's hereditary cerebellar ataxia is rarely associated with pes cavus. Menzel's hereditary ataxia is a familial form of olivo-ponto-cerebellar atrophy in which pes cavus can occur.

Acquired non-hereditary pyramidal conditions of the central nervous system

Hemiplegia, paraplegia and infantile encephalopathy tend to produce a varus equinus rather than a true varus deformity.

Primary pes cavus

Primary pes cavus is diagnosed by elimination in more than half the cases. Most authors believe that it is caused by a minimal muscle deficiency, which is the consequence of a latent neurologic involvement. The presence of one of the previously mentioned neurologic disorders must therefore be looked for in the family, pes cavus being sometimes the only sign of the disease.

● Clinical diagnosis

Reasons for consultation

Pain is the main reason for consultation. This is caused either by metatarsalgia due to excessive pressure on the metatarsal heads, present in all the anatomic forms of pes cavus, or arises in the heel, particularly in posterior pes cavus. Some patients have local tenderness when wearing shoes, at the uppermost point of the deformity. Callosities on clawed toes caused by rubbing on the shoe are often painful. Finally, at a more advanced stage, there is diffuse arthritic pain, which may affect various foot joints.

Discomfort while wearing shoes can result from many different factors: the clawed toes do not have enough space at the end of the shoe, as it is not high enough; the lump on the dorsum of the foot rubs against the upper of the shoe, and tightening of the laces does not bring the upper parts of the shoe together over the dorsum of the foot; the hunched receding heel is not properly supported against the counter of the shoe. Flat-heeled shoes are very poorly tolerated; high heels are more easily accepted [33].

Walking is disturbed by cramp and dull aching in the calf, by contraction of the muscles of the plantar arch during prolonged walking, and through difficulty in climbing slopes and by instability of the ankle, resulting in repeated sprains in varus. Some young active patients with isolated pes cavus dislike the unpleasant appearance of the deformity.

Clinical examination

The deformity, maintained by shortening of the triceps surae muscle, calcaneal tendon and plantar aponeurosis, consists of three components which are easy to see in the weight-bearing foot.

Cavus of the foot

A lump appears on the dorsum of the foot, which is larger medially than laterally. In the sole of the foot there is an increase in the concavity of the medial arch and exceptionally of the lateral edge, which does not have complete contact with the ground. Abnormal pressure points are observed causing hyperkeratosis, with corns and callosities at the heel and over the metatarsal heads. From the side, the difference in level between the forefoot and hindfoot is assessed after the calcaneus has been placed horizontally [33].

Calcaneal varus

When examined from the rear during weight-bearing, the heel is malaligned in varus (5 to 10°) by the premature adduction-supination action of the contracted triceps surae muscle. If the varus deformity spreads to the mid-tarsal region, hyperkeratosis is sometimes seen on the lateral side of the foot, or even a callosity under the cuboid bone.

Clawing of the toes

Clawing is mostly proximal, with hyperextension of the first phalanx and flexion of the second. The third phalanx may stay in the neutral position or be in flexion (complete clawing) or extension (Z toe). The pulp frequently remains at some distance from the ground level.

Clinical examination also looks for restriction of dorsiflexion of the ankle, which is nil or negative when the knee is in extension, but increases when the knee is flexed.

Study of the footprint is of limited use, but allows the deformity to be classified into three stages, depending on the width of the isthmus; (1) simple narrowing of the isthmus of the foot, (2) disappearance of the isthmus in the midplantar region, its tip being present in the anterior and posterior heel, (3) total disappearance of the isthmus with excessive weight-bearing on the anterior and posterior pillars [3].

Radiology

Weight-bearing X-rays of the ankle and foot include at least three views:

- a lateral view of the weight-bearing ankle and foot allows the cavus to be demonstrated and measured (fig. 16.2);
- a frontal view of the ankle, with a wire around the heel, demonstrates the frontal deformity of the hindfoot;
- a dorsoplantar view of the forefoot shows adduction of the forefoot and opening of the metatarsal plate.

Additionally, the lateral view of the non-weight-bearing heel and foot visualizes the difference in the level between the forefoot and hindfoot; the Walter-Müller view shows up any malalignment of the metatarsal heads, especially in anteromedial pes cavus.

Numerous geometric measurements have been proposed on weight-bearing X-rays to quantify the

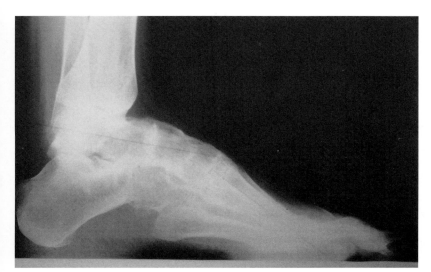

Fig. 16.2. Lateral X-ray film of weight-bearing ankle and foot showing the angle obtuse below at the intersection point of both sagittal axes of talus and 1st metatarsal

cavus deformity. The angle of the medial arch is widely used; in all types of pes cavus it is less than 120°. Also, in order to analyze the deformity of the forefoot, the diaphyseal axis of the first metatarsal and the sagittal axis of the talus are traced; they intersect with an angle obtuse below, the intersection point corresponding to the apex of the deformity.

Calculation of the pitch of the line between the five metatarsals allows an anteromedial pes cavus to be distinguished from a complete pes cavus. The deformity of the hindfoot is measured by the calcaneal pitch; in posterior pes cavus this calcaneal pitch exceeds 30°. An associated equinus deformity of the ankle is shown by an increase in the tibio-talar angle to more than 105°.

Treatment

Treatment with orthoses (insoles)

The deformity can be corrected using orthoses if it is reducible. Fixed deformities can be compensated for by orthoses. Orthoses should ideally be able to treat all types of deformity; however, in some cases they can only treat the part of the deformity causing a problem or complement another type of treatment, usually surgical. Orthoses can be plantar, for the heel, or distal for the toes.

Plantar orthoses

Their aim is to settle the heel at the proper level on the ground and to elevate and balance the forefoot. The heel-piece places the heel at the proper level. The reducible varus deformity is corrected by a posterior pronating lift; valgus is left uncorrected if it is not excessive: the posterior concave cup-shaped part of the orthosis that lifts the heel remains in a neutral position. Equinus is compensated by raising the heel of the shoe by about 2 cm for men and 4 cm for women, or sometimes with a heel-piece, whose height must be restricted to avoid the patient losing his shoe.

A support situated behind the metatarsal heads reduces the pressure on them. This is produced by an oblique metatarsal bar, which extends from the forefoot metatarsal area to the tarso-metatarsal space, if the forefoot is transversely cavus, or by a midline metatarsal support or pad. Excess local overloading of one or more of the heads requires a hollow situated under that area.

In practice, in varus pes cavus, the orthosis includes a hollow pronating heel-piece and a metatarsal bar. In valgus pes cavus, it consists of a neutral heel-piece and a median metatarsal support or pad.

Toe orthoses

These may be used for reduction, or may be merely protective. An orthosis of the first ray or a kidney-shaped orthosis is used if the hallux sticks up. This orthosis extends the plantar orthosis under the first phalanx of the hallux, making the pulp of this toe touch the ground.

Standard or made-to-measure orthoses, which are separate from the plantar orthosis and situated around the interphangeal joints of the small toes that are clawed, have the same aim.

Surgical treatment

Operations on the soft tissues

These aim to restore the truss of the foot and so consist either of lengthening the contracted tiebeams (plantar capsules, triceps surae muscle, calcaneal tendon and plantar aponeurosis), or of making the main rafters horizontal (metatarsals and calcaneus) by muscle transplantation.

Lengthening of the achilles-plantar system (triceps surae muscle, calcaneal tendon and plantar aponeurosis)

Transection of the soft tissues was recommended by Steindler [35] in 1920. This consists of detachment of all the structures attached to the plantar surface of the calcaneus, from the most superficial to the deepest level: the plantar aponeurosis, flexor digitorum brevis muscle, abductor hallucis muscle, quadratus plantae muscle and plantar calcaneocuboid ligament.

More recently, Meary [27] in the adult and Paulos [29] in the child, have recommended radical plantar release, which consists of bisection of the plantar aponeurosis, the calcaneocuboid and calcaneoscaphoid ligaments, the expansions of the tibialis posterior tendon and the plantar capsules of the tarsal joints. At the heel, the contracted calcaneal tendon requires lengthening.

Tendon transplantation

The various operations proposed for anterior pes cavus correspond to different aims.

Reduction of cavus can be obtained in two ways: (1) removal of the elements supporting the truss of the foot by passing the tendon of the peroneus longus muscle through the interosseous membrane and reinserting it on the lateral cuneiform bone, or onto the tendons of the tibialis anterior or peroneus brevis muscles [1]; or (2) flattening of the metatarsals by transplantation of the tendon of the extensor hallucis longus muscle onto the head of the first metatarsal and/or transplantation of each of the common extensor tendons of the toes onto the corresponding metatarsal. Active elevation of the foot can be restored by transplantation of the tibialis posterior tendon through the interosseous membrane onto the lateral cuneiform bone [17, 40] or onto the lateral cuboid at the anterior surface of the heel [23].

Reduction of clawing of the toes can be obtained by transplantation of the extensor tendons onto the lateral cuneiform bone, or by transplantation of the extensor tendons onto the flexor tendons [15].

In posterior pes cavus, flattening of the calcaneus may be obtained by transplantation of the tibialis posterior tendon onto the calcaneal tendon [31], of the tibialis anterior tendon onto the calcaneus [30, 39], or of the peroneus longus tendon onto the calcaneus [26].

To correct associated deformities, transplantation of the split lateral third of the tendon of the tibialis anterior muscle has been suggested, to correct the varus tendency in the hindfoot [12].

Bone operations

Anterior pes cavus

Bone resection aims to realign the axes of the talus and first metatarsal. This can involve several sites and is performed at the apex of the deformity. Anterior tarsectomy, described by Cole [7], has been widely used by Meary [27]. The operation is centered on the naviculo-cuneiform space and the cuboid, and consists of a dorsomedial closing wedge osteotomy, which corrects the cavus deformity that predominantly affects the medial rays, but increases adduction of the forefoot (fig. 16.3).

To avoid arthrodesis, Japas [21] proposed an inverted-V osteotomy, with the narrow end in the back of the navicular bone and the two limbs crossing the cuboid bone on the outside and the cuneiform bones on the inside. Wilcox and Weiner [44] and later Denis [10] proposed intracuneiform tarsectomy with cuboid impaction, but the small size of the cuneiform bones only permits minimal resection and causes problems with stability, with the necessary staples encroaching on the adjacent joint spaces.

Midtarsal tarsectomy was recommended by Imhäuser [18] and Steinhäusser [36]. The operation, centered on the midtarsal joint-space, removes a dorsolateral bone wedge, which allows the cavus and adduction of the forefoot to be corrected. If the cavus is marked, the bone wedge can include removal of the whole of the navicular bone and also encroach on the cuneiform bones (fig. 16.2). Steinhäuser showed that, because of the interdependence of the forefoot and hindfoot, adduction and supination of the forefoot cause varus of the heel. Also, blocking the midtarsal joint, the key joint of the foot, in a correct position abolishes the frontal swinging of the calcaneus. This suggestion is only feasible if the subtalar deformity is not fixed. Conversely, this operation totally suppresses mobility of the torsional couple.

Tarsometatarsal resection was recommended by Jahss [19]. This is centered on the tarsometatarsal joint. All of these tarsectomies are fixed by staples and immobilized in a plaster boot for about 6 weeks. Weight-bearing is allowed after 8 weeks.

Metatarsal osteotomy, popularized in France by Lelièvre [25], has been recommended in the USA by Swanson [37] and more recently by Watanabe [43]. It is centered on the metatarsal bases and involves removal of 5 dorsal bone wedges, whose height is calculated according to the pitch of the metatarsals on the ground (fig. 16.3). It respects the tarsometatarsal space. Additionally, it is not essential to fix with staples; within a week of weight-bearing the weight itself adjusts the position of the metatarsals, which flatten naturally and are consolidated by hypertrophic bone formation. This operation does not, however, allow major corrections to be made.

Posterior pes cavus

Osteotomy of the calcaneus is the universally accepted operation. It attempts to obtain a satisfactory calcaneal pitch of about 30°. Mitchell's upwards transfer of the pronated great tuberosity [28],

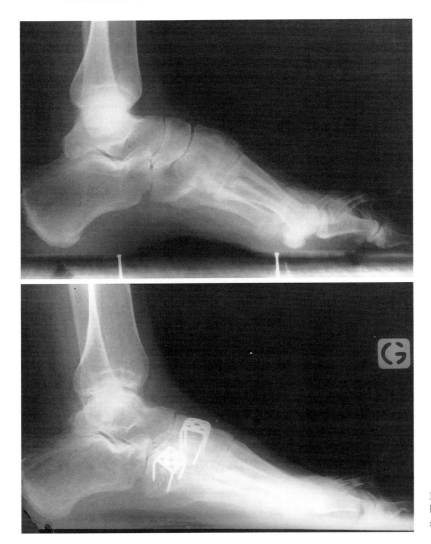

Fig. 16.3. Combined pes cavus corrected by anterior tarsectomy. Before and after surgical treatment

following posterior plantar aponeurectomy, reduces the cavus by elevating the calcaneal weight-bearing area of contact with the ground.

Dwyer's resection of a lateral bone wedge [11] additionally corrects the varus deformity of the hindfoot. It may be an advantage to replace this by a frontal transfer of the great tuberosity outwards, as recommended by Giard [13] or by Bradley and Coleman [4]. The osteotomy is fixed by a compression screw, which is inserted at the apex of the heel. Immobilization in a plaster boot is optional, and weight-bearing is allowed after 4 to 6 weeks.

In all cases, subtalar and midtarsal arthrodesis allows all the components of the deformity to be corrected simultaneously, but there is an ankylosis of the torque joint [34, 38].

In adults, the associated fixed deformities are treated by lengthening the calcaneal ligament when there is an equinus deformity of the heel, a closed wedge resection osteotomy to correct the varus in the hindfoot, and arthroplastic resection of the proximal interphalangeal joints, with or without metatarsophalangeal arthrolysis, when there is toe clawing.

Therapeutic indications

Jahss [20] insists that treatment for adult pes cavus must only be considered when the deformity has become symptomatic, i.e., when it has caused painful plantar callosities. Its aim is to allow almost normal shoes to be worn and, less important, to improve the cosmetic appearance of the foot. The initial treatment for complicated pes cavus in the adult is always conservative, using orthoses with a metatarsal bar and a posterior sole wedge. Chiropody may be required for callosities under the metatarsal heads and on the dorsal surface of the toes.

Surgery is considered only if conservative treatment fails. Under these circumstances, a systematic neurologic examination is performed to detect a progressive neuropathy, which would formally contraindicate the operation. If the neurologic condition is stabilized however, it is possible to operate, keeping in mind that prognosis is difficult in these conditions, and this may require operation to be delayed to observe how the disease progresses. Weight-bearing X-rays of the foot localize the deformity, specify its components in the three planes, confirm the irreducibility and measure its severity. In adults, tendon transplants are rarely performed, because of the irreducibility of the deformities. On the other hand, plantar aponeurectomy and section of the plantar capsules form an integral part of any corrective operation for pes cavus. Bone resection depends on the type and the site of the deformity [6].

Posterior pes cavus

In posterior pes cavus, osteotomy of the calcaneus is the best treatment because it produces global correction of the deformity. Jahss, however, prefers a tendon transfer [20].

Anterior pes cavus

In anterior pes cavus, the choice depends on the site of the apex of the deformity. This is usually in the naviculo-cuneiform or mid-tarsal areas; anterior or mid-tarsal tarsectomy are therefore indicated. More rarely, the deformity is situated in the tarsometatarsal area; metatarsectomy, or intracuneiform tarsectomy, or even arthrodesis of the tarsometatarsal joints is indicated.

Three important points should be underlined:
• when there is a callosity under the cuboid bone, the osteotomy must be situated proximal to the hyperkeratosis, never distal to it, to avoid increasing the pressure on the area of abnormal weight-bearing;
• whenever correction of the cavus reaches or exceeds 30°, midtarsal tarsectomy must be preferred to any other technique;.

• the resection should leave the foot as much as possible in a normal position, or even slightly over-corrected, because an iatrogenic flat foot is tolerated better than a residual cavus deformity.

Mixed pes cavus

In mixed pes cavus, most authors treat only the anterior component.

However, calcaneal osteotomy and tarsectomy can be combined with the same operation. In very deformed or arthritic pes cavus, subtalar and midtarsal arthrodesis allows correction in three planes. However, according to Steinhäuser [36], midtarsal arthrodesis alone, a simpler technique, can produce the same result.

Arthritic or neurologic pes cavus

In pes cavus with associated flexion-extension paralysis of the heel and/or talocrural arthritis, panarthrodesis or even talectomy, with or without tibio-calcaneal arthrodesis, may be indicated [20].

In patients whose general condition is poor, a partial procedure such as trimming a painful subcuboid callosity or isolated treatment for clawing of the toes, is sufficient.

In any case, the surgeon must consider if the operation is effective in treating the entire foot deformity. In practice, automatic correction of associated deformities of the toes or of the hindfoot is only seen near the site of the bone resection. Thus, only osteotomy of the calcaneus acts on the equinus deformity of the hindfoot and only metatarsal osteotomy can correct the clawing of the toes. On the other hand, operations on the mid-tarsal area have no influence away from the operation site. It is often necessary to perform in addition a lengthening of the calcaneal tendon, a closing wedge resection osteotomy of the calcaneus, and/or surgical treatment for clawing of the toes.

References

1. Bentson PGK (1933) The cavus and the muscle peroneus longus. Acta Orthop Scand 4: 50
2. Boike AM, Johng B, Hetherington VJ (1990) Pes cavus. In: Levy LA, Hetherington VJ (eds) Principles and Practice of Podiatric Medicine. Churchill Livingstone, Edinburgh, p 931

3. Bouysset M, Lejeune E, Bouvier M, Schnepp J, Carret JP (1987) L'examen de l'empreinte plantaire est-il désuet? Med Chir Pied 3: 89-91

4. Bradley GW, Coleman SS (1981) Treatment of the calcaneocavus deformity. J Bone Joint Surg 63A: 1159-1166

5. Braun S (1993) Le pied creux décompensé médical et ses orthèses. Rhumatologie pratique 7: 1-4

6. Butin E (1989) Le traitement chirurgical du pied creux de l'adulte. Thèse pour le Doctorat en Médecine, Lille N° 12

7. Cole WH (1940) The treatment of claw foot. J Bone Joint Surg 22: 895-908

8. Coleman SS, Chestnut WJ (1977) A simple test for hindfoot flexibility in cavovarus foot. Clin Orthop 123: 60-62

9. De Doncker E, Kowalski C (1970) Le pied normal et pathologique. Acta Orthop Belg 36: 386-559

10. Denis A, Piat C, Goutallier D (1988) Résultats de la tarsectomie distale extraarticulaire. Actualités en Médecine et Chirurgie du Pied 3: 152-156

11. Dwyer FC (1959) Osteotomy of the calcaneum for pes cavus. J Bone Joint Surg 41B: 80-86

12. Feiwell E (1977) Paralytic calcaneus in meningomyelocele. In : Mc Lauwin RL (ed) Myelomeningocele. Grune and Stratton, New York

13. Giard H (1984) L'ostéotomie de Dwyer dans le traitement du pied creux de l'enfant et de l'adolescent. Thèse pour le Doctorat en Médecine, Lille, N° 274

14. Green DR, Lepow GM, Smith T (1987) Pes cavus. In: Comprehensive Textbook of Foot Surgery, vol 1. Williams & Wilkins, Baltimore, p 27

15. Hibbs RA (1919) An operation for claw foot. JAMA 73: 1583-1585

16. Hicks J (1951) The function of the plantar aponeurosis. J Anat 85: 414-415

17. Hsu JD, Hoffer MM (1978) Posterior tibial tendon transfer through the interosseous membrane. Clin Orthop 131: 202-204

18. Imhäuser G (1984) Die Behandlung des schweren Hohlklumpfusses bei der neuralen Muskelatrophie. Z Orthop 122: 827-834

19. Jahss MH (1980) Tarsometatarsal truncated wedge arthrodesis for pes cavus and equinovarus deformity of the fore part of the foot. J Bone Joint Surg 62A: 713-722

20. Jahss MH (1983) Evaluation of the cavus foot for orthopedic treatment. Clin Orthop 181: 52-63

21. Japas MK (1968) Surgical treatment of pes cavus by tarsal V osteotomy. J Bone Joint Surg 50A: 927-944

22. Jarret BA, Manzi JA, Green DR (1980) Interossei and lumbricates muscles of the foot. J Am Podiatr Assoc 70: 1-13

23. Karlholm S, Nilsonne U (1968) Operative treatment of the foot deformity in Charcot-Marie-Tooth disease. Acta Orthop Scand 39: 101-106

24. Lapidus (1946) Spastic flat foot. J Bone Joint Surg 2 : 126-132

25. Lelièvre J, Maschas A (1956) La métatarsectomie. Technique, Indication. Rev Orthop 42: 886-887

26. Makin M, Yossipovitch Z (1966) Translocation of the peroneus longus in the treatment of paralytic pes calcaneus. J Bone Joint Surg 48A: 1541-1547

27. Meary R, Mattei, Tomeno B (1976) Tarsectomie antérieure pour pied creux. Rev Chir Orthop 62: 231-243

28. Mitchell GP (1977) Posterior displacement osteotomy of the calcaneus. J Bone Joint Surg 62A: 942-953

30. Peabody CW (1938) Tendon transposition. J Bone Joint Surg 20: 193-205

31. Poyle ND (1927) A new conception in the etiology of claw foot and associated talipes equinus. J Bone Joint Surg 9: 465-468

32. Samilson RL, William Dillin (1983) Cavus, cavovarus and calcaneovarus. Clin Orthop 177: 125-132

33. Schnepp J (1979) Le pied creux essentiel. Rappel anatomoclinique. Méthodes et indications thérapeutiques. Cahiers d'enseignement de la SOFCOT 10: 73-92

34. Siffert RS, Ugo del Torto MD (1983) Beak triple arthrodesis for severe cavus deformity. Clin Orthop 181: 64-67

35. Steindler A (1920) Stripping of the os calcis. Am J Orthop Surg 2: 8-12

36. Steinhäuser J (1978) Die Arthrodesen der Chopart's Schen Gelenklinie. Ferdinand Enke Verlag, Stuttgart

37. Swanson AB, Browne HS, Coleman JD (1966) The cavus foot concept of production and treatment by metatarsal osteotomy. J Bone Joint Surg 48A: 1019

38. Tomeno B (1981) Le pied creux essentiel. Rev Prat (Paris) 31: 1019-1029

39. Turner JW, Cooper RR (1971) Posterior transposition of tibialis anterior through the interosseous membrane. Clin Orthop 79: 71-74

40. Turner JW, Ciioer RR (1972) Anterior transposition of tibialis posterior through the interosseous membrane. Clin Orthop 82: 241

41. Viladot A (1985) Anatomie, physiologie et physiopathologie du système suro-achilléo-calcanéo-plantaire. Médecine et Chirurgie du Pied 2: 69-74

42. Vinken PJ, Bruin GW (1982) Handbook of clinical neurology. Elsevier, Amsterdam

43. Watanabe RS (1990) Metatarsal osteotomy of the cavus foot. Clin Orthop 252: 217-230

44. Wilcox PG, Weiner DS (1985) The Akron midtarsal osteotomy in the treatment of rigid pes cavus: a preliminary review. J Pediatr Orthop 5: 333-338

17. Pathology of the first ray

A. Hallux valgus

Y Tourné, F Picard and D Saragaglia

Introduction

Hallux valgus is the most frequently encountered pathology in surgical podiatry and was so named by Hueter, quoted by Schnepp [59] in 1871.

Particular neurologic, traumatic, and inflammatory etiologies will not be dealt with here. Instead, only static hallux valgus as a multifactorial disorder with numerous clinical and anatomic aspects will be discussed. Knowledge of the mechanisms which trigger hallux valgus, the factors which favor its development, and its self-aggravating patterns allows the current debate over therapeutic methods, although these remain numerous, to be based on fundamental medical and surgical principles.

Anatomy of the first ray

The first ray is composed of the medial cuneiform, the first metatarsal, and the two phalanges of the hallux along with the sesamoids. It plays a determining role in walking, and is particularly important in ambulatory propulsion.

Descriptive anatomy

The metatarsophalangeal joint of the hallux

The metatarsophalangeal joint of the hallux includes the base of the proximal phalanx, the head of the first metatarsal, the inferior aspect of which presents a blunt median ridge and two lateral concavities which hold the sesamoids. The sesamoids are integrated into a fibrocartilaginous structure which is the glenosesamoid ligament. The position of the sesamoids with reference to the intersesamoid metatarsal ridge is subject to anatomic variations [43, 55]. Muscles maintain balance between the first metatarsal head and the sesamoid sling, which extends from the proximal phalanx to which it is attached.

Malorientation of the metatarsal head, hypoplasia or actual agenesis of the intersesamoid ridge, and non-parallelism of the base of the proximal phalanx and the phalangeal head are among the probable congenital anatomic predisposing factors.

The cuneiform-metatarsal joint

The medial cuneiform presents an anterior convex articular surface that is reniform, oblique upward medially. The first metatarsal fits into the first cuneiform bone. The orientation and form of this joint-space can vary [46, 47] and in certain cases a very convex, oblique joint-space predisposes to malposition of the first metatarsal [2].

Intrinsic muscles of the first ray

These muscles are exclusively plantar except for the extensor digitorium brevis muscle, which is dorsal. Along the medial border, the medial bellies of the flexor hallucis brevis and abductor hallucis muscles run to the medial sesamoid and the base of the proximal phalanx. The abductor hallucis muscle originates from the calcaneus and is a major support for the medial arch.

Along the lateral border, the lateral sesamoid and proximal phalanx form the insertion of the adductor hallucis muscle (transverse head) as well as the main lateral belly of the flexor hallucis brevis.

Extrinsic muscles of the first ray

These are long muscles. The flexor hallucis longus muscle is inserted ventrally at the distal phalanx of the hallux. The extensor hallucis longus muscle is inserted dorsally at the base of the distal phalanx of the hallux.

Functional anatomy

The range of movement of the metatarsophalangeal joint of the hallux in the sagittal plane is very considerable and can attain 90° of dorsiflexion and 30° of plantarflexion, which may seem paradoxical since the intrinsic muscles are essentially plantar and therefore flexors.

Following the first phase of gait (ground contact) comes the second phase where the sole of the foot is in maximum contact with the ground. The ankle is passively carried from extension to flexion. The plantar muscles brace the medial arch. The long and short flexor muscles (hallucis longus and brevis) stabilize the hallux during this phase.

The third phase corresponds to the first thrusting motion, with contraction of the gastrocnemius muscle and resistance of the plantar muscles acting to absorb the shock. The forefoot spreads out on the ground. Lastly, the fourth phase corresponds to the second thrusting motion and the plantar muscles of the toes (notably the abductor hallucis, adductor transversus hallucis and flexor hallucis longus) add to the impetus provided by the gastrocnemius. These muscles fix the sesamoid sling and the proximal phalanx, allowing the step to end with dorsiflexion of the metatarsophalangeal joint of the hallux.

Finally, the abductor hallucis muscle is the only antagonist to outward deviation of the proximal phalanx. Its position respective to the first ray determines the position of the sesamoid sling and the proximal phalanx [43]. The strength of the abductor hallucis decreases with the length of the proximal phalanx. The metatarsophalangeal joint of the hallux and the muscles attached to it cannot be dissociated from the medial arch of the foot, running from the head of the first metatarsal to the posterior tuberosity of the calcaneus.

The flexor hallucis longus tendon forms a cord which suspends much of the medial arch, aided by the flexor digitorum longus muscle of the toes. The flexor hallucis longus stabilizes the talus and calcaneus. The abductor hallucis provides suspension along the whole medial arch.

Morphotypes of the foot [42, 53]

The anatomic and radiologic aspects of the forefoot allow definition of a digital and a metatarsal formula.
• The **digital formula** depends on the length of the hallux.
    - the forefoot is Egyptian if the hallux is longer than the second toe;
    - the forefoot is square if the first two toes have the same length with progressively decreasing lengths of the 3rd to 5th toes;
    - the forefoot is Greek if the first toe is shorter than the second with progressively decreasing lengths of the 2nd to 5th toes.
• The **metatarsal formula** allows distinction of a morphotype, where the first metatarsal is shorter than the second (index minus); a morphotype, where it is as long as the 2nd metatarsal (index plus minus); and a morphotype where it is longer than the 2nd (index plus). The protruding metatarsal heads describe a curve (Lelièvre's parabola).

Anatomy and pathology of hallux valgus

Hallux valgus is a dynamic and progressive deformity of the hallux combining osseous, muscular, and capsular-ligamentous lesions (fig. 17.1).

The osteo-articular lesions
[23, 33, 47, 59]

The osseous deformity combines outward deviation of the proximal phalanx (superior to 10°), pronation of the hallux, and inward deviation of the first metatarsal; the medial part of the metatarsal head progressively thrusts against the soft tissues and creates an exostosis. If there is medial capsular and

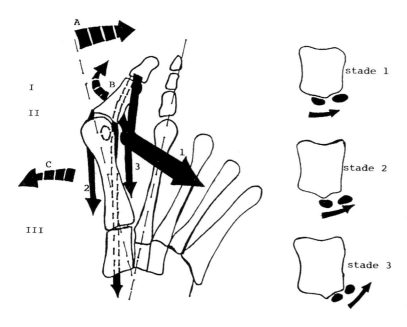

Fig. 17.1. Hallux valgus is a dynamic progressive deformity of the hallux combining osseous, muscular and capsulo-ligamentous lesions. *1* Adductor hallucis muscle, *2* abductor hallucis muscle, *3* extensor hallucis longus muscle, *4* flexor hallucis longus muscle. *A* Phalangeal valgus, *B* phalangeal pronation, *C* metatarsus varus. *I* Hallomegaly, *II* articular surface of the metatarsophalangeal joint, *III* articular surface of the cuneiform-metatarsal joint. Grade 1, 2 or 3 in relation to the "translocation" of the sesamoids

ligamentous stretching, lateral contracture occurs which results in progressive permanent deformity. The lateral base of the proximal phalanx pushes on the lateral part of the metatarsal head, which accentuates the inward deviation of the metatarsal and leads to a lateral metatarsophalangeal arthrosis. The sesamoids move laterally into the first inter-metatarsal space in a movement which combines inward deviation of the first metatarsal and pronation of the proximal phalanx.

The lateral sesamoid moves onto the lateral edge of the first metatarsal head. The lateral glenosesamoid ligament contracts and makes the deformity permanent. The progressive wear on the intersesamoid ridge predisposes to translocation of the sesamoids.

Muscular dysfunction

[1, 10, 43, 45, 47]

The hypermobility of the metatarsophalangeal joint of the hallux and the fragile muscular balance explain the self-perpetuating tendency of the deformities.

• The abductor hallucis tendon follows the lateral translocation of the sesamoids and becomes plantar. Thus, the only "antivalgus" muscle loses its proper function and only serves to flex the hallux. This plantar migration of the abductor tendon explains

the pronation of the proximal phalanx of the hallux. When the abductor tendon becomes plantar, it displaces the first metatarsal away from the second, causing the first metatarsal to move inward.

• The flexor hallucis brevis and adductor hallucis tendons migrate into a lateral position and accentuate the outward deviation of the hallux.

• The long muscles also contribute to the outward deviation of the proximal phalanx: the flexor hallucis longus and extensor hallucis longus muscles shorten and maintain the arc created by the deformity.

Associated lesions [10, 19, 28]

A shortened first ray, (whether congenital or because of metatarsus varus secondary to hallux valgus) and dislocation of the sesamoids cause abnormality of support under the first metatarsal head. This metatarsal splaying overloads the middle metatarsals, particularly the second. Lateral metatarsal dynamics are altered by the hyperlaxity of the tarsometatarsal joint-space, which adds to the overload on the middle metatarsals. Moreover, these middle metatarsals tend to become more vertical, thus augmenting their pitch in relation to the ground. This is due to a rupture of the balance between the interosseous and longus muscles which favors the latter. This phenomenon is accentuated in the 2nd ray since the valgus of the hallux is often plantar and maintains hyperextension of the 2nd toe.

The proximal phalanx is retracted in dorsiflexion with a plantar metatarsophalangeal dislocation, which encourages lowering of the corresponding metatarsal head. The claw-like retraction of the toe means that it loses its function of support, increasing the load on the metatarsal head. Metatarsophalangeal dislocation is often the end result of the progress of the deformity.

● Etiology and pathogenesis of hallux valgus

Hallux valgus is a deformity which occurs more often in women, as testified by the Kelikian series (98%), cited by Jahss [35], Barouk (97%) [6], Hardy (88%) [30] and Mann (64%) [45, 47]. This predominance is less overwhelming for congenital hallux valgus, in which 15% of the patients are males [24].

The role of shoes

Feminine footwear, which is often too small and with pointed toes, concentrates leverage on the proximal phalanx which is maintained in valgus.

High heels can excessively elevate the first ray and create adduction and supination of the first metatarsal, thus accentuating the metatarsus varus and the splaying of the forefoot. High heels overload the middle rays and aggravate the static metatarsalgia caused by hallux valgus and ineffectiveness of the first ray [10, 59].

Narrow shoes alone can also worsen exostoses, so that even a moderately deviated hallux can show large exostoses.

The role of footwear in the development of hallux valgus is corroborated by studies done in Japan [40] where the incidence of hallux valgus increased significantly with the use of Western-type shoes instead of traditional footwear. Nonetheless, the absence of hallux valgus in certain women who wear pointed shoes, and its development in men and children, means that other etiologic factors must be sought, which also represent some of the determining factors in the incidence of valgus linked to feminine footwear.

Predisposing anatomic factors

Length of the hallux

The metatarsal formula is independent of the formula for the toes. The Egyptian foot, in which the hallux is longer than the second toe, but where the first metatarsal is shorter than the second (formula index minus) is the anatomic situation which most predisposes to development of hallux valgus, notably if narrow shoes with pointed toes are worn. The excessive length of the hallux goes with hallomegaly [5, 25, 57].

Metatarsus varus

Occasionally, this is congenital and it corresponds to the atavistic foot described by Morton, with a first metatarsal which is short, mobile, and in varus [35].

More often, it is acquired and secondary to the appearance of hallux valgus [47] and becomes more prominent with the accentuation of the phalangeal valgus. It is fostered by an oblique cuneo-metatarsal joint-space [45] and by horizontalization and supination of the first metatarsal, but is even more proportional to the obliqueness of the cuneo-metatarsal joint [33].

Valgus flat foot

The relationship between valgus flat foot and hallux valgus remains controversial. Pronation of the forefoot is essential according to Inmann [33], yet totally fortuitous for Lelièvre [42] and Mann [47]. It does not seem to accord with certain mechanical theories about the genesis of hallux valgus.

For others, valgus flat foot promotes passive elevation of the first metatarsal and its movement towards a horizontal plane, which has the effect of lengthening the medial arch [58, 53]. In walking, passive valgus of the hallux takes place especially when there is weight-bearing on the medial aspect of the hallux.

This horizontalization of the first metatarsal is more pronounced when the cuneo-metatarsal joint is more oblique and/or mobile, as is seen in ligamentous hyperlaxity. This is particularly true in the case of obese individuals.

Congenital factors

Hallux valgus is of congenital origin in 1 out of 4 cases [6, 52]. It presents some specific anatomic features:
• excessively oblique cuneo-metatarsal joint-space,
• the first metatarsal is longer than in acquired hallux valgus,
• dysplasia of the metatarsophalangeal joint,
   - the metatarsal head is more round [6, 45] and sometimes laterally oriented,
   - dysplasia, or even aplasia, of the intersesamoid ridge which does not oppose deviation of the axis from the sesamoid sling,
   - sesamoid hypoplasia;
• metatarsus varus appears secondarily in most cases, and should not be considered as the element which triggers metatarsophalangeal instability.

Other factors

• The 2nd toe acts as a buttress and in the case of the hallux, after its functional disappearance (amputation or clawing) phalangeal valgus is accentuated [59].
• Interphalangeal valgus (lateral curvature between the first and second phalanges) causes a cam effect and provokes development of hallux valgus [59].
• Intermetatarsal bone: certain authors consider this to be an ossification of the tendon distal to the first cuneiform bone, while others maintain that it is an extra metatarsal. It accentuates the metatarsus varus by crowding the first space and deviates the hallux by its retractile attachment to the lateral base of the proximal phalanx [62].

Clinical considerations

Reasons for consultation

They are numerous, but they combine to cause patients to accept surgical intervention:

Exostosis

Popularly called a "bunion", this refers to an excessive outgrowth of the distal medial part of the first metatarsal causing pain when shoes are worn, while its unsightly appearance is often distasteful to young female patients.

Pain

This is the usual motive for consultation. Causes and localization are variable.

When narrow shoes are worn, pain is caused by the pressure on the exostosis, which irritates a sensory branch of the medial dorsal cutaneous nerve [47]. The patients are often young, with a moderate deformity, but reactive bursitis often develops and increases the pain, which makes shoes more and more difficult to tolerate.

Metatarsophalangeal pain can increase joint deformity, which may become permanent if the bursitis becomes aggravated and a sinus is formed.

Exceptionally, the pain may reveal a purulent metatarsophalangeal arthritis or even an osteitis. The deformity is marked and the patients tend to be aged.

Narrow shoes can trigger neuralgia of the first intermetatarsal space, which is often edematous [53].

Pain is often situated beneath the heads of the middle metatarsals and is aggravated by walking and heeled shoes, causing hot feet, plantar burning sensations and contractures. Pain may also be present on the dorsum of the proximal interphalangeal joint of a clawed toe which rubs against the shoe. This often concerns the 5th metatarsal head, which rubs against the side of the shoe when there is a triangular forefoot.

Problems with footwear

These problems occur early in young women who wear narrow, high-heeled shoes with pointed toes. The deformity is moderate, but the exostosis is poorly tolerated.

Male patients may also have problems when reinforced protective shoes are worn and in some sports (cycling, running, hiking, etc.).

They occur later in elderly patients who have chosen footwear adapted to the developing deformity. Problems come from the rubbing of shoes on the exostosis, the middle metatarsal heads, and clawed toes secondary to rounded forefeet.

Anatomic and radiographic studies (fig. 17.2)

These depend on a careful clinical examination of the foot, i.e., non-weight bearing, weight-bearing, footprint studies and specific weight-bearing X-rays completed in three spatial planes:

• the frontal dorso-plantar forefoot view in 10° ascension,
• the medial profile view,
• the axial view of the sesamoids (Güntz, Walter-Muller).

Circled views of the ankle in the weight-bearing foot by Meary's technique are also necessary to evaluate the position of the hindfoot relative to the talocrural joint.

Osteo-articular axial deviation

The proximal phalanx is deviated in the horizontal plane, but is also pronated by the faulty action of the abductor tendon of the hallux; this rotation of the phalanx is increased during weight-bearing and positions the end of the hallux upwards and outwards, while the toenail is oblique and faces inwards.

The physiologic metatarsophalangeal valgus of the first ray measured between the axes of M1 and P1 on the dorsoplantar view in weight-bearing is 8° to 12° (fig. 17.3a). The existence of a phalangeal curvature with interphalangeal valgus, associated with a medial interphalangeal callosity, can be identified both radiographically and clinically.

The lateral radiographs of the forefoot show a lack of parallelism of the two joint surfaces proximal and distal, of the proximal phalanx. This is quantifiable by calculating the Distal Articular Set Angle (DASA) or the Proximal Phalangeal Articular Angle (PPAA), both of which measure the angle between the proximal joint surface of P1 and the medio-diaphyseal axis of P1 (fig. 17.3b). Phalangeal rotation is evaluated clinically by measuring the angle between the phalangeal axis and the ground on weight bearing.

Varus of the first metatarsal is evaluated by measurement of the angle between M1 and M2, which is normally less than 10° (fig. 17.3a). This varus of the first metatarsal increases on weight-bearing, and becomes worse if there is laxity of the ligamentous structures and when the cuneo-metatarsal joint line is oblique, facing towards the medial aspect of

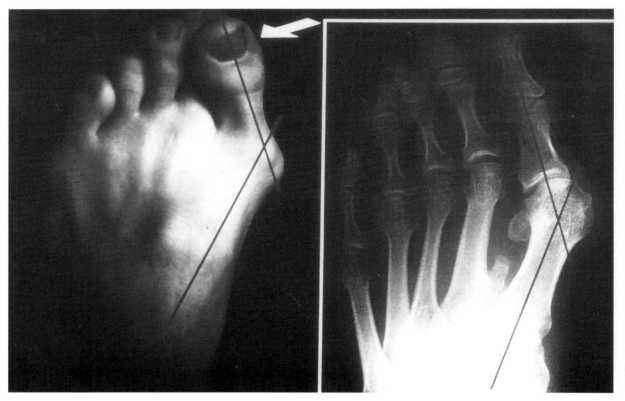

Fig. 17.2. Anatomic and radiographic correlations in the foot in weight-bearing: the hallux valgus, rotation of the phalanx, exostosis, metatarsus primus adductus and spreading of the metatarsal bones are assessed

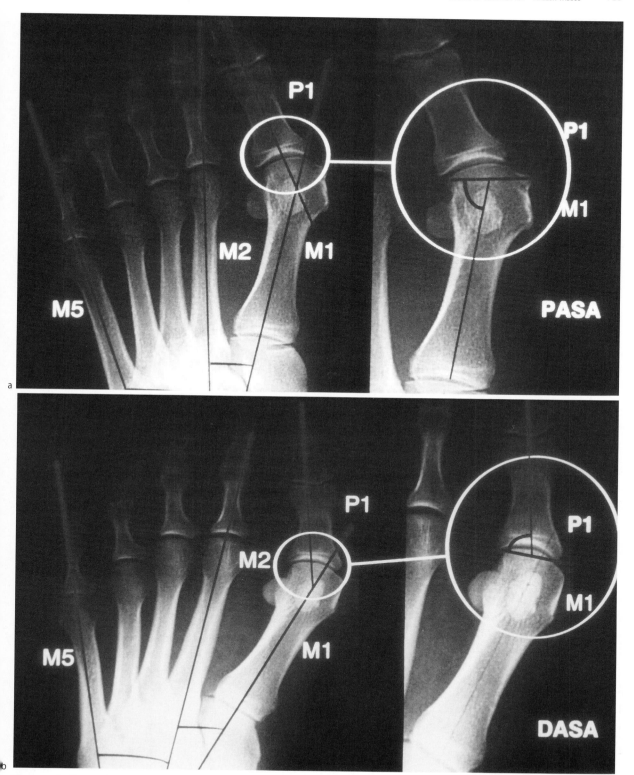

Fig. 17.3. Radiographic measurement of the deformities of the first ray in a dorso-plantar view. **a** Metatarsophalangeal valgus: M1P1 angle; metatarsus varus of the first ray: M1M2 angle; spreading of the metatarsal bones: M1M5 angle; deviation of the first metatarsal head = PASA or DMAA. **b** Radiographic measurements of deformities of the first ray in a dorso-plantar view: deviation of the base of the first phalanx: DASA or PPAA

the foot [45]. This varus is correlated with the width of the metatarsal fan as measured by the open angle of the foot between the M1 and M5 axes (20 to 28°) (fig. 17.3a). Weight-bearing side views show the malorientation of the metatarsal head which faces outwards. This may be congenital, or due to the acquired progressive deformity. Either the Proximal Articular Set Angle (PASA) or the Distal Metatarsal Articular Angle (DMAA) can be used to measure the angle between the articular surface of the head of M1 and the medio-diaphyseal line of M1 [66] (fig. 17.3b).

Plantar palpation coupled with examination of footprints is used to confirm the defective support beneath the first metatarsal head and its functional inadequacy.

Muscle and tendon imbalance

The lateral decentering of the metatarsophalangeal joint causes the development of the exostosis. It is overestimated on clinical examination because of the bursitis frequently associated with the deviated metatarsal head. Its real size can be estimated by lateral views of the forefoot which show the demarcation groove from the normal metatarsal head.

The axial view identifies the position of the sesamoids with respect to the sesamoid metatarsal ridge and the position of the sesamoid sling, which variably dislocates towards the outer side, proportional to the muscle imbalance.

Classically, three stages of displacement of the sesamoid sling are described:
• stage I, where the lateral sesamoid invades the intermetatarsal space, and the medial sesamoid straddles the intersesamoid ridge;
• stage II, where the lateral sesamoid is entirely in the intermetatarsal space;
• stage III, where both sesamoids are in the intermetatarsal space and even glide along the lateral aspect of the first metatarsal head.

Libotte and Blaimont [43] describe 5 situations, with a physiologic stage I, where the sesamoids are symmetric with respect to the ridge, a stage II where the medial sesamoid grazes the median ridge, a stage III where the medial sesamoid is beneath the ridge, a stage IV where the medial sesamoid passes lateral to the ridge, and lastly, a stage V where the medial sesamoid moves into the lateral sesamoid's place. The axial view confirms the congenital character of the deformity in adolescents or young adults by showing the hypoplasia of the median intersesamoid crest. There progressively follow wear of the crest which is

concomitant with the progressive stages of dislocation, accentuation of phalangeal valgus, and metatarsal varus [2, 59]. On the other hand, this view made postoperatively reflects the quality of sesamoid recentering and muscular rebalancing, and therefore the correction of the phalangeal valgus and metatarsus varus.

Morphotypes of the foot

The clinical assessment allows determination of the digital formula mentioned above.

Dorsoplantar views in weight-bearing confirm a Greek foot in 23% of cases, a square foot in 27%, and an Egyptian foot in 50%. The Egyptian foot with hallomegaly is present in more than 70% of cases of hallux valgus [42].

The dorsoplantar view in weight-bearing is absolutely necessary to determine the metatarsal formula which describes Lelièvre's parabola [in which the summit of the curve is the 2nd metatarsal head $(1 < 2 > 3 > 4 > 5)$] in physiologic conditions. The constitutional or acquired shortness of the first metatarsal $(2 > 3 > 4 > 1 >> 5)$ found in hallux valgus is associated with the Egyptian digital formula.

Associated lesions

Overloading of the middle rays

This usually begins in the 2nd ray with overlapping or underlapping clawing of the 2nd toe and metatarsalgia, with a painful plantar callosity under the head of the 2nd metatarsal. It can concern the 3rd and 4th rays and evolve to a rigid flat forefoot with painful plantar callosities. Clinically, there is hyperextension of the proximal phalanges, or even dorsal dislocation of the middle rays.

Dorsoplantar views done together with medial profile studies can confirm possible dislocation and an oblique lateral view at an angle of 40° confirms the overloading of the middle metatarsal heads.

Foot statics

Footprint examination gives precise information on the state of the plantar arch, and notably reveals the pejorative nature of valgus flat foot, which some authors continue to consider as a factor that may contribute to hallux valgus relapse.

A weight-bearing medial profile study supplies more details from studying the talo-first metatarsal line and Fick's angle of pitch, which amplifies the information obtained from the plantar prints.

Circled films of the hindfoot will clarify clinical impressions regarding varus or valgus of the hindfoot.

Reducing deformities of the first ray

In considering deformities in valgus of the proximal phalanx and in varus of the first metatarsal, the duration of the deformities and the associated capsular-ligamentous and muscular contractures must also be kept in mind. It is evident that reduction of the deformities is more likely to succeed if they are recent, and if the patient is young.

Simple reduction of deformities, however, is not an end in itself because in the case of severe deformity, reduction may abolish pre-existing mobility of the metatarsophalangeal joint. Indeed, adaptation of joint function occurs at the same time as aggravation of the deformities. It is a fundamental principle to avoid surgical transformation of a deformed but mobile joint into a joint with a more normal axis, but which is ankylosed and useless with an added risk of rapid relapse and degenerative arthrosis.

There is no single phenomenon of static hallux valgus because mechanical diversity is the rule [1, 66]:
• Congenital hallux valgus, in which the deformity appears before the age of 15, has its own anatomopathologic characteristics as discussed above. The problem appears during adolescence and corresponds to changes in footwear.
• Hallux valgus of the tonic foot in which the phalangeal valgus is moderate and the discomfort is really due to the size and progressive exposure of the metatarsal head (these subjects are frequently male).
• Hallux valgus of the lax foot with triangular forefoot, which is the case of most hallux valgus in young women. Hyperlaxity of the ligaments increases deformation but also allows for reduction. This type, however, can also be worsened by the appearance of a valgus of the hindfoot. The risk of postoperative relapse is high if this last deformity is neglected.
• Severe hallux valgus in the elderly: deformities of the first ray are severe, but they are long-standing and consultation is sought because of the associated lesions, which means that it may be difficult for the patient to understand why a surgical intervention on the first ray is advised.

• Hallux valgus of the arthrotic type with pain provoked on forced plantarflexion of the hallux.
• Hallux valgus which relapses: the state of the metatarsophalangeal articular cartilage plays an important role in deciding treatment.

At the end of this clinical and paraclinical survey, a diagnosis of static hallux valgus is established, with or without a congenital factor as determined by the criteria mentioned above. The patients' general condition as well as their neurovascular status will have been reviewed. The severity of deformities of the first ray and adjacent rays, the age of the patient, the duration and history of the problem, and contributory factors (footwear, professional activity, sports, etc.) remain the fundamental elements in choosing a therapeutic strategy.

Treatment

Objectives

The treatment objectives in static hallux valgus are clear and are based on several rules:
• to re-establish a physiologic metatarsophalangeal axis along the first ray,
• to establish physiologic and balanced muscular function with satisfactory support on the pulp of the great toe by recentering the tendons, capsules, muscles and sesamoids,
• elimination of problems due to chafing from footwear (exostosis, metatarsalgia, clawed toes).

The treatment of hallux valgus is therefore oriented towards completely reharmonising the forefoot.

Conservative treatment

Given the above rules, hopes for successful nonsurgical treatment are modest but include certain valuable elements, particularly following surgery [14]:
• Physical therapy, and sometimes added autotherapy, can permit recovery of active and passive mobility by relaxing the hallux, forefoot massage, and use of an antivalgus brace at night.
• Footwear that is wide over the forefoot and made of soft leather must be prescribed, while high-heeled shoes with pointed toes should be worn only briefly and infrequently.

• Plantar orthoses to correct a rounded forefoot or a valgus flatfoot can also be of use.

Surgical treatment

Since Morton in 1876 and Reverdin in 1881, surgical methods of treatment have multiplied, and now number around 200. The techniques that are commonly used will be discussed with regard to their effectiveness.

Surgical methods

Principles for surgical intervention are determined by the physiologic disorders involved [1, 10, 11, 59]; they are:
• elimination of the lateral fibrous knot, release of the sesamoid sling, and tightening of the medial capsular ligaments to correct phalangeal valgus and metatarsus varus by establishing a correct axis of the first ray;
• osteotomies to establish a correct axis along the first ray in the case of severe deformities, cuneo-metatarsal joint stiffness or hyperlaxity, and congenital axial deviations. These osteotomies interrupt bony continuity at different levels and allow osseous reorientation during re-establishment of continuity. Fixation usually implies the use of screws, pins, or plates;
• interventions on joints when metatarsophalangeal arthrosis is present;
• correction of flat forefoot and its consequences on the toes.

We use Groulier's classification system [26, 28] which distinguishes conservative and radical methods.

Bunionectomy

This should never be an isolated procedure, but should be associated with the other therapeutic options. It eliminates problems due to the rubbing of shoes. A medial buttress should be left in place so as to avoid hypercorrection and phalangeal subluxation in varus [26, 59].

Conservative methods

Recentering the sesamoid sling [42, 44]

Disinsertion of the tendon of the adductor hallucis muscle from the phalangeal base, and possibly from the lateral sesamoid as well, is associated with a sesamoid-metatarsal horizontal arthrotomy and sometimes with a metatarsophalangeal vertical lateral arthrotomy. Medial capsular ligament tightening recenters the sesamoid sling while correcting the phalangeal valgus and metatarsal varus.

McBride's procedure [25, 45, 60]

In addition to the operations mentioned above, transfer of the adductor hallucis tendon muscle from the phalangeal base and the lateral sesamoid to the neck of the first metatarsal permits dynamic correction of metatarsus varus. Although ablation of the lateral sesamoid was part of the original technique, this is no longer done. This intervention is completed by medial retightening, which corrects a reducible metatarsal. Technical variations proposed by certain authors [25, 45] have not modified the fundamental principles of this surgical procedure.

Shortening the proximal phalanx

Removal of 3 to 5 mm of the phalangeal diaphysis is an inevitable element for durable retightening of the capsular-ligamentous medial plane in the Egyptian foot morphotype. This shortening of a hallomegaly plays an important part in relaxing the lateral soft tissues before sesamoid recentering [25, 42, 57]. This can be a trapezoidal cuneiform osteotomy with a medial base when the hallomegaly is associated with interphalangeal valgus [23].

Finally, this phalangeal osteotomy, combined with medial capsular-ligamentous retightening and metatarsal osteotomy, helps to correct phalangeal rotation.

Metatarsal osteotomies

Although these cannot serve as the only method for metatarsophalangeal realignment, they aresometimes employed as adjuncts to interventions on the soft tissues and the proximal phalanx in several situations:
• the metatarsophalangeal alignment is incomplete
• when metatarsus varus is important (often > 15°)
• when cuneometatarsal stiffness makes it irreducible
• the metatarsal head presents an orientation defect (PASA) and phalangeal realignment alone may cause joint incongruence.
• forefoot hyperlaxity, which could lead to secondary interventions on the soft tissues.

Metatarsal osteotomy diminishes pressure on the soft tissues, ensuring that one part of the correction is durable, and so reduces risk of relapse while relieving difficulties with footwear.

Osteotomy of the base of the metatarsal (fig. 17.4)

• Most often, this is a medial addition operation [25, 26, 27, 28], necessitating a cortico-cancellous bone mini-graft (taken from the exostosis and by shortening P1) and a stable fixation (screwed mini-plates). This corrects only the metatarsus varus deviation and so is effective only in the horizontal plane. Advocates of this procedure specify its use for metatarsus varus of more than 16°.

• Lateral subtraction osteotomy is sometimes used [66], and aims at correction in both the frontal and sagittal planes. Fixation is simpler since a compression screw can be used.

• The osteotomy line can be curved (or sometimes V-shaped) and can be adjusted as desired since, unlike the two described above, nothing is either added or removed (fixation is made with 1 or 2 separate screws in compression [16], or even 2 crossed pins). This operation is principally indicated for severe metatarsus varus deviations.

Distal osteotomies

Some of these concern the epiphysial-metaphysal region and are derived from Austin's technique, elaborated by Kenneth-Johnson. They are V-shaped [3, 56] and produce a lateral relocation of the metatarsal head. Advocates of this procedure reserve its use for metatarsus varus of less than 16° and most often for subjects under 50 years [36, 38, 39, 51].

The other distal osteotomies are done on the metaphysial-diaphysial region (Mitchell) and reorientate the metatarsal head with a possible multidirectional effect. However, there is sometimes afterwards an untoward shortening of the 1st meta-

tarsal. These osteotomies must also be restricted to metatarsus varus of less than 16° [68].

Technical variations of these juxtacephalic osteotomies exist such as Hohman's osteotomy, revised by Copin, which obtains multidirectional correction of the metatarsal head [15].

Bipolar osteotomy

This is advocated in France by Schnepp [58] and associates distal medial subtraction with a proximal medial addition. It is used in metatarsus varus superior to 16° (proximal osteotomy) with metatarsal cephalic dysplasia (distal osteotomy).

Diaphysial osteotomies

Only the long oblique osteotomy will be discussed here, as described by Burutaran [13], revised by Gudas [29], and particularly by Weil in the USA [67] and introduced into France by Barouk [7]. It is known by the name of SCARF, this osteotomy allows 8 displacements of the 2 fragments, plantar (joined to the metatarsal head) and dorsal (joined to the metatarsal base).The essential features which its advocates stress are:

• lateral relocation to correct the metatarsus varus,
• medial rotation to correct the metatarsal cephalic dysplasia and the PASA,
• lowering of the head which is automatically part of the reorientation of the longitudinal axis and is produced by overlapping the two fragments like shingles on a roof,
• modifications of the length of the first metatarsal (shortening or lengthening) requiring prudent manipulation.

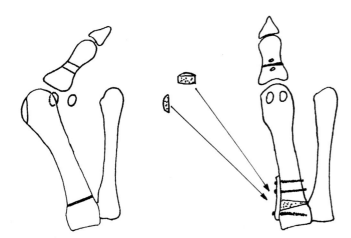

Fig. 17.4. Basi-metatarsal osteotomy with a medial addition and a screwed mini-plate stabilization

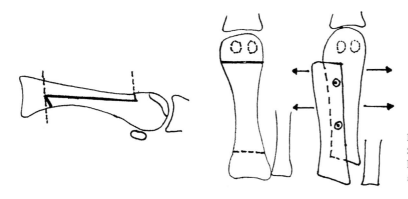

Fig. 17.5. Longitudinal shaft osteotomy: SCARF procedure. The osteotomy is stabilized by 2 dorsoplantar screws in compression

The osteotomy is stabilized by 2 dorso-plantar compression screws in compression (fig. 17.5). All cases of metatarsus varus and metatarsal cephalic dysplasia are indications for this osteotomy.

Operations on the cuneo-metatarsal joint

• *Cuneo-metatarsal arthrodesis*

Advocated by Lapidus, followed by Myerson [50], this is indicated in hypermobility of the cuneo-metatarsal joint with a marked metatarsus varus. The metatarsal head is depressed at the same time, to free the metatarsophalangeal joint. This technique seems useful mostly in young patients.

• *Osteotomy of the first cuneiform*

Advocated by Groulier [28], this consists of an opening wedge osteotomy by medial addition, which is self-stabilizing. Its aim is to reorientate the metatarso-cuneiform joint line and advocates reserve it for metatarsus varus inferior to 22°. It is an alternative to osteotomy of the base of the metatarsal.

Radical methods

The Keller-Brandes technique as modified by Lelièvre [42] combines resection of the base of the first phalanx with sesamoid recentering and medial capsular retightening.

Excessive resection at the base of the first phalanx, however, can result in mutilations with a floppy toe and aggravation of the middle metatarsalgia; therefore the existence of more reliable techniques means that this intervention is practiced less and less.

Implanted prostheses: the Swanson prosthesis

These are implanted in the phalanx, where they replace the base. They are combined with the Keller-Lelièvre technique and are indicated for metatarsophalangeal arthrosis. Swanson monoblock implants unite the phalanx and metatarsus. Complications, due to biomechanical inadequacy of the material (silicone), which offers little resistance to pressures at the first metatarsophalangeal space, have led to their being abandoned in France [19, 20, 26].

Interposition prostheses [8, 34]

These are button shaped and made of metal. They are inserted between the first metatarsal and the phalanx after resection of the base, and are indicated in arthroses of the metatarsophalangeal joint. Used in conjunction with osteotomies, they promote better realignment of the first ray.

Resurfacing prostheses

Some of these are total prostheses [8, 34, 41, 48], while others are purely metatarsal. They are indicated when a metatarsophalangeal arthrosis is associated with phalangeal valgus. They are sometimes used with metatarsal osteotomy as an adjunctive measure to reduce metatarsus varus. These are still under evaluation as a useful alternative to metatarsophalangeal arthrodesis.

Metatarsophalangeal arthrodesis

Technical variations are numerous [17, 26, 61, 63], although the screwed plate is the most satisfying method from a biomechanical point of view [54]. The accepted position is in 10 to 20° of valgus of the first phalanx on the first metatarsal axis and 25 to 35° of dorsiflexion of the first phalanx on the first metatarsal, so as to avoid overloading both the head of M1 and the interphalangeal joint and to prevent shoe rubbing [46].

Arthrodesis is indicated for metatarsophalangeal arthrosis of the hallux, for severe hallux valgus in the elderly and during revision procedures. Provided that biomechanical requirements are respected and that both the talocrural joint and the interphalangeal joint of the hallux are mobile, normal walking can be restored.

Surgical indications

Considerations

• the age of the patient and therefore his functional and socioprofessional needs,
• the duration of the deformity and hence the acquired or congenital nature of the static hallux valgus,
• reducibility of the different elements of the deformity both pre- and postoperatively,
• the severity of the deformity, the morphotype of the foot, and the state of the cartilage of the different joints as seen in pre-operative radiographs.

Congenital static hallux valgus

After fusion of the epiphysis, surgical treatment becomes a possibility for adolescents and adults. When metatarsus varus is absent in early deformities, the technique selected must combine a soft tissue intervention and phalangeal shortening osteotomy (Egyptian foot) for varisation and derotation [4, 6, 52].

In deformities with true metatarsus varus, a metatarsal osteotomy must be combined with phalangeal and capsular procedures to secure a metatarsus varus of between 8 and 10°. The osteotomy must correct both the overall metatarsus and the metatarsophalangeal dysplasia (PASA). A combination of proximal osteotomy and cephalic or SCARF osteotomies may be indicated [6, 7].

Deterioration of the lesions and ligamentous hyperlaxity is always possible and may finally impose a radical procedure on the bone to avoid relapse.

Acquired static hallux valgus with healthy articular cartilage

Phalangeal shortening is indicated whenever an Egyptian foot with hallomegaly is present [5, 26, 57].

If the metatarsus varus is less than 12°, capsular retightening usually suffices except when there is metatarsophalangeal incongruence or when the foot is lax. In such cases, a juxtacephalic or SCARF osteotomy is indicated.

If the metatarsus varus is between 12 and 16° a metatarsal osteotomy seems to be generally preferred with a choice of either a juxtacephalic or SCARF osteotomy.

If the metatarsus varus is more than 16°, juxtacephalic osteotomy is no longer indicated and the choice is reduced to proximal osteotomies with a medial wedge or in V-shape, particularly for metatarsus varus of over 20°, and the SCARF procedure (fig. 17.5).

Cartilaginous lesions

Certain authors propose the same interventions, evoking the biomechanical benefits of decompression on cartilage [7, 18].

Others, however, specify metatarsophalangeal arthrodesis if strict technical considerations are observed, and the proximal and distal joints are free [17, 26, 62].

Silicone implants have been abandoned, since they result in too many complications [19, 20].

Total or partial metallic implants remain useful, in association with freeing of the soft tissues and tightening of the medial capsular ligaments. Metatarsal osteotomy is sometimes added [41, 48].

Treating surgical complications

Trophic disturbances

Complications are more often edematous than algodystrophic, but they may continue for several months and necessitate a complete care program which includes elastic support therapy, promotion of lymphatic drainage and physiotherapy.

Metatarsophalangeal joint stiffness of the hallux

This results from the arthrotomy, soft tissue stripping and capsular retightening. Usually moderate, this tends to diminish when ambulation is restarted. Stiffness can resist physiotherapy, with no plantarflexion and dorsiflexion inferior to 60°, in cases of excess residual length of the first ray, i.e., without first phalangeal shortening in an Egyptian foot [28]. Stiffness of the metatarsophalangeal of the hallux evolves rapidly towards arthrosis.

Complications linked to osteotomy

Phalangeal osteotomy

Pseudarthrosis is quite rare [5, 57]. The presence of osteoporosis, however, should alert the surgeon to avoid repeated procedures due to degeneration of the osteotomy site. Necrosis of the phalangeal base is often due to an osteotomy made too proximally [19].

Metatarsal osteotomies

The risk of pseudarthrosis is less than 10%, and even less when the position is very stable (screwed plate) [25] or the osteotomy line very long (Scarf) [7]. Proximal osteotomies carry a risk of exaggerated elevation of the first metatarsal head, with overloading of the middle metatarsal heads. Although juxtacephalic osteotomies present a risk of cephalic necrosis, recent series do not confirm this [12, 49].

Relapses

Deformity reappears within 2 years following the initial intervention in 10 to 12% of cases according to the series consulted [26]. Four causes are frequently found:
- inadequate freeing of the lateral capsular ligaments,
- inadequate retightening of the medial capsular ligament,
- metatarsus varus over 15° left uncorrected,
- uncorrected hallomegaly.

If the recurrent deformity is not rigid, an appropriate conservative intervention will suffice. If the deformity is rigid, with arthrosis, and especially if there is stiffness in aged subjects, arthrodesis seems the best alternative.

Overcorrection

Acquired postoperative iatrogenic hallux varus is not tolerated as well as the original hallux valgus since a shoe cannot be worn. Dorsiflexion of the first phalanx is associated with the varus, with clawing of the interphalangeal joint in some cases. This occurs in about 5% of patients according to the series consulted [27, 65]. Causes include excessive lateral freeing and medial over-tightening, particularly when associated with McBride's procedure or with excessive bunionectomy.

Treatment includes obligatory complete arthrolysis: medial, with resection of the abductor hallucis muscle, lateral with removal of the intercapital fibrosis.

When the deformity is not rigid, and without interphalangeal clawing, a mobilizing intervention is necessary:
- tendon transfers: of the extensor hallucis longus [21, 37], abductor hallucis [31], or first dorsal interosseous tendons [65].

- reconstruction of the lateral ligament (LigaproR of 1.5 mm diameter) [64].
- sometimes a medial wedge is added when the exostectomy has been excessive [27].

If deformities are old, rigid, and with clawing of the interphalangeal joint, metatarsophalangeal arthrodesis remains the best solution [26, 63].

Postoperative metatarsalgia

Surgery on the first ray may unfortunately create new stresses on the forefoot.

The Hueter-Mayo or Keller-Brandes procedures eliminate pressure on the first ray and overload the middle rays.

Lengthening, shortening, elevation or depression of the first metatarsal can modify the biomechanics of anterior support. Stiffness of the metatarsophalangeal joint induces reflex supination of the foot and so lateral hyperpressure.

Treatment of associated lesions

When deformities are moderate, i.e., limited to callosities and minimal supple clawing without tendon contracture, they disappear in 2/3 of cases after reduction of the metatarsus varus and repositioning the sesamoids. Surgical treatment of hallux valgus alone may suffice, aided by plantar insole supports.

When clawing of the proximal interphalangeal joints is rigid, excision arthroplasty can be done on the head of the first phalanx with temporary stabilization by axial pinning. However, the metatarsophalangeal imbalance is usually irreversible and rigid, as is the clawing. It is sometimes so predominant that even the hallux valgus symptoms are overshadowed.

Metatarsal surgery is then required:
- some experts advocate a basal lift osteotomy, with possible shortening [19, 28],
- Helal's diaphysial osteotomy [32] still lacks precision and may lead to pseudarthrosis,
- the cervical osteotomy of Gauthier's dorsal cuneiform resection combats phalangeal hypertension, but does not shorten the metatarsus and so does not combat excessive tension on the capsule [66],
- Weil's capito-cervical osteotomy [9] allows metatarsal shortening and osteoarticular relaxation of the forefoot, with lateral or medial translation of the toes, when combined with an intervention on the extensor tendons, i.e., the extensor brevis.

When the metatarsophalangeal joint is dislocated, certain authors recommend Gauthier's or Weil's osteotomies, while others prefer Swanson's or Gauthier's ball-shaped implants when dislocations are old and rigid [22].

References

1. Allieu Y (1984) L'hallux valgus. Étiopathogénie et formes cliniques. Rhumatologie 40: 21-25
2. Ameil M, Gérard Y (1983) Quelques précisions anatomiques sur le premier rayon du pied. Med Chir Pied 9: 23-26
3. Austin D, Leventen E (1981) A new osteotomy for hallux valgus. Clin Orthop 157: 25-30
4. Banks AS, Yu Scheng HSU, Marias HS, Zirm R (1994) Juvenile hallux abductor valgus. Association with metatarsus adductus. J Am Podiatr Med Assoc 84: 219-224
5. Barouk LS (1988) Indication et technique des ostéotomies extra-articularies du gros orteil. Med Chir Pied 4: 147-154
6. Barouk LS, Diébold P (1991) Hallux valgus congénital, symposium. Med Chir Pied 7: 65-112
7. Barouk LS (1992) Notre expérience de l'ostéotomie SCARF des premier et cinquième métatarsiens. Med Chir Pied 8: 67-84
8. Barouk LS (1982) Utilisation de la prothèse bouton au niveau du premier rayon. Med Chir Pied 8: 125-136
9. Barouk LS (1994) L'ostéotomie cervico-capitale de Weil dans les métatarsalgies médianes. Med Chir Pied 23-33
10. Bénichou M, Allieu Y (1990) Hallux valgus: bases physiopathologiques et étiopathogéniques. In: Claustre J, Simon L (eds) Les métatarsalgies statiques. Monographie de podologie. Masson, Paris, pp 111-117
11. Bénichou J (1990) Quel traitement chirurgical pour quel hallux valgus ? In: Claustre J, Simon L (eds) Les métatarsalgies statiques. Monographie de podologie. Masson, Paris, pp 127-129
12. Blum JL (1994) The modified Mitchell osteotomy. bunionectomy. Indications and surgical considerations. Foot Ankle 15: 97-141
13. Burutaran JM (1976) Hallux valgus y cortedad anatomica del primar metatarsano (correcion quirurgica). Actualités de Médecine et de Chirurgie du Pied. Masson, Paris, pp 261-266
14. Claustre JE (1990) Y-a-t-il un traitement médical de l'hallux valgus ? In: Claustre J, Simon L (eds) Monographies de podologie. Masson, Paris
15. Copin G. (1991) L'opération de Hohmann: ostéotomie sous capitale du 1er métatarsien. Orthop Traumatol 1: 40-46
16. Coughlin JM (1994) Proximal first metatarsal osteotomy. In: Foot and Ankle. Raven Press, New York, pp 85-105
17. Coughlin MJ, Abdo RV (1994) Arthrodesis of the first metatarso-phalangueal joint with vitallium plate fixation. Foot Ankle 15: 18-28
18. Delagoutte JP, Peltre G, Becker JM, Erb C, Reynier A (1987) La chirurgie à visée biomécanique dans l'hallux valgus est-elle licite au-delà de 60 ans ? Med Chir Pied 3: 187-189
19. Delagoutte JP (1989) L'hallux valgus. In: Delagoutte JP, Bonnel F (eds) Le Pied: pathologie et techniques chirurgicales. Masson, Paris
20. Denis A (1992) Le point sur les interpositions d'implants en élastomère de silicone dans la chirurgie du premier orteil. Med Chir Pied 8: 121-124
21. Diébold PF, Delagoutte JP (1988) À propos du traitement de l'hallux varus post-opératoire. Med Chir Pied 4: 41-43
22. Gauthier G (1984) 178 prothèses monobloc en élastomère de silicone mises à l'avant-pied. Résultats à la 5e année. Rev Chir Orthop (suppl II) 70: 167-169
23. Gianestras NJ (1972) Modified Akin procedure for the correction of hallux valgus. Am Acad Orthop Surg 21: 254-262
24. Goldcher A (1991) Fréquence sexe et hérédité. In: Symposium hallux valgus congénital. Med.Chir Pied 7: 65-112
25. Groulier P, Curvale G, Prudent MP, Vedel F (1988) Résultats du traitement de l'hallux valgus selon la technique de Mc Bride modifié avec ou sans ostéotomie phalangienne ou métatarsienne complémentaire. Rev Chir Orthop 74: 539-548
26. Groulier P (1990) Traitement chirurgical de l'hallux valgus et des métatarsalgies associées du 2e rayon. Table ronde avec la participation de JP Carret, G. Curvale, JP Delagoutte, A. Denis, O. Jardé, JF. Lelièvre, MP Prudent, P. Vichard, A. Zeil. Rev Chir Orthop 76: 116-131
27. Groulier P, Curvale G, Coillard JY, Franceschi JP (1992) Hallux varus acquis post-opératoire. traitement chirurgical. Rev Chir Orthop 78: 449-455
28. Groulier P (1993) Du traitement chirurgical de l'hallux valgus et de ses complications. In: Duparc J (ed) Cahiers d'enseignement de la SOFCOT. Conférences d'enseignement. Expansion Scientifique Française, Paris, pp 13-30
29. Gudas CJ, Laros GS, Zygmunt KM (1989) A bunionectomy with internal screw fixation. J Am Podiatr Med Assoc 79
30. Hardy RH, Claphan JCR (1952) Hallux valgus. Predisposing anatomical causes. Lancet 1: 180
31. Hawkins FB (1971) Acquired hallux varus: cause, prevention and correction. Clin Orthop 76: 169-176
32. Helal B (1975) Metatarsal osteotomy for metatarsalgia. J Bone Joint Surg 57B: 187-193
33. Inman VF (1973) Surgery of the foot. Mosby, St Louis
34. Jarde O, Trinquier JL, Filloux JF, Tranvan F, Vives P (1993) La prothèse métatarso-phalangienne Sixtine du premier rayon. Résultats préliminaires à propos de 74 cas. Med Chir Pied 9: 143-147
35. Jahss MH (1991) Disorders of the Foot and Ankle, 2nd edn. Saunders, Philadelphia

36. Johnson K, Cofield R, Morrey B (1979) Chevron oste-otomy for hallux valgus. Clin Orthop 142: 44-47

37. Johnson KA, Spiegel PV (1984) Extensor hallucis longus transfer for hallux varus deformity. J Bone Joint Surg 66 A: 681-686

38. Johnson JE, Clanton TO, Baxter DE, Gottlieb MS (1991) Comparison of chevron osteotomy and modified Mc Bride bunionectomy for correction of mild to moderate hallux valgus deformity. Foot Ankle 12: 61-68

39. Johnson KA (1994) Chevron osteotomy, masters technique in orthopedic surgery.In: Thompson RC (ed) Foot and Ankle. Raven Press, New York, pp 31-48

40. Kato T, Watanabe S (1981) The etiology of hallux valgus in Japan. Clin Orthop 15: 78-81

41. Koenig RD (1990) Koenig total great toe implant: preliminary report. J Am Pediatr Med Assoc 80: 462-468

42. Lelièvre J, Lelièvre JF (1981) Pathologie du pied. Masson, Paris

43. Libotte M, Lusi K, Blaimont P, Bourgeois RA (1985) Condition d'équilibre de la première articulation métatarso-phalangienne. Acta Orthop Belg 51: 28-45

44. Libotte M, Blaimont P (1985) Traitement de l'hallux valgus par la mise en place de l'adducteur du gros orteil. Acta Orthop Belg 51: 46-51

45. Mann RA (1978) Du Vries' Surgery of the foot. Mosby, St Louis

46. Mann R, Oattes JC (1980) Arthrodesis of the first metatarsophalangueal joint. Foot ankle 1: 369-374

47. Mann RA, Coughlin MJ (1981) Hallux valgus. Etiology, anatomy, treatment and surgical considerations. Clin Orthop 157: 31-41

48. Merkl PF, Sculco TP (1989) Prosthesis replacement of the first metatarsophalangueal joint. Foot Ankle 9: 267-271

49. Mitchell CL, Flemming JJ, Allen R, Glenney C, Sandford GA (1958) Osteotomy bunionectomy for hallux valgus J Bone Joint Surg 40: 41-58

50. Myerson M, Allon S, Mc Garvey W (1992) Metatarso-cuneiform arthrodesis for management of hallux valgus and metatarsus primus varus. Foot Ankle 12: 107-115

51. Pochatko DJ, Schlehr F, Murphey MD, Hamilton JJ (1994) Distal chevron osteotomy with lateral release for treatment of hallux valgus deformity. Foot Ankle 15: 457-461

52. Pontious J, Kieran DMP, Mahan T, Carter S (1994) Characteristics of a adolescent hallux abducto-valgus. A retrospective review. J Am Podiatr Med Assoc 84: 208-218

53. Regnauld B (1986) Les désaxations du premier orteil. In: Le Pied. Springer Verlag, Paris

54. Rong-Stad KM, Miller GJ, Vander Grieud RA, Cowin D. (1994) A biomechanical comparison of four fixation methods of first metatarso-phalangueal joint arthrodesis. Foot Ankle 15: 415-419

55. Rosembaum de Britto S (1982) The first metatarso-sesamoïd joint. Int Orthop 6: 61-67

56. Rossi WR, Ferreira JCA (1992) Chevron osteotomy for hallux valgus. Foot Ankle 13: 378-381

57. Saragaglia D, Bellon-Champel P, Soued I, Tourné Y, Butel J (1990) Place de l'ostéotomie d'accourcissement de la 1ere phalange associée à la libération des parties molles dans le traitement chirurgical de l'hallux valgus. Rev Chir Orthop 76: 245-252

58. Schnepp J (1983) Traitement de l'hallux valgus avec métatarsus varus irréductible du premier métatarsien. L'ostéotomie bipolaire. Rev Chir Orthop (suppl II) 69: 113-115.

59. Schnepp J. (1986) L'hallux valgus: bases pathogéniques et anatomopathologiques. Thérapeutique et indications. In: Duparc J (ed) Cahiers d'enseignement de la SOFCOT. Expansion scientifique Française, Paris, pp 269-277

60. Tomeno B, Emani A (1980) Le traitement de l'hallux valgus par la technique de Mc Bride. Rev Chir Orthop 66: 399-400

61. Tomeno B, Kademm SE (1982) L'arthrodèse métatarso-phalangienne du gros orteil. Réflexions à propos de 93 interventions. Rev Chir Orthop 68: 379-384

62. Tourné Y, Leroy JM, Maire JP, Saragaglia D (1991) Os intermétatarsien et hallux valgus. Med Chir Pied 7: 117-121

63. Tourné Y, Leroy JM, Maire JP, Saragaglia D (1993) L'arthrodèse métatarso-phalangienne du premier rayon. À propos de 62 cas. Med Chir Pied 9: 161-171

64. Tourné Y, Saragaglia D, Montbarbon E, Picard F, Charbel A (1994) L'hallux varus iatrogénique: tactique chirurgicale. À propos de 14 cas. Med Chir Pied 10: 249-255

65. Valtin B (1991) Le transfert du premier interosseux dorsal dans le traitement chirurgical de l'hallux varus iatrogène. Med Chir Pied 7: 9-10

66. Valtin B (1994) Table ronde sur les ostéotomies du premier métatarsiens dans le traitement chirurgical de l'hallux valgus. Med Chir Pied 10: 71-128

67. Weil LS (1991) Modified Scarf bunionectomy: our experience in more than 1000 cases. J Foot Surg 30: 609-622

68. Wu KK (1994) Wu's buniectomy: a clinical analysis of 150 personal cases. J Foot Surg 31: 288-297

17. Pathology of the first ray

B. Hallux rigidus

D Saragaglia, Y Tourné and F Picard

Introduction

The term "hallux rigidus" seems to have been used for the first time in 1888 by Cotterill [4] and refers to a more or less complete loss of mobility of the first metatarsophalangeal (MTP) joint. Dorsiflexion without axial deviation of the first ray is particularly compromised. This stiffness evolves in the context of arthrosis-type degenerative lesions with narrowing of the joint-space and dorsal osteophytosis. The term hallux rigidus is therefore synonymous with metatarsophalangeo-sesamoid arthrosis of the first ray.

After hallux valgus, hallux rigidus is the second most frequent lesion of the first ray and its consequences on functional capacity are far from negligible.

Physiopathology

Normal motion range for the MTP varies between 30° of plantarflexion and 90° of dorsiflexion. Normal walking requires 65 to 75° of dorsiflexion for adequate propulsion of the foot during walking. At the end of a step, the first metatarsal rolls on the sesamoids and comes vertically onto the proximal phalanx of the hallux. During this phase, the plantar side of the proximal phalanx remains pressed against the ground. Progressive loss of MTP dorsiflexion causes supination of the forefoot at the end of gait to avoid pressure on the first metatarsal head and provokes a dorsal interphalangeal hypermobility

of the hallux which gives a characteristic "canoe" [3] appearance.

The biomechanical and clinical consequences of this lesion are overloading of the head of the 5th metatarsal causing the appearance of a plantar callosity and overloading of the head of the first phalanx, which also provokes a plantar callus. Muscle contractures along the lateral aspect of the leg and of the flexor hallucis brevis muscle which controls flexion of the proximal phalanx (hallus flexus) are sometimes associated.

Pathogenesis

The exact cause of hallux rigidus is not entirely understood. Nonetheless, two major etiologies can be distinguished [7, 11]: primary or idiopathic, and secondary. Among the secondary causes are identified:
• morphologic abnormalities, which may show an unusually long first metatarsal contributing to excessive weight-bearing on the MTP, or a dorsiflexion of the first metatarsal, termed "metatarsus primus elevatus" by Lambrinudi [9] in 1938,
• dystrophic lesions, especially osteochondritis dissecans of the first metatarsal head. At the beginning of its evolution this lesion is hard to see in radiographs and is often masked in later stages by secondary degenerative lesions,
• lesions of the metatarsosesamoid joint, particularly when the sesamoids are too far posterior, since this contributes to overload on the metatarsal head

during weight-bearing, leading to post-traumatic avascular necrosis and degenerative arthrosis,
• post-traumatic lesions, whether due to inadequate footwear such as undersized shoes, excessive immobilization, or a secondary algodystrophy. Moreover, articular fractures of the first metatarsal head or metatarsophalangeal dislocations often lead to eventual arthrosis.
• arthritis of the MTP, whether of inflammatory, infectious, or microcrystalline in origin,
• postsurgical lesions are mostly seen following a Keller-Lelièvre procedure, when excessive freeing of soft tissues leads to a chondrolysis of the metatarsal and phalangeal aspects of the joint.

In many cases, several factors probably interact, but the incidence is greater in two populations: young adults (under 40) and the elderly (over 60).

Clinical observations

The features of hallux rigidus classically present in two different ways depending on the stage of evolution:

At an early stage (stage I), hallux dolorosus is identified. Pain is the primary symptom. It is most often manifested at the MTP but can be masked by pain along the lateral side of the foot (callusing beneath the head of the 5th metatarsal) or along the outer aspect of the leg simulating a radiculalgia.

Clinical examination seeks to identify limited MTP dorsiflexion, which may reach only 30°. Radiologic examination shows narrowing of the MTP joint with moderate osteophyte formation.

At a later stage (stage II), hallux limitus (fig. 17.6) is identified. Pain is still present, but has diminished somewhat, while limited dorsiflexion is the main feature. The hallux may be "canoe-shaped" or may be plantarflexed because the head of the first metatarsal is elevated. A large dorsal exostosis is often present with an overlying bursitis making footwear difficult to tolerate. Calluses are also frequently present beneath the head of the 5th metatarsal and in some cases, when the hallux is "canoe-shaped", callusing may occur under the proximal phalangeal head. When the interphalangeal joint (IP) is in flexion, an overlying dorsal callus is often found. Radiologic views are often characterized by major narrowing of the joint space with medial, dorsal, and lateral osteophytosis at the head of the first metatarsal.

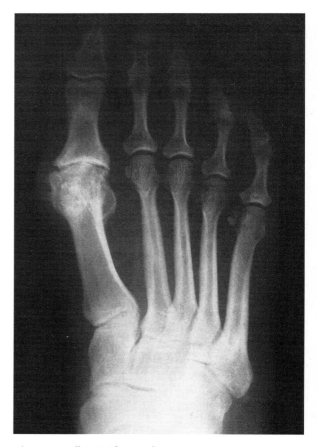

Fig. 17.6. Hallux rigidus at a limitus stage

Treatment

Conservative treatment

This uses corticoid injections, plantar insoles and orthopedic footwear, as well as physiotherapy:

Corticoid injections. 2 to 3 injections of corticoids are made by the posterolateral route, depending on the improvement noted.

Plantar orthoses and orthopedic footwear. Flexible insoles are used which are reinforced under the first metatarsal head and with a gap under the hallux. This is intended to compensate for insufficient dorsiflexion of the hallux during the last phase of gait. A gap can also be made under the 5th metatarsal head to protect it from painful callosities. Shoes equipped with a rigid outer sole beneath the forefoot can also be prescribed by adding a simple thickness of leather under the metatarsophalangeal joint.

Physiotherapy. This may include foot and leg massage, postural exercises by patient or therapist, active mobilization, walking rehabilitation, hydrotherapy and occupational therapy [3].

Surgical treatment

Conservative methods

• Periarticular "trimming" is an old technique, the results of which are variously assessed.
• Keller's technique (resection of the base of the proximal phalanx) is no longer often used to correct hallux rigidus. It has several drawbacks which justify abandoning this technique even though some authors [7] still consider it to be a useful procedure.
• Osteotomy to shorten the proximal phalanx [5, 6]: although the biomechanics seem useful (reduction of pressure on the MTP), long-term results need further evaluation before the procedure can be routinely recommended.
• A dorsal closing wedge osteotomy of the base of the phalanx is advocated by Moberg [12] with the aim of restoring some degree of dorsiflexion.
• The Valenti hinge arthroplasty [2] also attempts to restore dorsiflexion by dorsal resection of the base of the proximal phalanx and of the first metatarsal head.

Radical methods

Metatarsophalangeal arthrodesis is a valuable alternative in many cases, but has the disadvantage of permanent joint stiffness. Its advantage, however, is that it immobilizes the joint in a functional position (25 to 35° of dorsiflexion) and eliminates pain [14].

Prosthetic placements use several different types of prostheses, including silicone elastomer, ball-shaped total prostheses [5, 10, 13], interposed prostheses whether in silicone elastomer (spacer prosthesis) or metal [1, 8], and finally gliding surface total prostheses. Since fractures of silicone ball-shaped spacers are frequent and long-term problems with "siliconitis" appears frequently with these and with spacer prostheses, it seems reasonable to discourage their use in the first ray.

Interposed or gliding surface total prostheses have been recently developed as implants which require further long-term evaluation. Unfortunately, the considerable pressure exercised on the first ray in walking, combined with the tendency in hallux rigidus to stiffening after any attempts to restore mobility, may lead to failure with these implants sooner or later.

Indications

Conservative treatment seems to be indicated in stage I (hallux dolorosus). This is frequently quite effective and often permits stabilization of the lesion for several years. Only in the rare case of failure of this method should osteotomy to shorten the first phalanx [6] be considered, provided that the first ray is longer than the second.

Surgical treatment is suggested in stage II when there is pain and major limitation of mobility. The choice of procedure depends on age, sex and functional needs. Metatarsophalangeal arthrodesis is a reliable technique when correctly performed and establishes dorsiflexion of between 25 to 35°. As to "mobilizing" procedures, it must be kept in mind that hallux rigidus has a spontaneous tendency to recurrent stiffening so that surgery may have to be repeated. This means that mutilating interventions must be completely avoided since the long-term consequences could be disastrous.

References

1. Barouk LS (1992) Utilisation de la prothèse bouton au niveau du 1er rayon. Med Chir Pied 8: 125-136
2. Bonnel F, Fauré P, Nicoleau P, Claustre J (1993) Chirurgie de l'hallus rigidus: technique de Valenti. Med Chir Pied 9: 3-6
3. Claustre J, Delagoutte JP, Simon L (1982) Hallux rigidus. In: Claustre J, Simon L (eds) Troubles congénitaux et statiques du pied. Orthèses plantaires. Masson, Paris, pp 145-153
4. Cotterill JM (1988) Stiffness of the great toe in adolescents. Br Med J 1: 1158
5. Delagoutte JP, Bonnel F (1989) Le pied: Pathologie et techniques chirurgicales. Masson, Paris, pp 166-170
6. Delagoutte JP, Mainard D (1992) L'ostéotomie de la première phalange du gros orteil dans le traitement de l'hallux rigidus. Med Chir Pied 8: 137-138
7. Hawkins BJ, Haddad RJ (1988) Hallux rigidus. Clin Sports Med 7: 37-49
8. Jardé O, Trinquier JL, Filloux JF, Tran Van F, Vives P (1993) La prothèse métatarso-phalangienne sixtine du premier rayon. Résultats préliminaires, à propos de 74 cas. Med Chir Pied 9: 143-147
9. Lambrinudi C (1938) Métatarsus primus elevatus. Proc R Soc Med 31: 1273

10. Mac Auliffe TB, Helal B (1990) Replacement of the first metatarsophalangeal joint with a silicone elastomer ball-shaped spacer. Foot Ankle 10: 257-262

11. Mann RA, Coughlin MJ, Du Vries HL (1979) Hallux rigidus. A review of the literature and a method of treatment. Clin Orthop 142: 57-63

12. Moberg E (1979) A simple operation for hallux rigidus. Clin Orthop 142: 55-56

13. Swanson AB, De Groot Swanson G, Maupin BK, Shi Sho-Min, Peters JG, Alander DH, Cestari VA (1991) The use of a grommet bone liner for flexible hinge implant arthroplasty of the great toe. Foot Ankle 12: 149-155

14. Tourné Y, Leroy JM, Maire JP, Saragaglia D (1993) L'arthrodèse métatarso-phalangienne du premier rayon. À propos de 62 cas. Med Chir Pied 9: 161-171

18.

Disorders of the sesamoid bones

F Gaillard

The sesamoid bones of the hallux, so-called because they resemble a sesame seed, are small but constant bones located on the plantar aspect of the first metatarsophalangeal joint (MTP). Their pathologic aspects are often unrecognized clinically or radiologically. During antiquity, they were supposed to be the starting-point for resurrection at the Last Judgment because of their great strength [13]. Other myths depicted them as the "seat of the soul" [11].

Anatomy and physiology

The sesamoids appear at nine years of age in girls and at eleven in boys. They are single or bipartite, sometimes with several fragments joined. Their cortex is very hard and strong.

The medial and lateral sesamoids are embedded in the plantar part of the capsule of the first MTP joint, within the tendon of the flexor hallucis longus muscle. They are ovoid; the medial bone is bigger. They are embedded in the thickness of the glenoid ligament at the inferior part of the first MTP joint. Their upper surface is covered with articular cartilage, which glides on the longitudinal groove in the inferior surface of the first metatarsal head. There is a ridge under this head between the two grooves, which keeps the sesamoids in position and gives them stability. They are separated by a groove where the FHL tendon glides, surrounded by a synovial sheath [2, 10].

The sesamoids have a static function: they protect, by their solidity, the first MTP joint and the tendon of the flexor hallucis longus muscle. They are themselves protected by the very thick underlying tissues (cellulo-adipose tissue with a serous bursa). They also have a dynamic function, by providing anteromedial support in the terminal phase of gait, when the first metatarsal head rotates on the bisesamoid capsule [4, 7]. They guide the forces that lead, at the end of the step, to verticalization of the first metatarsal. At this moment, they receive 60% of the body weight.

The intersesamoid ligament is the mediator of propulsion, giving it maximal efficiency. The transverse intermetatarsal ligament is connected to the sesamoids and any dysfunction of these bones, especially luxation, affects general MTP stability.

Clinical features

The clinical symptoms of a sesamoid lesion are often the same, whatever their origin: medial metatarsalgia with localized pain, especially at the terminal phase of gait, relieved by rest, with a very localized point of tenderness. Sometimes there is a local swelling or a painful callosity.

Static or microtraumatic pathology

Many conditions lead to microtraumatisms or static overload:
- anteromedial pes cavus, with overload of the first metatarsal bone, now verticalized, and calcaneus valgus;

- retro-position of the sesamoids;
- sports: soccer (cramp under the shoe sole), athletics, tennis (direct stress);
- vocational overuse;
- too high heels

Clinical signs are not specific, often with a swelling due to a bursitis. Radiography is generally normal. Treatment must be preventive, but for bursitis an insole to decrease the load is used, sometimes combined with aspiration of the bursa. An injection of corticosteroids is rarely necessary [1, 3].

Necrosis of the sesamoids (Renander's disease)

This affection occurs in teenagers or young adults, often female, involving the lateral sesamoid as much as the medial. The favoring circumstances are the same as above. Clinical features are either chronic and nonspecific, with localized pain and gait in varus, or acute, with sudden onset, night pain and inflammatory signs simulating a microcrystalline episode. Sometimes extension of the hallux is very painful, and diffuse pain may be associated with swelling.

Radiographic study must include dorsal, lateral and tangential views (Walter-Muller and Güntz). It is possible to find characteristic modifications of one bone: demineralization and irregular patchy sclerosis which can be isolated or associated with flattening, irregular fragmentation into two or more parts, sometimes with a cloud of bony fragments [1, 5, 6, 8].

Scintigraphic examination is very useful at the beginning, when the radiographs are normal. Bone scintigraphy is characteristic, with early and quite localized hyperfixation in one sesamoid. MRI can also provide an early diagnosis [1].

Histopathology shows bone necrosis, with lesions of the medullary spaces followed by lesions of the bony matrix.

Initially, treatment is conservative: it is essential to limit the load on the sesamoids to avoid worsening of the lesion with fragmentation. With early diagnosis and relief from weightbearing, the lesion is often limited and the sesamoids retain good shape and function. Thus the initial treatment involves principally a lessening of the load, at first complete, and after that an orthosis with support behind the metatarsal head and total exclusion of stress under the affected sesamoids. If diagnosis or treatment is

late, the sesamoids become flattened and then fragmented. Persistent pain after 6 months and marked fragmentation can lead to a sesamoidectomy with good results. This must always be limited to one sesamoid and respect the tendinous insertion to avoid unbalancing the forefoot [1, 17].

Reflex sympathic algodystrophy

Reflex sympathic algodystrophy of the sesamoids is very rare but can exist separately, or at least predominate in an affection of the entire forefoot. Clinical manifestations are not specific, except a severe tenderness with cutaneous hyperesthesia. Children and adolescents can be affected [9].

Bone scintigraphy shows characteristic hyperfixation (except for children, who normally have frequent hypofixation), very early before radiographic signs appear.

Radiographic findings are the extent and specificity of this reflex sympathic algodystrophy site, with multicavitary demineralization, or a "target" appearance of the sesamoids [9]. These characteristic features are specific, and only found in reflex sympathic algodystrophy. Both sesamoids are affected.

The disease course is variable: recurrent, migratory, but generally regressive with a good outcome.

The treatment is the same as for all reflex sympathic algodystrophy.

Differential diagnosis from necrosis is sometimes difficult, with similar clinical findings and scintigraphic hyperfixation; but reflex sympathic algodystrophy involves both bones, the radiographic findings are different over time, and reflex sympathic algodystrophy is generally less localized and spreads to the entire forefoot.

Fractures of the sesamoids

The medial bone is the most commonly involved. Diagnosis is often difficult, because of the nonspecificity of the clinical picture and complementary examinations, and because of the numerous normal radiographic variants [6, 15, 16].

An acute form appears after direct or indirect trauma, generally during sport (jumping), with crushing by a vertical compression force on a sesamoid, locked under the first MTP joint by the contraction of the flexor hallucis brevis muscle [15,

16]. Pain is severe, increased by pressure or palpation, usually with swelling.

Stress fracture follows repeated microtraumatisms, unaccustomed exertion and predisposing anatomy (subluxation or hypermobility of the sesamoid, dysplasia of the metatarsal head).

Radiographic diagnosis needs special views (Walter-Muller, Güntz). Sometimes it is very difficult to differentiate a fracture (irregular, sinuous, usually unilateral) from a congenitally bipartite sesamoid bone (regular, median, usually bilateral) [12, 15, 17]. Scintigraphy with a very early hyperfixation or MRI can be very useful [1].

Treatment is generally conservative: strapping, a hollowed-out insole, sometimes a plaster cast for 6 weeks. Union is not always obtained, even when the clinical outcome is good. Surgery is possible in painful forms after 6 months with ablation of the fragments; for some authors, earlier unilateral sesamoidectomy has given good results [17].

Arthritis

Sesamoid abnormalities are encountered in rheumatoid arthritis and other forms of chronic arthritis [3, 4, 5].

The sesamoids can be the initial lesion of rhumatoid arthritis , but they are generally involved during its course, with local swelling, tenosynovitis or bursitis. In long-standing disease, rheumatoid pannus destroys the cartilage and invades the subchondral bone. Radiographic lesions are nonspecific, principally destructive (cavities, erosions, narrowing of the joint space)[14], and resemble those of the 5th MTP head (initial demineralization, cavities, erosions, variably destructive lesions). Dislocation of the sesamoids from the 1st MTP leads to a progressive hallux valgus deformity.

In spondylarthropathies, the clinical findings are generally very similar, with sometimes some particular radiologic signs: sesamoid periostitis or "whiskering" with an irregular osseous outline is a conspicuous feature, especially in psoriasic arthritis [14].

Microcrystalline pathology

In gout the typical acute episode involves the 1st MTP joint, but can involve the sesamoid region. Sometimes, it is the only site of the inflammatory process, with crystal deposition within synovium, cartilage and bone. Shallow and deep erosions of the sesamoid bones can be seen, specially in chronic gout with tophi, particularly in the medial sesamoid: erosions may be noted with subchondral cysts and reactive sclerosis [14].

Pseudogout episodes may be related to chondrocalcinosis with calcium pyrophosphate deposition, and, in the young adult, to hydroxyapatite deposition. Radiographs show periarticular or tendinous calcification [5].

Septic pathology

Sesamoid osteomyelitis and adjacent septic arthritis are very unusual, but may complicate trauma or septicemia. The clinical signs are initially very acute, with the formation of abscesses, and then more chronic with destructive osteomyelitis. Sometimes, chronic bone infection follows neglected sepsis in a simple callosity, with sinus formation [5].

Other pathologies

• Osteoarthrosis of the sesamoids is frequent, usually asymptomatic and of little consequence [14]. Joint narrowing with sclerosis, osteophyte production, bony eburnation and flattening of part of the sesamoid also occurs. For pain, a de-stressing insole, NSAI, or, rarely, local corticosteroid injections are generally helpful.
• Any disorder of the 1st MTP joint can affect the sesamoids, which are therefore involved in hallux valgus with dislocation and hallux rigidus (cf. corresponding chapters).

● Conclusion

Clinicians and radiologists often overlook the sesamoids, which are important in forefoot function and the process of walking. The sesamoids cannot be considered in isolation since specific diseases have consequences for the entire foot. It must not be forgotten in all foot diseases that the sesamoids can be affected by recurrent mechanical stress, sometimes with specific lesions.

References

1. Benamou P.H, Chevrot A, Dupont AM, Godefroy D, Montagne J, Morvan G (1993) Pathologie du premier rayon. Rhumatologie pratique 99: 1-3
2. Bonnel F, Canovas F, Braun S (1996) Anatomie de l'avant-pied. In: Valtin B (ed) Chirurgie de l'avant-pied. Expansion scientifique française, Paris, pp 1-21
3. Braun S, Tomeno B, Kieffert P (1991) Heurts et malheurs du premier rayon. Rhumatologie pratique, 56, 1-6
4. Claustre J, Simon L (1982) Pathologie sésamoidienne du premier rayon. In: Claustre J, Simon L (eds) Troubles congénitaux et statiques du pied. Orthèses plantaires. Masson, Paris, pp 152-163
5. Claustre J, Simon L (1978) Aspects de la pathologie sésamoidienne du premier métatarsien. Rev Rhum 45: 479-485
6. Daum B (1996) Pathologie sésamoidienne. A paraître
7. David R, Delagoutte JP, Renard M (1988) Etude anatomique fonctionnelle des os sésamoides du premier métatarsien. Etude comparative avec os grands sésamoides du cheval. Med Chir Pied 4: 195-206
8. Denis A (1975) L'osteonécrose aseptique des sésamoides du premier orteil. Maladie de Renander. Rhumatologie 27: 113-117
9. Doury P, Eulry F, Pattin S (1984) L'algodystrophie des sésamoides du gros orteil. Med Chir Pied 1: 55-58
10. Giannini S, Catani F (1996) Biomécanique de l'avant-pied. In: Valtin B (ed) Chirurgie de l'avant-pied. Expansion scientifique française, Paris, pp 22-38
11. Helal B (1979) Sésamoides du pied du sportif. In: Claustre J, Simon L (eds) Le pied du sportif. Masson, Paris, pp 116-117
12. Legrand-Isambert A (1979)Contribution à l'étude du diagnostic des fractures des sésamoides du gros orteil. Thèse Medecine, Paris, 71 p
13. Lelièvre J, Lelièvre JF (1981) Pathologie du pied. Masson, Paris
14. Resnick D, Niwayama G, Fiengold M L (1977) The sesamoid bones of the hands and feet: participators in arthritis, Radiology 123: 57-62
15. Viladot A (1979) Traumatismes de l'avant-pied. In: Expansion scientifique francaise (ed). Paris. Pathologie de l'avant-pied.Viladot A. 321
16. Voutey H (1978) Fractures phalangiennes. In: Voutey H (ed) Manuel de chirurgie orthopédique et de rééducation du pied. Masson, Paris, pp 251-253
17. Voutey H, Mirbey J (1986) Traitement des fractures et nécroses sésamoidiennes de l'hallux. In: Claustre J, Simon L (eds) Actualités en médecine et chirurgie du pied. Masson, Paris, pp 46-54

19.

Some reflections on the first ray

P Groulier and A Rochwerger

Hallux abducto-valgus is a common deformity, affecting women far more often than men. It is an exaggeration of the physiologic angle of the first ray, which leads to a pathologic deviation because of an anatomic predisposition. The apex of the deviation is at the metatarsophalangeal joint. This joint has a wide range of motion and is characterized by its weakness and its tendency to become disorganized by the combined effects of phalangeal valgus distally and metatarsus adductus proximally.

Excessive length of the hallux has an unfavorable action. It increases the phalangeal lever arm and the valgus deformity of the first toe, which is under pressure from the shoe. The hallux presses, through its base, on the first metatarsal head and displaces it medially because of accomodating movement at the first metatarsocuneiform joint proximally. Thus, disorganization of the metatarso-sesamoido-phalangeal joint of the first ray develops. The metatarsal head deviates from its physiologic sesamoid support. The soft tissues over the joint become irritated by shoe pressure, at the level of the so-called "bunion", (an incorrectly termed exostosis).

The deviation is doomed to become progressively worse through the action of the long and short muscles of the toe. With a single exception, all these muscles exert a deforming force through their bowstring effect. The deviation is self-perpetuating and finally becomes irreducible.

Stiffening of the first metatarsocuneiform joint makes the metatarsus adductus angle definitive. Lateral contracture fixes the metatarsosesamoidal luxation and anchors one of the sesamoids to the lateral side of the metatarsal head. This disorganization of the metatarso-sesamoido-phalangeal joint affects the function of the first ray during stance and the propulsive phase of gait.

The first metatarsal head deviates from the longitudinal axis of the foot. In the sagittal plane the head is elevated. The hallux deviated in valgus is rotated around its axis, lying on its medial side. Participation in weight-bearing and the propulsive activities of the first ray decreases. Consequently, the toe and metatarsal head are moved passively. Disorders occur because of transfer of the load onto the adjacent rays, first to the second ray and later to the whole forefoot. This explains the metatarsalgia as a symptom of hallux abducto-valgus.

The therapeutic principles can be deduced from an analysis of the lesions and their course. For the success of any operative procedure, the treatment should act on the source of the deviation and on perpetuating and aggravating factors.

The first ray can only be reconstructed by a total lateral release. The more effective the release of the conjoined tendon of the adductor hallucis muscle and section of the lateral fibrous node, the greater the restoration of the sesamoid apparatus to its anatomic position beneath the metatarsal head.

It is fundamental to correct the excessive length of the hallux by shortening the first phalanx. This is the guarantee for a good long-term result. A wedge-shaped phalangeal osteotomy seems necessary when the valgus deformity is located either in the phalanx or at the metatarsophalangeal joint. The metatarsus adductus, when moderate and without stiffness of the metatarso-cuneiform joint, can be reduced by procedures on the soft tissues. Otherwise a metatarsal osteotomy is required. This may be distal, diaphyseal, or proximal. It allows correction of the deviation in one or several planes. Whatever procedure is used, it should be done with moderation. Excessive resection of the bunion is useless and only leads to loss of stability in the metatarsophalangeal joint. After osteotomy of the first ray, some degree of divergence between the first and second rays should be retained.

The shortening of the first phalanx should transform an Egyptian-pattern forefoot (hallux longer than the toe) into a standard-pattern forefoot (the first toe equal to the second toe) but not into a Greek pattern (the second longer than the first) to avoid a hammer deformity of the second toe.

Joint preservation procedures are preferable to destructive operations. But when the deformities are significant with evidence of degenerative changes, especially in older patients, fusion of the first metatarsophalangeal joint gives a lasting functional result. The treatment of coexisting problems in the forefoot depends on the course of the disease.

Usually, treating the hallux abducto-valgus abolishes the metatarsalgia. Nevertheless, irreversible lesions such as luxation or subluxation of the metatarsophalangeal joints of the second ray need specific surgical treatment.

Finally, as has been said, there is no such thing as one type of hallux valgus or one type of treatment.

Repair should be thought of in terms of making a choice between several methods, and in the light of coexisting lesions, with regard for the patient's age and the evolution of the deformities.

Hallux rigidus is the arthritic degeneration of the metatarsophalangeal joint of the first ray. Sometimes the joint is totally stiffened. When it is in correct position, nothing needs to be done. However, pain sometimes occurs in the first metatarsophalangeal joint due to shoe pressure on the exuberant juxta-articular bone.

Removal of the juxta-articular bone alleviates the pain. When stiffness is accompanied by severe deformity, the symptoms call for a surgical procedure. Sometimes motion is limited, so that the joint aches at full stretch. This functional discomfort makes surgical treatment necessary. Arthrodesis of the first metatarsophalangeal joint in the corrected position is preferable to an arthroplasty, with or without implant.

To prevent the development of arthrosis, it is possible to deal surgically with excess length of the phalanx or deviation of the first metatarsal in the sagittal plane. These procedures do not interfere with subsequent and more destructive surgical procedures.

20.
Static pathology of the forefoot
(Morton syndrome excluded)

P Diébold, R Meyer and M Bonjean

Static pathology of the forefoot, as a cause of so-called "static" metatarsalgia, represents the most frequent reason for consultation in pathology of the foot. Such metatarsalgia can originate from a wide range of affections; any static disruption will bring about an imbalance of the metatarsal row and an uneven distribution of pressures and will thus cause podalgia.

● Biomechanical considerations

For many years, the forefoot was described as a downwardly concave anterior arch. Since the clinical examination was done in decubitus and since anatomic descriptions dealt with the feet of corpses, classical theories never took into account the foot as it is in weight-bearing. They considered the foot as a tripod with only the heel and the first and fifth metatarsal heads resting on the ground. In reality, this tripod only exists in very rare and abnormal circumstances. The "concave anterior arch" exists only in decubitus and disappears as soon as the foot bears weight because, when in contact with the ground, the weight is distributed between the five metatarsal heads. Therefore, the foot has one posterior pillar and one adaptive anterior pillar.

No situations, and therefore no disorders, are purely static when weight-bearing exists. The patient never remains motionless, so the pressures vary uninterruptedly from the lateral to the medial border of the foot, from one foot to the other, and from the heel to the forefoot.

Kowalski and De Doncker [9] have described the forefoot as a tricycle with two fixed central rays. The first metatarsal represents the inner wheel and the two lateral metatarsals represent the outer wheel. In reality, the metatarsal keyboard can be described as an adaptable range, in which the forefoot acts as a spring. Pisani [33] defines two aspects of the foot: the calcaneal foot (calcaneus, cuboid and two lateral metatarsals) for support and the talar foot for adaptation.

When a person is walking or standing, all the metatarsals support part of the weight, but the first metatarsal in a normal situation supports twice as much weight as each lateral ray. The distribution of the weight depends on the anatomy of the metatarsals. The five metatarsals have a length and an orientation that are variable in relation to the ground. Study of their position and of the statics of the metatarsal keyboard allows an analysis of the metatarsalgia: in the sagittal plane, the alignment occurs with an outwardly decreasing inclination to the ground; the first metatarsal pitch in relation to the ground is approximately 18 to 25°, whereas that of the fifth metatarsal is only 5°. Any increase of this pitch between the metatarsal and the ground will cause an excess load on the corresponding metatarsal head. This is the case with the anterior cavus foot, high-heeled shoes, etc.

In the horizontal plane, the metatarsal spread follows a curve which can be drawn by a line joining the metatarsophalangeal interspaces. This curve of Hoffman-Lelièvre (metatarsal protrusion distance) (fig. 20.1) which is concave backwards was studied by Viladot [36]. It depends on both the length of the metatarsals and the space between them. When

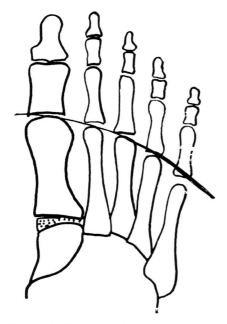

Fig. 20.1. Lelièvre parabola (or metatarsal protrusion distance)

M1 = M2, the foot is called "index plus minus"; when M1 is longer than M2, the metatarsal morphotype is called "index plus"; and when M1 is clearly smaller than M2, this type is called "index minus". A short first metatarsal (index minus), whether of congenital or iatrogenic origin, will cause a transfer of weight onto the lateral metatarsals.

The angle between the metatarsals, and particularly the angle between the 1st and 2nd metatarsals is just as important: metatarsus varus of the 1st ray (metatarsus primus adductus) accounts for insufficiency of that first ray. This forefoot, when of congenital origin, is called the "atavistic foot" or "embryonic foot". In its most pronounced form, it is Morton's triangular forefoot [31].

The morphotypes of the toes and of metatarsal spread can explain some static metatarsalgias and some disorders of the first ray: a longer hallux combined with a longer 1st metatarsal predisposes to hallux rigidus; a longer hallux combined with a metarsus varus of the first ray predisposes to hallux valgus. The ideal or perfect form would be a first metatarsal as long as the second with a second toe longer than the hallux.

During walking, the weight is distributed not only on the metatarsal heads but also on the toe pulp. At the end of gait all the toes bear weight, relieving the metatarsal heads of part of the body weight. Any affection that reduces the pulp contact with the ground causes overloading of the corresponding metatarsal head and consequently provokes a metatarsalgia.

Actually, the whole foot from hindfoot to forefoot is involved in the development of a metatarsalgia. If one refers to the biomechanical model of the helix, one can easily understand the effect of the hindfoot on the forefoot: if a pes cavus overloads the metatarsal heads, then a varus-type hindfoot may equally overload the "front heel".

The metatarsodigital complex must be analyzed in terms of its dynamics. Any reduction of metatarsal mobility (rigidity of the tarsometatarsal, metatarsophalangeal or interphalangeal joints) can modify the distribution of metatarsal weight-bearing on the ground. Thus, in the overloaded medial rays syndrome (round forefoot or insufficiency of the first ray) the metatarsals remain on the ground longer during gait. The first phalanx goes from a normal horizontal position to a slight extension, which causes flexion of the distal phalanges. A "thrust" of the metatarsal head against the phalanx then occurs, the latter being maintained on the ground by the flexor muscles. This thrust causes progressive stretching of the capsule. It must be recalled that the metatarsophalangeal joint presents two aspects, a fragile dorsal one and an extremely sturdy plantar one which extends lengthwise under the lower face of the metatarsophalangeal joint, allowing the metatarsal head to glide forward. In the case of an excess load on the metatarsal head with the proximal phalanx in extension, the lateral repercussion causes a reduction in the function of the interosseous and lumbrical muscles and consequently their atrophy. Their initially plantar axis of movement becomes lateral and then dorsal. These muscles will then take part in the tendency toward luxation created by the dorsal capsular stretching. At this stage, the plantar plate splays out and this phenomenon increases whenever there are overweight problems or endocrine disorders, etc. Thus all the conditions obtain to facilitate the development of a rupture of the plantar capsule, with a permanent and fixed luxation of the first phalanx on the dorsal face of the metatarsal head, which is an additional factor aggravating over-pressure on the ground of the metatarsal head. This is the pathomechanics of the second ray syndrome.

A remaining unclear point is the exact etiology of the metatarsalgia, in other words, of the metatarsal pain: is it only a matter of excess load on the plantar tissues? In reality, the trophicity of the plantar pad, the bony weight-bearing surface, and the duration of weight-bearing are all involved here. When the plantar hyperkeratosis, which is the initial reaction to excessive weight-bearing is stressed, a bursa will form and will be painful, especially when it becomes a true metatarsal bursitis. Accordingly, the following elements all take part in the appearance of pain: the bony element, the shock-absorbing element of the plantar pad, and the element resisting pressure represented by the thickness of the skin. Any weakening of the plantar pad will accelerate the occurrence of pain and complications. This explains the aggravating effect of diabetes or arteritis, but also the effect of mere excess weight and postmenopausal "trophostatic" changes. Among the causes of non-static metatarsalgia, traumatic or microtraumatic causes and inflammatory arthritis also need to be mentioned.

Moreover, "static" metatarsalgia has at times been contrasted with "dynamic" metatarsalgia, which is particularly provoked by a disharmony between the second and third metatarsal lengths, mainly when running (even in the absence of pes cavus).

● Clinical examination

Diagnosis of metatarsalgia is based on clinical examination. This consists of 5 stages: anamnesis, examination of the patient standing with bare feet, analysis of gait, examination in decubitus, examination of the foot with the shoe on, and examination of the shoe. The anamnesis will specify the exact localisation of the pain, the circumstances of its appearance, when the foot is shod or barefoot, its evolution since the onset, the presence or absence of a limp, or of discomfort in putting the shoe on. Traumatic or microtraumatic factors will be looked for, particularly in sports, and help to detail the medical or surgical history. Possible venous insufficiency or a metabolic disease such as diabetes is sought.

The unclothed patient must be examined while standing: the examiner will not only look for a static podologic problem but will also examine the statics of the lower limbs in their entirety, and even those of the spine. Then, walking allows study of the different stages of the gait and any modification of gait due to the metatarsalgia, even if minor. Walking

on tiptoe and on the heels is observed. A complete study of the statics of the hindfoot is made. The areas of excessive plantar loading are thus defined in weight-bearing, as well as any problems of plantar statics.

The examination of the dorsum of the foot specifies the orientation of the forefoot in relation to the hindfoot and of the foot in relation to the axis of the leg, and especially any deformities of the forefoot: the position of the metatarsal spread and of the toes, presence of clawed toes, defects of pulp contact with the ground, callosities or disorders of the nails.

In dorsal decubitus, the examination is completed with the bare foot in the hand [4]. The length of the rays and the angle between the toes and metatarsals are observed, especially for the first ray; the reducibility of the deformities and any contractures of the metatarsophalangeal joints are systematically assessed by pinching between the thumb and index finger from the second to the fifth joint; the metatarsal interspaces, plantar pads and mobility of the metatarsophalangeal joints are reviewed in a search for the podal sign of Lachman which shows joint hyperlaxity, reducibility of the clawed toe or luxation of a metatarsophalangeal joint.

After having placed the patient in ventral decubitus, with flexed knee and ankle at 90°, further attention is given to the axis of the foot (with the hindfoot in neutral position) in relation to the leg, the plantar skin and the presence and size of callosities, skin atrophy (sometimes unrelated to the site of the pain) and the presence or absence of a bursitis.

The shoe will also be examined as to the type and symmetry of its deformation. If the patient wears plantar orthoses, it can also be very useful to examine these in order to validate the orthotic therapy.

● Etiology

The classification of causes of metatarsalgia is difficult. They are described, from medial to lateral: first ray insufficiency, 2nd ray syndrome, Freiberg's disease, round forefoot, insufficiency of one lateral metatarsal, intractable hyperkeratosis, lateral metatarsalgia (excessive lateral plantar weight-bearing and bursitis at the 5th head). Finally, the pathology of the toes will be considered.

First ray insufficiency (fig. 20.2)

This is a physiopathologic entity with multiple components. The fundamental function of the 1st ray and hallux in propulsion is evident. Its insufficiency may be secondary to the horizontalization of the 1st metatarsal found in constitutional hyperlaxity and in flat foot (where the pronation of the hindfoot is associated with supination of the forefoot). The depressor muscles of the first ray, such as the peroneus longus muscle, become insufficient. Horizontalization of the 1st metatarsal is found in shortness of this ray which can be congenital or surgical or functional. When it is congenital, it is the "atavistic foot", described by Morton, or "embryonic foot". The metatarsal morphotype in this case is usually of the type: 2 > 3 > 4 > 1 > 5, which Arandes and Viladot named "index minus". More rarely, this constitutional insufficiency of the 1st ray can be the outcome of isolated hypertrophy of the 2nd metatarsal.

Shortness of the 1st ray can have an iatrogenic origin. The Mayo procedure with resection of part of

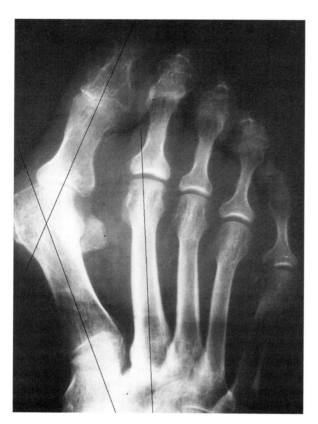

Fig. 20.2. Congenital shortening of the first metatarsal

the metatarsal head in the surgery of hallux valgus is a tremendous example; it leads to a short first metatarsal with a transfer of weight onto the 2nd ray and therefore metatarsalgia. In the Keller-Lelièvre procedure, with excessive resection of the 1st phalanx, the recession of the sesamoid changes the weight-bearing under the first head causing functional shortness of the first ray and in this case also, transfer metatarsalgia appears. This functional insufficiency of the 1st ray is found in the pathogenesis of hallux valgus, with a loss of the harmonious metatarsal curve (metatarsal protrusion distance).

Second ray syndrome

This syndrome was described by Denis et al [11] in 1979, in France, and by Mann [27] in the United States. We have here the most frequent cause of static metarsalgia, apart from pathology of the 1st ray. This 2nd ray syndrome is characterized by painful instability of the 2nd metatarsophalangeal joint. It evolves in 3 stages: a stage of simple instability of the 2nd toe, a stage of subluxation or reversible luxation, and a stage of definitive luxation of the phalangeal base onto the dorsum of the 2nd metatarsal head.

• **The 1st stage** is simply called the painful stage. The pain is characteristic. It is localized at the 2nd metatarsophalangeal joint, generally on its dorsal face, sometimes on its plantar face under the 2nd MT head. On examination, dorsiflexion of the 2nd toe is often painful but the painful instability of the 2nd metatarsophalangeal joint is more characteristic: with one hand (generally the left) the examiner holds the 2nd metatarsal head in place while the other takes the 1st phalanx between the thumb and index, imposing vertical movements on it; these movements can be compared to the search for the Lachman sign in the knee region. The vertical instability thus elicited is painful and reproduces the pain felt by the patient in ambulation. The remainder of the 2nd ray examination is normal. The 1st ray is generally painless. Above all, this maneuver allows us to eliminate the painful syndrome of the 2nd intermetatarsal interspace, in which bidigital vertical pressure at the interspace is much more painful. Claustre et al [7] noted that the footprint can at this stage be abnormal, with elective excess weight-bearing under the 2nd metatarsal head, even though X-ray examination remains normal.

• **The 2nd and inflammatory stage** corresponds to subluxation of the 2nd metatarsophalangeal joint, causing an inflammatory synovial reaction. This micro-traumatic synovitis can sometimes mimic inflammatory arthritis but this can be excluded if the rest of the clinical and para-clinical assessment is normal. During the examination, a greater mechanical instability is found, though this is less painful than during the 1st stage, and with a dorsal subluxation of the metatarsophalangeal joint which may be fixed. Actually, the joint is only painful during the last stages of subluxation. A callosity under the 2nd metatarsal head is usually noted. The dorso-plantar X-ray view shows narrowing of the joint space; the oblique view may show dorsal subluxation of the 1st phalanx.

• **The 3rd stage** is that of permanent luxation of the 2nd metatarsophalangeal joint. This luxation, which can be felt by bidigital palpation, is the origin of the characteristic deformity with a thickening of the 2nd toe base. There is proximal interphalangeal clawing of this toe, with a loss of pulp loading in weight-bearing. The clawed toe often shows a dorsal callosity which causes painful rubbing on the shoe. Though the irreducible dorsal luxation of the phalangeal base is obvious on palpation, the pain is generally of less importance; discomfort due to the clawing, felt when putting on a shoe, constitutes the major complaint (fig. 20.3). The X-ray shows the luxation of the 2nd metatarsophalangeal joint and sometimes already a narrowing of the 3rd joint. According to Denis, the origin of this instability is the imbalance between the long muscles and the short and lumbrical muscles, whose strength decreases. Bonnel and Claustre [7] consider that the metatarsophalangeal luxation is the consequence of stretching, followed by rupture of the plantar capsule, this rupture being favored by pre-existing degenerative lesions of the capsule.

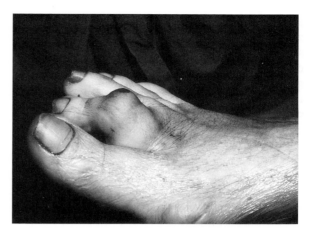

Fig. 20.3. Second ray syndrome

Course

This is variable: some patients will very quickly reach the luxation stage whereas others will complain for several years about a stubborn painful instability.

Treatment

The treatment is conservative for the first two stages of the syndrome and surgical afterwards. During the 1st and 2nd stages a plantar orthosis is necessary, provided with a bar behind the metatarsal heads and often with a hollow under the second metatarsal head. The treatment includes nonsteroidal anti-inflammatory drugs. Intra-articular corticosteroid injection is strictly contraindicated, because it accelerates the development of luxation of the second metatarsophalangeal joint. The value of periarticular infiltration is very debatable. Periarticular use of a short-acting cortisone derivative may at most be considered when there is acute inflammatory and painful involvement of the joint. Weight-bearing must be avoided for some days after the injection. During the first and second stages, symptomatic physiotherapy can be suggested, for its analgesic effect and also to maintain some flexibility in the second ray.

Surgical treatment is indicated when conservative management fails, or when the luxation is irreducible. Some authors [8] have advocated synovectomy through a lateral approach with dorsal capsulotomy, synovectomy and release of the collateral ligaments. The extensor tendon must be elongated by Green's method. The toe length must be carefully considered. In the case of a congenital or postoperative lesion with the second toe longer than the hallux, an interphalangeal joint arthroplasty is performed with shortening of the 2nd ray. At the stage of irreducible luxation the narrowing of the metatarsophalangeal joint demands an intervention on the metatarsal, i.e., a distal or basal osteotomy to elevate or shorten it.

The basal metatarsal osteotomy is rather imprecise and brings about adhesion to the tendon and the skin and does not allow access to the joint. It is indicated in the case of a very short first metatarsal. The distal osteotomy of Gauthier [19] can serve for the 2nd ray syndrome. After arthrolysis of the metatarsophalangeal joint and synovectomy, this osteotomy of the metaphysis with a dorsal wedge allows the metatarsal head to tilt backward. The patient's foot is placed in a posterior support shoe or he uses crutches in order to avoid weight-bearing for 4 weeks, which is the usual time needed for consolidation. This surgical procedure brings about excellent results; the few cases in which the metatarsal head necroses seem due to residual hyper-pressure on an over-long metatarsal.

Barouk introduced Weil's osteotomy in France [1], i.e., an almost horizontal oblique osteotomy allowing total recession of the metatarsophalangeal joint and stretching of the extensor tendinous and muscular system. It is indicated when M2 is too long; the recession must be substantial enough to ensure that M1 = M2 and M3 is 3 mm shorter. This recession settles the problems related to the interphalangeal clawing. In simple pathology of the second ray, the resection-reinsertion of Regnault [34] is contraindicated, as are simple resection of the metatarsal head or the insertion of a silicone prosthesis, which has the same effects on the 2nd ray as on the 1st and leads to transfer metatarsalgia under the 3rd and 4th metatarsal heads.

Arthroplasty by the plantar route, described by Brahms [3], which resects the base of P1, is dangerous in the 2nd ray syndrome. Helal's osteotomy of the distal metatarsal metaphysis [21] in no way resolves the metatarsophalangeal luxation, the verticalization of the 1st phalanx and the contracture of the collateral ligaments. In the irreducible stage, when it has become necessary to treat the rigid clawing of the 2nd toe, simple arthroclasis is often insufficient and arthroplasty or arthrodesis of the interphalangeal joint is indicated.

Freiberg's disease

Freiberg's disease is described by some authors as an osteochondritis, by others as an aseptic osteonecrosis of the metatarsal heads, most often affecting the 2nd head (some 70% of cases), rarely the 3rd (about 25%), and only exceptionally the 4th. In athletes, microtraumatic osteochondritic changes in the 1st metatarsal have been described, akin to those of Freiberg's disease. The first description of this affection by Freiberg goes back to 1914. When affecting the 2nd metatarsal head, it is also called

Köhler's disease. The aseptic osteonecrosis of the 3rd metatarsal head, studied by Panner in 1921, is sometimes named after him. Erlacher also described lesions of bony necrosis of the 4th and 5th metatarsal heads in 1922.

It mostly affects female patients, and mainly during adolescence before fusion of the epiphysis and diaphysis occurs. The actual metatarsalgia often only appears in adult life and is to be considered as the outcome of Freiberg's disease, asymptomatic and unnoticed during adolescence. Nevertheless, true cases of acute Freiberg's disease have been described in adults [13]. It is difficult to postulate a single physiopathologic mechanism in adolescents and adults but the hypothesis of micro- or macrotraumatism is currently the prevailing one. This hypothesis has been defended by Cameron [5], among others, and explains the most frequent necrosis in the upper part of the metatarsal head. There is a subchondral fissure associated with secondary bony necrosis of vascular origin. An over-long second metatarsal thus constitutes a predisposing factor. Stress fractures of the metatarsal heads, recently described [25], may thus be related to these cases of Freiberg's disease in adults, or may at least constitute one of its causes.

Clinical features

In the first stage, the pain is often plantar, starting and ascending from the 2nd MT head and often described as radiating backwards the dorsum of the foot, provoked by weight-bearing and walking and relieved by rest. On examination, a dorsal non-inflammatory swelling of the joint, without vertical metatarsophalangeal instability, may be noted. Passive dorsiflexion is painful. At this stage, the X-ray is normal; only technetium scanning may show an isolated hyperfixation. An exploratory aspiration may yield a few drops of fluid due to mechanical irritation.

Course

The onset, though sometimes acute, is in reality often gradual and is the cause of the metatarsalgia, but the first stage often passes unnoticed. Later, the pains are rather dorsal and related to the presence of intra-articular loose bodies. The pain is often quite mild, more a discomfort which sometimes only appears while running.

The advanced stage is that of static metatarsalgia. The dorsal swelling is more marked and reveals, as does the overall stiffening of the joint, the development of metatarsophalangeal arthrosis with palpable dorsal osteophytosis. Discomfort when putting on the shoe is then considerable and may be the main reason for consultation.

Radiographic signs

These can be described in 4 stages: Initially the X-ray is normal; then slight subchondral sclerosis of the metatarsal head appears; later this image of necrosis may assume a heterogeneous or mottled aspect, (fig. 20.4a). At this stage the diagnosis of a stress fracture or even of a patchy algodystrophy may be posed, since a localized fracture can lead to algodystrophy and conversely, an algodystrophy can itself be complicated by a stress fracture.[25, 30]

At the 2nd stage the deformations become characteristic. The metatarsal head, often better viewed in a 3/4 oblique radiograph, loses its sphericity and becomes centrally flattened (fig. 20.4b). The joint-space is preserved, sometimes even widened. There is no phalangeal abnormality. The deformation of the metatarsal head increases progressively and is associated with the presence of intra-articular loose bodies corresponding to detached necrotic fragments.

The last stage (3rd or 4th, depending on the classification) is that of metatarsophalangeal arthrosis with compression of the joint space and arthrotic deformations affecting the phalangeal base (subchondral sclerosis, osteophytosis).

Diagnosis

In an acute or subacute onset, one must exclude arthritis, a 2nd ray syndrome, and a stress fracture of

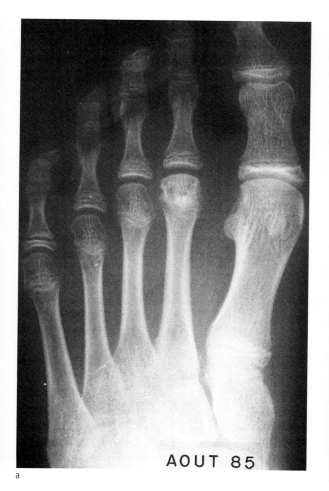
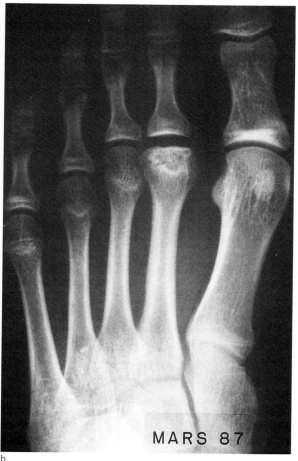

a   b

Fig. 20.4. a Freiberg's disease, stage 1 (13-year-old girl); **b** same patient, one year and seven months later, Freiberg's disease, stage II: observe the loss of sphericity of the second metatarsal head and the widening of the joint space

the 2nd metatarsal head which may actually, as has been said, be a cause of Freiberg's disease.

Treatment

The treatment is conservative at the first stage, before the detachment of a fragment into the joint. The forefoot must not be allowed pressure over for 4 weeks, with anti-inflammatory and analgesic treatment, followed by the prescription of a plantar orthosis to relieve the painful metatarsal heads. This treatment may lead to complete recovery, especially if there is no true aseptic osteonecrosis but rather a stress fracture of the metatarsal head. Most often, the patients are examined at a later stage when they are adults for whom the first stage has passed unnoticed.

At the later stage, the treatment is surgical; removal of the loose fragments in the joint, synovectomy and trimming may be sufficient. Nevertheless, Gauthier's surgical procedure, a wedge osteotomy with dorsal base after removing the necrotic part, may oppose a zone of healthy cartilage to the phalanx by tilting the MT head backward. This procedure gives good results as long as the patient engages in a short re-education program in order to avoid any limitation of dorsiflexion of the metatarsophalangeal joint. If the phalangeal base is deformed, it will have to be remodeled. The procedure described by Helal (a bone graft replacing the necrotic tissue) risks recreating an over-long 2nd ray, which is a factor in metatarsophalangeal joint stiffness.

The round forefoot or anterior round foot

This is the consequence of overloading of the middle metatarsal heads and represents about 60% of cases of static metatarsalgia. The flat or triangular forefoot represents a less developed or intermediate stage of this overloading of the middle MT heads.

Mechanism

The round forefoot is favored by 1st ray insufficiency, often in the context of an "atavistic foot", and by hallux valgus, hyperlaxity of the ligaments and generally by inadequate footwear. This pathology most often concerns women during or after the menopause, often in the context of "trophostatic" complications in which overweight contributes at least as much as endocrine disorders to the decompensation of preexisting static problems. The ball of the foot collapses and splays out. The intermetatarsal ligaments become overstretched. Most often this is combined with clawing of the toes, favored by the equinus of the forefoot, the consequence of high-heeled shoes. The shoe is also often too tight and it worsens the hallux valgus and the varus of the fifth toe, thus contributing like the toe clawing, to excess loading of the middle metatarsal heads.

Clinical features

The patient (usually a woman) consults because of plantar pain in the forefoot like a permanent burning or scorching feeling, especially when walking, sometimes as if there were a foreign body or a stone in the shoe. After walking, this burning sensation may take some hours rest to disappear.

Examination reveals the deformities of the ball of the foot and toes and whether or not it is possible to correct them. The forefoot appears to be convex downwards. The severity of the plantar callosities is also assessed (fig. 20.5); with worsening of the clinical picture, the maximal hyperkeratosis is under the 2nd and especially the 3rd metatarsal heads. On the contrary, the skin remains normal under the 1st and 5th metatarsal heads. The crushing of the plantar pad may lead to the appearance of a bursa under the 2nd or 3rd metatarsal heads with episodes of acute metatarsal bursitis, often very sensitive to the least pressure. Increasing crushing of the plantar pad of the forefoot and dorsal hyperflexion of the metatarsophalangeal joint with clawing explain the later appearance of a metatarsophalangeal subluxation, or

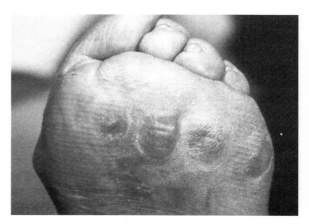

Fig. 20.5. Round forefoot; callosities under the metatarsal heads

even a luxation, related to overstretching of the dorsal capsule.

This static metatarsalgia due to overload of the middle heads should not be confused with a Morton's syndrome, the pain of which is more acute, more sudden, intermittent and quickly relieved by removing the shoe and massaging of the forefoot. The physical examination findings are also very different. Actually, in the stage of evolved anterior round foot, there is a complex involvement of the metatarsophalangeal joints and therefore of the plantar pads, as well as the intermetatarsal spaces.

Treatment

Conservative treatment includes adequate footwear, plantar orthoses, and rehabilitation. Advice about footwear concerns the width and pliability of the toe-cap and the abandonment of high heels.

Plantar orthoses are prescribed as long as the deformations of the metatarsophalangeal joints remain reducible. The sole of the shoe includes a metatarsal bar with a median heightening [4]. The shaping of this bar must be precise in order to obtain real efficiency in relieving the middle metatarsal heads. Martorell [29] suggested a plantar orthosis including a raise in front of the metatarsal heads and under the interphalangeal joints, in order to reduce the clawing and restrict the displacement of the forefoot. Forestier's metatarsal pad and garter has been criticized by Lelièvre [26]. Finally, toe orthoses may be a useful addition for a corn or painful clawing.

Rehabilitation is too often neglected, or postponed until the postoperative stage. In fact, it is an integral part of conservative treatment and even as a preoperative measure if surgery turns out to be necessary. "Limbering-up" exercises for the metatarsophalangeal joints should be taught to the patient, to be performed daily at home. The purpose of this re-education is to elevate the metatarsal heads while depressing the 1st phalanges and is done from the medial to the lateral side of the foot. This re-education is not only passive but also active, using the flexor and extensor muscles in order to restore equilibrium. The abductor and adductor muscles of the 1st ray are also exercised. Postural exercises in plantarflexion of the metatarsophalangeal joints are often easier to practice. Tiptoeing in order to obtain pulp bearing of all the toes may be tried but is often more difficult to achieve. Exercises using a towel, a small ball, a marble or a pencil in order to reinforce the function of the toes are well-known.

Surgical treatment

This occurs after treatment of the 1st ray; it is the treatment of all the middle rays, as it seems illogical in a round forefoot to treat only one ray. It can only be considered for moderate degree of pes cavus, since in a very pronounced cavus foot some metatarsal osteotomies may lead to iatrogenic insufficiency of the middle rays, with the overload being transferred under the 1st and 5th heads, causing other types of metatarsalgia.

The soft tissues

A method of total dorsal tenocapsular release was described by Voutey [37] in the static forefoot, and adopted by de Stoop [12] in rheumatoid arthritis. It is a complete release of the metatarsophalangeal joints with lengthening of the extensor digitorum longus tendons, section of the tendons of the extensor digitorum brevis, transverse section of the metatarsophalangeal joint capsules and release of the collateral ligaments. Walking is allowed after 48 hours, with "self re-education". Perrin [32] reports 80% of good and excellent results for this type of procedure. Judet has described transplantation of the extensor tendons onto the metatarsal necks: the tendon of the extensor digitorum longus is cut at the metatarso-phalangeal joint, passed through the metatarsal head and sutured to itself. This procedure assumes the metatarsophalangeal joint to be flexible but the transferred tendon tends to stretch and the elevating effect on the metatarsal quickly disappears.

Osseous procedures

• Condylectomy consists of removal of the plantar aspect of the metatarsophalangeal head. Its results are very unreliable.

• Metatarsal osteotomies may be proximal, distal or diaphyseal [22]. The procedure always begins with total arthrolysis of the metatarsophalangeal joint and of the corresponding interphalangeal joint.

Osteotomies of the metatarsal bases may be oblique, as described by Delagoutte [10], or V-shaped as described by Denis and in the USA by Giannestras [20], or semi-circular or wedge-shaped with a dorsal base. All these osteotomies can shorten the metatarsal. Their major disadvantage is that they are extremely difficult to adjust precisely, as regards both the relative lengths of the metatarsals and their elevation.

Elevation osteotomies are described by Helal at the distal ends of the metatarsal shafts. There is no attempt at fixation; walking adjusts the elevation of the osteotomized metatarsals. Complications such as persistent deformities of the toes or nonunion of the metatarsals frequently appear. Gauthier described a wedge-shaped distal osteotomy with a dorsal base, easily performed but ineffective in correcting excessive length of the metatarsal. Regnault suggested an osteotomy to re-embed the heads, which is more difficult and may lead to necrosis of the metatarsal head if the length correction is insufficient. Weil's osteotomy, introduced in France by Barouk [2] is an oblique osteotomy from front to back, with virtually no angulation. It is done on the three middle metatarsals and it allows good recession of the metatarsal heads; it resolves the problem of the clawed toe. Resection of the metatarsal heads, commonly attributed to Lelièvre, has very little place in so-called static pathology, unlike rheumatoid polyarthritis. These resections often result in "too short" metatarsals with excess pressure under the stumps and metatarsalgia recurs in the short or long term. This metatarsal realignment may however, be considered for the serious after-effects of forefoot surgery [28]. The published results of the numerous metatarsal osteotomies, whether proximal or distal; show between 75 and 80% of good results. Failures seem mostly due to the appearance of transfer metatarsalgia in an adjacent non-osteotomized metatarsal, to pseudarthrosis, frequently to algodystrophy, to skin complications (necrosis), or to rare cases of sepsis.

• Transfer metatarsalgia. This may complicate osteotomies of one or two metatarsals, or can appear when the surgical procedure has caused an over-correction. A plantar callosity appears under the head of the osteotomized metatarsal or of the adjacent metatarsal which was not present before the operation. The treatment consists of a relieving plantar orthosis, sometimes with a local hollow under a metatarsal head to relieve weight-bearing. It may sometimes be necessary to do another osteotomy.

• Pseudarthrosis of the metatarsals is relatively common after osteotomy [14]. It is due to the non-immobilization of the osteotomy, or to premature resumption of forefoot weight-bearing, or finally to hypermobility of the osteotomy site. It is more frequently a complication of basi-metatarsal osteotomies than of distal osteotomies. It must be considered when there is persistent metatarsalgia even though plantar calluses have disappeared. The contracture of the soft tissues and the surgical scarring make clinical examination difficult. If the X-ray in oblique view does not show anything, technetium bone scan hyperfixation, if persisting long after the operation, will suggest a pseudarthrosis, confirmed by CT. Reoperation is often necessary, with osteosynthesis by a pin or a dorsal plate. Relief of the forefoot by means of a shoe with a posterior weight-bearing support will be necessary for 5 or 6 weeks.

Insufficiency of a middle metatarsal

In ambulation, all the metatarsal heads contact the ground. Partial or total loss of support on the ground of one of the metatarsal heads will bring about transfer metatarsalgia under the adjacent heads. Such a disorder can be of congenital, iatrogenic or neurologic origin.

Congenital shortness of the metatarsals

The syndrome of middle metatarsal insufficiency appears in aplasia or hypoplasia of one or several parts of the bone. This hypoplasia with insufficiency can affect the toe, the metatarsal or the whole ray. The metatarsal shortness (brachymetatarsus) brings about recession of the toe giving the impression of a toe implanted on the dorsum of the foot. There is dorsal friction between the toe and the shoe and lateral friction against the adjacent toes. The most common form is hypoplasia of the 4th ray. During the growth period, the 4th toe remains behind the others at the level of the other MT heads. A deviation of the adjacent toes then occurs with camptodactyly and clawing of the 5th toe, also elevation of the 3rd toe and overloading of the 3rd and 5th heads linked with static metatarsalgia. A 3rd metatarsal hypoplasia is much more uncommon. The metatarsal hypoplasia is often associated with a large anteroposterior sulcus on the sole of the foot, also showing hypoplasia of the intrinsic muscles. Such an abnormality is in fact well tolerated for a long time and only decompensates during adult life. Its treatment is predominantly symptomatic, by plantar and digital orthoses.

Iatrogenic metatarsal insufficiency

This complicates some operations for metatarsalgia by resection of one metatarsal head or it's replacement with a silicone implant. The metatarsal recession also leads to transfer metatarsalgia with callosities under the adjacent heads, especially the 3rd when the 2nd head has been resected.

Metatarsal insufficiency of neurologic origin

Some very pronounced neurogenic cavus feet are associated with a convex forefoot. Such transverse cavus explains why only the 1st and 5th metatarsal heads contact the ground. The neurologic disorder leads to the cavus because it provokes muscular imbalance with a predominance of the transverse adductor muscle, the hallux and the peroneus (fibularis) longus muscle. Acute metatarsalgia appears under the 1st and/or 5th heads, with hyperkeratosis, bursitis and even, in some rare cases, a perforating ulcer.

Treatment of metatarsal insufficiency

Usually a plantar orthosis and re-education in its various forms will be sufficient. The lower limb will be treated in its entirety, especially in the neurologic cavus foot. There is frequently a shortness of the calcaneal tendon which needs to be taken into account by re-education of the triceps surae muscle and calcaneal tendon (stretching).

Surgical treatment can be considered in two ways: either by lengthening a metatarsal bone which is too short, or by shortening the adjacent metatarsals. Lengthening of a metatarsal has been used since Illizarov's work, and is performed after a shaft osteotomy by distraction with an external fixator. This technique, which is often painful, may only be considered for a young patient. The technique of shortening the adjacent metatarsals is generally opted for; it was introduced by Barouk and has been described earlier. Recentering of the metatarsal heads according to Regnauld is sometimes preferred. The insertion of a metatarsal head prosthesis on the short metatarsal and amputation of the dorsal toe have now both been abandoned. With a chronically painful neurologic cavus foot one may resort to lengthening procedures on the calcaneal tendon, combined with various osteotomy techniques to correct the cavus of the foot.

Intractable plantar hyperkeratosis

This condition is akin to the round forefoot. It affects some neurogenic cavus feet and some ischemic or post-traumatic feet. In addition to the metatarsalgia, the patient may complain of this increasing hyperkeratosis, with recurring and increasingly disabling callosities. Pedicure, which removes the callosities, more and more often becomes insufficient. It is important to explain to the patient that the hyperkeratosis and callosities are only the consequences of overloading of the area, which provokes the dermatitis with cutaneous ischemia. Removal of this hyperkeratosis, which is a scar made of poorly vascularized tissue, does not prevent increasingly rapid recurrence. The differential diagnosis from a plantar wart is sometimes difficult: the callosity is always located on a weight-bearing area but a wart may have the same localization. A callosity is painful only in ambulation unless it is superinfected. The diagnosis becomes obvious during careful surgical resection; the dark purpuric focus usually seen in a wart, is not seen here. Moreover, the dermoglyphs are preserved on a callosity, but not on a wart. The differential diagnosis is essential because a callosity must never be treated by excision or diathermy.

The treatment of these callosities comprises reeducation, suitable foot-wear and appropriate plantar orthoses. If proper conservative treatment is ineffective, surgical treatment may be proposed according to the etiology, especially for the neurogenic cavus foot.

Lateral plantar overloading with secondary pathology

Lateral plantar overloading has been well described by Claustre and Bonnel [7]. It is a static dysfunction with hyperpressure on the 5th metatarsal head. Most often, this lateral overload reveals or complicates a lesion located elsewhere in the foot.

The patient generally complains of lateral metatarsal pain, occurring only when standing or walking; sometimes the main problem is difficulty in wearing shoes, chiefly due to the lesions which provoke the overload.

On examination, the fifth metatarsophalangeal joint is painful when mobilized and especially on plantar pressure. A reduction of the vertical mobility of the 5th metatarsal is noted. A hypercallosity due to overloading is also noted under the 5th head, sometimes a bursa or an actual bursitis. There may be difficulty in walking, with avoidance of weight-bearing on the lateral side of the foot.

The etiologic inquiry must include a complete assessment of the foot. One must enquire about previous trauma or surgery. X-rays in weight-bearing complete the physical examination. This etiologic inquiry is generally easy: the rare localized lesions of the fifth ray are a quintus varus deformity or more rarely a dislocation of the 5th metatarsophalangeal joint.

The more remote causes are:

- a painful hallux rigidus leading to avoidance of support on the first ray and a gait with varus of the forefoot. The assessment of the first ray allows the diagnosis (c.f. first ray pathology);

- sometimes a calcaneus varus is observed, either alone or associated with a pes cavus.

• Lateral overloading may complicate an insufficient anteromedial plantar loading, whatever the causal first ray pathology may be. It may be an isolated horizontalization of the first metatarsal as it is seen in some neurogenic feet or in equino-varus club-foot. The reduction of anteromedial plantar support with a lateral metatarsalgia is also frequently of iatrogenic origin, especially in case of subtalar arthrodesis with permanent, painful fixed varus.

The treatment must be based on the etiology if possible: hallux rigidus or sesamoid disorders for the first ray; treatment of an arthritis or a bursitis of the 5th metatarsophalangeal joint which may be a manifestation of rheumatoid arthritis. The plantar orthosis must have a retrocapital support and a recess under the stressed area and a pronator heel counter if there is a reducible varus of the hindfoot.

Metatarsophalangeal subluxation and quintus varus deformity often need surgical treatment.

Lateral bursitis of the 5th metatarsal head

This lateral bursitis of the 5th metatarsal head or "tailor's bunion" (bunionette) is the consequence of painful friction between the protuberance of the 5th metatarsal head and the shoe. This protuberance is the result of a deformation with angulation of the 5th ray: it is either an acquired deformity or the complication of a congenital quintus varus. When acquired, it is observed more often in females; the deformity starts at about the age of 10 or 12 but becomes painful only in adult life when it is associated with a hallux valgus in a triangular but unfixed forefoot, as is often the case. Of course, it is the pressure of the shoe that transforms the prominence of the metatarsal head into a bursitis. This bursitis is sometimes one of the first signs of a rheumatoid arthritis.

Clinical features

The female patient generally complains of a painful thickening revealing the bursitis or of major discomfort when wearing shoes, more rarely for a lateral metatarsalgia.

On examination one observes the angle of the 5th ray, possible clawing of the 5th toe, or a lateral or dorsolateral plantar callus [15]. A bursa on the lateral side of the 5th metatarsal head (bunionette) and sometimes a true bursitis are frequently noted. There is tenderness over the 5th head. The 5th toe is deviated medially and can cross above or below the 4th toe. Progress may be towards a medial subluxation of the 5th metatarsophalangeal joint; the palpable protuberance then corresponds exclusively to the 5th head, which rubs against the shoe and provokes first a bursa, and then an often secondarily-infected bursitis. This course is quite similar to that of congenital quintus varus deformity (see below) but also to that of hallux valgus, with which disorders of the 5th ray are often associated.

Radiographic features

A dorso-plantar view in weight-bearing, and a 3/4 oblique view to show the lateral metatarsal heads better, are performed. The dorso-plantar view permits measurement of the intermetatarsal angle between M4 and M5 (normally 12°-15°) and of the angle of metatarsal spread between M2 and M5 (16°-18°). Two types of metatarsus valgus can be distinguished [7]: a simple deviation of a morphologically normal metatarsal or a deformation with a lateral concavity, usually situated at the junction of the middle and distal thirds of the shaft. This explains the protuberance of the 5th head, which is twisted outward. According to Jahss [23], this deformity is usually associated with a brachymetatarsus.

Conservative treatment

This includes adjustment and particularly widening of the shoe. High heels are forbidden. Stretching of the shoe by the shoe-maker, opposite the area where the 5th head presses, is very helpful. A plantar orthosis to relieve the fifth metatarsal head but above all a toe orthosis to protect it are also useful, but these measures are effective only if the shoe is wide enough. Chiropody, especially for the hyperkeratosis, has a place in this conservative treatment.

Surgical treatment

This is performed for recurrent bursitis or obstinate lateral metatarsalgia. The choice of surgical procedure depends on the radiologic findings. If there is widening of the intermetatarsal M4M5 angle, a metatarsal osteotomy is performed: a V-shaped basimetatarsal osteotomy fixed during consolidation with a pin between M4 and M5 leads to complete correction of the intermetatarsal angle and corrects, if necessary, any equinus of the fifth metatarsal by dorsal elevation [15].

In cases with deformation of the shaft, the osteotomy is more distal. Barouk [1] recommends then a Weil's osteotomy with medial displacement and without metatarsal recession. Kitaoka H [24] suggests a distal osteotomy of the Johnson type, displacing the metatarsal head medially and fixing the osteotomy with two pins: this procedure is accompanied by arthrolysis, lengthening of the tendon of the extensor muscle in order to reduce the clawing and release of the abductor muscle of the 5th ray. More limited procedures on the metatarsophalangeal joint such as removal of the bursa, resection of the lateral side of this metatarsal head, or fibrotendinous cerclage are insufficient and lead to rapid recurrence.

With proper technique, a correctly performed osteotomy generally provides a complete cure of the bursitis over the 5th metatarsal head.

Metatarsalgia: conclusion

Static metatarsal pathology has shown to be extremely diverse. The diagnosis of a static metatarsalgia needs assessment of the whole foot, both forefoot and hindfoot. It is not always easy to exclude commencing inflammatory rheumatoid disease, or an intermetatarsal lesion such as Morton's syndrome, particularly since the latter may be associated with true static metatarsalgia, as described above. Acute metatarsalgiae: inflammatory, traumatic, or micro-traumatic (stress fracture, plantar plate rupture) are diagnoses that are often difficult to exclude and have been detailed above.

The surgical treatment of static metatarsalgia is considered only after the failure of thorough and prolonged conservative treatment, and especially after analysis of the statics of the foot as a whole. Correction of any pathology of the 1st ray, and particularly of a hallux valgus, must always precede any other procedure on the forefoot, whose destabil-ization is often only due to the abnormality of the first ray.

Toe disorders (excluding the first ray)

In walking, the toes play an important part during the last phase of the gait cycle; during running, their propulsive function being predominant, any pathology of the toes may affect the gait cycle, forefoot function and especially the function of the metatarsophalangeal joints. Therefore, in this chapter, the mechanical dysfunction and deformities of the toes will be dealt with to the exclusion of neurogenic and inflammatory disorders.

Pathogenesis of clawed toes

Deformation of the lateral toes is extremely common, especially in women. Well tolerated for a long time, particularly by patients who do no sport, it often becomes uncomfortable after the age of fifty. Clawing is most frequently acquired, occurring in static disorders facilitated by a feminine shoe which is too short, too tight, and with a high heel: it is more rarely a congenital malformation (clinodactyly, quintus varus supradductus).

The acquired claw-toe is provoked, as seen earlier, by the footwear. An artificial insufficiency of the 1st ray is created and an overloading of the lateral metatarsals, which remain longer in contact with the ground in ambulation. The 1st phalanx moves from a horizontal position to slight extension and hence a major flexion of the distal phalanx is noted because of contracture of the flexor digitorum longus muscle. The metatarsal head, pressing on the base of the 1st phalanx, provokes progressive overstretching of the dorsal capsule and the plantar plate. The 1st phalanx remains in hyperextension and the lumbrical and intrinsic muscles move from a plantar to a lateral position in relation to the metatarsal head, and then from this lateral position become dorsal. From being flexors, they become extensors, which increases the tendency to luxation. This mechanism has already been described in the 2nd ray syndrome. The ligamentous hyperlaxity, the overweight problem and the "trophostatic" postmenopausal context facilitate this physiopathologic sequence. Once established, the clawing makes wearing shoes very difficult. By rubbing against the shoe an irreducible clawing provokes cutaneous lesions such as dorsal callosities and dorsal, subungual and pulpar corns of the toes.

The difficulty in wearing shoes is often the main complaint of the patient.

The horizontal equilibrium of the metatarsophalangeal joint is due to the extensor muscle opposing the action of the flexor muscle, but dorsiflexion of the metatarsophalangeal joint is mainly related to the pressure of the toes on the ground during walking. The interosseous tendons are situated on the dorsal side of the transverse intermetatarsal ligament, the lumbrical muscles on its plantar aspect. Both are situated under the axis of the curve of dorsiflexion of the metatarsophalangeal joint, facilitating flexion of this joint. These muscles thus stabilize the toe [33, 35]. Permanent shoe-wearing provokes atrophy of the intrinsic muscles with imbalance of their activity. Thus, the sequence described above will be set into motion and one of three deformities may develop: hammer-toe, clawing and the swan-neck toe (figs. 20.6 & 20.7). When the flexor digitorum longus contracts with no resistance, the toe becomes a hammer-toe with permanent flexion of the distal interphalangeal joint. When the flexor digitorum brevis muscle contracts without contraction of the flexor digitorum longus muscle beyond the distal interphalangeal joint, swan-neck deformity of the toe develops. Finally, simultaneous contraction of the flexor digitorum longus beyond the distal interphalangeal joint and of the flexor digitorum brevis brings about a completely clawed toe. When acquired, these deformities become fixed only if there is an unstable metatarsophalangeal joint due to overstretching of the plantar plate; during walking, the action of the intrinsic muscles (interossei and lumbricals), combined with the resistance of the capsule leaves the 1st phalanx in a neutral position. The involvement of the plantar plate may lead to a lasting dorsiflexion of the proximal phalanx and a clawed toe. Of course, clawing of the 2nd toe occurs more often when the second toe is longer than the hallux (Greek type of forefoot). The exact mechanism of congenital toe clawing, is not well-known. These toes are generally reducible in childhood and develop a fixed swan-neck deformity in adult life.

Clinical features

The patient complains of discomfort with shoes and in walking, metatarsalgia, or a recurrent painful corn. The early onset and course of these disorders are noted as well as shoe-wearing habits, previous treatment, the possible role of sport and especially of

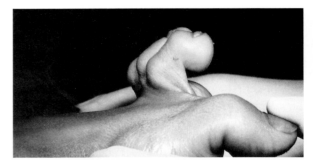

Fig. 20.6. Clawing of the toes

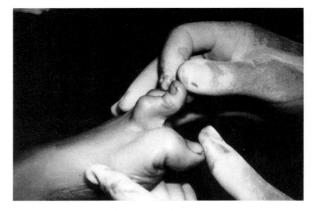

Fig. 20.7. Swan-neck deformity of the second toe

running. The possible role of these factors in the context of the woman's mode of life and choice of footwear is assessed.

The examination of the feet when weight-bearing, in walking and in decubitus, must be global. In the toes, the appearance of the skin and nails is noted, the digital formula, toe harmony, pulp contact with the ground. In the standing patient the horizontal deformities (hallux valgus, quintus varus) or vertical deformities ("canoeing" of the metatarsophalangeal joint in a hallux rigidus, a clawed toe and its type, dorsal or pulpar corns) are evaluated. With the podoscope one assesses the statics of the foot and the degree of pulp-bearing on the ground (insufficient support in some fixed clawed toes, excess load on the fifth ray); if necessary, the support force may also be tested, e.g., with a sheet of paper that the toe must hold on the floor under its pulp.

The dynamics of the toes are noted when walking and even when jumping or running.

In decubitus, each toe is examined separately with the foot held in the hand (Braun). Any nail or skin abnormality is noticed; the interdigital spaces are carefully and precisely examined (corns between toes, intertrigo). The articular function is analyzed in the clawed toes and also in the normal toes. Vertical instability of the metatarsophalangeal joints and stiffness of the interphalangeal joint, especially the proximal one, are sought. Muscle testing, especially of the intrinsic muscles (approximation and separation of the toes) as well as a test of toe sensation are performed, and even a complete neurologic examination in cases of neurogenic foot anthropathy.

We must remember, as usual, the importance of a detailed examination of the shoe (which is often unsuited to the patient's foot), its deformation and how it wears.

General treatment of clawed toes

Conservative treatment is based primarily on the wearing of suitable shoes; the patient must be made aware of the deformation of the forefoot, the conflict between container and content in the shoe and the necessity of changing some shoe-wearing habits, which is sometimes difficult. Asking the shoemaker for some slight modifications of the shoe will often be very helpful. Chiropodal treatment is given for corns, calluses and nails, supplemented by skin protectors. A toe orthosis can decrease the problems of clawing, if this is still flexible. An interdigital separating orthosis, made to measure, prevents rubbing of the 4th against the 5th toe and allows an interdigital corn to disappear for the time being.

A plantar orthosis is often necessary to treat some overloaded areas under the metatarsal heads: a subcapital recess is sometimes added to the bar behind the heads to relieve a painful joint by transferring the load to an adjacent joint. When there is a clawed toe, an antecapital component under the toe can sometimes be used to restrict the recession of the 2nd phalanx in walking.

Re-education of the toes must not be neglected; massage including auto-massage, mobilization, stretching exercises of the forefoot, possibly supplemented by exercises in the swimming-pool, retraining of the intrinsic muscles and also of the whole foot, all have their place while the clawing is still reducible.

Surgical treatment

This is performed under local or loco-regional anesthesia. Three procedures are available.

Tendon transfer according to Girdlestone

The flexor digitorum longus tendon is removed from the plantar side of the third phalanx. Through a small incision under the metatarsophalangeal joint, it is split into two bands which are then sutured together on the dorsum of the first phalanx or onto the tendon of the long extensor. When the proximal interphalangeal joint is rigid, this procedure does not release this joint.

For *arthroplasty*, a transverse incision over the proximal interphalangeal joint is better than a lateral longitudinal one. This procedure brings about excellent results, especially for pain [16], but because of the risk of recurrence some surgeons prefer to perform a proximal interphalangeal arthrodesis rather than an arthroplasty. They need only freshen the base of the second phalanx and sharpen the first phalanx, before driving it into the second phalanx. The consolidation of this arthrodesis is not always very good. The arthroplasty itself does not allow much residual mobility (10 to 20° of plantarflexion is possible). After the operation, edema may often persist for 2 or 3 months which makes shoe-wearing difficult and the patient should be warned of this. A permanent fixed dorsal hyperextension of the first phalanx may give trouble.

Then a *lengthening of the extensor muscle* on the dorsum of the forefoot by Green's technique is necessary to reduce its pulling power. Sometimes simple percutaneous tenotomy is sufficient. Some authors prefer lengthening of the flexor tendons with transplant of the tendons of the flexor digitorum longus muscle onto those of the flexor digitorum brevis. This procedure is logical when the first toe is longer than the second with a normally aligned 1st ray. We stress once more the effectiveness of metatarsal osteotomies for reducible clawed toes, such as Gauthier's osteotomy, where the dorsiflexion of the MT head restores plantarflexion of the phalanx; or Weil's osteotomy, in which recession of the metatarsal head allows the capsulo-ligamentous system to be released and the clawing to disappear.

Total clawing

This consists of dorsiflexion of the proximal phalanx associated with a hammer-toe. It often affects all the toes. The deformation may be flexible or fixed. It is due to an imbalance between the intrinsic and extrinsic muscles (fig. 20.6). It may be observed in some types of neurogenic pes cavus (poliomyelitis, Charcot-Marie-Tooth disease).

The patient may complain of a pulpar or subungual corn or a corn on the dorsum of the proximal interphalangeal joint, or of metatarsalgia. The difficulty in wearing shoes due to the corns is often very serious.

The conservative treatment of these completely clawed toes is possible if the clawing is still flexible, in children or teenagers. An operation is often preferred in childhood in order to prevent permanent deformation of the phalanx, which may appear during growth. In this case Girdlestone's procedure is chosen: it includes a disinsertion of the tendon of the flexor digitorum longus muscle combined with an arthroplasty of the distal interphalangeal joint and a lengthening of the extensor tendon. This reduction is held by a pin for 6 weeks.

For the adult patient, the operation comprises lengthening of the extensor longus tendon, arthrodesis of the proximal interphalangeal joint, and arthroplasty of the distal interphalangeal joint using several different transverse incisions. The result is generally a stiffened toe but without corns, especially the painful subungual ones.

In cases of swan-neck deformity (fig. 20.7), characterized by the dorsiflexion of the first phalanx, plantarflexion of the second phalanx and hyperextension of the third phalanx, an arthroplasty of the proximal interphalangeal joint may give predominance to the flexor muscle and thus a distal clawing. Therefore an arthrodesis of the proximal interphalangeal joint and a lengthening of the extensor tendon are performed.

Clinodactyly, the supradducted 2nd toe and the quintus varus supradductus are described separately because of their clinical and surgical characteristics.

Clinodactyly

Clinodactyly is a congenital lateral deformity which is the most frequent, situated usually at the 4th toe. It also generally includes deviation in flexion or extension. It is particularly troublesome when the abnormal toe lies in adduction, above or beneath the 3rd toe. In infradductus particularly, this clinodactyly of the 4th toe causes clawing of the 3rd toe with a dorsal corn. Sometimes a hammer-toe is present at the 4th toe.

In babies, an adhesive bandage may sometimes correct the deformity. If it does not, only surgical correction can be considered, in childhood or when growth has ceased.

Suppradductus of the second toe

This deformity differs from a clawed toe by its association with an unstable second metatarsophalangeal joint, a lateral deviation of the first ray and a medial deviation of the third toe. Most often, the 2nd toe is medially deviated but it can overlap the 3rd toe. At a further stage, complete overlapping of the first toe by the second in an elderly patient is often difficult to treat.

The possibilities for conservative treatment are very limited; when the clawing and overlap are permanent, an orthopedic shoe must be prescribed. But when the clawing is still reducible a properly molded toe orthosis can sometimes lower the 2nd toe, this inverted U-shaped orthosis being itself supported by the adjacent toes. When the deformity has been present for a long time, and even if it still reducible, a corrective toe orthosis is often so poorly tolerated in the shoe that surgical treatment is justified.

A global procedure on two or even three contiguous rays is usually desirable. On the 2nd toe, the tendon of the extensor muscle is lengthened with capsulotomy and release of the metatarsophalangeal joint. If recently ruptured, the lateral ligaments can be sutured. If hyperextension of the first phalanx persists, the long flexor tendon muscle may be transferred by Girdlestone's technique to stabilize the 2nd toe between the 1st and 3rd toes. For a more severe lesion, this procedure has to be associated with either the radical cure of a hallux valgus or, if the patient refuses, a varization osteotomy of the proximal phalanx of the first ray, creating a wide space for the 2nd ray. Such a procedure excludes weight-bearing on the forefoot for 4 weeks. If the clawing is severe and irreducible, a wide resection of the first phalanx and syndactylization of the 2nd and 3rd toes are sometimes necessary.

Amputation of the 2nd ray, as sometimes suggested to release the metatarsal head, may rapidly increase the metatarsalgia and particularly the hallux valgus and any clinodactyly. These amputations of the second toe are poorly tolerated and need a simultaneous arthrodesis of the first metatarsophalangeal joint to maintain good equilibrium of the forefoot.

Quintus varus supradductus

This congenital deformity has to be distinguished from a protrusion of the 5th metatarsal head with a lateral bursitis (tailor's bunion), an acquired condition described above.

It is marked by medial deviation of the fifth toe, which overlaps the fourth toe. This deformity is often bilateral but is usually well tolerated by the child. In the adult, there is discomfort in shoe wearing; a dorsal corn may appear on the 2nd phalanx; sometimes an interdigital corn is present in the 4th interspace; and lastly there is frequently a callosity on the plantar aspect of the 5th metatarsal head and a bursitis over this head. The 5th toe is deviated and in external rotation, supported on the outer side of the 4th toe.

Conservative treatment is indicated only in children: an elastic adhesive bandage sometimes allows reduction of this quintus varus, provided it is worn for a long time.

In the adult, the efficiency of a toe orthosis is limited and temporary. Surgical treatment may be suggested if symptoms are troublesome. Procedures on the soft tissues only seem to be insufficient. Amputation of the 5th toe must be avoided because it brings about pain under the fifth metatarsal head and clawing of the fourth toe. Syndactylization with the 4th toe is generally unsatisfactory cosmetically and functionally. It seems preferable to choose a procedure [17] which combines transfer of the long extensor tendon according to Lapidus, complete medial tenoarthrolysis with reduction of the dorsal subluxation, resection of the lateral side of the 5th metatarsal head to reduce its bulk, and performance of a rotational skin-flap to counter the contracture, which is always marked. Such a correction eliminates the painful pressure on the 5th MT head and makes shoe-wearing easier by reducing the thickness of the outer side of the forefoot.

Conclusion

The static pathology of the forefoot, reviewed here, seems varied and often complex, especially if associated with pathology of the 1st ray. A meticulous clinical analysis is essential to identify the cause of the symptoms (pain, callosities, difficulty in wearing shoes). Any pathology bringing about dysfunction of the articular chains in the forefoot, or any lesion in the midfoot or hindfoot, may give rise to metatarsalgia. The anterior "heel" represented by the metatarsal heads resting on the ground works harmoniously with the posterior heel. The global analysis of the foot must imperatively take into account the dynamics of the foot and not merely the static disturbances, morphologic abnormalities and inequalities of loading.

Conservative treatment, primarily prophylactic, consists mainly of advice on shoe-wearing. If the usual city shoe is still largely subject to fashion, this is often quite contrary to the physiology of the foot. The sports shoe has greatly improved, allowing better step, adaptation of its shape to the type of foot, and the correction of some static or dynamic problems. Using modern plantar orthoses, more adequate and better tolerated, or sometimes toe orthoses, makes the prescription of orthopedic shoes less necessary.

The indication for surgical treatment is the fixed and intolerable lesion which benefits from modern procedures such as the V-osteotomy or of the Scarf osteotomy of the 1st ray, as well as the Gauthier and Weil osteotomies on the lateral rays.

References

1. Barouk LS (1994) Les ostéotomies métatarsiennes. (Symposium) Bordeaux
2. Barouk LS (1994) L'ostéotomie cervico-céphalique de Weil dans les métatarsalgies médianes. Med Chir Pied 1: 23-23
3. Brahms MA (1967) Common foot problems. J Bone Joint Surg 49A: 1653-1664
4. Braun S (1971) Comment examiner un pied. Vie Médicale 21: 2593-2615
5. Young MC, Fornasier VL, Cameron HV (1987) Osteochondral Disruption of the second metarsal: a variant of Freiberg's infraction? Foot Ankle 8: 103-109
6. Chou L, Mann R (1994) Rheumatoid-type repair in the non rheumatoid patient for intractable plantar pain following failed previous surgery of the forefoot. AOFAS 24th meeting, New Orleans
7. Claustre J, Simon L (1990) Les métatarsalgies statiques. Masson, Paris
8. Cracchiolo A. III Surgical procedures of the lateral metatarsals. In: Jahss MH (ed) Disorders of the Foot and Ankle. Saunders, Philadelphia
9. De Doncker E, Kowalski C (1979) Cinésiologie et rééducation du pied. Masson, Paris
10. Delagoutte JP, Bonnel F (1989) Le pied pathologique et techniques chirurgicales. Masson, Paris
11. Denis A, Huber-Levernieux CL, David A (1979) Syndrome douloureux du 2e rayon métatarso-phalangien. In: L'actualité rhumatologique présentée au praticien. Expansion Scientifique Française, Paris
12. De Stoop N, Suykens S, Veys EM (1987) Le pied psoriasique. In: Claustre J, Simon L (eds) Actualités en médecine et chirurgie du pied, 2e série. Masson, Paris

13. Diébold PF, Daum B (1990) Les métatarsalgies dans la maladie de Freiberg. In: Claustre J, Simon L (eds) Les métatarsalgies statiques. Masson, Paris

14. Diebold PF, Daum B (1991) Pseudarthrose des métatarsiens. In: Hérisson C, Claustre J, Simon L (eds) Le pied post-traumatique. Masson, Paris

15. Diébold PF, Bejjani FJ (1987) Basal osteotomy of the fifth metatarsal with intermetarsal pinning: a new approach to tailor's bunion. Foot Ankle 8: 40-45

16. Diébold PF, Daum B (1992) Stratégie thérapeutique dans la pathologie du pied du vieillard. In: Hérisson C, Simon L (eds) Le pied du sujet âgé. Masson, Paris

17. Diébold PF, Daum B, Delagoutte JP (1988) À propos du traitement du quintus supradductus. Expansion Scientifique Française, Paris

18. Freiberg AH (1926) The so-called infraction of the second metatarsal bone. J Bone Joint Surg 8: 257-261

19. Gauthier G (1974) Maladie de Freiberg ou 2e maladie de Kohler: proposition d'un traitement de reconstruction au stade évolué de l'affection. Rev Chir orthop 60 (suppl 2): 337-342

20. Giannestras NT (1967) Foot disorders. Medical an surgical management. Lea and Fediger, Philadelphia

21. Helal B (1975) Metatarsal osteotomy for metatarsalgia. J Bone Joint Surg 57: 187-192

22. Helal B, Jeeb P (1987) Diseases suggested pattern of management. Foot Ankle 8: 94-102

23. Jahss MH (1982) Disorders of the foot. WB saunders, Philadelphia

24. Kitaoka HB, Holiday AD, Campbell D (1991) Distal Chevron osteotomy for bunionette. Foot Ankle 12: 80-85

25. Lechevalier D, Magnin J, Crozes P, Dellestable F, Eulry F (1994) Huit fractures par insuffisance osseuse des têtes métatarsiennes. Med Chir Pied 10: 1-43

26. Lelièvre J (1981) Pathologie du pied, 5e edn. Masson, Paris

27. Mann RA, Mizel MS (1985) Monoarticular non traumatic synovitis of the metatarsophalangeal joint: a new diagnostis? Foot Ankle 6: 18-21

28. Mann RA (1986) Surgery of the foot. Mosby, St. Louis

29. Martorell-Martorell J (1973) Concept et étude sur la métatarsalgie et son traitement. In: Actualité de médecine et chirurgie du pied. Masson, Paris

30. Meyer R, Kieffer D, Durkel J, Kuntz JL (1995) Fractures de contrainte multiples des métatarsiens; à propos de deux observations. Med Chir Pied 11: 107-112

31. Morton D (1948) The human foot. Columbia University Press, New York

32. Perrin M (1989) La subluxation des orteils et son traitement. Med Chir Pied 52: 59-63

33. Pisani G (1993) Pieda astragalico e piede calcaneale. In: Trattato di chirurgia del piede. Edizioni Minerva Medica, Torino, pp 37-54

34. Régnauld B (1986) Le pied. Springer Verlag, Paris

35. Sarrafian SK (1993) Anatomy of the foot and ankle. J B Lippincott, Philadelphia

36. Viladot A (1979) Pathologie de l'avant-pied. Expansion Scientifique Française, Paris

37. Voutey H (1978) Manuel de chirurgie orthopédique et de rééducation du pied. Masson, Paris

21.

Morton's metatarsalgia

C Huber-Levernieux

Morton's metatarsalgia is the commonest nerve entrapment syndrome in the foot. Clinical diagnosis may be easily made from its typical presentation. Imaging investigations should be reserved for uncommon cases or failure of surgery. Correlations between static disorders, intermetatarsal bursitis and interspace neuroma are still debated and have a certain implication for the failure of surgery, which should only be chosen after attempting conservative treatment.

Morton's metatarsalgia results from interdigital nerve compression in the intermetatarsal space. The precise etiology and treatment of this common and disabling lesion are not entirely resolved.

The common plantar nerve (fig. 21.1) with the plantar metatarsal vessels crosses under the deep transverse metatarsal ligament, which is stretched between the metatarsal heads. When it divides into the proper plantar digital nerves, it inclines upwards and forwards to pass over the superficial transverse ligament [1], particularly individualized at the middle part of the forefoot and stretched during weight-bearing and dorsiflexion of the toes. This crossing from the plantar area to the adjacent sides of the toes occurs in a sensitive area where the nerve may be trapped between the two ligaments. The risk increases in the third space where the nerve is closer to the third metatarsal head [5]. The involvement of the intermetatarsal bursa, located dorsal to the transverse metatarsal ligament and close in its anterior part to the division of the nerve, is suggested by many authors [2, 6], as much as this bursa, present

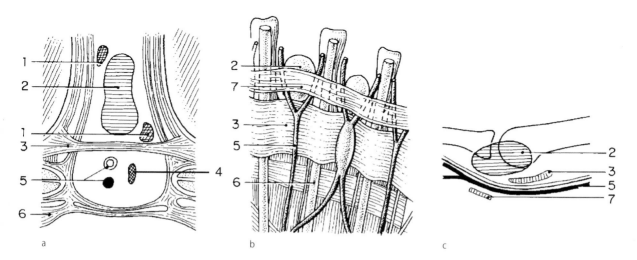

Fig. 21.1. a Web space. **b** Plantar view of transverse superficial ligament. **c** Section of third metatarsal interspace. *1* Interosseous muscles, *2* intermetatarsal bursa, *3* transverse metatarsal ligament, *4* lumbrical muscle, *5* interdigital nerve and artery, *6* flexor tendon, *7* transverse superficial ligament

in each intermetatarsal space, is enlarged forwards and extends 10 mm beyond the distal edge of the transverse metatarsal ligament [7] in the second and third intermetatarsal spaces and may communicate with the metatarsophalangeal joint.

Pathologic anatomy

At macroscopic examination, the lesion appears as a fusiform thickening of the common plantar digital nerve, extending sometimes to the digital branches, or as widened and flattened nerve, embedded in local fibrosis, which may adhere to the intermetatarsal bursa or metatarsophalangeal capsule.

The histologic study confirms the presence of pseudoneuroma which includes three kinds of lesions:
• nerve changes: edema of the endoneurium [24] detected by the electron microscope, first isolated, then associated with fibrosis; axonal degeneration occurs much later without degeneration of the myelin sheath;
• vascular changes: fibro-elastosis reducing the diameter of endoneural and perineural vessels;
• connective tissue changes: dense collagenous sclerosis without inflammatory infiltration.

According to most authors, these changes confirm the hypothesis of nerve entrapment in the crossing between the deep and superficial transverse intermetatarsal ligaments.

Diagnosis

The clinical symptoms of Morton's metatarsalgia, recognized so long ago [4, 19], are often so typical that diagnosis is suspected as soon as interviewing the patient. However, less suggestive cases can require use of modern imaging techniques.

Metatarsalgia occurs most often in women aged about fifty years (range 18 to 80 years) and involves classically the third interspace, although Mann and Reynolds [18], have found an equal number of neuromas in the second and third interspaces. For these authors, neuromas of the first and fourth interspaces are exceedingly rare, whereas among 300 patients operated on by one of us, or in the series of

Claustre and Bonnel [11], 2% of neuromas were situated in each of these intermetatarsal spaces. The presence of two or more neuromas in the same foot is not admitted by some authors [27], but is recorded in other studies.

In typical cases, the pain, the sole symptom, occurs as a paroxysmal attack combining localized plantar metatarsalgia and irradiation to contiguous toes, perceived as intense burning, shooting or cramping pains. They can be so acute that they are "sickening", and compel the patient to take off her shoe, which can sometimes induce transitory exacerbation. This sharp pain is relieved by rest, ranging from a few minutes to several hours but sometimes numbness persists in the toes. The pain may be limited to an acute metatarsalgia or become localized exclusively in the toes; it may radiate up the foot or the leg. In most cases the attack is caused by walking wearing tight-fitting shoes, although spontaneous or rest pain have been noted. A history of previous trauma is referred to in 15% of cases [18].

The diagnosis, suspected on interview, must be confirmed by clinical examination demonstrating the nerve compression features. The spontaneous pain can be reproduced by pressure on the interspace between the thumb and index or transverse metatarsal pressure (Mulder's sign), or passive toe dorsiflexion (Lasègue's toe sign). On the contrary, plantar pressure on the metatarsal heads situated near the painful intermetatarsal space does not reproduce the pain.

Sensory changes such as hyper- or hypoesthesia to pinprick may be noted in the nerve territory, either in the depth of the space or in the toes. The most typical finding is a hypoesthesia in the shape of a "page of a book" on the adjacent sides of the toes at the painful intermetatarsal space.

The movement of the adjacent metatarsophalangeal joints remains normal and inflammatory changes remain absent. Other symptoms may suggest the etiologic diagnosis. Static disorders not reported by Mann [18], are frequently mentioned by other authors [1]: cavus (68%), malalignment of the metatarsal heads and inadequate padding, flattened forefoot (round forefoot) (60%), hallux valgus (10%). These static disorders provoke metatarsalgia often associated with clinical findings suggesting minor nerve compression.

Involvement of an intermetatarsal bursitis is stressed by many authors. The bursitis may be clinically evident, either by protruding on the dorsal aspect of the involved interspace or by widening the toe gap, sometimes perceived by the patient as a fullness in the sole when walking. The palpation of the bursitis can reproduce the spontaneous pain. This bursitis may have a mechanical origin or may be an inflamed bursal cyst or a rheumatoid bursitis in patients who subsequently develop rheumatoid arthritis (Awerbuch) [3].

The diagnosis of neuroma is therefore based on clinical findings, which may also suggest the etiology [9], either primary in a normal foot and probably furthered by tight-fitting fashion shoes and microtrauma, or secondary to static disorders or bursitis.

The differential diagnosis from other lesions may be obvious, but sometimes the interplay between nerve compression, static disorders and bursitis makes this difficult. Static metatarsalgia has no physical signs of nerve compression. Metatarsophalangeal joint involvement associated with joint effusion may cause nerve compression, due to inflammatory synovitis or subluxation of the second metatarsophalangeal joint with the bursitis already mentioned, as in Morton's syndrome.

Other diagnoses must be excluded: Freiberg's disease, stress fracture, particularly of the metatarsal head [17], localized reflex sympathetic algodystrophy, sensory neuropathy or tumoral pathology.

In patients whose features are unusual, or when it is necessary to identify the reasons for surgical failure, sensitive and specific imaging procedures may be desirable for morphologic diagnosis. The reliability of their results has still to be proven.

Conventional radiographs are normal. Measurement of sensory conduction velocity [2, 8], which is operator-dependent, is not very specific. The same reservation affects ultrasonography [10, 21, 22]: false negative findings at ultrasound vary according to the authors. The ultrasound findings may depend on the stage of the symptoms: hypoechogenic if they are at an early stage, hyperechogenic (rosette image) if of longer duration.

At computed tomography (CT) [20], the neuroma, when identifiable, is shown as a homogeneous opacity of about 60 HU which is 4 to 5 mm in diameter, well circumscribed in the plantar aspect of the interspace and some mm behind the metatarsophalangeal joint. It is poorly differentiated from the muscles or subcutaneous tissue and poorly enhanced by contrast injection.

MRI is more accurate in soft tissue diagnosis. In T1-weighted sequence, the neuroma is shown as a grayish mass, sometimes pear-shaped, of intermediate signal intensity in relation to the surrounding hyperintense fatty tissue, visible in both the coronal plane and horizontal sections, with the same topography as in CT. In T2-weighted sequence, the mass exhibits moderate hypersignal intensity, enhanced by gadolinium injection [26]. Technical devices have been suggested to improve MRI accuracy: solenoid coil [12], signal enhancement by gadolinium injection with suppression of the fat signal [25]. The MRI findings are sometimes difficult to interpret and may vary with the stage of evolution.

Evaluation of the correlation between imaging and surgical findings is restricted to a few series. A recent study [22] shows that false negatives are common at MRI (3 cases in 8) but less than in ultrasonography (5 cases in 8). In summary, none of the different modalities for detecting plantar neuromas are certain. These expensive procedures must be reserved for the cases in which the diagnosis is unsure and for those with recurrent pain after surgery.

● Treatment

Conservative treatment

Conservative treatment must be instituted in all cases before making a decision about surgery. Success is more likely if the symptoms are recent, not more than six months to a year, and when there are static disorders which may be corrected by orthoses. Conservative treatment includes three possibilities: hygiene, insoles and local corticosteroid injections.

Hygienic measures consist of relative rest, at least avoiding hiking and long walks; foot-wear must be comfortable with a wide flexible upper, thick sole and a stable heel of reasonable height. Finally, physical exercises to strengthen the intrinsic muscles can improve hyperpressure on the splayed metatarsal heads of a hypotonic forefoot.

Insoles must be prescribed even when static disorders seem minimal. Their design must be simplified to be efficient: a localized pad (fig. 21.2) to relieve the metatarsal heads bordering the involved interspace is preferred to a metatarsal bar, except in cases of major pes cavus. These supports must be worn permanently if justified by static disorders.

Local intermetatarsal space injection of corticosteroids is recommended at once for repeated attacks of pain, or secondarily when insoles improve

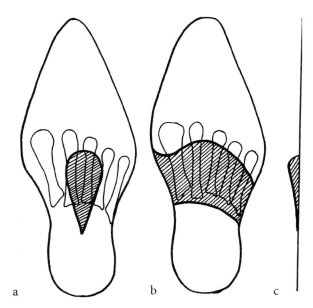

Fig. 21.2. Orthosis. **a** Anterior heel. **b** Metatarsal bar. **c** Cross section

poorly the condition. Injection technique is easy: the metatarsal heads bordering the involved interspace are located on the dorsum of the foot and the injection point is located between them, one cm behind the interdigital commissure. The needle is introduced perpendicular to the skin to a depth of about 15 mm. After control aspiration the injection of hydrocortisone 1 ml must be made without encountering resistance. If acute pain is elicited by pricking the nerve, the needle must be withdrawn a few mm. If the improvement obtained in a few days does not last, a second injection is suggested 15 days later. Then the rate must not exceed one or two injections, a year.

Most authors report failure of conservative treatment in 70% of cases. Only Greenfield [14], in a study of 76 cases, found 30% with immediate and lasting complete relief; after 2 years, 48% of his patients were asymptomatic and 41% experienced only slight discomfort.

Surgical treatment

Surgery must be chosen only after failure of conservative management. Several techniques are proposed. Most authors [15, 18, 23], prefer a longitudinal incision on the dorsal aspect over the affected interspace, transection of the transverse metatarsal ligament and resection of the neuroma. Only Gauthier [13], describes a method used for other peripheral nerve entrapments, i.e., simple division of the compressive transverse metatarsal ligament and neurolysis without neuroma resection.

The neuroma may be removed through a plantar approach by a curved transverse incision in front of the pressure area, allowing the exploration of adjacent interspaces. Johnson [16] suggests a longitudinal incision on the plantar aspect for the surgery of recurrent neuroma.

All the authors who resect the neuroma recommend wide resection of the proximal part of the nerve behind the intermetatarsal ligament to allow retraction of the digital nerve into the intrinsic muscles and avoid a symptomatic scar neuroma. Associated procedures, according to the operative findings, consist of resection of the intermetatarsal bursa and correction of forefoot deformities. The operative results are reported in Table 21.1 and classified as excellent if the patient has complete relief, uses regular shoes and walks normally; fair, if a slight pain persists without dysfunction; failure, if there is no improvement or pain as severe and disabling as before operation. This failure can occur at once or after a transitory remission.

The reasons for surgical failure are not totally clear; specific imaging may offer substantial advances. Wrong localization of the interspace is difficult to assess because typical images of asymptomatic neuroma have sometimes been found during investigation for some other forefoot pathology. For Mann, besides insufficient resection, the presence of an accessory nerve trunk passing under the transverse metatarsal ligament in a third of his cases may explain a recurrent neuroma, if damaged at the time of primary surgery. This assumption seems to be confirmed by excision of fibrosis and recurrent neuroma in reoperated cases. In all of these cases, Mann found that the transverse metatarsal ligament had reconstituted itself, thus invalidating Gauthier's technique. Finally, the longer duration of pre-operative symptoms, the greater the probability of recurrence.

For Johnson [16], the pathologic specimens obtained at reoperation showed residual tissue of the primary interdigital neuroma in association with fibrosis and a residual stump neuroma. For this author and in our cases, 33% of the reoperations were disappointing.

Table 21.1. Surgical evaluation of Morton's neuroma

	Technique	Cases	Average follow-up (years)	Excellent /Good (%)	Fair (%)	Failure (%)
Gauthier [13] 1975	Dorsal incision Transverse metatarsal lig. section Neurolysis	304	(0,3 à 2,5)	83	14,5	2,5
Mann [18] 1983	Dorsal incision Transverse metatarsal lig. section Neuroma resection	56	1,8 (0,5-6,5)	80	6	14
Ruuskanen [23], 1994	Dorsal incision Transverse metatarsal lig. section Neuroma resection	58	6 (2-12)	57	24	11
Denis 1995	Transversalplantar incision Neuroma resection	300	(2-8)	60	20	20
Jardé [15] 1995	Dorsal or plantar incision Transverse metatarsal lig. section Neuroma resection	46	(4-15)	74,5	21,2	4,3

Conclusion

The diagnosis of a Morton's neuroma is based on clinical findings. The etiology and pathogenesis are still debated. The hypothesis of entrapment and microtrauma is currently the most popular, stressing the critical role of the transverse metatarsal ligament in compressing the interdigital nerve. The role of intermetatarsal bursitis remains unclear. MRI investigation must be reserved for unusual cases and for recurrent symptoms. The failures of surgery must encourage the initial use of conservative treatment.

References

1. Abberton MJ (1982) Anatomical factors in causation of Morton's metatarsalgia. Actual Med Chir Pied 13: 181-197

2. Alexander IJ, Johnson KA, Parr JW (1987) Morton's neuroma. A review of recent concepts. Orthopedics 10: 103-106

3. Awerbuch MS, Shephard E, Vernon-Roberts B (1982) Morton metatarsalgia due to intermetatarsophalangeal bursitis as an early manifestation of rheumatoid arthritis. Clin Orthop 167 : 214-221

4. Betts LO (1940) Morton's metatarsalgia: neuritis of the fourth digital nerve. Med J Aust 1: 514-515

5. Bonnel F, Claustre J (1989) Espace intercapito-métatarsien en avant-pied. Structure anatomique. Med Chir Pied 5: 97-100

6. Bossley CJ, Cainrey PC (1980) The intermetatarsophalangeal bursa: its significance in Morton's metatarsalgia. J Bone Joint Surg 62 B: 184-187

7. Claustre J, Bonnel F (1990) L'espace intercapito-métatarsien. Anatomie et biomécanique. In: J. Claustre, L. Simon (eds) Monographie de Podologie 11. Les métatarsalgies statiques. Masson, Paris, pp 41-48

8. Dapres G, Claustre J, Bonnel F, Georgesco J, Cadhilac J (1987) Place de l'exploration électro-myographique dans le diagnostic de la maladie de Morton. In: Claustre J, Simon L (eds) Actualités en médecine et chirurgie du pied. 2e série. Masson, Paris, pp 64-68

9. Denis A, Huber-Levernieux C, Voisin MC (1983) Nouveau regard sur la métatarsalgie de Morton. In: S. de Sèze, A. Ryckewaert (eds) L'actualité rhumatologique. Expansion Scientifique Française, Paris, pp 99-109

10. Denis A, Ollivier L, Kowalski E (1987) Apports de l'échographie pour le diagnostic de la maladie de Morton. In: Claustre J, Simon L (eds) Actualités en médecine et chirurgie du pied. 2e série. Masson, Paris, pp 68-70

11. Enjalbert M, Claustre J, Bonnel F, Simon L, Baldet P (1990) Maladie de Morton et métatarsalgies. In: Claustre J, Simon L (eds) Monographies de Podologie 11. Les métatarsalgies statiques. Masson, Paris, pp 237-244

12. Erickson SJ, Canale PB, Carrera GF, et al (1991) Interdigital neuroma: high resolution MR imaging with a solenoid coil. Radiology 181: 833-836

13. Gauthier G, Dutertre P (1975) La maladie de Morton: syndrome canalaire. 74 opérés sans résection du névrome. Lyon Médical 223: 917-921

14. Greenfield J, Rea J, Ilfeld FW (1984) Morton's interdigital neuroma. Indications for treatment by local infections versus surgery. Clin Orthop 185: 142-144

15. Jardé O, Trinquier JL, Pleyber A, Meire P, Vives M (1995) Traitement du névrome de Morton par neurectomie. À propos de 43 observations. Rev Chir Orthop 81: 142-146

16. Johnson JE, Johnson KA, Krishnan K (1988) Persistant pain after excision of an interdigital neuroma. Results of reoperation. J Bone Joint Surg 70A: 651-657

17. Le Chevalier D, Magnin J, Crozes P, et al (1994) Huit fractures par insuffisance osseuse des têtes métatarsiennes. Med Chir Pied 1: 40-43

18. Mann RA, Reynolds JC (1983) Interdigital'neuroma. A critical clinical analysis. Foot Ankle 3: 238-243

19. Morton TG (1876) A peculiar and painful painful affection of the fourth metatarsophalangeal articulation. Am J Med Sci 71: 37-45

20. Morvan G, Busson J, Wybier M (1991) Tomodensitométrie du pied et de la cheville. Masson, Paris, 185 p

21. Redd RA, Peters VJ, Emery SF, Branch HM, Rifkin MDK (1989) Morton's neuroma: a sonographic evaluation. Radiology 171: 415-417

22. Resch S, Stenstrom A, Jonsson A, Jonsson K (1994) The diagnostic efficacy of magnetic resonance imaging and ultrasonography in Morton's neuroma: a radiological-surgical correlation. Foot Ankle 15: 88-92

23. Ruuskanen MM, Niinimaki T, Jalovaara P (1994) Results of the surgical treatment of Morton's neuralgia in 58 operated intermetatarsal spaces followed over 6 (2-12 years). Arch Orthop Trauma Surg 113: 78-80

24. Shereff MJ, Grande DA (1991) Electron microscopic analysis of the interdigital neuroma. Clin Orthop 271: 296-299

25. Terk MR, Kwong PK, Suthar M, Horvath BC, Colleti PM (1993) Morton neuroma: evaluation with MR imaging performed with contrast enhancement and fat suppression. Radiology 189: 239-241

26. Theodoresco B, Lalande G (1991) Résonance magnétique et névrome de Morton. Rev Chir Orthop 77: 273-275

27. Thompson FM, Deland JT (1993) Occurence of two interdigital neuromas in one foot. Foot Ankle 14 : 15-17

22.

Painful heel syndromes of mechanical origin

G Guaydier-Souquières

Painful heel syndromes of mechanical origin are a common reason for consultation in disorders of the foot, but it should not be forgotten that heel pain may be the presenting sign of an inflammatory rheumatic disease. The exact mechanism of this type of heel pain is complex and debated and several causes may be associated. It is generally due to tendon or ligament enthesopathies of mechanical origin, i.e., to lesions at their osseous attachments, but may sometimes be a consequence of nerve entrapment.

Anatomic review

The wide plantar tuberosity of the calcaneus is divided into a large medial process and a smaller lateral process. This tuberosity gives origin to various fascial, muscular and tendinous structures [31]:

• the plantar aponeurosis, an extension of the triceps surae muscle and the calcaneal tendon. Anteriorly, five pretendinous bands are attached to the tendon sheaths of the flexor muscles at the level of the metatarsophalangeal joints,

• the abductor hallucis muscle, which runs anteriorly from the medial process of the tuberosity and terminates on the medial sesamoid and the base of the first phalanx of the hallux. It abducts and above all flexes the hallux, and also plays a role in stabilizing the foot [4],

• the abductor digiti minimi muscle, which runs from the lateral process toward the lateral aspect of the base of the first phalanx of the fifth toe. It not only abducts this toe but also stabilizes the foot and plantarflexes the first phalanx of the fifth toe,

• the flexor digitorum brevis muscle runs from the middle part of the tuberosity toward the lateral aspect of the second phalanx of the lateral four toes. It plantarflexes the second phalanges on the first, then the first phalanges on the metatarsals.

Beneath the calcaneus is an areolar fat pad, divided by fibrous septa, which encloses the subcalcaneal bursa and a dense venous network which forms part of the plantar cutaneous venous plexus.

Sensory nerves

The medial calcaneal nerve which supplies the greater part of the heel arises from the tibial nerve, generally above the tarsal tunnel but sometimes within it. The tibial nerve then divides, within the tarsal tunnel, into lateral and medial plantar nerves. Some branches arise from the medial plantar nerve to supply the skin of the heel. A branch to the abductor digiti quinti muscle arises near the origin of the lateral plantar nerve. It passes deep to the abductor hallucis muscle and then runs obliquely between the thick fascia of the latter and the quadratus plantae muscle, changing direction around the underside of the tuberosity of the calcaneus and then running transversely towards the abductor digiti minimi muscle. In addition to its motor function, this nerve contains sensory fibers to the calcaneal periosteum and the plantar fascia [3, 37]. Lastly, the sural nerve gives rise to sensory branches supplying the lateral surface of the heel and a small lateral area of its undersurface.

Physiologic review

In the first phase of gait, the heel strikes the ground in supination, then the foot passes into pronation, while the motion of the subtalar joint controls the stability of the forefoot and the longitudinal arch of the foot. Impact on the ground is distributed and absorbed, first by the plantar structures of the heel, above all the fat pad and fascia, then by the midfoot and lastly by the forefoot [10]. In the last phase of gait, when the weight is borne by the toes, dorsal hyperflexion of the metatarsophalangeal joints stretches the complex formed by the triceps surae muscle, calcaneal tendon, calcaneus and plantar fascia. In particular, the triceps surae, abductor hallucis and flexor digitorum brevis muscles also contract until the foot leaves the ground [48]. The last two muscles then help propulsion by the triceps surae muscle by anchoring the toes to the ground and they also prevent collapse of the plantar arch [10, 20, 32].

While walking, and even more while running, the plantar muscular, tendinous and fascial structures attached to the tuberosity of the calcaneus obviously undergo considerable stress, accentuated by excessive weight or by static deformities [41, 47, 48]. For instance, the hindfoot valgus component of flat foot (pes planus) excessively everts the subtalar joint and stretches the complex formed by the triceps surae muscle, calcaneal tendon, calcaneus and plantar fascia [32, 44, 47]. Conversely, the rigid cavus foot is accompanied by excessive inversion and decreased mobility of the subtalar joint, leading to poor distribution of loading forces and increased strain on the plantar structures [32].

Clinical presentation

Symptoms

The patient complains of pain, usually progressive, located at the undersurface of the heel and above all at the anteromedial part. Typically, the timing of the pain indicates its mechanical origin, i.e., it is alleviated by rest and aggravated by walking, running, prolonged standing or climbing stairs. Pain can also return during the night or on renewed weight-bearing after a long period of rest. It is sometimes compared to the feeling of a nail or a piece of gravel in the shoe. In other cases, it is likened to a burn or an electric shock. This suggests an entrapment neuropathy, especially if numbness and paresthesia of the heel are also present and if pain becomes more severe during the day [1], or if there are nocturnal paresthesiae [24].

Pain progressively worsens and may be stabbing, even excruciating, resembling a nail driven into the foot or a red-hot iron and causing marked functional disability. The patient walks on the back of the heel or takes short steps on tiptoe, causing calf cramps. Therefore climbing stairs becomes impossible or extremely difficult, giving a sensation of avulsion of the back of the heel [9].

Clinical examination

On examination, pressure on the medial anterior part of the undersurface of the heel generally elicits sharp pain in an area which may be diffuse or on the contrary very limited, generally in the medial part of the heel. This suggests enthesopathy of the plantar fascia or the abductor hallucis muscle.

Lateral or central heel pain is more rarely felt. Posterior heel pain may also sometimes be produced by grasping the heel in the palms of both hands; this is due to excessive traction on the complex composed by the calcaneal tendon, calcaneus and plantar fascia, and is specifically related to pes cavus [9].

Elicited pain may be accentuated during movements which stretch the plantar fascia and the plantar muscles attached to the tuberosity of the calcaneus: dorsiflexion of the foot and toes, resisted plantarflexion, walking on the heel or on tiptoe.

The medial calcaneal nerve may be compressed if heel pain or paresthesiae are elicited by pressure or percussion of the tarsal canal behind the medial malleolus, or more rarely by pressure on the central aspect of the calcaneus, along the course of the calcaneal nerve between the medial malleolus and the heel, where sometimes a small, hard and mobile mass can be felt [1, 24]. Hypo- or hyperesthesia of the heel should be sought. If pressure on the medial edge of the anterior part of the heel is painful and produces paresthesiae, the nerve to the abductor digiti quinti muscle may be compressed [3].

A static or dynamic deformity is often found: flat foot, which causes heel pain due to excessive pronation [36], or above all cavus foot, which is accompanied by shortening of the complex consisting of the

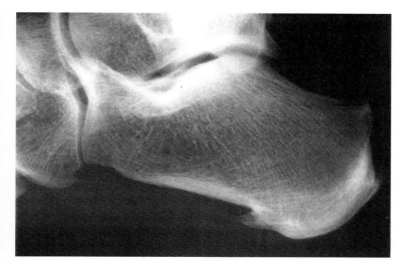

Fig. 22.1. Inferior calcaneal spur of mechanical appearance

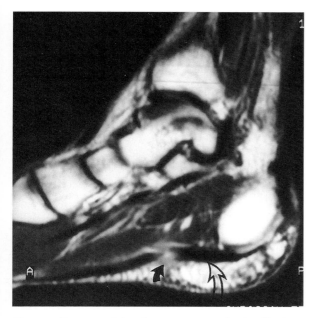

Fig. 22.2. Rupture of the plantar aponeurosis visualized on sagittal MRI image (courtesy of Dr. T. Tavernier). Area of rupture enhanced by gadolinium (*black arrow*). Overall thickening of the fascia indicating chronic fasciitis (*white arrow*)

triceps surae, calcaneal tendon and plantar fascia, and which causes excessive inversion [9].

The patient's shoes should be examined; if they are misshapen, this will indicate either poor choice of footwear or the consequences of a static or dynamic deformity, or both.

Finally, thorough investigation is necessary to look for excessive weight, prolonged standing at work, or practice of a sport increasing liability to heel pain, in particular jumping or dancing. Any factor suggesting a cause other than mechanical should also be sought, in particular a spondylarthropathy, which will be dealt with below.

Supplementary investigations

No investigation is routinely requested; the choice of technique is dictated by the clinical picture and suspected diagnosis or by a protracted course. If the diagnosis of heel pain of mechanical origin is uncertain after clinical examination, radiographs of the foot (anteroposterior, lateral and oblique) should be obtained. A profile of the medial side of the weight-bearing foot will often reveal a osseous spur of the lower calcaneus. A spur which is well-defined, pointed, of uniform appearance and small or moderate in size indicates a mechanical origin (fig. 22.1).

Other investigations such as ultrasound, computed tomography (CT) or magnetic resonance imaging (MRI) may be useful in some cases, in particular if rupture of the plantar aponeurosis is suspected [40] (fig. 22.2). Technetium bone scan is indicated to detect spondylarthropathy or stress fracture [14, 16, 19], nerve conduction and electromyographic studies to seek for a tarsal tunnel syndrome or an S1 radiculopathy, and in other cases doppler or other techniques may be informative.

Clinical forms

Acute form

This generally occurs after a jolt on landing in an athlete (a runner or jumper) or after a violent injury. Sudden and extremely acute pain makes it impossible to put the heel to the ground or even to bear any weight on the forefoot [27]. This acute form should be distinguished from true rupture of the plantar aponeurosis at its attachment. Features suggestive of the latter are a tearing sensation felt by the patient and above all major functional disability; examination reveals localized swelling, sometimes even bruising, exquisite tenderness and sharp pain on dorsiflexion of the foot [27]. A depression can be felt at the site of an aponeurotic rupture, or a hard and painful mass. In addition to ultrasound, MRI is then particularly useful in confirming rupture as the plantar aponeurosis is clearly depicted and even loss of continuity may be visualized [40] (fig. 22.2). Posteromedial rupture seems to be more frequent and to have a better prognosis than the central and lateral form, which may lead to residual pain on running or even walking and inability to continue athletic activities at the previous level. In such cases MRI demonstrates fusiform thickening or cyst-like folds of the aponeurosis [4, 40].

As discussed later, calcaneal fracture is a possibility which should also be considered in this acute context.

Forms related to a specific terrain

Liability to mechanical heel pain is greater in:
• the athlete, especially if he or she practices running, jumping, dancing, or more rarely tennis, the martial arts, rugby, etc. Heel pain of mechanical origin is frequent in these sports and often occurs after repeated heavy landings, especially on hard ground or with unsuitable footwear (heels which are too flat or with poor shock absorption), especially if there is a static deformity such as valgus heel or cavus foot [32, 41],
• the elderly person or the postmenopausal woman, especially if accompanied by a vascular disorder or increased body weight [21, 45],
• occupations involving prolonged standing (cooks, waiters, hairdressers); here again, obesity is frequently an aggravating factor,

• lastly, children, where the diagnosis may be Sever's disease or epiphysitis of the calcaneus, which is not a tendon enthesopathy but a disorder affecting the calcaneal growth plate.

Etiologies

There is now almost unanimous agreement that heel pain of mechanical origin most often corresponds to a plantar muscular and fascial insertional disorder involving one or more of the plantar structures attached to the plantar tuberosity of the calcaneus, in particular the plantar aponeurosis and the abductor hallucis muscle. Susceptibility to such a disorder is increased by a static deformity such as calcaneus valgus or, on the contrary, cavus and excessive inversion, sometimes with forefoot pronation [9, 36, 41, 42].

But these may be combined with other mechanisms [5]:
- subcalcaneal bursitis,
- sequelae of injury to the sole of the foot,
- thinning of the fat pad of the heel, leading to impaired shock absorption,
- above all, entrapment neuropathy, which may be the only cause and requires specific therapeutic management. The medial calcaneal nerve may be compressed either in the tarsal tunnel, if it arises at this level, or along its course to the heel. A neuroma has sometimes even been discovered during surgery [1]. A more frequent possibility is compression of the nerve to the abductor digiti minimi muscle by the edge of the abductor hallucis muscle, as this muscle is subjected to stress and becomes hypertrophied by overuse, especially if there is a calcaneal varus [38]. Electrodiagnostic testing is very difficult in such cases; although often no abnormality is detected, it may sometimes help in diagnosis [43] The incidence of nerve compression is debated: for some authors, it is frequently involved [3, 37], whereas others think it uncommon [45]. It is often difficult to differentiate from a plantar muscular and fascial attachment disorder [41].

As for the plantar calcaneal spur, it is currently admitted that this is not in itself a cause of pain but only a normal manifestation of the process of aging. Moreover, many calcaneal spurs are asymptomatic or are an incidental finding [44]. While a spur is more frequently found in patients with inferior heel pain than in asymptomatic patients, it is actually due to the pull of the muscles on the tuberosity of the calcaneus [31]. This pull is greater if there is a valgus deformity of the calcaneus, especially if the patient is overweight [36, 41, 47]. However, an osseous spur may compress the nerve to the abductor digiti minimi muscle as the nerve winds round the spur [3, 5].

Lastly, heel pain may be present in the sinus tarsi syndrome, but the principal site of pain suggestive of this syndrome is the lateral orifice of the sinus tarsi, anterior to the lateral malleolus, and the pain is often associated with a sensation of instability.

Differential diagnosis

Before confirming the diagnosis of common heel pain of mechanical origin, it is important to eliminate other causes of heel pain [3, 13, 39].

Inflammatory rheumatic diseases

Inflammatory rheumatic diseases, in particular the spondylarthropathies (ankylosing spondylitis, Reiter's syndrome, psoriatic arthropathy), where heel pain is frequent and sometimes the initial symptom, related to inflammatory enthesitis (see Chapter 12). This possibility should be borne in mind in particular in a young patient, especially male, and if pain is associated with posterior heel pain and morning stiffness. The timing of the pain may be deceptive and may not be only inflammatory in nature but also present while weight-bearing and walking. A thorough clinical examination should be carried out to search for psoriasis of the skin or nails, back pain and cervical or lumbar stiffness, or pain in one or both sacroiliac joints, whether spontaneous or elicited by pressure and movement. Radiographs of the feet (anteroposterior, lateral and oblique views) may show images of calcaneal inflammation with a large, irregular, uneven, poorly-defined spur, or even a proliferative erosive periostitis [22, 39]. Such lesions are particularly marked in Reiter's syndrome [15] and are proliferative rather than destructive in psoriatic arthropathy. Involvement of the subtalar joint is much rarer [18, 22]. HLA typing for the B27 antigen should be done and radiographs of the sacroiliac joint should be obtained together with spinal radiographs to seek for syndesmophytes, which begin at the dorsolumbar junction. A radio-isotope bone scan [14, 19] and a CT scan of the sacroiliac joints may also be requested. We shall not detail diagnostic criteria further here.

In rheumatoid arthritis, on the other hand, heel pain is rare and not severe. It is often felt only on local pressure and is located posteriorly and superiorly due to pre-achilles bursitis, rather than inferiorly [7, 8, 22]. Even in the absence of pain, lateral radiographs may reveal osteoporosis, erosion of the lower or rather the posterior calcaneus, or even an osseous spur which is not always inflammatory in appearance, especially as static deformities are often present in advanced forms [7]. Pre-achilles bursitis provides a more suggestive image of posterosuperior erosion sparing the upper part of the cortical margin. This lesion is very often clinically silent [8, 22, 46]. Rheumatoid involvement of the subtalar joint may also cause pain in the heel area and give rise to valgus deformity [22, 46].

Lastly, gout can also cause heel pain but this is more likely to be located above or behind the calcaneus. Calcaneal spurs are frequent in this disease.

Other systemic disorders

Other systemic disorders, such as diffuse idiopathic skeletal hyperostosis, may be accompanied by large bony excrescences below and behind the calcaneus. The diagnosis can be confirmed by radiographs of the dorsolumbar spine [12, 39]. Heel pain due to insertional disorder may also occur in the course of fibromyalgia. Degenerative osteoarthritis of the subtalar joint is mainly of traumatic origin.

Bone lesions

• Fracture of the calcaneus must be considered if heel pain is acute. On the other hand, stress fracture, which preferentially affects military recruits or athletes after excessive training, has a more insidious course and may be difficult to diagnose as radiographs are initially normal. CT scan is then very helpful [16, 33],
• calcaneal fracture may also occur in postmenopausal women, suggesting the presence of osteoporosis. Lastly, cases have been reported of acute post-traumatic heel pain due to fracture of the calcaneal spur [28],

• more rarely, pain may be due to osteitis, Paget's disease, reflex sympathetic dystrophy or a calcaneal tumor. If images of bone destruction are present, surgical biopsy must be done to seek a malignant tumor. Osteoid osteoma causes very sharp pain increasing at night and usually alleviated by salicylates. Both conventional radiographs and CT show a characteristic rosette image and technetium bone scan demonstrates marked localized increased uptake.

Soft tissue lesions

• A tumor, plantar wart, or hyperkeratosis due to localized microtrauma such as a nail protruding from the sole of the shoe. Ledderhose's disease causes plantar pain under the midfoot, but not under the heel.

Nerve lesions

• Lesion of the S1 sciatic root or peripheral neuropathy: pressure on the undersurface of the heel is not painful in this case. Electrodiagnostic testing is useful if any doubt persists,
• tarsal tunnel syndrome: calcaneal nerve entrapment at this level can, as already mentioned, cause lower heel pain, while compression of the tibial nerve or of one or both of its branches gives a different clinical picture, with plantar pain which radiates to the toes or may be only distal and partial, accompanied by slight motor deficiency and sometimes by objective sensory disorders [11, 17] (see chapter 25). Here again, electromyographic study may be useful when clinical features are not typical or when conservative treatment fails. It should also be noted that in leprosy and diabetes mellitus hypertrophy of the nerves makes them more susceptible to entrapment within the tunnel,
• the association of a tarsal tunnel syndrome with sciatic nerve root pain has also been described [43].

Arterial lesions

Arterial insufficiency may cause burning pain in the heel. The diagnosis is confirmed by the doppler technique.

● Treatment

Treatment of heel pain is primarily conservative, and often conservative only, and in most cases the patient will be pain-free within a few weeks [5, 35, 42, 45, 47]. The extent of the therapeutic measures taken will depend on the clinical picture.

Rest

Depending on the intensity of the pain, this may range from limitation of activity to strapping or sometimes even complete bed rest if the heel pain is acute.

Heel supports

These are simple visco-elastic heel supports, commercially available, preferably with a flexible area under the medial part of the tuberosity of the calcaneus [30], or soles in a shock-absorbing material such as sorbothane. Custom-made plantar supports with a firm heel wedge and a recessed anteromedial part are even more effective and are of course also designed to aid balance and compensate for any static or dynamic deformity. The device must not be high enough to come into contact with the zone of impingement [9]. Custom-made orthoses appear to be more effective than standard devices, especially as static or dynamic deformities are frequent [9, 34, 42]. In the United States, whole-foot insoles are often prescribed which are custom-made from a mold to correct static deformities and reduce the pull on the plantar aponeurosis [10].

Advice on footwear

Shoes should have thick rubber or crepe soles for better shock absorption, a 2 or 3 cm heel and a firm shank. For an athlete, the sole beneath the heel should be thick, made of polyurethane or with an air cushion. Any training errors should be corrected and training done on suitable terrain [48]. Alternative training activities such as cycling or swimming may be suggested [41].

Other therapeutic measures

• Systemic nonsteroidal anti-inflammatory drugs, though these are often not very effective in these cases,
• physical therapy (ultrasound, laser), exercises to stretch the plantar aponeurosis, passive mobilization, deep transverse massage,
• weight-loss if the patient is obese,
• followed by physiotherapy if there is a static or dynamic deformity,
• local steroid injection at the most painful point of the anteromedial part of the underside of the heel, repeated once or twice if necessary [13]. This is decided on if other conservative measures prove inadequate, or earlier if the pain is acute. Some authors recommend prior anesthesia of the tibial nerve at the tarsal tunnel, halfway between the medial malleolus and the calcaneal tendon [29]. Corticosteroids are injected here if there are signs suggesting entrapment of the tibial or calcaneal nerves.

Surgery

Surgery is exceptionally indicated and should be considered only in rare cases which do not respond to rest and conservative treatment. It would seem wise to wait several months before deciding on operation [5, 41, 45]. Although it generally results in relief from pain, the consequences of failure may be serious in athletes practicing sports at a highly competitive level. The procedure chosen is dictated by the causal mechanism. Spur resection alone is insufficient, and even useless in certain cases [47]. The most usual procedure is resection of the calcaneal attachments of the plantar aponeurosis [41] and release of the muscle origins [23, 47]. Other procedures have been suggested [2, 25].

Surgery is more often indicated if nerve entrapment is present, but here again only after conservative treatment has failed. Neurolysis or section of the calcaneal nerve at the tarsal tunnel or along its course between the medial malleolus and the heel [1] or neurolysis of the nerve to the abductor digiti minimi muscle is performed, either together with spur resection and muscular and fascial release, or alone. These procedures seem effective in many cases [3, 5]. The success previously attributed to spur resection alone can be explained by decompression of the nerve to the abductor digiti minimi muscle.

Whatever type of surgical procedure is performed, the use of plantar insoles will facilitate weight-bearing and progressive return to physical activity, which should be complete after about three months [23], the duration of absence from work depending on the patient's occupation [47].

If the plantar aponeurosis is ruptured, healing will generally be obtained by conservative treatment: complete rest, local application of ice, nonsteroidal anti-inflammatory agents, crutches and strapping [27, 41]. Progressive return to weight-bearing after about three weeks is made easier by plantar insoles, and a gradual return to sporting activity may be allowed after six weeks, running and jumping being permitted only when standing on tiptoe is no longer painful. Surgery should be considered only if conservative measures fail [27].

● Conclusion

While heel pain of mechanical origin is most often related to an insertional lesion, in particular of the plantar aponeurosis or the abductor hallucis muscle, other mechanisms such as nerve compression may be involved. In order to establish a diagnosis, other causes of heel pain must be eliminated, in particular S1 radiculopathy and spondylarthropathies. The acute forms, frequent in the athlete, may be due to rupture of the plantar aponeurosis or calcaneal fracture. Surgery is only considered in the rare cases in which heel pain persists in spite of rest and conservative treatment.

References

1. Altman MI, Hinkes MP (1984) Heel neuroma. A case history. J Am Podiatr Med Assoc 72: 517-519
2. Baerg RH (1991) Calcaneal decompression for heel pain. Clinics Pod Med Surg, 8, 1: 197-202
3. Baxter DE, Pfeffer GB (1992) Treatment of chronic heel pain by surgical release of the first branch of the lateral plantar nerve. Clin Orthop 279: 229-236
4. Berkowitz JF, Kier R, Rudicel S (1991) Plantar fasciitis: MR Imaging. Radiology, 179: 665-667
5. Bordelon RL (1983) Subcalcaneal pain. Clin Orthop 177: 49-53
6. Bourrel P, Rey A, Blanc JF, Palinacci JC, Bourges M, Giraudeau P (1976) Syndrome du canal tarsien. A propos de 15 cas "purs" et de 100 cas "associés" à la lèpre ou au diabète. Rev Rhum 43: 723-728

7. Bouysset M, Tebib J, Weil G, Noel E, Colson F, Llorca G, Lejeune E, Bouvier M (1989) The rheumatoid heel: its relationship to other disorders in the rheumatoid foot. Clin Rheum, 8: 208-214

8. Braun S (1975) Les calcanéites de la polyarthrite rhumatoïde. In: Simon L and Claustre J (eds) Le pied inflammatoire. Maloine, Paris, pp 43-47

9. Braun S (1986) La talalgie plantaire commune: du diagnostic au traitement. In: Claustre J and Simon L (eds) Pathologie du talon, Masson, Paris, p 153-159

10. Campbell JW, Inman VT (1974) Treatment of plantar fasciitis and calcaneal spurs with the UC-BL shoe insert. Clin Orthop 103: 52-62

11. Cimino WR (1990) Tarsal tunnel syndrome: review of the litterature. Foot Ankle 11: 47-52

12. Claustre J, Simon L (1982) Le pied hyperostosique. Rev Rhum, 49: 629-633

13. Claustre J, Simon L (1984) Talalgies. Appareil locomoteur. Encycl Med Chir, Paris, 14 116 A 10. p 1-14

14. Claustre J, Rossi M, Sirven A, Chevalier J, Simon L (1986) Apport de la scintigraphie dans les talalgies. Med Chir Pied 6: 53-56

15. Doury P, Pattin S (1979) Le calcaneum dans le syndrome de Fiessinger-Leroy-Reiter. Rev Rhum 46, 12: 705-709

16. Doury P (1988) Les fractures de fatigue (ou maladie de Pauzat) chez les sportifs. J Traumatol Sport 5: 218-225

17. Delagoutte JP, Bonnel F, Claustre J (1989) Syndrome canalaires. In: Delagoutte JP, Bonnel F (eds) Le Pied. Masson, Paris, p 255-259

18. Dromer C, Richardi G, Nourhashemi F, Vedrenne C, Sixou L, Leguennec P, Railhac JJ, Fournié B (1995) Les atteintes de l'articulation sous-talienne dans les spondylarthropathies inflammatoires. Med Chir Pied 11, 2: 97-100

19. Eulry F, Lechevalier D, Gaillard JF, Crozes P, Magnin J, Doury P (1995) La scintigraphie osseuse du calcaneum a-t-elle une place dans le diagnostic des arthrites réactionnelles. Med Chir Pied 11: 102-106

20. Fournié B, Fournié A, Martinez C (1986) Talalagie plantaire ou tendinite de l'abducteur du gros orteil. In: Claustre J, Simon L (eds) Pathologie du talon. Masson, Paris, p 160-165

21. Furey JG (1975) Plantar fasciitis. J Bone Joint Surg, 57: 672-673

22. Gerster JC, Vischer TL, Bennani A, Fallet GH (1977) The painful heel. Ann Rheum Dis, 36: 343-48

23. Gormley J, Kuwada GT (1992) Retrospective analysis of calcaneal spur removal and complete fascial release for the treatment of chronic heel pain. J Foot Surg 31: 166-69

24. Jackson DL, Haglund B (1991) Tarsal tunnel syndrome in athletes. Am J Sports Med 19: 61-65

25. Jay R M, Davis BA, Schoenhaus HD, Beckett D (1985) Calcaneal decompression for chronic heel pain. J Am Podiatr Med Assoc 75: 535-537

26. Klein MA, Sreitzer AM (1993) MR Imaging of the tarsal sinus and canal: normal anatomy, pathologic findings, and features of the sinus tarsi syndrome. Radiology 186: 233-240

27. Leach R, Jones R, Silva T (1978) Rupture of the plantar fascia in athletes. J Bone Joint Surg 60: 537-539

28. Leis SB, Burnett O, Harkless LB (1986) Painful heel syndrome. J Am Podiatr Med Assoc 76: 518-521

29. Lelièvre J (1981) Talalgies. In: Lelièvre J, Lelièvre JF (eds) Pathologie du pied. Masson, Paris, p 561-571

30. Levitz SJ, Dykyj D (1990) Improvements in the design of visco-elastic heel orthoses. J Am Podiatr Med Assoc 80: 653-656

31. Mc Carthy DJ, Gorecki GR (1979) The anatomical basis of inferior calcaneal lesions. J Am Pod Med Assoc 69: 527-536

32. Mann RA, Baxter DE, Lutter LD (1981) Running symposium. Foot Ankle J, 1: 190-224

33. Meltzer EF (1989) A rational approach to the management of heel pain. J Am Podiatr Med Assoc, 79: 89-92

34. Nigg BM, Herzog W, Read LJ (1988) Effect of viscoelastic shoe insoles on vertical impact forces in heel-toe running. Am J Sports Med, 16: 70-76

35. O'Brien D, Martin WJ (1985) A retrospective analysis of heel pain. J Am Podiatr Med Assoc, 75: 416-418

36. Prichasuk S, Subhadrabandhu T (1994) The relationship of pes planus and calcaneal spur to plantar heel pain. Clin Orthop 306: 192-196

37. Przylucki H, Jones CL (1981) Entrapment neuropathy of muscle branch of lateral plantar nerve: cause of heel pain. J Am Podiatr Assoc 71: 119-125

38. Radin EL (1983) Tarsal tunnel syndrome. Clin Orthop 181: 167-170

39. Resnick D, Niwayama G (1983) Entheses and enthesopathy. Radiology 146: 1-9

40. Roger B, Christel P, Poux D, Saillant FG, Cabanis EA (1987) Imagerie par résonnance magnétique (IRM) des lésions de l'aponévrose plantaire. J Radiol 68: 749-753

41. Schepsis AA, Leach RE, Gorzyca J (1991) Plantar fasciitis. Clin Orthop 266: 185-196

42. Scherer PR (1991) Heel spur syndrome. J Am Podiatr Med Assoc 81: 68-72

43. Schon LC, Glennon TP, Baxter DE (1993) Heel pain syndrome: electro-diagnostic support for nerve entrapment. Foot Ankle 14: 129-135

44. Shama SS, Kominsky SJ, Lemont H (1983) Prevalence of non-painful heel spur and its relation to postural foot position. J Am Podiatr Med Assoc 73: 122-123

45. Shikoff MD, Figura MA, Postar SE (1986) A retrospective study of 195 patients with heel pain. J Am Podiatr Med Assoc 76: 71-75

46. Vidigal E, Jacoby RK, Dixon ASJ, Ratliff AH, Kirkup J (1975) The foot in chronic rheumatoid arthritis. Ann Rheum Dis 34: 292-297

47. White DL (1994) Plantar fascial release. J Am Podiatr Assoc, 84: 607-613

48. Wu KK (1990) Foot orthoses, sport shoes and sports medicine. In: Wu KK. Foot Orthoses. William and Wilkins, Baltimore, Hong Kong, London, Sydney, p 353-357

23.

Tendinopathy of the calcaneal tendon

M Bouysset

The calcaneal tendon (Achilles tendon) is the common terminal part of the gastrocnemius and soleus muscles (triceps surae muscle), and is the biggest and strongest tendon of the body; its chief role is plantarflexion. The vascularization of the tendon itself is very poor but the peritenon areas have an important blood supply, a source of inflammatory reaction in chronic overuse conditions [29]. Athletic tendinopathy will be emphasized in this chapter. It appears at different levels of physical activity depending on the athlete concerned and the causes are often numerous.

Pathology

It is commonly considered that the term tendinitis is synonymous with tendinous tears; the inability of the tendon to resist repetitive strain results in tears, sometimes microscopic without palpable modifications in the tendon, or macroscopic with presence of obvious nodules at inspection and/or a palpable rupture of continuity [45]. The lesion classically appears 2 cm to 6 cm proximal to the insertion of the calcaneal tendon, in the zone of relative ischemia subject to the maximal mechanical stresses [2, 46]. Degenerative involvement appears common in the tendons of persons older than 35 and sometimes provokes spontaneous rupture [25].

The degeneration of the tendon, usually of microtraumatic origin, progresses through well-defined stages which depend on the site of the involvement [1, 6, 12, 21, 29, 45, 51]:
• peritendinitis: inflamed tendon sheath, diffuse edema and thickening of the fatty areolar tissue of the sheath, with fat necrosis and connective tissue proliferation [21, 30];
• tendinosis: degenerative changes within the tendon substance itself. Tendon failure occurs when great loads are applied to a normal tendon or when a defective tendon yields under normal loading. Tendinosis includes focal degeneration with possible separation of the tendon fibers, infiltration of granulation tissue and possible calcification [1, 2, 21, 40, 45, 46];
• the pathology of the calcaneal insertion site includes:

- retro-calcaneal bursitis, often difficult to differentiate from achilles tendinitis [18, 45], is often thought to be secondary to compression of the retro-calcaneal bursa between the calcaneal tendon and a prominent superior angle of the calcaneal tuberosity;

- retro-achillean bursitis;

- true insertional lesions of the tendon (enthesitis) appear secondary to degenerative modification at the site of insertion of the tendon fibers into the calcaneum;

- complete tendon rupture, the most serious structural lesion, is sometimes observed without any symptoms preceding the injury [1].

Finally, tendinopathies secondary to inflammatory or metabolic diseases must always be kept in mind.

Predisposing and precipitating factors

Among factors predisposing to tendinous involvement, hyperpronation is commonly cited. It increases internal rotation of the tibia and deviates the tendon medially because its insertion is laterally located due to calcaneal valgus; therefore the stresses on the medial side of the tendon increase [2, 8, 15, 21, 22, 23, 30].

Other predisposing factors must be considered: the cavus foot does not absorb shock well and the stress on the calcaneal tendon increases, especially on the lateral side; forefoot varus, which leads to compensatory hyperpronation also strains the tendon [8]; dynamic muscular imbalance with weakness of the anterior muscles, or on the contrary, stronger posterior muscles, can lead to a calcaneal tendinopathy. Other possible etiologic factors are: stiffness of the musculotendinous system of the calf, limb-length discrepancy, knee joint malalignment, or even lack of elasticity of the tendon.

Some pathologic conditions intensify the stresses on the posterior musculature of the leg: anterior impingement syndrome of the talocrural joint, hallux rigidus [46].

Factors precipitating overuse of the triceps surae muscle must also be sought; they are of extrinsic origin and include [30]:

• Inappropriate training schedules [1, 13]: sudden increase in the duration, intensity or specificity of training; bad techniques, especially inappropriate or no warm-ups or stretching [21, 45]. The type of sport itself plays a part, since sports causing violent or repeated contact with the ground promote calcaneal tendinopathy (running, basketball, volleyball);

• the nature of the surface: ground unsuited to practice of the sport (uneven, too soft, too hard), change of terrain without gradual adaptation. Every cause of imbalance which increases either plantarflexion or dorsiflexion forces at the talocrural joint increases the stresses on the calcaneal tendon and on the posterior muscles of the leg;

• the shoes or equipment may be inappropriate or faulty: inability of the shoe heel to dissipate weight-bearing stresses; a shoe stiffener which does not properly support the hindfoot; too worn or too heavy shoes; shoes with over-rigid soles, which increase the tension in the triceps surae muscle and tendon during heel take-off.

Finally, some classical causes must be eliminated: direct blows on the calf, insufficient fluid intake, hyperuricemia, hypercholesterolemia, xanthomatosis of the calcaneal tendon (see below), recent taking of fluoroquinolones [43, 52].

● Clinical features and supplementary tests [45]

The pain is the main feature and generally develops gradually. Often it appears initially during walking or effort and disappears with warming, only to reappear after sport. This pain may be a slight discomfort at first; then it may increase in intensity and duration and can become permanent and severe with almost total functional disability. The precipitating role of some circumstances must be looked into (walking, going up or down stairs).

The physical examination, always comparing both feet, is made first in the standing position [45]. It looks for pain during contraction of the triceps surae muscle in tests with increasing exertion: standing on tiptoe, walking on tip-toe, jumping on both legs, and then on one. Likewise, pain during passive stretching of the tendon must be searched for (squatting is often restricted and painful). In the prone position, with the feet clear of the end of the examination couch, inspection and palpation confirm possible local inflammatory features (warmth, crepitus, bursitis), and evaluate the pre-achillean area and the tendon itself (particularly around 6 cm proximal to its insertion). Palpation identifies the most tender area, any modifications of tendinous consistence (localized thickening of a tendinosis with a nodule, thinning or even a gap) and their localization [45].

A combined clinical, radiologic and laboratory assessment is made when there is the slightest doubt. It inquires about the presence of the predisposing and precipitating factors already cited, which are incriminated in 60 to 70% of cases and must exclude other more general causes of tendinopathy [23] (see below). Standard lateral X-ray views in weight-bearing searches for insertional calcaneal periostosis and/or intratendinous calcification. Ossification has been observed [41]. Ultrasonography may reveal tendinous nodules and demonstrate possible pre-achillean bursitis or a partial rupture [24]. CT is not useful, and MRI is rarely necessary in the common tendinopathy though it seems to be the best procedure for accurate assessment of the calcaneal tendon. Four types of lesions are identified: type I, inflammatory reaction; type II, degenerative changes; type III, partial rupture; and type IV, complete rupture [50].

Anatomo-clinical types

Among the anatomo-clinical types of calcaneal tendinopathies, overall two main types may be specified:

Peritendinitis

Peritendinitis, is often apparently of microtraumatic origin, with a diffuse thickening of the sheath which impairs the gliding-function of this tissue. Rest, nonsteroidal drugs and physiotherapy are usually efficient at the beginning; the peritendinitis can heal without complications. When overuse persists (when an athlete tries to continue through pain) chronicity of the lesion may develop with scarring of the tendon and its sheath.

Tendinopathy of the tendon itself (tendinosis)

It may occur as a result of traumatism or microtraumatisms in athletes or in some occupations [12, 40]. Palpation reveals one or more tender nodules to be often present in patients with chronic symptoms; there may be a palpable soft tissue defect due to partial rupture, the most common site being 3 to 6 cm proximal to the insertion of the tendon. Secondary complete rupture of the tendon is not rare after tendinosis [6, 12]. Peritendinitis and tendinosis are frequently combined to give the chronic tendinopathy of the athlete [12, 46].

Several other clinical types of tendinopathy may occur [10, 11, 12, 14, 22, 34, 38]: retrocalcaneal bursitis, often with Haglund's deformity; pre-achillean bursitis ("pump bump") with a tender swelling over the insertion of the tendon usually results from irritation due to unsuitable footwear.

Tendinopathies secondary to inflammatory, infectious [47] or metabolic diseases

They sometime appear during athletic or other physical activities which may reveal the systemic disease in some cases [16, 37]. Spondylarthropathy must be thought of when there is nocturnal low back pain in a young man who also has morning lumbar stiffness, or associated arthritis of one or several joints, or psoriatic lesions; in case of doubt, X-ray of the sacro-iliac joints and testing for the HLA B27 antigen are indicated (Chapter 12). Often, inflammatory tendinopathy is bilateral [11]. Other diseases must also be excluded: gout, chondrocalcinosis, hypercholesterolemia, sometimes with tendon xanthoma [26, 31] (fig. 23.1); calcifying tendinitis. Recent treatment with fluoroquinolones must be considered [43, 52]. Rheumatoid arthritis is another possibility [33].

Rupture of the calcaneal tendon

This most serious clinical picture is usually diagnosed by the clinical features [48]. Recreational sports requiring sudden acceleration or jumping play an important part in its incidence (badminton, basketball, tennis) [4, 28]. Long-term corticosteroid treatment favors rupture, particularly in systemic diseases where bilateral rupture appears more frequently [39]. Typically, clinical evaluation of calcaneal tendon rupture includes a history of sudden acute pain at the back of the ankle, often associated with an audible snap or crack, followed by swelling and tenderness around the tendon. Standing on tiptoe is impossible, but other causes of a painful foot and ankle may also have this effect and

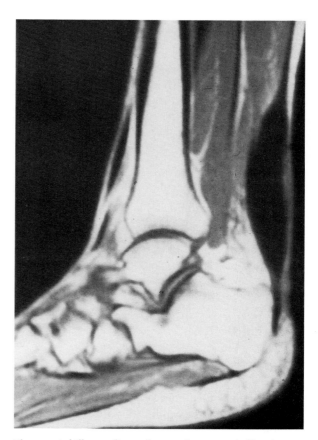

Fig. 23.1. Achilles tendinopathy: xanthomatous infiltration

therefore false-positives may occur. The presence of a palpable or visible gap in the tendon may be observed which is the point of maximal tenderness. Thompson's test is 100% reliable in acute and 80% in chronic ruptures; in spite of this, the diagnosis is reportedly missed in 18 to 25% of cases by the initial examiner [28]. The patient lies prone with both feet clear of the end of the couch; when the calf muscle is gently squeezed, the ankle will move into plantar-flexion if the calcaneal tendon is intact. If the tendon has ruptured, this movement will be absent or very slight; the injured ankle must be compared with the uninjured one. Other clinical tests are described (needle-test and knee-flexion examination) [36, 48]. Radiographic abnormalities may include decrease or disappearance of Kagger's clear pre-achillean triangle, exemplified by an increased opacity around and within the triangle. Often ultrasonography is used to confirm the clinical findings but this procedure is not always reliable if a hematoma is present [5, 24]. MRI is rarely necessary for a typically recent rupture, but effectively demonstrates old lesions and their type and site. These misdiagnosed old ruptures are not rare, when the initial clinical picture has been followed by little pain or functional incapacity.

Differential diagnosis

The differential diagnosis of calcaneal tendinopathy must exclude [4, 30, 45, 49] the os trigonum syndrome; stress fracture of the calcaneus, whose diagnosis is sometimes difficult initially; and Sever's disease (which can be seen in the lateral radiograph). Other causes may be listed: adjacent tendinopathies [30], osteomyelitis of the tibia or calcaneus, adjacent bone or soft tissue tumors. As in 20 to 30% of cases the rupture is diagnosed at a late stage, other lesions must be excluded: severe talocrural strain, calcaneal fracture, subtalar strain or disinsertion of the medial head of the gastrocnemius (digitigrade walking is observed in this last case) [4].

● Treatment

The treatment of calcaneal tendinopathy initially remains conservative [5, 8, 30, 45, 46] and any causal general disease must be treated as well as the tendinopathy itself. It will be all the more efficient if the possible association of several causes is kept in mind (gout, fluoroquinolone treatment, etc.). Reduction of

physical activity must be continued for a variable time, depending on each case. Complete rest may be necessary in the acute painful stage; strapping which decreases ankle dorsiflexion, immobilization with a removable cast [46] or complete plaster immobilization are sometimes useful. Several analgesic measures may be used: nonsteroidal anti-inflammatory drugs, decreasing doses of oral steroids when there is a very severe local inflammatory reaction [46]; cold therapy is the time-honored way of modifying the acute inflammatory response. Intratendinous corticosteroid injections are prohibited and peritendinous injections must be avoided. They mask the pain, and expose the tendon to further injuries [32, 45], even though, in some precise treatment studies, these complications do not appear [42]. Physical therapy is commonly used, chiefly ultrasound; dynamic balancing exercises are prescribed to work on the strengthening and stretching of the various muscles of the lower extremity (particularly the triceps surae and hamstring muscles) [45, 46]. Eccentric rehabilitation exercises may be used [2, 20].

Wearing a soft heel-lift decreases the impact of the heel on the ground. The treatment of predisposing factors prevents recurrences; particularly, the biomechanic control of static disorders by plantar orthoses avoids overstrain of the tendon [5, 18, 46]. Substitute aerobic exercises including cycling and swimming are encouraged. Once the pain and inflammation are stabilized with conservative treatment, analysis of walking and running may be performed to decrease the role of precipitating factors and a program of gradually increased activity helps to avoid recurrences [1, 46]. The conservative treatment of Haglund's syndrome emphasizes the role of proper well-padded shoes (molded achilles pad). Although the majority of patients respond favorably to conservative management, excision of the calcaneal prominence decompresses the affected area and provides relief in refractory cases [45, 46]. As a general rule, Subotnick thinks that surgical correction is needed for chronic paratenon pathology that has not responded to a year of physical therapy or rest; however, some cases of chronic peritendinitis have favorably responded, after up to 2 years, to physical therapy and orthoses which redistribute the weight load [46].

Surgical treatment

There is a place for surgical treatment in the care of calcaneal tendinopathy but the number of relevant cases is very small [45]. Surgery excises the inflamed or scarred tendon sheath and, when necessary, debrides the degenerative tendon. If a partial rupture is seen, excision of the frayed ends is carried out. Reinforcement of the tendon may be performed.

Tendinosis responds less well to conservative treatment and the surgery more frequently needed in this lesion depends on the degree of tendon involvement and the severity of the symptoms.

Treatment of tendon rupture

The non-surgical treatment of acute tendon rupture consists of a plaster cast in full equinus without weight-bearing for one month, then in half equinus with weight-bearing for the second month, finally, with the foot dorsiflexed to the neutral position for the third month. This, or slightly different programs of care, leads to lengthening of the tendon and therefore a decrease of the strength of the triceps surae muscle. The main disadvantage of this method is the possibility of recurrence, which can certainly be decreased by longer cast immobilization (ten weeks), and the wearing of a heel lift with a strict hygiene of life during the months which follow the removal of the cast [44]. This treatment of the recent rupture is an acceptable solution for patients who do not want surgical treatment or for patients who present contraindications [4, 5, 9, 12, 19, 27, 28, 35, 44].

Surgical treatment of the rupture allows a quicker recovery of sporting activities. Recurrent ruptures are exceptional but local complications (infection, necrosis of the skin or of the tendon), are more frequent. It is suitable with precise indications: age (a young high-level athlete); the site of rupture (distal rupture and bony disinsertion are indications for surgery); the observation of a tendon gap on palpation, either in old ruptures, or after full equinus immobilization during conservative treatment [4, 48].

Percutaneous methods of repair under local anesthesia have been described [7, 17]. The rate of recurrence is greater than in classical surgery for some authors [3].

● Conclusion

Calcaneal tendinopathy is a matter for conservative treatment in the majority of cases. As important as the treatment of the tendinopathy itself is that of its causes, which are either mechanical, or secondary to a systemic disease.

References

1. Allenmark C (1992) Partial Achilles tendon tears. Clin Sports Med 11: 759-769
2. Ambrosia (D') RD, Drez D Jr (1989) Prevention and treatment of runnning injuries, 2nd edn. Slack, New Jersey
3. Aracil J, Pina A, Lozano JA, Torro V, Escriba I (1992) Percutaneous suture of Achilles tendon ruptures. Foot Ankle 13: 350-351
4. Benazet JP, Saillant G, Lazennec JY, Roy-Camille R (1991) Ruptures récentes et anciennes du tendon d'Achille. Rhumatologie pratique 64:2-5
5. Blake R.L, DPM, MS, Ferguson H.J (1991) Achilles tendon rupture. A protocol for conservative management. J Am Podiatr Med Assoc 81: 486-489
6. Bonnel F, Baldet P, Claustre J, Fauré P (1993) Tendinopathies mécaniques de surcharge au pied et à la cheville. Med Chir Pied 9: 191-201
7. Bradley JP, Tibone J (1990) Percutaneous and open surgical repairs of Achilles Tendon Ruptures: a comparative study. Am J Sports Med 18: 188-195
8. Brody M (1981) La pathologie du jogging. Clinical symposia. Ciba
9. Campbell P, Lawton JO (1993) Spontaneous rupture of the achilles tendon: pathology and management. Br J Hosp Med 50: 321-325
10. Chauveaux D, Liet P (1990) Diagnostic de la maladie de Haglund: un nouvel angle radiologique. Med Chir Pied 6: 175-178
11. Claustre J (1984) Les syndromes de surmenage du pied du sportif. In: Claustre J, Bénézis C, Simon L (eds) Le pied en pratique sportive. Masson, Paris, pp 105-116
12. Claustre J, Bonnel F, Simon L (1985) Les tendinopathies de la jonction achilléo-calcanéenne: démembrement nosologique. Med Chir Pied 2: 93-98
13. Clement DB, Taunton JE, Smart GW (1984) Achilles tendinitis and peritendinitis etiology and treatment. Am J Sports Med 12: 179-184
14. Delagoutte JP, Peltre G, Becker JM (1987) La maladie de Haglund. Med Chir Pied 3: 21-23
15. Donatelli R (1990) The biomechanics of the Foot and Ankle. F.A Davis Company, Philadelphia, pp 153-170
16. Eulry F, Verrière D, Dellestable F, Haguenauer D, Crozes Ph, Lechevalier D, Magnin J (1993) Tendinopathie d'Achille inaugurant un syndrome de Fiessinger-Leroy-Reiter. Med Chir Pied 4: 224-226
17. Fitzgibbons RE, Hefferon J, Hill J (1993) Percutaneous achilles tendon repair. Am J Sports Med 21: 724-727
18. Frey C, Rosenberg Z, Shereff MJ, Kim H (1992) The retrocalcaneal bursea: anatomy and bursography. Foot Ankle 13: 203-207
19. Fruensgaard S, Helmig P, Riis, Stovring JO (1992) Conservative treatment for acute rupture of the Achilles tendon. Int Orthop 16: 33-35
20. Fyfe I, Stanish WD (1992) The use of eccentric training and stretching in the treatment and prevention of tendon injuries. Clin Sports Med 11: 601-624

21. Galloway M.T, Jokl P, Dayton OW (1992) Achilles tendon overuse injuries. Clin Sports Med 11: 771-782

22. Hintermann B, Holzach P (1992) Die Bursitis sub-achillea - eine biomechanische Analyse und klinische Studie. Z Orthop 130: 114-119

23. Järvinen M (1992) Epidemiology of tendon injuries in sports. Clin Sports Med 11: 493-50

24. Kälebo P, Allenmark C, Peterson L, Swärd L (1992) Diagnostic value of ultrasonography in partial ruptures of the Achilles tendon. Am J Sports Med 20: 378-381

25. Kannus P, Jozsa L (1991) Histopathological changes predecing spontaneous rupture of a tendon. A controlled study of 891 patients. J Bone Joint Surg 73: 1507-1525

26. Kenan S, Abdelwahab IF, Klein M.J, Aaron A (1992) Case report 754. Skeletal Radiol 21: 471-473

27. Krüger-Franke M, Scherzer S (1993) Langzeitergeb-nisse operativ behandelter Achillesshnenrupturen. Unfallchirurgie 96: 524-528

28. Landvater SJ, Renström P (1992) Complete Achilles tendon ruptures. Clin Sports Med 11: 741-758

29. Leadbetter WB (1992) Cell-matrix response in tendon injury. Clin Sports Med 11: 533-578

30. Lemm M, Blake RL, Colson JP, DPM, Ferguson H (1992) Achilles peritendinitis. A literature review with case report. J Am Podiatr Med Assoc 82: 482-490

31. Liem MSL, Gevers Leuven JA, Bloem J.L, Schipper J (1992) Magnetic resonance imaging of Achilles tendon xanthomas in familial hypercholesterolemia. Skeletal Radiol 21: 453-457

32. Mahler F, Fritschy D (1992) Partial and complete ruptures of the Achilles tendon and local corticos-teroid injections. Br J Sports Med 26: 7-14

33. Matsumoto K, Hukusa S, Nishioka J, Asajima S (1992) Rupture of the Achilles Tendon in Rheumatoid Arthritis with histologic evidence of Enthesitis. Clin Orthop 280: 235-240

34. Maynou C, Delobelle JM, Urvoy Ph, Mestdagh H (1993) Traitement des talalgies postérieures d'origine morphostatique par ostéotomie de Zadek. Med Chir Pied 9: 149-156

35. Nistor L (1981) Surgical and non-surgical treatment of Achilles tendon rupture. A prospective randomized study. J Bone Joint Surg 63A: 394-399

36. O'Brien T (1984) The needle test for complete rupture of the Achilles tendon. J Bone Joint Surg 66A: 1099-1101

37. Olivieri I, Cantini F, Napoli V, Braccini G, Padula A, Pasero G (1993) Seronegative spondylarthropathy without spine involvement in Behcet's Syndrome. Clin Rheumatol 12: 396-400

38. Pavlov H, Heneghan MA, Hersh A, Goldman AB, Vigorita V (1982) The Haglund syndrome: initial and differential diagnosis. Diagn Radiol 144: 83-88

39. Price AE, Evanski PM, Waugh TR (1986) Bilateral simultaneous achilles tendon ruptures, a case report and review of the literature. Clin Orthop 213: 249-250

40. Puddu G, Ippolito E, Postacchini F (1976) A classifica-tion of Achilles tendon disease. Am J Sports Med 4: 145-150

41. Raynor KJ, Mc Donald RJ, Edelman RD, Parkinson DE (1986) Ossification of the Achilles tendon. J Am Podiatr Assoc 76: 688-690

42. Read MTF, Motto SG (1992) Tendon Achillis pain: steroid and outcome. Br J Sports Med 26: 15-21

43. Ribard P, Audisio F, Kahn MF, De Bandt M, Jorgensen C, Hayem G, Meyer O, Palazzo E (1992) Seven Achilles tendinitis including 3 complicated by rupture during fluoroquinolone therapy. J Rheumatol 19: 1479-1481

44. Rodineau J, Sabourin F, Middleton P (1984) Le traite-ment orthopédique des ruptures du tendon d'Achille. In: Claustre J, Simon L (eds) Le pied en pratique spor-tive. Masson, Paris, pp 78-80

45. Saillant G, Rodineau J, Thoreux P, Roy-Camille R (1991) La tendinite d'Achille. La revue du praticien 18: 1644-1649

46. Subotnick S, Sisney P, (1986) Treatment of Achilles Tendinopathy in the Athlete. J Am Podiatr Med Assoc 76: 552-557

47. Thomas E, Leroux JL, Senegas A, Tinseau E, Bonnel F, Baldet P, Blotman F (1993) Les ténosynovites tubercu-leuses du pied. Med Chir Pied 9: 227-230

48. Tomassi, FJ (1992) Current diagnostic and radio-graphic assessment of tendon Achillis Rupture. J Am Podiatr Med Assoc 82: 375-379

49. Von Lohrer H (1991) Seltene ursachen und differen-tialdiagnosen der achillodynie. Sportverletz Sportschaden 5: 182-185

50. Weinstabl R, Stiskal M, Neuhold A, Aamlid B, Hertz H (1991) Classifying calcaneal tendon injury accor-ding to MRI findings. J Bone Joint Surg 73B: 683-685

51. Williams JGP (1986) Achilles tendon lesions in sport. Sports Med 3: 114

52. Zabraniecki L, Bouyssou ML, Brosset A, Lesort A, Arnaud M, Bonnet C, Bertin P, Treves R (1993) Tendinopathies aux fluoroquinolones: étude de 5 cas. Revue du Rhumatisme 752

Additional references

Berg EE (1992) Percutaneous Achilles Tendon Lengthening Complicated by Inadvertent Tenotomy. J Pediatr Orthop 12: 341-343

Cetti R, Christensen SE, Ejsted R, Jensen NM, Jorgensen U (1993) Operative versus nonoperative treatment of Achilles tendon rupture. Am J Sports Med 21: 791-799

Gaillard F, Calmet G, Echard JP, Schernberg F (1995) Intérêt de l'analyse du triangle de Kajer. Journées Provinciales de la Société Française de Médecine et Chirurgie du pied. 12 et 13 mai, Grenoble

Lohrer VH (1991) Seltene Ursachen und Differential-diag-nosen der Achillodynie. Sportverletz Sportschaden 5: 182-185

Railhac JJ, Holley P, Barbut JP, Assoun J, Aziza R, Trochard J Imagerie du Tendon d'Achille. In: Chevrot A, Kahn MF, Morvan G (eds) Imagerie des parties molles de l'appareil locomoteur. Sauramps médical, Montpellier, pp 169-174

Thermann H, Hoffmann R, Zwipp H, Tscherne H (1992) The use of ultrasonography in the foot and Ankle. Foot Ankle 13: 386-390

24.

Ankle tendon pathology
(excluding calcaneal tendon disorders)

M Bonnin

Ankle tendon disorders were for a long time obscure entities, largely restricted to disorders of the calcaneal tendon. Progress in imaging techniques, in particular the advent of magnetic resonance imaging, has led to improved classification of ankle pain and improved analysis of tendon lesions. Growing popular enthusiasm for the practice of sports, in particular for running, has increased the incidence of tendon disorders and revealed lesions which had previously remained asymptomatic.

● Tibialis posterior tendon pathology

Lesions of the tendon of the tibialis posterior muscle are common but are sometimes overlooked. Over the last ten years, considerable advances have been made in their diagnosis, imaging and treatment, but nevertheless their true incidence is still poorly known.

The tendon of the tibialis posterior muscle may be damaged in three quite different contexts:
• in rheumatoid arthritis, where tenosynovitis of the tendon is chronologically one of the earliest lesions of the hindfoot;
• in the athlete, rupture due to trauma in a healthy tendon is rare: 3 in 1000 tendon ruptures [1, 33]. Traumatic displacement of the tendon anterior to the medial malleolus may also be observed [30, 48];
• the most frequent pathology is a gradual tear of degenerative origin. This lesion appears preferentially in women in their fifties, in a context of excess weight, diabetes and arterial hypertension [22].

Anatomy

The tibialis posterior muscle originates from the posterior aspect of the interosseous membrane and the adjacent bony surfaces of the tibia and fibula. The muscle fibers converge onto the tendon in the distal third of the leg. The tendon runs along the posterior aspect of the medial malleolus, as the most anterior element in the tarsal tunnel. It is related anteriorly to the medial malleolus, laterally to the deltoid ligament, medially to the flexor retinaculum and posteriorly to the flexor digitorum longus and then the posterior tibial neurovascular pedicle. It curves under the tip of the medial malleolus and ends in multiple insertions.

Its main insertion is on the navicular tuberosity and the naviculocuneiform joint capsule. Plantar expansions reach the inferior aspect of the second and third cuneiform bones, the base of the second, third and fourth metatarsals and the cuboid bone. A posterior expansion reaches the sustentaculum tali [19, 57]. Only the principal ending of the tendon is mobile. The tendon expansions are fixed and their role seems to be restricted to static stabilization [43]. The tendon is encased in a synovial sheath as it runs below and behind the malleolus and no true mesotendon has been demonstrated in this zone.

The vascular supply of the tibialis posterior tendon comes from three sources [17] (fig. 24.1):
• muscular arteries arising from the tibialis posterior artery supply the musculotendinous junction;
• further blood supply to the musculotendinous junction comes from the proximal mesotendon and adjacent tissues;

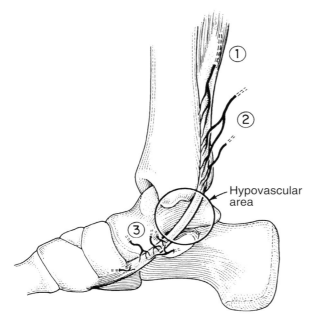

Hypovascular area

Fig. 24.1. The arterial supply of the tibialis posterior tendon: *1* muscular origin, *2* vessels from the vincula, *3* periosteal origin. The extent of the hypovascular area is 14 mm [17]

• the junction of tendon and bone receives its blood supply from the periosteum. The vessels run lengthwise along the surface of the tendon.

There is a hypovascular zone in the middle part of the tendon due to the absence of anastomoses between the ascending and descending arterioles. This zone starts 40 mm from the navicular insertion (10 to 15 mm from the tip of the medial malleolus) and extends proximally for 14 mm.

Biomechanics

The tibialis posterior muscle is the main dynamic stabilizer of the hindfoot against valgus motion. It is a powerful supinator, leading to varus of the hindfoot and adduction of the midfoot. The tendon expansions act as passive stabilizers of the midfoot.

The motion of the hindfoot and the role of the tendon during the gait cycle have been the subject of numerous studies [23, 36, 68]. The stance phase extends from 0% (heel-strike) to 62% (toe-off) of the gait cycle:
• from 0 to 15%: the heel strikes the ground in slight varus and then, under the effect of body weight, the hindfoot shifts to valgus. This change in position takes place in the subtalar joint and increases

throughout this phase. It is a passive phenomenon. The tibialis posterior tendon is inactive;
• from 15 to 40%: the tibialis posterior tendon (as well as the triceps surae, flexor digitorum and intrinsic muscles of the foot) becomes active and the hindfoot progressively assumes a varus position to reach a neutral position at 30% of the cycle. The axis then becomes varus;
• from 40 to 62%: the degree of varus of the hindfoot progressively increases and the heel leaves the ground. The tibialis posterior tendon is active; it continues to increase the degree of varus and participates in plantarflexion of the ankle. It rapidly becomes inactive again after toe-off (62%). The overall range from varus to valgus during the stance phase is 6° for a foot with a normal axis [68].

Ruptures of the tibialis posterior tendon

Pathogenesis

Tenosynovitis of the tibialis posterior muscle in rheumatoid arthritis will be dealt with separately.

The most frequent lesions are of degenerative origin. Several etiologies have been proposed:
• mechanical attrition of the tendon where it curves round the medial malleolus, which acts like a pulley. This wear is increased by aging and obesity and is the most classic hypothesis [22, 25, 26]. The role of mechanical overuse to which the tendon may be subjected by a pre-existing flat foot is debatable [28]. Mann, however, observed that if rupture were due to purely mechanical causes, it should occur exclusively at the level of the medial malleolar pulley, whereas in fact rupture is generally more distal [26];
• the role of pre-existing stenosing tenosynovitis which progressively damages the tendon has been suggested [31, 67];
• the hypothesis of rupture due to localized hypovascularity has recently been defended [17]. Several arguments favor this etiology: ruptures are generally located in the avascular zone and there is a high incidence of diabetes and arterial hypertension in patients with tendon rupture [22]. The tendinopathy worsens; the tendon becomes elongated and then ruptures completely. The loss of this stabilizer gradually leads to stretching of the calcaneonavicular ligament, then the foot tilts into planovalgus.

The resulting deformity consists of three components: in the frontal plane, the calcaneus assumes a valgus position; in the sagittal plane, the talus becomes vertical; in the horizontal plane, the forefoot is abducted.

From a clinical and anatomic point of view, three stages have been described by Johnson and Jahss [6, 26, 54]:
• stage I: partial rupture of the tendon with multiple fissural lesions in elective areas and synovitis; the tendon is often thickened. There is no hindfoot deformity;
• stage II: fraying and elongation of the tendon, which is very adherent to adjacent tissues. There is a periosteal reaction with spur formation on the posterior aspect of the medial malleolus. The talonavicular ligaments become stretched. The hindfoot assumes a valgus attitude but the deformity is supple and reducible;
• stage III: complete tendon rupture, fixed deformity of the hindfoot which may extend to subtalar dislocation. The condition progresses to subtalar arthrosis.

Clinical features

These vary according to the clinical stage (table 24.1, fig. 24.2). Examination shows loss of power of the tibialis posterior muscle and characteristic ankle deformity.

Two methods are used to test for loss of power:
• **resisted supination:** with the patient lying supine, the examiner immobilizes the forefoot with one hand and asks the patient to actively invert the foot. This test assesses the strength of the tibialis posterior by comparison with the other foot. The tendon is palpated with the other hand to look for a painful area. Sometimes, the outline of the tendon can no longer be perceived. Assessment can be misleading because the movement of inversion can be aided by the tibialis anterior or flexor digitorum muscles. In order to neutralize their effect, some authors suggest that the test should be done with the foot in a neutral position with maximum eversion [25, 26, 55]. Others prefer to carry out the test in maximum equinus [19]. Whatever technique is used, this test is difficult to interpret. Comparison with the other foot and palpation of the tendon are essential;
• **standing on tiptoe:** in this position, tension of the tendon of the tibialis posterior muscle locks the hindfoot in varus. If the tendon is ruptured, the calcaneus shifts out of varus and the subject is unable to remain on tiptoe on one foot. During this maneuver the patient's knees must remain fully extended as simple knee flexion makes it easier to raise the heel from the ground. However, this test is positive only in long-standing, rigid forms of rupture of the tendon.

Ankle deformity is the main element of diagnosis. Rupture of the tendon of the posterior tibial muscle is in fact the first cause that should be considered in an acquired asymmetric planovalgus foot in adults in their fifties:
• hindfoot valgus is assessed by viewing the patient from behind when standing still and while walking;
• forefoot abduction can be assessed by viewing the patient from in front while walking, or from behind when the patient is standing still. This is Johnson's "too many toes" sign: in a patient standing symmetrically and viewed from behind, more toes can be seen outside the leg on the affected side than on the

Table 24.1. Clinical and anatomic classification of tibialis posterior tendon dysfunction (from Johnson [25] and Jahss [6, 49])

Stage	Anatomy	Biomechanics	Period after onset of symptoms	Clinical findings
I	Peritendinitis Synovial proliferation Partial tear	No deformity	6-18 months	Medial pain Loss of power No deformity
II	Elongation Marked degeneration Retromalleolar osteophyte	Valgus hindfoot Supple deformity	18-30 months	Medial pain Valgus deformity Reducible deformity Flattening of the medial arch
III	Marked elongation or complete rupture Subtalar arthritis	Forefoot abduction Valgus hindfoot Rigid deformity Lateral impingement	> 30 months	Lateral pain Moderate medial pain Marked rigid deformity

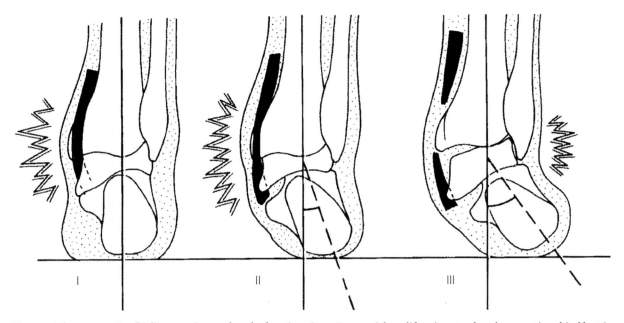

Fig. 24.2. The 3 stages in tibialis posterior tendon dysfunction. Stage I: synovial proliferation, tendon degeneration, hindfoot in normal alignment. Stage II: atrophic and elongated tendon, hindfoot in reducible valgus deformity. Stage III: elongated or ruptured tendon, hindfoot in nonreducible valgus deformity

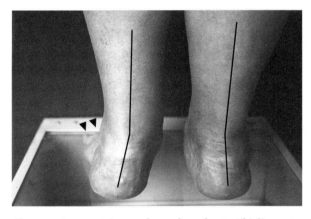

Fig. 24.3. Asymmetric pes planovalgus due to tibialis posterior tendon dysfunction; the "too many toes" sign

opposite side (fig. 24.3) because of depression of the medial arch and the valgus attitude of the foot.

Examination evaluates the reducibility of the deformity and residual supination of the forefoot when the hindfoot is maintained in neutral position.

On palpation, tenderness is located exclusively in the medial sub- and retromalleolar region in the early stages. Once a certain degree of subluxation of the subtalar joint has been exceeded, tenderness appears on palpation of the lateral orifice of the

sinus tarsi and the fibular tendons. This lateral pain is related to impingement between the calcaneus and the lateral malleolus.

Plain radiographs make it possible to assess the degree of planovalgus deformity and to look for subtalar arthrosis.

Magnetic resonance imaging (MRI) reveals the tendon lesion itself. Three stages have been described as seen on MRI [6, 54], corresponding to the anatomic stages: Stage I, tendon thickening with longitudinal splitting; Stage II, hourglass thinning of the tendon at the level of the lesion; Stage III: complete rupture with interposition of fibrous tissue. MRI is more reliable than surgical exploration for the analysis of intratendinous lesions [6].

The presence of an accessory navicular bone may cause symptoms similar to those of disorders of the tibialis posterior tendon. It is a cartilaginous nucleus adjacent to the navicular bone, which after ossification may remain at some distance from that bone (type I), become attached to it by synchondrosis (type II), or become totally fused (type III) [59]. A type II accessory bone may become symptomatic if there is a fracture of the bony bridge which links it with the navicular bone. The patient complains of localized pain at the insertion of the tendon and the foot may progress to pes planus.

Diagnosis is based essentially on clinical examination and plain radiographs. CT scan may show fracture of the bony bridge (fig. 24.4).

Treatment

Therapeutic management of disorders of the tendon depends on the degree of functional disability and the clinical stage. If discomfort is minimal, the first line of treatment is conservative, whatever the pathologic stage:

• **Stage I:** treatment is primarily conservative and is based on the following measures:

- use of a heel wedge and supinator insoles with a medial arch support in order to reduce strain on the tendon;

- reduced activity, in particular in the athlete;

- local physical therapy to reduce pain and inflammation;

- exercises to strengthen the flexor digitorum longus and flexor hallucis longus muscles;

- corticosteroid injections within the tendon sheath have been proposed but these weaken the tendon and make secondary rupture more likely.

In acute tendinitis, it may be necessary to protect the tendon with a splint or even a plaster cast for a few weeks.

If conservative treatment is a failure after six months, a surgical procedure may be proposed. This consists of exploration of the tendon, synovectomy and repair or excision of the damaged areas.

• **Stages II and III:** at this stage of deformity it is too late for conservative treatment, which can only be considered as long as discomfort is minimal. Two surgical techniques can be used:

- tendon transfer using the tendon of the flexor digitorum longus muscle (FDL). This may consist of either simple tenodesis [6, 24], bony reinsertion of the FDL in the navicular bone [35], or suture of the FDL to the distal stump of the posterior tibial tendon [25, 26, 55]. Some authors carry out calcaneal osteotomy at the same time for better correction of the valgus [19];

- subtalar arthrodesis with the aim of replacing the calcaneus in a neutral position under the talus.

In advanced cases, after the axis of the hindfoot has been corrected, fixed supination of the forefoot may be revealed and associated mediotarsal arthrodesis must also be carried out. The choice of surgical technique is difficult. Tendon transfer can be used if the deformity is moderate, supple and easily reduced [19, 24, 25, 26, 35].

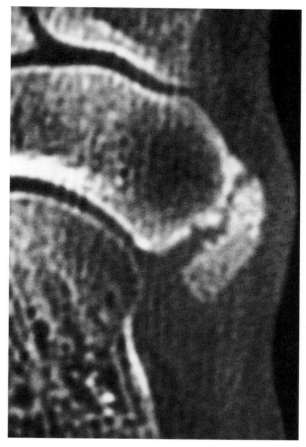

Fig. 24.4. 32-year-old patient: pain in an accessory navicular bone after eversion trauma

For Conti and Jahss [6], conservative procedures only give good results if there are no serious intra-tendinous lesions and should be restricted to lesions which are stage I on MRI.

Arthrodesis is unavoidable in certain circumstances: marked deformity (more than 10° of valgus) or deformity which cannot be completely corrected, clinical signs of impingement between the calcaneus and the lateral malleolus, or the presence of subtalar arthrosis [19]. The choice between isolated subtalar arthrodesis or combined subtalar and mediotarsal arthrodesis depends on whether or not there is residual supination of the forefoot.

If there is a painful accessory navicular bone, and when discomfort persists in spite of supinator insoles, surgical excision of the accessory bony fragment with reinsertion of the tibialis posterior tendon (Kidner's operation) is mandatory [59].

Acute rupture of the tendon in an athlete whose tendon is presumably healthy, requires emergency surgical repair by end-to-end suture.

Dislocation of the tibialis posterior tendon

This is a rare pathologic condition occurring in the young subject (10 to 50 years) as a sequel to ankle injury. The mechanism is not clearly explained in the literature [30, 48]. It is generally diagnosed late, an average of nine months after the initial injury [48].

The diagnosis of dislocation of the tendon must be considered if medial ankle pain persists several months after injury. Sometimes the patient complains of a jolting sensation. Diagnosis is primarily based on clinical examination and is easy if the dislocation can be reproduced by a movement of resisted inversion of the foot, or if the tendon can be palpated in front of the medial malleolus. Sometimes, diagnosis is difficult if the whole region is swollen and no tendon can be felt.

Plain radiographs are generally normal. An anteroposterior view in slight external rotation may show a bony fragment on the edge of the medial malleolus, indicating avulsion of the flexor retinaculum [30].

CT scan and above all MRI can demonstrate the tendon in an abnormal position or an erosion of the medial malleolus [48].

Treatment in the acute stage is debatable. The foot can be simply immobilized in a plaster cast but some authors, observing systematic recurrence after immobilization, recommend immediate surgical treatment [48]. At a late stage, surgery is the only possibility. The procedure consists of reducing the tendon into anatomic position and attaching the flexor retinaculum. Sometimes, the gutter must be deepened and a new retinaculum must be created using the periosteum [30] or the deltoid ligament.

Fibular tendon pathology

This was long limited to tendon dislocation after injury, but the field has recently been enlarged to include other pictures, notably subluxation and fissural lesions.

Anatomy

The fibularis brevis and longus muscles each end in a tendon which runs within a synovial sheath on the posterior aspect of the lateral malleolus in a fibro-osseous tunnel [53, 57].

• The fibro-osseous tunnel is formed by the posterior aspect of the lateral malleolus and by the superior fibular tendon retinaculum. The posterior aspect of the lateral malleolus forms a true groove in 82% of cases, it is flat in 11% and convex in 7% [57].When this groove is present, it is on average 7 mm deep. The lateral edge of this posterior surface sometimes forms a bony or cartilaginous ridge which helps to stabilize the tendons. This ridge is present in 70% of cases and absent in 30% [14].

The superior fibular retinaculum is attached to the posterolateral ridge of the lateral malleolus and divides into two bands; one inserts into the sheath of the calcaneal tendon, the other into the posterior part of the lateral surface of the calcaneus. The latter band runs parallel to the calcaneofibular ligament [18]. Because of its direction, this ligament limits varus motion of the ankle. It is the main stabilizer of the fibular tendons in their sheath.

• The fibularis brevis muscle (FB) has a thick, fleshy belly and descends further distally. The tendon generally emerges at the level of the tibiotalar joint space [7]. It runs anteriorly under the tip of the lateral malleolus, passes above the fibular trochlea of the calcaneus and reaches the styloid process of the fifth metatarsal, into which it inserts.

• The tendon of the fibularis longus muscle (FL) issues from the muscle belly in the distal third of the leg. It runs on the posterior aspect of the fibularis brevis behind the lateral malleolus. At the tip of the lateral malleolus, it curves and runs downwards and forwards. It passes beneath the fibular trochlea of the calcaneus and the inferior fibular retinaculum in a second fibro-osseous tunnel. It then curves again and runs inward and distally. It changes direction for the third time at the cuboid bone, curving inwards on the anterior aspect of the cuboid tuberosity to insert into the first metatarsal base and sometimes into the first cuneiform bone. At the turning point, it courses in a rigid fibro-osseous tunnel. A sesamoid bone or fibrocartilage, the fibular bone (os peroneum), is found within the tendon in 75% to 95% of cases [45, 52].

• Anatomic variations: three supernumerary muscles may run with the PB and the PL [8, 34, 57, 63, 65]:

   - The fibularis quartus muscle, described in 1816 [47], is found in 21% of cases [63]. It generally arises from the proximal part of the PB with an insertion on a hypertrophic fibular trochlea. It may also arise from the PL and rejoin the tendons of the PL or PB.

   - The fibularis digiti quinti muscle is a more distal anomaly. This accessory muscle is present in

34% of cases [34]. It is a tendon expansion arising from the PB just before its insertion to reach the extensor of the fifth toe or the base of its proximal phalanx, sometimes the fifth metatarsal.

- The fibularis tertius muscle does not belong to the posterolateral region of the ankle. It runs outside the extensor digitorum muscle and inserts into the fifth metatarsal base. It is present in 91.5% of cases [34].

• The fibular synovial sheath starts 2.5 to 3.5 cm above the lateral malleolus and ends 2 cm from its insertion in the case of the PB and at the cuboid for the PL [57]. The fibular (peroneal) synovial sheath never communicates with the talocrural articulation [4].

Split lesions of the fibularis brevis tendon

These are longitudinal fissures of the tendon which occur in its retromalleolar part. The lesion starts at the tip of the lateral malleolus and may extend for 5 cm. The lateral band of the PB may be luxated or subluxated outside the lateral ridge of the malleolus [56, 61]. Sobel [62] described four grades: grade I: splayed-out tendon, grade II: partial thickness fissure; grade III: full-thickness fissure less than 2 cm long; grade IV: full-thickness fissure more than 2 cm long (figs. 24.5b, c).

Splits of the tendon of the fibularis (peroneus) brevis generally occur after an injury in equinovarus and are sometimes associated with chronic ankle laxity [4]. An injury in dorsiflexion may sometimes be incriminated [32].

Two possible mechanisms are postulated: repeated compression of the FB against the lateral malleolus by the FL, or subluxation of the FB leading to tendon tear at the posterolateral ridge of the lateral malleolus. These two mechanisms can be associated.

For some authors, compression by the FL is the main factor [3, 44]. For others, the initial factor is lateral subluxation of the FB: in addition to the classic ligamentous lesion, an injury in inversion can damage the fibular retinaculum, allowing subluxation of the FB [18, 62]. If a fibularis quartus is also present within the tendon sheath, this increases the risk of a fissure. In a cadaver study, Sobel observed 18% of FB lesions when there was an accessory fibular muscle [63]. Such lesions are more likely if the hindfoot is varus.

Clinically, patients complain of lateral retromalleolar pain, sometimes radiating onto the lateral aspect of the leg, associated with a sensation of the ankle giving way or true ankle instability. Snapping or a lateral jolting sensation may sometimes be perceived by the patient. The history generally reveals a previous "sprain", and sometimes repeated sprains. On palpation, tenderness is precisely localized behind the lateral malleolus. The painful area becomes more evident in resisted eversion of the foot. A jolting sensation or a feeling of dislocation may be perceived by the examiner. Usually the strength of the foot in eversion is not reduced. Ankle laxity should be sought. Plain radiographs are normal.

The key investigation is MRI [60]. The axial plane is the most useful. It may reveal only splaying of the FB at the posterior aspect of the lateral malleolus, sometimes a true fissure and subluxation of a lateral band of the FB. Effusion in the tendon sheath or an accessory muscle may be observed (fig. 24.5a).

However, the MR image should be interpreted with caution and in the light of clinical examination, as a certain number of fissural lesions visible on MRI are totally asymptomatic.

The first line of treatment should always be conservative, combining systemic and topical anti-inflammatory agents, physical therapy and sometimes immobilization in a plaster cast. If functional signs persist and if lesions are visible on MRI, surgical treatment is indicated, associating several procedures:

• repair of the tendon of the fibularis brevis with excision of necrotic areas, suture of the tear and tubulization of the splayed tendon. Sometimes, simple excision of a band of the tendon or a large nodule should be carried out. If there is no remaining healthy tissue, the damaged area is resected and the remaining segments of the FB are fixed to the FL by tenodesis;

• resection of an accessory muscle;

• reinsertion of the fibular retinaculum;

• ligamentoplasty in the case of associated talocrural and/or subtalar laxity.

Pathology of the fibularis longus tendon

These disorders are rarer and more distally located, generally between the tip of the lateral malleolus and the cuboid tuberosity, where the FL changes direction. Several factors make the tendon vulnerable in this area:

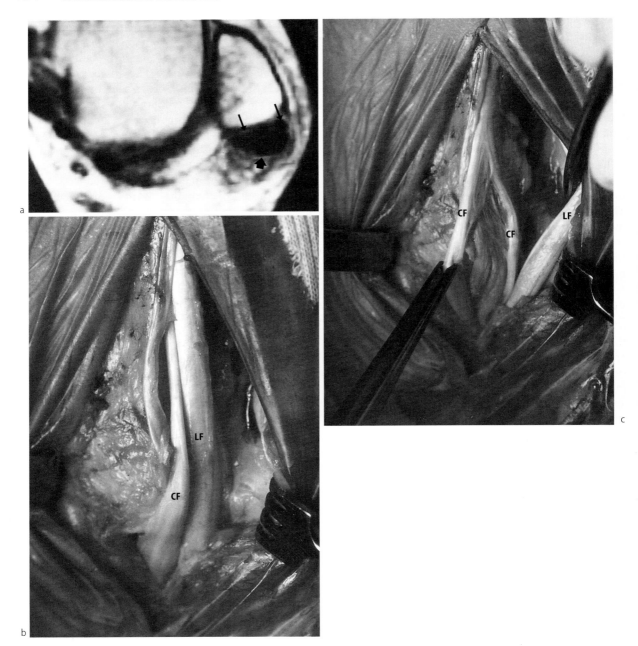

Fig. 24.5. 51-year-old woman: posterolateral pain at the left ankle.

a MRI - axial plane - fissure of peroneus brevis. The tendon is separated into two parts (*small arrow*). The peroneus longus is intact just behind (*large arrow*).

b Operative view: the FB is trapped between the lateral malleolus and the FL tendon. The lateral portion of the FB tendon is subluxated.

c After retraction of the FL, fissured FB is visible. CF: fibularis brevis. LF: fibularis longus

• friction against the fibular trochlea of the calcaneus, which may be hypertrophic and cause impingement [50];
• the FL courses in a narrow tunnel on the lateral aspect of the calcaneus;
• an accessory fibular bone or os peroneum within the tendon, where it curves round the cuboid bone, may be fractured.

Here again, a varus hindfoot is a predisposing factor for such injury.

Sobel recently regrouped these pathologic conditions under the name of "painful os peroneum syndrome" [64]. Anatomically, there may be tendon laceration which can proceed to rupture [66] or fracture of the accessory fibular bone. Inversion injury is usually the cause of these symptoms.

Clinically, the patient complains of pain on the lateral aspect of the ankle between the lateral malleolus and the cuboid. On examination, palpation of the FL and inversion of the foot produce pain. Resisted plantarflexion of the first ray may produce pain, as may resisted eversion.

Imaging may reveal a fracture of the accessory fibular bone in oblique views [49] and a hypertrophic fibular trochlea may be seen in CT scan.

Treatment is primarily conservative: anti-inflammatory agents, physical therapy, discontinuation of sports activities, pronation insoles if the calcaneus is in varus.

Failure of conservative treatment leads to surgical treatment. This can consist of tendon repair, resection of the fibular trochlea and removal of an os peroneum. In some cases, the damaged area must be resected, with tenodesis between the stumps of the FL and the FB [49, 50, 64].

Extrinsic pain in the fibular tendons

Pain in the sheath of the fibular tendons may occur in the absence of anatomic tendon lesions. It may be due to simple adhesive post-traumatic synovitis [8, 42] which generally resolves with medical treatment. Pain may be linked to the presence of an accessory muscle and in this case the cure is surgical excision.

Dislocation of the fibular tendons

Displacement of the fibular tendons to the lateral aspect of the lateral malleolus is rare. It was described for the first time in 1803 by Monteggia [40]

and is generally caused by a sports injury, in particular while skiing (71% of cases) [15]. Such dislocation represents 0.5% of ski injuries [15] but this incidence is decreasing since the use of higher ski boots [45].

Dislocation occurring in the neonatal period [29] and voluntary dislocation [16] have been described.

The mechanism most often incriminated is forced dorsiflexion with violent contraction of the fibular muscles [2, 13, 15, 69]. Inversion or eversion in slight plantarflexion may be incriminated when they are associated with violent contraction [37].

During skiing, dislocation always occurs in the foot on the downhill ski, which is in forced eversion when turning to come to a halt. If the ski tip is subjected to rotation or abrupt plantarflexion, dislocation follows [15].

Forced eversion puts tension on the calcaneofibular ligament and thrusts the tendons back against the fibular tendon retinaculum [18].

Several anatomic types of dislocation have been described [13, 45]: type I, subperiosteal dislocation; type II, subcutaneous dislocation due to tear of the retinaculum; type, III bone avulsion; and type IV, posterior tear of the retinaculum.

Clinically, the patient presents with severe posterolateral pain after an ankle injury. Generally, the tendons have spontaneously reduced into the correct position and a sprain is diagnosed after perfunctory examination. At this stage, diagnosis is based on precise analysis:
• pain located exclusively behind the lateral malleolus,
• mechanism different to that of an ordinary sprain,
• no pain along the course of the anterior talofibular ligament,
• violent pain on resisted eversion of the foot; moreover, this maneuver may reproduce the dislocation.

Radiographically, avulsion at the tip of the lateral malleolus can be observed in type III dislocations (15 to 50% of cases according to the series) [5, 41].

The initial diagnosis is often missed and the condition progresses towards recurrent fibular-tendon dislocation. The patient complains of a snapping sensation and ankle instability. Here again, diagnosis is based on meticulous examination which shows no laxity and reproduces the tendon dislocation. CT scan or MRI are rarely required to reveal subluxation.

In emergency, the dislocation can be treated conservatively: immobilization in a plaster cast for six weeks without weight-bearing. Escalas observed recurrence in 74% of cases after such treatment and several authors advise surgical treatment in the acute stage [12,13, 37, 45, 46]. The procedure consists of repair or transosseous reinsertion of the fibular retinaculum.

If dislocation becomes recurrent, surgery is the only treatment. It may be complicated by the presence of fissural tendon lesions. Several types of procedure have been described:
• simple repair of the retinaculum [38],
• bone-block procedures [11],
• ligamentous repair using a band of the calcaneal tendon [27],
• transfer of the fibular tendons beneath the calcaneofibular ligament [51, 58].

Pathology of the tendon of the flexor hallucis longus muscle (FHL)

FHL injury mainly affects those taking part in activities requiring repetitive movements of flexion and extension on tiptoe. Dancers are the most frequent sufferers and the FHL "is considered to be the dancer's calcaneal tendon" [20]. The FHL is vulnerable where it passes at the posterior aspect of the talus, since it runs within a rigid fibro-osseous tunnel between the posteromedial and lateral talar tuberosities. Any tendon inflammation leads to impingement at this level.

Clinically, the athlete complains of medial retromalleolar pain during sporting activity. In ballet dancers, "pointes", "demi-pointes" and "pliés" increase pain and are sometimes impossible. Sometimes, the great toe may lock due to stenosing tendovaginitis of the FHL in its tunnel, a condition known as "pseudo-hallux rigidus" [20, 21].

On examination, pain is produced by palpation of the medial retromalleolar portion of the FHL and is aggravated if the hallux is mobilized at the same time. Passive forced plantarflexion of the ankle does not increase the pain unless there is associated posterior impingement against an os trigonum.

Diagnosis is essentially clinical and it is unusual to have recourse to other investigations such as MRI.

Differential diagnosis must be made from other causes of posterior ankle pain, recently grouped together as the "posterior crossroads syndrome" [9]: impingement on the os trigonum or the posterolat-

eral tuberosity of the talus (Chapter 28), tibiocalcaneal impingement, impingement on the distal band of the posteroinferior tibiofibular ligament.

The initial treatment is usually conservative: ice, rest, anti-inflammatory agents and sometimes orthopedic insoles (medial arch supports, heel wedges, rigid soles [15]). If there is no response, surgical tenolysis may be necessary. If posterior impingement is also present, the os trigonum is excised in association with tenolysis [19].

Pathology of the tendon of the tibialis anterior muscle

The tibialis anterior muscle arises from the anterolateral surface of the proximal half of the tibia and from the adjacent part of the interosseous membrane. The tendon originates at the distal third of the leg, passes under the extensor retinaculum of the tarsus and inserts into the medial surface of the first cuneiform and the first metatarsal base. It is the main dorsiflexor of the foot. At the ankle, it is surrounded by a synovial sheath.

Except in the context of rheumatoid arthritis, chronic disorders of this tendon are rare. Rupture is the most frequent pathology [10, 39, 52], generally occurring in patients aged over 50, spontaneously or during minimal trauma. The most frequent mechanism is forced plantarflexion causing eccentric contraction of the muscle. The rupture occurs a few cm above the tendon insertion [52].

Diagnosis is often made late since pain is moderate. The patient presents steppage but gait is nearly normal because of compensation by the toe extensors. Walking on the heel is impossible and the outline of the tendon can no longer be felt in resisted dorsiflexion of the foot. The differential diagnosis of steppage of neurologic origin must be excluded. Electromyography can be useful in doubtful cases. Treatment is surgical if the rupture is recent. Most authors advise abstention from surgery if the injury is long-standing.

References

1. Anzel FH, Covey KW, Weiner AD, Lipscomb PR (1959) Discruption of muscles and tendons: an analysis of 1014 cases. Surgery 45: 406-414

2. Arrowsmith SR, Fleming LL, Allman FL (1983) Traumatic dislocations of the peroneal tendons. Am J Sports Med 11: 142-146

3. Basset FH, Speer KP.(1993) Longitudinal rupture of the peroneal tendons. Am J Sports Med 21: 354-357

4. Bonnin M, Tavernier T, Bouysset M (1997) Split lesions of the peroneus brevis tendon in chronic ankle laxity. Am J Sports Med 25: 699-703

5. Church CC (1977) Radiographic diagnosis of acute peroneal tendon dislocation. AJR 129: 1065-1068

6. Conti S, Michelson J, Jahss M (1992) Clinical significance of Magnetic Resonnance Imaging in pre-operative planning for reconstruction of posterior tibial ruptures. Foot Ankle 13: 208-214

7. Coudert X, Kouvalchouk JF (1991) Conflit musculaire dans la goutière rétro-malléolaire par faisceaux musculaires surnuméraires du court péronier latéral: à propos de 2 cas. Rev Chir Orthop 77: 260-262

8. Coudert X, Kouvalchouk JF, Dufour O (1992) Causes rares de syndromes des péroniers latéraux. J Traumatol Sport 9: 188-193

9. Cusimano A, Gandon D, Segal P (1993) Images particulières évoquant des lésions du ligament péronéo-tibial inférieur à sa partie postérieure au cours de syndromes post-traumatiques du carrefour postérieur de la cheville. J Traumatol Sport 10: 220-229

10. Dooley BJ, Kudelka P, Menelaus MB (1980) Subcutaneous rupture of the tendon of tibialis anterior. J Bone Joint Surg 62B: 471-472

11. Duvries HL (1959) Surgery of the foot. Mosby-Year Book, St Louis, pp 252-255

12. Earle AS, Moritz JR, Tapper EM (1972) Dislocation of the peroneal tendons at the ankle-An analysis of 25 ski injuries. Northwest Med 71: 108-110

13. Eckert WR, Davis EA (1976) Acute rupture of the peroneal retinaculum.J Bone Joint Surg [Am] 58: 670-673

14. Edwards ME (1928) The relations of the peroneal tendons to the fibula calcaneus and cuboideum. Am J Anat 1: 213

15. Escalas F, Figueras JM, Merino JA (1980) Dislocation of the peroneal tendons-Long term results of surgical treatment. J Bone Joint Surg [Am] 62-A, 451-453

16. Frey C, Shereff MJ (1988) Tendon injuries about the ankle in athletes. Clin Sports Med 7: 103-117

17. Frey C, Shereff MJ, Greenidgen N (1990) Vascularity of the posterior tibial tendon. J Bone Joint Surg [Am] 72A: 884-888

18. Geppert MJ, Sobel M, Bohne WHO (1993) Lateral ankle instability as a cause of superior peroneal retinacular laxity: Anatomic and biomechanical study of cadaveric feet. Foot Ankle, 14: 330-334

19. Hall RL (1994) Injuries of the posterior tibial tendon. In: Pfeffer GB, Frey C (eds) Current Practice in Foot and Ankle Surgery, Vol 2. McGraw Hill Inc, New York, pp 124-156

20. Hamilton WG (1982) Stenosing tenosynovitis of the flexor hallucis longus tendon and posterior impingement upon the os trigonum in ballet dancers. Foot Ankle 3: 74-80

21. Hamilton WG (1988) Foot and ankle injuries in dancers. Clin Sports Med 7: 143-173

22. Holmes GB, Mann RA (1992) Possible epidemiological factors associated with rupture of posterior tibial tendon. Foot Ankle 13: 70-79

23. Inman VT, Ralston HJ, Todd F (1981) Human walking. Williams and Wilkins, Baltimore

24. Jahss M (1991) Tendon disorders of the foot and ankle. In: Jahss M (ed) Disorders of the Foot and Ankle Medical and Surgical Management. Saunders Compagny, Philadelphia, pp 1461-1513

25. Johnson KA (1982) Tibialis posterior tendon rupture. Clin Orthop 177: 140-147

26. Johnson KA, Strom DE (1989) Tibialis posterior tendon dysfunction. Clin Orthop 239: 196-206

27. Jones E (1932) Operative treatment for chronic dislocation of the peroneal tendons. J Bone Joint Surg 14: 574-576

28. Keenan MA, Peabody TD, Gronley JK, Perry J (1991) Valgus deformities of the fat and characteristics of gait ion patients who have rhumatoid arthritis. J Bone Joint Surg 73A: 237-247

29. Kojima Y, KataokaY, Susuki S, et al (1991) Dislocation of the peroneal tendons in neonates ans infants. Clin Orthop 266: 180-184

30. Delabareyre H, Saillant G (1994) Luxations et ruptures du jambier postérieur. J Traumatol Sport 11: 20-25

31. Langenskiold A (1967) Chronic non specific tenosynovitis of the tibialis posterior tendon. Acta Orthop Scand 38: 301

32. Larsen E (1987) Longitudinal rupture of the peroneus brevis tendon. J Bone Joint Surg [Br] 69B: 340-341

33. Leach RE, Dilorio, Harney RA (1982) Pathologic hind foot conditions in the athlete. Clin Orthop 177: 116-121

34. Ledouble J (1897) Traité des variations du système musculaire de l'homme. Schleides Frères, Paris, pp 334-342

35. Mann RA (1992) Flatfoot in adults. In: Mann RA, Coughlin MJ (eds) Surgery of the Foot and Ankle. Mosby, St Louis, pp 757-784

36. Mann RA (1993) Biomechanics of the Foot and Ankle. In: Mann RA, Coughlin MJ (eds) Surgery of the Foot and Ankle. Mosby, St Louis, pp 3-44

37. Marti R (1977) Dislocation of the peroneal tendons. Am J Sports Med 5: 19-22

38. Meary R, Tomeno B (1979) Luxation récidivante des tendons péroniers. Encycl Med Chir, Paris, Techniques Chirurgicales Orthopédie 3-23-10, 44 900,

39. Mensor MC, Ordway GL (1953) Traumatic subcutaneous rupture of the tibialis anterior tendon. J Bone Joint Surg 35A: 675-680

40. Monteggia GB (1803) Instituzini chirurgiche, Parte secondu, Milano, pp 336-341

41. Moritz JR (1959) Ski injuries. Am J Surg 98: 493-505

42. Mounier Khun A, Marsan C (1968) Le syndrome des tendons péroniers. Ann Chir 22: 641-649

43. Mueller TJ (1991) Acquired flat foot secondary to tibialis posterior dysfunction: Biomechanical aspects. J Foot Surg 30: 1-11

44. Munk RL, Davis PH (1976) Longitudinal rupture of the peroneus brevis tendon. J Trauma 16: 803-816

45. Oden RR (1985) Tendon injuries about the ankle resulting from skiing. Clin Orthop 216: 63-69

46. Orthner E, Polcik J, Schabus R (1989) Die luxation der peroneussehnen. UnfallChirurgie 92: 589-594

47. Otto WA (1816) Neve seltene Beobachtungen zur anatomie physiologie und pathologie Gehörig, p 40

48. Ouzounian TJ, Myerson MS (1992) Dislocation of the posterior tibial tendon. Foot Ankle 4: 215-219

49. Peterson DA, Stinson W (1992) Excision of the fractured os peroneum: A report of five patients and review of the literature. Foot Ankle 13: 277-281

50. Pierson JL, Inglis AE (1992) Stenosing tenosynovitis of the peroneus longus tendon secondary to hypertrophy of the peroneal tubercule and an associated os peroneum. J Bone Joint Surg [Am] 74: 440-442

51. Pozo JL, Jackson AM (1984) A rerouting operation for dislocation of peroneal tendons -operative technique and case report. Foot Ankle 5: 42-44

52. Rimoldi RJ, Oberlander MA, Waldrop JI, Hunter SC (1991) Acute rupture of the tibialis anterior tendon: A case report. Foot Ankle 12: 176-177

53. Rouvière H (1962) Anatomie humaine descriptive et topographique TIII. Masson, Paris, pp 366-368

54. Rosenberg ZS, Cheung Y, Jahss MH, Noto AM, Norman A, Leeds NE (1988) Rupture of posterior tibial tendon: CT and MR Imaging with surgical correlation. Radiology 169: 229-235

55. Saillant G, Delabareyre H, Roy Camille R (1990) Les ruptures du tendon du jambier postérieur: Étude clinique et thérapeutique à propos de 13 cas. Rev Chir Orthop 76: 559-567

56. Sammarco GJ, Di Raimondo CV (1989) Chronic peroneus brevis tendon lesions. Foot Ankle 9: 163-170

57. Sarrafian SK (1993) Anatomy of the Foot and Ankle. Lippincott Compagny, Philadelphia, pp 283-293

58. Sarmiento A, Wolf M (1975) Subluxation of peroneal tendons: Case treated by rerouting tendons under calcaneofibular ligament. J Bone Joint Surg [Am] 57: 115-116

59. Sella EJ, Lawson P, Ogden JA (1986) The accessory navicular synchondrosis. Clin Orthop 209: 250-262

60. Sobel M, Bohne WHO, Makisz JA (1991) Cadaver correlation of peroneal tendon changes with Magnetic Resonnance Imaging. Foot Ankle 11: 384-388

61. Sobel M, Dicarlo EF, Bohne WHO, Collins L (1991) Longitudinal splitting of the peroneus brevis tendon. An anatomic and histologic study of cadaveric material. Foot Ankle 12: 165-170

62. Sobel M, Geppert MJ, Olson EJ, Bohne WHO, Arnoczky SP (1992) The dynamics of peroneus brevis tendon splits: A proposed mechanism-Technique of diagnosis and classification of injury. Foot Ankle 13: 413-422

63. Sobel M, Levy M, Bohne WHO (1990) Congenital variation of the peroneus quartus muscle: an anatomic study. Foot Ankle 11: 81-89

64. Sobel M, Mitzel MS (1993) Peroneal tendon injury . In: Pfeffer GB, Frey C (eds) Current Practice in Foot and Ankle Surgery , vol 1. McGraw-Hill, New York, pp 30-56

65. Testut L (1884) Les anomalies musculaires chez l'homme, expliquées par l'anatomie comparée: Leur importance en anthropologie. Masson, Paris, pp 588-744

66. Thompson FM, Patterson AH (1989) Rupture of the peroneus longus tendon Report of three cases. J Bone Joint Surg [Am] 71A: 293-295

67. Trevino S, Gould N, Korson R (1981) Surgical treatment of stenosing tenosynovitis at the ankle. Foot Ankle 2: 37

68. Wright DG, Desai ME, Henderson BS (1964) Action of the subtalar and ankle joint complex during the stance phase of walking. J Bone Joint Surg [Am] 46A, 361

69. Zoellner G, Clancy WJ (1979) Recurrent dislocation of the peroneal tendons. J Bone Joint Surg [Am] 61: 292-294

25.

Entrapment neuropathies
(excluding Morton's neuroma)

G Guaydier-Souquières

Introduction

A nerve entrapment syndrome is defined as mechanical irritation of a peripheral nerve as it passes through an inelastic bony, ligamentous and muscular tunnel. It includes mechanical compression of nerve branches. These syndromes give rise to subjective sensory disorders such as pain or paresthesiae, while motor disorders are minor and may often even be absent. Diagnosis is made on clinical grounds but is often difficult and requires a thorough knowledge of sensory distribution in the foot and of the course of the nerve branches, bearing in mind that there is considerable anatomic variation in the division of nerve trunks.

In the foot, entrapment syndromes are uncommon. The best-known and most frequent are Morton's syndrome, or compression of the digital nerve (dealt with in Chapter 21), and the tarsal tunnel syndrome. However, other forms of nerve compression exist and will be reviewed.

Tarsal tunnel syndrome

Anatomic and physiologic review

The tarsal tunnel syndrome in the foot is comparable to the carpal tunnel syndrome in the hand, but is much less frequent. It results from compression of the tibial nerve or of one or several of its branches as it passes through the fibro-osseous tunnel which lies behind and below the medial malleolus. Its limits

and contents have been detailed in Chapter 1. We merely note here that along its distal course the flexor hallucis longus tendon comes forward closer to the flexor digitorum longus tendon and displaces superficially the neurovascular bundle contiguous to the flexor retinaculum. The tibial nerve typically divides into medial and lateral plantar nerves in the distal part of the tarsal tunnel, but this bifurcation may be more proximal and this would appear to increase the risk of compression [21]. The plantar nerves then exit from the tarsal tunnel by passing under the fibrous arch of the abductor hallucis muscle and may also be compressed at this point [14].

The distribution of the tibial nerve and its branches can vary greatly [4], but the sensory area supplied by the medial plantar nerve can be approximated to a triangle on the sole of the foot with an anterior base and extending to the first three toes and medial half of the fourth toe, overlapping onto the dorsal aspect of the third phalanges of these toes (fig. 25.1). The lateral plantar nerve supplies the lateral part of the sole, extending over the dorsal aspect of the third phalanges of the fourth and fifth toes.

In addition, the medial calcaneal nerve, which usually arises above the tarsal tunnel, may arise in the tunnel and be compressed within it. This nerve supplies almost all the plantar surface of the heel, except for a small lateral area which is innervated by branches of the sural nerve.

The medial and lateral plantar nerves also supply all the intrinsic muscles of the foot except the extensor digitorum brevis muscle.

Compression of a nerve causes local ischemia or axonal demyelinization, to a degree which depends

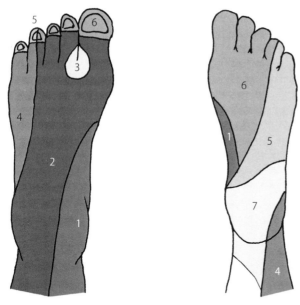

Fig. 25.1. Sensory nerve distribution in the foot. **a** Dorsal aspect. **b** Plantar aspect. *1* Saphenous n (branch of the femoral n.), *2* superficial peroneal n., *3* deep peroneal n., *4* sural n., *5* lateral plantar n., *6* medial plantar n., *7* medial calcaneal n.

on the severity and duration of compression. Sensory signs are the earliest and most frequent as sensory fibers are less tolerant of ischemia than motor fibers [8, 38]. Clinical signs also appear to be directly related to the pressure on nerve fibers [14]. Lastly, it should be noted that neuropathies, diabetic neuropathy in particular, make nerves more vulnerable to any type of compression [7, 24].

Clinical features

The patient complains of pain and paresthesiae, described as burning sensations, pins and needles, numbness or "wooden feet" [8, 11, 14, 34]. These symptoms are localized in the sole of the foot, radiating from behind or below the medial malleolus to the area of distribution of one or both plantar nerves or even of the medial calcaneal nerve. This distal radiation is often partial and may affect only one or two toes or even the pad of a single toe. Irritation of the medial plantar nerve should be suspected if the first three toes are affected, of the lateral plantar nerve if the last two toes are affected, and of the medial calcaneal nerve if the heel is affected [37]. Sometimes pain radiates proximally towards the ankle and leg (Valleix phenomenon) [8].

Pain or paresthesiae are worsened by walking, prolonged standing or sports activity, running in particular, and are alleviated by rest [23, 34, 36]. They may however also be present at night or during rest, especially if compression is long-standing [14, 31, 38]. Gentle massage and elevation or movement of the foot readily give relief. Symptoms may be bilateral, especially in obesity or neuropathy [19].

Physical examination

Physical examination confirms the diagnosis if it reproduces pain or paresthesia similar to the patient's symptoms on percussion or firm pressure on the tarsal tunnel, along the medial retromalleolar sulcus or at its exit (this is the analog of Tinel's sign). This maneuver may also elicit proximal pain [8, 11]. Production of pain or paresthesia should also be sought when the foot is held in forced dorsiflexion-eversion, which stretches the tibial nerve [8].

Objective sensory signs are less common, generally hypoesthesia or more rarely hyperesthesia in the area of distribution of the tibial nerve or one of its branches; here again signs may be partial, limited to a single toe-pad.

Motor loss is slight or absent and does not give rise to spontaneous complaints by the patient. However, the physician should routinely search for motor signs by comparing the symptomatic with the asymptomatic limb [8, 14]: clawing of one or several toes due to weakness of the interosseous or lumbrical muscles, impaired flexion or spreading of the toes, difficulty in harmoniously flexing the toes when standing, and above all a partial or total lack of pressure under the extremity of one or several toes. The latter can be objectively tested by the "paper sign": the examiner places a sheet of paper under the toes of each foot and then attempts to pull it away; on the affected side, this can be done without tearing the paper. This test also determines whether the medial plantar nerve is involved (the sheet of paper is placed under the pad of the hallux) or the lateral plantar nerve (paper under the fourth and fifth toes). Lastly, overlap of the hallux is sought: in plantar-flexion, the hallux passes under the second toe due to weakness of the abductor hallucis muscle, indicating involvement of the medial plantar nerve

The other clinical signs are rarer: increase in local temperature, diffuse soft tissue swelling behind and below the medial malleolus which is primarily suggestive of tenosynovitis, especially if accompanied by crepitus [25]. Trophic skin changes are very rare and remain minor: excessive perspiration or dryness of the sole of the foot, thinning of the skin.

The following should also be sought: a static disorder increasing the likelihood of strain on the nerve [34], excessive weight, venous insufficiency, intensive sports activity, in particular running, or previous injury.

Supplementary investigations

Supplementary investigations are not routinely requested as the diagnosis is made on clinical grounds. However, they may be useful if the diagnosis remains uncertain, which is frequently the case as the functional signs often tend to be atypical. They may also help to determine the cause of nerve compression and guide the surgical procedure if this is decided upon.

Radiographs include bilateral comparative views: lateral view of the weight-bearing foot, anteroposterior view of the weight-bearing talocrural joint with a circled view of the ankle, and a retrotibial projection of the calcaneus.

Computed tomography (CT) and moreover magnetic resonance imaging (MRI) can be of value, once again in comparison with the uninvolved side. Axial and sagittal T1-weighted high-resolution MRI depicts the nerve and its branches as well as the adjoining soft tissues and often reveals the compressive lesion, such as adenopathy, tenosynovitis or tumor [16, 41, 42]. Because MRI is a costly investigation, it is only undertaken before a surgical procedure or if there is reason to suspect a tumor, especially in a child [40].

Nerve conduction and electromyographic studies can be most valuable in diagnosis [8, 11, 19, 40]. The symptomatic side is compared with the asymptomatic side with stimulation of the medial and lateral plantar nerves and the tibial nerve, first at the popliteal fossa and also distal and proximal to the tarsal tunnel. Slowing of motor conduction, a reduced pattern and fasciculation at rest are sought in the flexor digitorum brevis and abductor hallucis muscles [17, 23]. Sensory nerve conduction testing, which is more difficult in the foot than in the hand, can be carried out or somatosensory evoked potentials can be studied [9, 40].

Such tests can give an idea of the progressive nature of the nerve compression and help to distinguish between entrapment neuropathy and radiculopathy or peripheral neuropathy. They are also valuable in guiding a surgical procedure. Sometimes signs of compression may be found in two different locations [36]. It is in diagnosing tarsal tunnel syndrome that electromyographic study is most efficacious in the foot. However it is often difficult to perform and the results do not always appear to agree with peroperative observations [13]. Even if it is normal, this does not exclude the diagnosis, which remains clinical.

Laboratory tests, if requested, are normal unless a metabolic or inflammatory disorder is present. Lastly, if arteriopathy is suspected a doppler study is helpful.

Etiology

The possible causes are many [8, 14, 20, 23, 36]:
- sequelae of injury or fracture, particularly frequent in athletes [28] and fibrous scar tissue after surgical procedures such as arthrodesis,
- repetitive microtrauma, especially in runners,
- static disorders, particularly in athletes, such as heel valgus, forefoot supination or, on the contrary, heel varus and forefoot pronation [34], hypermobility of the first ray, tarsal fusion or joint stiffness,
- inflammatory tenosynovitis with swelling, increase in local temperature and sometimes crepitus [25],
- neuropathy in the course of systemic, metabolic or endocrine diseases. In such instances the syndrome may be bilateral [20]. The search for associated compression is difficult and requires careful electromyographic study with measurement proximal and distal to the site of compression,
- venous insufficiency, revealed by the presence of dilated veins adjacent to a nerve [18],
- flexor retinaculum or abductor hallucis muscle hypertrophy [14, 18],
- more rarely, a lipoma, synovial cyst, thrombotic vein or schwannoma, which can be diagnosed by MRI before the surgical procedure [18, 29, 41].

Although in many instances no cause is found, MRI has nevertheless reduced the incidence of these "idiopathic" forms.

Differential diagnosis

For the diagnosis to be made, numerous other disorders [20] must be excluded, in particular neurologic:

• S1 radiculopathy, which may be suspected in the presence of spinal cord and neurologic signs and confirmed by electromyography if necessary,

• nerve entrapment at a more proximal or especially a more distal level (interdigital neuroma),

• neuropathy, in particular due to diabetes mellitus or alcohol abuse, which may be suspected if there are distal sensory disorders with a symmetrical "stocking" distribution [24],

• amyotrophic lateral sclerosis, with muscle weakness, exaggerated reflexes and fasciculation.

The following must also be excluded:

• an adjacent pathology: a joint lesion, particularly of the subtalar joint, a tendon lesion or a tumor, a plantar muscular and fascial insertional disorder (cf. chapter 22), or an os trigonum syndrome. Sensory or motor nerve signs are absent in all these cases,

• reflex sympathetic algodystrophy [28],

• compartment syndrome, arteriopathy or Raynaud's phenomenon.

Treatment

Treatment is primarily conservative [14, 31]:

• rest, application of ice, limitation of motion by a basketweave taping system [31], while continuing regular active mobilization to prevent joint stiffening,

• nonsteroidal anti-inflammatory drugs and, if rheumatoid arthritis is present, treatment of the underlying disorder,

• advice on suitable footwear, in particular in the athlete, and if necessary a change of training surface,

• correction or compensation of any static disorder by custom-made plantar insoles or physical therapy,

• injection of corticosteroids within the tarsal tunnel, halfway between the medial malleolus and the calcaneal tendon and behind the posterior tibial artery, sparing the tendon structures. Steroids are less effective than in the carpal tunnel syndrome and failure does not mean there is no entrapment.

If the condition does not improve, as is frequently the case, surgery is proposed, and electromyography and if possible MRI are performed previously [18]. The flexor retinaculum is sectioned and neurolysis is performed with careful release of all the components of the tarsal tunnel and opening of the medial and lateral plantar compartments. This generally brings about improvement [14, 38], but is a delicate procedure and if the diagnosis is delayed there may be residual pain or paresthesiae alone,

accompanied by electromyographic anomalies [13, 30]. In certain refractory cases, MRI may be helpful in guiding a secondary surgical procedure [43].

Nerve branch entrapment distal to the tarsal tunnel

The branches of the tibial nerve may be compressed within the tarsal tunnel, but may also be compressed distally, making diagnosis even more difficult.

Nerve to the abductor digiti minimi muscle

This proximal branch of the lateral plantar nerve courses deep to the abductor hallucis muscle and then deviates between the thick fascia of this muscle and the quadratus plantae muscle, passing around the anterior aspect of the posteromedial tuberosity of the calcaneus and then running transversely towards the abductor digiti minimi muscle, which it penetrates after giving rise to some sensory branches to the plantar fascia and part of the calcaneal periosteum [4, 6, 33, 37] (fig. 25.2).

The frequency of this compression apparently increases with the proximity of the nerve to the posteromedial tuberosity of the calcaneus [33]. It causes heel pain on weight-bearing and walking, and burning paresthesiae. On physical examination, pain is elicited by pressure on the medial and

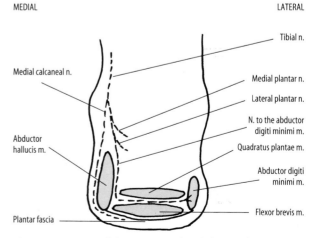

Fig. 25.2. Course of the nerve to the abductor digiti quinti muscle

anterior edge of the heel and there may be weakness of the abductor digiti minimi muscle [33, 37]. This compression is often related to repetitive microtrauma or to static disorders such as valgus flatfoot.

Treatment is primarily conservative: correction of the static disorder and corticosteroid injections. If this fails, surgical release or nerve resection can be considered and generally give good results [3, 6].

Lateral plantar nerve

Compression of this nerve has also been described distal to the tarsal tunnel and the fibrous arch of the abductor hallucis muscle in a fibrous tunnel between the flexor digitorum brevis muscle, which has a fibrous thickening, and the quadratus plantae muscle [39]. This distal compression is rare and may be attributed to a crush injury of the foot, repetitive microtrauma (frequent ladder climbing or use of poorly fitting orthoses) or a compressive lesion such as an adenopathy [25, 39].

The patient presents with pain in the plantar arch, aroused by pressure anterior to the pressure zone of the heel and sometimes radiating to the fourth and fifth toes. Hypoesthesia in the area of distribution of the lateral plantar nerve should be sought (fig. 25.1). Electrical studies may reveal slowed conduction over the painful area, sensory study being done by stimulation of the fifth toe.

Failure of conservative treatment leads to surgical release with resection of the fibrous thickening of the flexor digitorum brevis muscle [39].

Medial plantar nerve

Compression of this nerve at the level of the abductor hallucis muscle causes the condition known as "jogger's foot" [8, 36, 37]. Plantar pain is suggestive if it appears after exertion during sports, in particular a running race or a cycle race, and if it is accompanied by paresthesiae of the pad of the hallux, produced on walking but sometimes also present at rest. Examination may reveal hypoesthesia in the area of distribution of this nerve (fig. 25.1). Electrical studies may be helpful in diagnosis if they show slowed nerve conduction distal to the tarsal tunnel and weakness of the abductor hallucis muscle; sensory study is carried out by stimulation of the hallux [17, 40].

If conservative treatment fails, surgical release and resection of the fibrous arch of the abductor hallucis muscle are proposed. There have been some rare reports of other causes of compression such as schwannoma [44].

Superficial fibular nerve entrapment

The superficial fibular nerve (fig. 25.3) is a lateral branch of the common fibular nerve. It pierces the deep fascia in the distal third of the leg, at a varying level [5, 36]. Above the extensor retinaculum it bifurcates to form the intermediate and medial dorsal cutaneous nerves, which give rise to the dorsal digital nerves of the first three toes and sometimes of the fourth toe; numerous anatomic variations have been described [5] (fig. 25.4).

In the leg, the superficial fibular nerve supplies the fibular muscles but in the foot it is purely

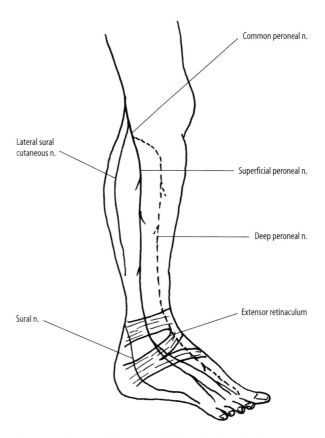

Fig. 25.3. Course of the superficial and deep fibular nerves

MEDIAL   LATERAL

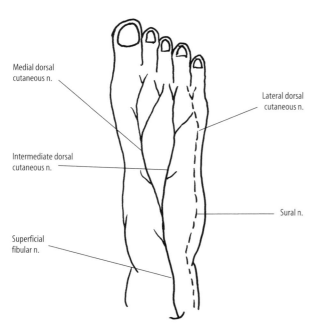

Medial dorsal
cutaneous n.

Lateral dorsal
cutaneous n.

Intermediate dorsal
cutaneous n.

Sural n.

Superficial
fibular n.

Fig. 25.4. Distal course of the superficial fibular nerve and the sural nerve

sensory. It provides sensation over the medial and middle dorsum of the foot and the dorsal aspect of the first two phalanges of the first three or four toes [15] (fig. 25.1).

This nerve may be compressed in several critical areas: not only at its origin or in the distal third of the leg, but also at the anterolateral aspect of the ankle, the tarsometatarsal junction, the base of the first metatarsal and the medial part of the first metatarsal head [15].

Symptoms

Compression of the superficial fibular nerve causes paresthesiae and numbness of the dorsum of the foot and of the first three or four toes and pain in the same area, suggesting the diagnosis to a varying degree. These signs tend to be accentuated by walking or running [36]. Involvement may be general or may only affect a single nerve branch.

The physician may find hypoesthesia or dysesthesia in the same territory and functional signs may be elicited during certain maneuvers such as passive inversion and plantarflexion of the foot, or on the contrary active dorsiflexion and resisted eversion. It

is important to look for pain on localized percussion of the various critical points or on palpation along the course of the nerve branches. A nerve which is mobile to the touch may even be found [15, 25, 26].

If the diagnosis is uncertain, and above all if surgical treatment is being considered, electrical studies may be helpful but this purely sensory nerve of the foot is difficult to investigate. The nerve trunks must be located by surface electrodes and bilateral comparisons with antidromic and orthodromic stimulation are necessary [40]. Compression at a more proximal level can also be sought by stimulation at the knee [27]. This investigation shows whether or not the response is prolonged or decreased in amplitude, or even whether there is a conduction block in the area where entrapment is clinically suspected or at a more proximal level, and can differentiate between total or partial involvement. The results may nevertheless be normal because of the various anastomoses with other nerves, in particular the deep fibular nerve. Fibrous scar tissue may make this investigation impossible and somatosensory evoked potentials can be helpful in such instances [9, 40].

Etiology

Several factors may co-exist, mainly traumatic:
- microtrauma during work or sports: cycling (due to impingement against the toe-clip or shoes), football, karate, running, tennis or dancing [10, 15, 36],
- injury involving direct impact on the instep, as in football, or a sharp sudden pull on the nerve (ankle sprain) [36],
- surgical procedure or ankle arthroscopy: a nerve branch may easily be damaged during the approach especially as anatomic variations are numerous [5],
- footwear which is too narrow or which fits high around the ankle, accounting for the predominance of this entrapment in women [15],
- static disorders: hallux valgus [26], or the prominent tarsal bones of the cavus foot [15],
- other lesions are more rarely involved: tenosynovitis, synovial cyst, arthrosis or neuropathy.

Differential diagnosis

Clinical signs of neuropathy or other nerve entrapments should be sought with the help of electrical studies [27]:

• compression of the superficial fibular nerve at a more proximal level, generally in the lower third of the leg, where it is compressed by the edge of the fascia and where a local swelling is sometimes found. Entrapment may more rarely be present in the lateral compartment, causing a compartment syndrome with pain after prolonged effort during sports, or at the neck of the fibula. This weakens the fibular muscles and leads to recurrent ankle sprains [15, 36],

• syndrome of the fibular neck, which often occurs after prolonged periods spent with the legs crossed: there is weakness of the extensor muscles of the foot as well as of the fibular muscles due to associated compression of the deep fibular nerve,

• L5 radiculopathy,

• compression of the saphenous nerve at the level of the subsartorial canal or injury of this nerve after venous stripping, causing distal paresthesiae which may radiate to the medial part of the ankle or even the foot [25].

Treatment

Conservative measures include:

• alteration of footwear to prevent any impingement on the dorsal aspect of the midfoot,

• correction or stabilization of static disorders by custom-made plantar insoles and physical therapy,

• rest, analgesics, application of topical anti-inflammatory agents,

• if pain persists in spite of this treatment, a corticosteroid can be injected locally at the site where entrapment is clinically suspected, allowing confirmation of the diagnosis [15].

If these measures fail, a surgical procedure may be considered, if possible after the diagnosis has been confirmed and the site of entrapment indicated by electrical studies. This procedure may be release or in some cases resection of the nerve after it has been carefully localized (since this nerve is purely sensory in the foot). Hallux valgus is of course also corrected if present [10, 26].

Deep fibular nerve entrapment

The deep fibular nerve, the medial branch of the common fibular nerve, arises at the neck of the fibula and runs downward, forward and medially,

descends to the leg with the anterior tibial artery and gives rise to branches to the anterior muscles of the leg (fig. 25.3). On the dorsal aspect of the lower part of the instep, beneath the extensor retinaculum, it divides into two branches: the muscular lateral branch to the extensor digitorum brevis muscle, and the medial branch which supplies sensation to the first web space and anastomoses with a branch of the superficial fibular nerve (fig. 25.1).

The most frequent entrapment of this nerve, known as the anterior tarsal tunnel syndrome, is located on the dorsal aspect of the ankle between the talonavicular joint and the inferior extensor retinaculum. The nerve may also be compressed distally on the dorsal aspect of the midfoot by the extensor hallucis brevis tendon, or proximally by the extensor hallucis longus tendon and the edge of the extensor retinaculum [1, 2, 36].

Symptoms

Entrapment of the deep fibular nerve causes mediotarsal pain which is readily aggravated by running but is often also nocturnal when the feet are in supination. The pain can then be alleviated by movements of dorsiflexion and eversion of the foot [25, 36]. It may be accompanied by paresthesiae of the first web space and numbness. On examination, pain may be produced on plantarflexion and inversion of the foot or by pressure on the anterior aspect of the ankle, and hypoesthesia of the first web space and the adjacent sides of the first two toes should be sought [1, 2]. If the site of compression is proximal to the bifurcation of the nerve, weakness of the extensor digitorum brevis muscle may be observed and decreased strength on extension of the first phalanx of the toes. This muscle may sometimes be atrophied [1].

Electromyographic study, which is certainly difficult in this case also, sometimes shows slowed conduction velocity but it may be normal [12], in particular if there is an accessory fibular nerve [2].

Etiology

Compression is often due to trauma [12, 36]:

• direct injury with forced inversion of the foot,

• recurrent ankle sprains, in particular in runners or those practicing football, skiing or dancing,

• compression by footwear such as ski-boots, or shoes with straps crossing the dorsal aspect of the foot.

Other possible causes are:
• tenosynovitis, especially rheumatoid tenosynovitis of the extensor hallucis longus muscle,
• osteoarthrosis and bone spurs of the talonavicular joint, exostosis, fracture callus, adenopathy, synovial cyst,
• a static disorder such as cavus foot,
• neuropathy.

Differential diagnosis

Diagnosis must exclude:
• nerve entrapment at a more proximal level at the neck of the fibula, accompanied by weakness of the levator muscles of the foot,
• compression of the common fibular nerve, accompanied by weakness of the fibular muscles,
• compression of an interdigital nerve,
• L5 radiculopathy,
• a disorder of the talocrural joint,
• a compartment syndrome with pain in the anterolateral compartment of the leg after prolonged exercise,
• distal arteriopathy.

Treatment

Treatment is primarily conservative [2, 36], by rest and physiotherapy, alteration of footwear, plantar orthoses for stabilization, or local injection of corticosteroids. If this fails, surgical release can be proposed but this is a delicate procedure [1]. Previously, injection of a local anesthetic can be attempted to confirm diagnosis [12].

● Sural nerve entrapment

The sural nerve arises from the popliteal fossa and pierces the fascia of the leg at the mid-third of the leg. It runs down superficially in the posterior region of the leg, then courses along the calcaneal tendon and curves around the lateral malleolus behind the fibular tendons. After giving rise to collateral branches to the talocrural joint and the region of the lateral malleolus and to calcaneal branches, it courses along the lateral edge of the foot where it becomes the lateral dorsal cutaneous nerve. This gives rise to the lateral collateral nerve of the fifth toe and to the last two or three dorsal collateral nerves by anastomosing with a branch of the superficial fibular nerve (fig. 25.4). It is a purely sensory nerve and its cutaneous distribution in the foot extends to the lateral aspect of the hindfoot and the heel and to the lateral part of the dorsal aspect of the foot along the fifth ray and fifth toe, and sometimes also to the fourth toe depending on the anastomosis with the superficial fibular nerve [32] (fig. 25.1).

Symptoms

Sural nerve entrapment causes paresthesiae and pain in this area of distribution. On examination, pressure and percussion along the course of this nerve may reproduce the functional symptoms, in particular on the lateral aspect of the calcaneus near the fibular trochlea [36]. The presence of a mass which is sensitive to palpation is suggestive of the diagnosis [32]. Hypoesthesia is sometimes present in the area supplied by the nerve. Lastly, pain may be produced by plantarflexion in inversion, whereas dorsiflexion alleviates the pain.

Among the radiographs requested, a retrotibial projection of the calcaneus is particularly helpful for better visualization of the fibular trochlea.

Electrical studies are done to search for a neuropathy.

Etiology

The causes of sural nerve entrapment are multiple, and are mainly traumatic [28]:
• wearing of shoes with an excessively rigid back stiffening, especially if the shoes also have high heels,
• post-traumatic malunion of a calcaneal fracture,
• fibrosis after recurrent ankle sprain or other injury,
• excessively prominent fibular trochlea,
• surgery involving the calcaneal tendon or submalleolar region,
• sequel of a diagnostic biopsy, as the sural nerve is the most usual biopsy site and there is a risk of neuroma [25],
• inflammatory tenosynovitis of the fibular tendons,
• synovial cyst,
• neuropathy, diabetic neuropathy in particular.

Differential diagnosis

In addition to neuropathies, the following should be excluded:

• proximal entrapment of the sural nerve where it pierces the deep fascia, especially if the patient wears tight socks, or in myositis ossificans [22, 35]; in this case there are also sensory disturbances on the lateral aspect of the leg and lateral malleolus,

• sinus tarsi syndrome, with pain at the lateral orifice of the sinus, often accompanied by a sensation of instability.

Here again treatment is primarily conservative: suitable footwear, physiotherapy and local injection of corticosteroids. But surgical release is often necessary, especially if there is calcaneal malunion or sequelae after previous surgery [28, 32, 36]. As the sural nerve is purely sensory, it can be excised [28], even up to its origin because of the risk of recurrence. However residual pain is to be feared and suture may be preferred.

● Conclusion

Entrapment neuropathies are certainly rare in the foot. Their diagnosis is difficult and often delayed, because pain and paresthesiae tend to be partial and atypical, the more so as there is great anatomic variation in the sensory distribution of these nerves. In the not uncommon event of failure of conservative treatment, electrical studies can confirm the clinical diagnosis, especially if the tibial nerve or its branches are entrapped at the tarsal tunnel. But this investigation is often very difficult and may be disappointing when entrapment involves a distal branch or a purely sensory nerve. MRI may show a compressive lesion. These investigations make it possible to guide surgical release, which is difficult but generally gives satisfactory results, at least in entrapment in the tarsal tunnel.

References

1. Adelman KA, Wilson G, Wolf JA (1988) Anterior tarsal tunnel syndrome. J Foot Surg 27: 299-302
2. Andresen BL, Wertsch JJ, Stewart WA (1992) Anterior tarsal tunnel syndrome. Arch Phys Med Rehabil 73: 1112-1117
3. Baxter DE, Pfeffer GB (1992) Treatment of chronic heel pain by surgical release of the first branch of the lateral plantar nerve. Clin Orthop 279: 229-236
4. Bonnel F, Briand D, Nicoleau F, Fauré P (1993) Anatomie et biométrie des nerfs sensitifs plantaires. Med Chir Pied 9: 79-84
5. Bonnel F, Janotta P, Briand D, Claustre J, Fauré P (1992) Le nerf fibulaire superficiel au pied (musculo-cutané). Med Chir Pied 8: 95-100
6. Bordelon RL (1983) Subcalcaneal pain. Clin Orthop 177: 49-53
7. Bourrel P, Rey A, Blanc JF, Palinacci JC, Bourges M, Giraudeau P (1976) Syndrome du canal tarsien. À propos de 15 cas "purs" et de 100 cas "associés" à la lèpre ou au diabète. Rev Rhum 43: 723-728
8. Cimino WR (1990) Tarsal tunnel syndrome: review of the literature. Foot Ankle 11: 47-52
9. Dang Vu V, Diébold P, Daemgen F, You B, Jesel M (1995) Intérêt des nouvelles techniques d'exploration électrologique dans le diagnostic des atteintes compressives canalaires ou post-traumatiques des nerfs des pieds. Med Chir Pied 11: 37-44
10. Delagoutte JP, Bonnel F, Claustre J (1989) Syndromes canalaires. In: Delagoutte JP, Bonnel F (eds) Le pied, pathologie et techniques chirurgicales. Masson, Paris, pp 255-259
11. De Lisa JA, Saeed MA (1983) The tarsal tunnel syndrome. Muscle Nerve 6: 664-670
12. Dellon AL (1990) Deep peroneal nerve entrapment on the dorsum of the foot. Foot Ankle 11: 73-79
13. De Stoop N, Suykens S, Goossens M, Coppens M, Badile N, Dewitte A (1989) Tarsal tunnel syndrome: clinical and pathological results. Acta Orthop Belg 55: 461-466
14. Edwards WG, Lincoln CR, Basset FH, Goldner JL (1969) The tarsal tunnel syndrome. JAMA 207: 716-720
15. Enjalbert M, Heerisson C, Claustre J, Bonnel F, Simon L (1988) Le syndrome du nerf musculo-cutané au pied. À propos de dix observations. Rev Rhum 55: 889-893
16. Erickson SJ, Quinn SF, Kneeland JB, Smith JW, Johnson JE, Carrera GF, Shereff MJ, Hyde JS, Jesmanowicz A (1990) MR Imaging of the tarsal tunnel and related spaces: normal and abnormal findings with anatomic correlation. AJR 155: 323-328
17. Felsenthal G, Butler DH, Shear MS (1992) Across-tarsal tunnel motor-nerve conduction technique. Arch Phys Med Rehabil 73: 64-69
18. Frey C, Kerr R (1993) Magnetic resonance imaging and the evaluation of tarsal tunnel syndrome. Foot Ankle 14: 159-164
19. Goodman CR, Kehr LE (1988) Bilateral tarsal tunnel syndrome. A correlative perspective. J Am Podiatr Med Assoc 78: 292-294
20. Grumbine NA, Radovic PA, Parsons R, Scheinin GS (1990) Tarsal tunnel syndrome. Comprehensive review of 87 cases. J Am Podiatr Med Assoc 80: 457-461
21. Havel PE, Ebraheim NA, Clark SE, Jackson WT, Di Dio L (1988) Tibial nerve branching in the tarsal tunnel. Foot Ankle 9: 117-119

22. Husson JL, Mathieu M, Briand B, Meadeb J, Barumbi O, Masse A (1989) Le syndrome de compression du nerf saphène externe (ou nerf suralis). Acta Orthop Belg 55: 491-497

23. Jackson DL, Haglund B (1991) Tarsal tunnel syndrome in athletes, case reports and literature review. Am J Sports Med 19: 61-65

24. Johnson EW (1993) Electrodiagnostic aspects of diabetic neuropathies: entrapments. Muscle Nerve 16: 127-134

25. Landry ME (1991) Peripheral nerve disorders. In: Levy LA, Hetherington VJ (eds) Principles and practice of podiatric medecine. Churchill Livingstone, Edinburgh, pp 377-421

26. Lee B, Crowhurst JA (1987) Entrapment neuropathy of the first metatarsophalangeal joint. J Am Podiatr Med Assoc 77: 657-659

27. Levin KH, Stevens JC, Daube JR (1986) Superficial peroneal nerve conduction studies for electromyographic diagnosis. Muscle Nerve 9: 322-326

28. Myerson M, Quill GE (1993) Late complications of fractures of the calcaneus. J Bone Joint Surg 75A: 331-341

29. Myerson M, Soffer S (1989) Lipoma as an etiology of tarsal tunnel syndrome: a report of two cases. Foot Ankle 10: 176-179

30. Oh SJ, Arnold TW, Park KH, Kim DE (1991) Electrophysiological improvement following decompression surgery in tarsal tunnel syndrome. Muscle Nerve 14: 407-410

31. Perlman P (1991) Podiatric sports medicine. In: Levy A, Hetherington VJ (eds) Principles and practice of podiatric medicine. Churchill Livingstone, Edinburgh, pp 647-666

32. Pringle RM, Protheroe K, Mukherjee SK (1974) Entrapment neuropathy of the sural nerve. J Bone Joint Surg 56B: 465-468

33. Przylucki H, Jones CL (1981) Entrapment neuropathy of muscle branch of lateral plantar nerve: cause of heel pain. J Am Podiatr Assoc 71: 119-125

34. Radin EL (1983) Tarsal tunnel syndrome. Clin Orthop 181: 167-170

35. Shaffrey ME, Jane JA, Persing JA, Shaffrey CI, Phillips LH (1992) Surgeon's foot: a report of sural nerve palsy. Neurosurgery 30: 927-930

36. Schon LC, Baxter DE (1990) Neuropathies of the foot and ankle in athletes. Clin Sports Med 9: 489-509

37. Schon LC, Glennon TP, Baxter DE (1993) Heel pain syndrome: electro-diagnostic support for nerve entrapment. Foot Ankle 14: 129-135

38. Stern DS, Joyce MT (1989) Tarsal tunnel syndrome: a review of 15 surgical procedures. J Foot Surg 28: 290-294

39. Valtin D, Azorin M, Meyer O, Bigot B (1992) La compression du nerf plantaire latéral, une cause de douleur plantaire. Med Chir Pied 8: 49-53

40. Vanderstraeten G (1989) Entrapment neuropathies of the foot. Electromyographic techniques. Acta Orthop Belg 55: 451-455

41. Zeiss J, Fenton P, Ebraheim N, Coombs RJ (1990) Normal magnetic resonance anatomy of the tarsal tunnel. Foot Ankle 10: 214-218

42. Zeiss J, Fenton P, Ebraheim N, Coombs RJ (1991) Magnetic resonance imaging for ineffectual tarsal tunnel surgical treatment. Clin Orthop 264: 264-266

43. Zuckerman JD, Powers B, Miller JW, Lippert F (1988) Benign solitary schwannoma of the foot. Clin Orthop 228: 278-280

44. Zuckermann JD, Powers B, Miller JW, Lippert F (1988) Benign solitary schwannoma of the foot. Clin Orthop 228: 278-280

Additional references

45. Carrel JM, Davidson DM, Goldstein KT (1994) Observations on 200 surgical cases of tarsal tunnel syndrome. Clin Podiatr Med Surg 11: 609-616

46. Day FN, Naples JJ (1994) Tarsal tunnel syndrome: an endoscopic approach with 4- to 28- month follow-up. J Foot Ankle Surg 33: 244-248

47. Galardi G, Amadio S, Maderna L, Meraviglia MV, Brunati L, Dal Conte G, Comi G (1994) Electrophysiologic studies in tarsal tunnel syndrome. Diagnostic reliability of motor distal latency, mixed nerve and sensory nerve conduction studies. Am J Phys Med Rehabil 73: 193-198

48. Klein MA, Sreitzer AM (1993) MR Imaging of the tarsal sinus and canal: normal anatomy, pathologic findings, and features of the sinus tarsi syndrome. Radiology 186: 233-240

49. Mahan KT, Rock JJ, Hillstrom HJ (1996) Tarsal tunnel syndrome. A retrospective study. J Am Podiatr Med Assoc 86: 81-91

50. Pfeiffer WH, Cracchiolo A (1994) Clinical results after tarsal tunnel decompression. J Bone and Joint Surg 76A: 1222-1230

51. Schon LC (1994) Nerve entrapment, neuropathy and nerve dysfonction in athletes. Orthop Clin North Am: 47-59

26.

Stress fractures of the foot and ankle

J Bernard, L Zabraniecki, A Constantin and A Thomas

Introduction

As early as 1887, before the era of radiology, Pauzat linked painful swelling of the dorsum of the foot, occurring after marching, with metatarsal lesions [34]. He was the first to describe "bone injury due to stress". A century later, in the era of MRI, diagnosis remains clinical.

In 1975, Devas published a book on stress fractures which is still a reference work [10]. This subject is topical because it is related to the present enthusiasm for physical and sporting activity in a Western population with a sedentary life-style, and because this pathology is a true "experimental model" for the study of bone tissue and its capacity to react to intense, repeated exertion.

These fractures are the late consequence of the pathology of adaptation of bone to stress. They have an important place in microtraumatology related to physical, sporting and military activity.

Although they may occur at any age, they are distinct from spontaneous fractures of the aged subject. The underlying bone is healthy, and the dominant etiologic factor is recent, repetitive and intensive physical activity. In certain circumstances, it is difficult to distinguish the roles played by physical activity on the one hand and by bone insufficiency on the other. This situates the limitations of the subject.

Pathophysiology

An essential quality of bone tissue is the capacity of adapting to the stresses to which it is regularly submitted (Wolff's law). Mechanical forces stimulate remodeling; locally, the resistance of the bone subjected to stress increases [Frost's "mechanostat", 19]. A stress fracture occurs when these capacities for local adaptation are exceeded; intensive, repetitive and unaccustomed physical activity leads to vascular lesions in the areas where stress is concentrated [4, 26], changes in the architecture of collagen fibers [7], osteocyte necrosis and primary osteoclastosis followed by periosteal and endosteal bone formation. It is imbalance between these destructive lesions due to overload and the capacity for bone repair which leads secondarily to a microfissure and then a stress fracture [2, 9, 15, 23].

Areas of stress concentration are specific to the kind of physical activity in a given morphologic type. Load distribution differs according to whether the subject has flat or high-arched feet, or is walking, running or jumping [2, 18]. No morphologic type is particularly at risk or is particularly immune from stress fractures [14]; it is the way in which the foot is used that causes injury.

Risk factors

Mechanical properties, together with bone mass and size, intervene in the occurrence of stress injury. These factors vary from one individual to another, and in the same individual during life. Sudden change in physical activity is the prime factor, but knowledge of the following factors help to determine those who, in a population living under the same conditions, are likely to be affected:

• in the child bone tissue is more elastic, so that this lesion is less frequent in children [15, 33];

• acquired cell insufficiency and low response of bone tissue to stimuli in aged subjects make them more liable to fracture, particularly if a new physical activity is undertaken [24];

• genetic studies have made it possible to determine differences in bone mass from one individual to another, within the same sex or the same race, or between sexes and between races [36]. In a sporting or a military setting, low bone mass is a risk factor; women are more at risk than men, and Caucasians more than blacks [5, 6, 32, 37, 38];

• narrow anteroposterior tibial width increases the likelihood of stress fractures [20];

• muscle and bone form a composite entity [39]. Muscle mass and its physiologic state contribute to bone resistance [16]. Low muscle mass is a risk factor [8];

• life-style, either sedentary or with regular physical activity, conditions the maintenance of muscle and bone mass and architecture. Sedentary life is a risk factor [6, 28];

• daily calcium intake plays an important role in building up maximal bone stock and in its maintenance, a major factor in its resistance to stress. It has been demonstrated that low calcium intake is an important risk factor [27].

Circumstances of occurrence

Increased physical activity

• Vigorous games learnt by the young child at school;
• young military recruits during the first six weeks of army physical training;
• rapid resumption of training by an athlete after a period of inactivity;
• the "aging athlete" keeping up a high level of training in spite of progressive age-related decrease in bone and muscle mass;
• the "active sedentary" person starting "active retirement".

Changes in load distribution

• The child who progresses from crawling to standing on both feet;
• stereotyped technical movements in the accomplished athlete (a jump, dance-step, rhythm of track running);

• change from a sport where there is relatively little stress on the skeleton to one with increased bone stress (e.g., from swimming to long distance running, from cycling to playing football);
• change in footwear or running surface;
• change in gait related to a foot injury;
• prescription of orthotic devices;
• overenthusiastic rehabilitation following a long period of immobilization of the leg or foot after corrective surgery or for a muscle-wasting disorder [17].

Clinical features

The clinical features of stress fractures of the foot and ankle are characteristic. Symptoms at onset are pain or mere discomfort, causing little disability and occurring on exertion; an impression of "narrow shoes" or "tightness round the ankle" has been reported. If exercise is continued, pain increases and appears as soon as weight-bearing is attempted, subsides with rest, and is regularly accompanied by swelling over the affected part. Functional disability is moderate.

The worried patient spontaneously reduces weight-bearing to some extent and healing is obtained after a month. Diagnosis is delayed if these initial symptoms, a true fracture prodrome with normal X-rays, go unrecognized. The soldier and the motivated athlete may disregard pain for the sake of performance. Sharp pain then sets in, preventing sleep, with major functional disability and ecchymosis, confirming the diagnosis of complete fracture with displacement. After some days of non-weight-bearing, the pain will no longer prevent sleep. Pain becomes chronic, preventing any sporting activity. Palpation at a later stage reveals bony callus, the sign of exuberant bone repair. This picture corresponds to the course of incomplete fractures.

Methods of diagnosis

Clinical

The history provides details of occurrence and functional symptoms.

Physical examination determines the morphologic type, and the presence of swelling or ecchymosis.

Careful palpation of each segment of all the bones of the lower limbs is essential for diagnosis: there is exquisite tenderness, comparable to that described when weight-bearing is attempted. Palpation frequently reveals associated tender points in the other bones of the foot, tibiae, femora and pelvis.

The joints adjacent to the painful point are free and symmetric; their movement is painful only if the fracture is adjacent to the joint (distal tibial epiphysis, talus). Later, the presence of callus completes the picture for superficial bones.

Conventional radiology

Normal radiographs at the onset of symptoms are a finding which contributes to the diagnosis. This is demonstrated in the prospective study of Greaney: only 28% of clinical and scintigraphy fractures in his series were confirmed by radiology at the outset, and 54% on repeat X-rays. X-rays continue to be normal if the condition is diagnosed early and if relief of the affected limb is rapid [21].

The fracture line is the first radiologic sign to appear. It is almost always impossible to reveal on plain X-rays in trabecular bones (navicular, base of the metatarsals, talus, calcaneus, cuboid, distal tibial epiphysis).

In cortical bone (metatarsals, fibula, distal tibial epiphysis) multiple views are required (oblique and partial), and when the fracture line is revealed it can be likened to a "hair lying on a piece of porcelain". A complete fracture, with or without displacement, bears witness to late diagnosis.

Images of fracture repair appear secondarily. They are often the only ones to be described, sometimes "pointing a finger" at the fracture line.

In cortical bones, there may be only slight periosteal layering if de-stressing is early. Conversely, massive irregular callus appears when the patient has continued walking on the fracture for a long period. After several months, the image evolves towards a spindle shape with regular thickening of the cortical bone.

In trabecular bone, a band of sclerosis appears perpendicular to the lines of force. It is even more evident when diagnosis is late and a long bone is involved.

Bone scintigraphy

Bone scanning with technetium-99m is extremely sensitive, but is indicated only if there is doubt as to clinical diagnosis, normal X-rays, and an at-risk location. All bones subjected to stress should be scanned; comparative images of the bones of the feet should be requested. At an early stage, scintigraphy reveals a poorly-outlined focal area of increased uptake over the painful segment of bone. At a later stage, the area of increased uptake delineates the fracture.

Asymptomatic focal areas of increased uptake in other zones where exercise-related stresses concentrate are often seen in association. These are a diagnostic argument. Maladaptation of bone to stress is most often multifocal [42]. Should one admit, like Greaney [21] and Milgrom [31], that these asymptomatic areas are stress fractures? Do they not simply reflect vascular phenomena involved in the adaptation of bone to stress? [4].

Modern imaging techniques

Recourse to modern imaging techniques such as CT and MRI should be exceptional.

They have two major advantages:
• they prevent one bone being hidden by another, increase spatial resolution and offer the possibility of multiple sections, thus more easily revealing the fracture line;
• they allow investigation of soft tissues and so are an essential element in differential diagnosis.

On CT the fracture line is seen as hypodense, often surrounded by a hyperdense area (trabecular bone) or periosteal apposition (cortical bone). MRI reveals the fracture line as a low signal intensity in T1- and T2-weighted images. There is also often swelling around the fracture, which is seen as decreased signal intensity in T1, becoming increased signal intensity in T2.

Bone densitometry

This reliable tool for determining bone mass, fat mass and lean mass is of particular interest in epidemiology, and has shown that low bone mass and low lean mass are two risk factors for stress fractures [8]. This measurement is of minimal value for the individual; it must be done when there are multiple stress fractures and long bones are involved, when there is little relation between the physical activity practiced and the injury incurred, or when, in a regular athlete, these injuries cannot be explained by the circumstances. This investigation detects demineralizing bone disorders and changes in bone status in the athlete, whether these arise from physical activity [5, 13], or are age-related [1].

Frequency and distribution of stress fractures

The incidence of stress fractures varies greatly from one study to another. This variation is related to differences in definition, which may be clinical and radiologic, or clinical and scintigraphic, or scintigraphic alone, and also linked to the type of physical activity undertaken, diagnostic techniques and the prospective or retrospective nature of the studies.

In an athletic context, all stress fractures taken together represent 6 to 10% of the injuries diagnosed. They are the fourth cause of disability in this group. No prospective study has been carried out [14, 22, 28, 33].

In a military context, comparison between the retrospective study of Brudvig (1.3 %) [6] and the prospective study of Milgrom (31%) [31] is very instructive. This marked difference in studies of populations with a comparable mode of life shows that these injuries are only rarely diagnosed. This is because the natural course of the disorder is towards spontaneous healing, and is also due to ignorance of the prefracture syndrome and to differences in diagnostic methods. Brudvig's retrospective study used scintigraphy only exceptionally. Milgrom used it routinely and also informed the recruits and training personnel, creating ideal conditions for early diagnosis. Thus Milgrom, and also Greaney, reported a large number of stress injuries in trabecular bones such as the talus, navicular and the base of the metatarsals, which are practically never reported in

Table 26.1. Ninety-eight young military recruits admitted to hospital for stress fracture: comparison of clinical, radiologic and scintigraphic locations

Painful area		Radiologic site		Scan-positive site
Proximal lower limb	18	Femoral neck	13	19
		Acetabulum	1	4
Buttock	3	Ischiopubic ramus	4	6
Thigh	1	Femoral diaphysis	0	3
Knee	7	Tibial plateau	8	10
Leg	33	Proximal 1/3 tibial diaphysis	8	2
		Mid 1/3 tibial diaphysis	15	28
Ankle	13	Distal 1/3 tibial diaphysis	2	4
		Tibial epiphysis	5	12
		Distal 1/3 fibula	3	3
		Talus	1	3
Heel	21	Calcaneus	24	36
Instep	10	Navicular bone	2	10
		Cuboid bone	0	2
Forefoot	17	1st metatarsal.	1	2
		2nd metatarsal	6	6
		3rd metatarsal.	7	7
		4th metatarsal	0	0
		5th metatarsal	1	1
		Sesamoid bone	1	1
TOTAL	123		102	177

retrospective studies. Similarly, these two studies, based on the same definition and the same diagnostic modalities, indicate that differences in footwear and training lead to the same pathology but at different sites. While calcaneal fractures predominate in Greaney's study, they are exceptional in Milgrom's work.

In the majority of these studies, while the tibia is most often involved, fractures of the foot and ankle taken together come in second place before the femur. The relative frequency of the various sites of the foot and ankle also varies considerably from one study to another [29]. McBryde [28], in long-distance runners, found that 55% of fractures were metatarsal; 30% involved the fibula and 9% the distal third of the tibial diaphysis. The remaining 4% comprised the calcaneus, talus, navicular and sesamoid bones.

In our military experience over three years, we report the clinical, scintigraphic and radiologic findings in 98 young recruits with stress fractures (table 26.1). These total 123 clinical lesions, 102 X-ray images and 177 scintigraphy scans. Distribution between lesions in the foot and ankle and those at higher levels was even. Calcaneal fractures represented one-third of all lesions, followed by the metatarsals and the navicular bone.

Fracture sites and characteristics

Metatarsals: this is the best-known location (fig. 26.1). The injury presents as pain on weight-bearing and pressure with swelling of the dorsum of the foot. The second and third metatarsals are most often affected; involvement of the fourth and fifth is rare but regularly described. Involvement of the first metatarsal usually goes unrecognized because it is situated at the base, in a trabecular area. Fractures of the diaphyses and necks of the metatarsals associate a fracture line and periosteal apposition, while fractures of the base appear late as a band of bone condensation [14, 29, 30].

Calcaneal injury is indicated by heel tenderness on pressure applied with two fingers to the submalleolar area. Swelling makes the wearing of shoes difficult. Such fractures are often bilateral and may also be multiple in the same calcaneus. X-rays show layered bands of bone condensation perpendicular to the lines of force [21].

Navicular bone: here, stress fracture was long overlooked but diagnosis is easy. On weight-bearing, the medial aspect of the instep is painful and swollen. Initial X-rays are routinely normal. Scintigraphy in prospective studies has shown its high incidence [21, 40].

Cuboid bone and cuneiforms: these locations have been described since the use and improved definition of CT technique.

Talus: the sign of a talar fracture is ankle pain with swelling of the anterior aspect of the talocrural joint. CT reveals images of trabecular bone reconstruction above the trochlea [12].

Sesamoid fracture leads to pain on weight-bearing with swelling below the head of the first metatarsal.

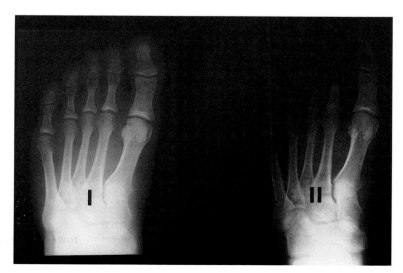

Fig. 26.1. Stress fracture of the left third metatarsal. Pain and swelling on the dorsal aspect. Point of exquisite tenderness in the distal third of the diaphysis of the third metatarsal. X-ray day 1: (**I**) no anomaly; X-ray day 45: (**II**) bony callus

In this location, scintigraphy is easy to use. At the stage of complicated fracture, the irregular fracture line, together with the pain and increased isotope uptake exclude the diagnosis of a bipartite sesamoid bone [11].

First phalanx: difficulties in revealing this fracture by radiography are the same as in all the trabecular bones of the foot [41].

Fibula: this fracture, the so-called fracture of the long-distance runner, is revealed by discomfort at the junction of the lower and middle thirds of the leg, with overlying swelling. The fracture line, which is oblique, cortical and often partial, is very difficult to demonstrate.

Tibia: involvement of the distal third of the tibial diaphysis is very similar to that of the fibula. It is revealed by pain in the upper ankle, difficult to locate on palpation but of frankly mechanical character. A band of late bone condensation perpendicular to the long axis of this bone confirms the diagnosis, which can sometimes be clinically difficult.

Clinical forms

Multifocal fractures (fig. 26.2): in a context of new, intensive and repetitive physical activity, lesions are frequently bilateral (calcaneus, metatarsal) and several sites are often involved (tibia, femur, pelvis). Often, the functional signs may be predominately local, but questioning and systematic palpation segment by segment of the bones under stress will reveal the multifocal involvement which, in this context, is an argument in favor of the diagnosis. Military recruits are typical of this clinical model.

Solitary fractures: the athlete who changes from a stereotyped technical movement to correct gait or stride will often present unifocal symptoms. This recent change in load distribution will alert the physician.

Latent forms: asymptomatic stress fractures are discovered in association with fractures which are both clinically and radiologically evident. They are scintigraphic and radiologic findings. The fact that latent forms exist is further proof that these fractures are greatly underestimated.

Differential diagnosis

Analysis of the circumstances in which injury occurred, together with the clinical and radiologic findings, will generally lead to a positive diagnosis. Use of scintigraphy in doubtful cases leaves little room for differential diagnosis.

• In traumatic fractures which were "undeserved", because trauma was slight and bone mass was normal, there may have been prior damage which led to secondary decompensation with fracture.

• Conversely, if fractures occur in sites with high resistance or after moderate physical exertion, the possibility of **insufficiency fractures** [9] should be considered. These are particularly frequent in elderly subjects. The clinical presentation is similar, but their primary cause is a marked decrease in bone mass and not intense physical activity. Location in the foot or ankle may be the first fracture leading to a diagnosis of osteoporosis, established after X-ray and bone density measurement. The underlying cause (corticotherapy, monoclonal gammapathy, endocrine disorder, postmenopause) should be sought in order to institute specific treatment [25]. It may be a new fracture site in known osteoporosis, an indication of inadequate treatment, or an iatrogenic complication in the case of fluoride treatment [33];

• In exceptional cases, the possibility of a tumor may be considered; an osteoid osteoma may be revealed in the course of intensive physical activity. Clinical study, a therapeutic trial with aspirin, scintigraphy findings and modern imaging techniques allow secure diagnosis.

• Thanks to the new imaging techniques for soft tissue investigation, any tumoral malignancy can be excluded.

Clinical course

If the presenting symptoms of involvement of the base of the fifth metatarsal and the medial sesamoid bone go unrecognized, the result will be complete fracture with displacement and no tendency to spontaneous consolidation. The pull of the ligamentous attachments hinders this [14].

Untreated fractures of the navicular bone progress towards pseudarthrosis. This is due to the vascular pattern peculiar to this bone [40]. In other locations, if

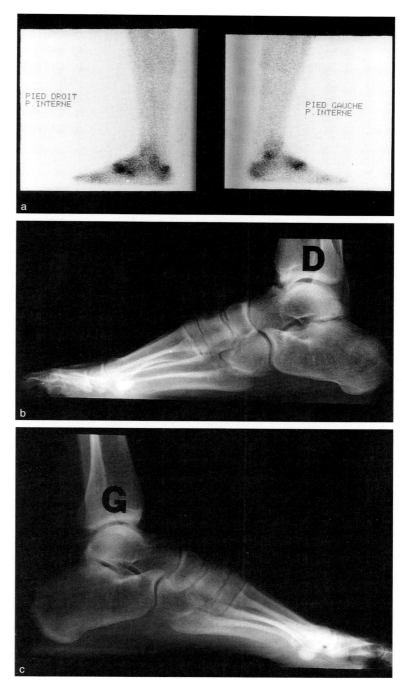

Fig. 26.2. Multiple stress fractures of both feet after ten days of intensive marching. Bilateral heel pain and pain at the antero-lateral aspect of the right mid-foot. **a** Scintigraphy: increased uptake in both calcanei and both cuboid bones, predominating on the right (+ 36 %). **b, c** Comparative X-rays of both feet: an isolated band of sclerosis in the right calcaneus

exercise is continued, healing will take place with pain and the formation of massive, irregular callus.

Because of the secondary appearance of underlying lesions in the large bones of the lower limbs, which can take a serious course, stress fractures of the foot and ankle have been called "sentinel locations" [3].

An algodystrophic syndrome in the sequelae of stress fractures is not exceptional. The revelation by MRI of microfissures in algodystrophic bones of primary appearance raises the question of cause or consequence.

Treatment

The treatment of overuse injury of the foot and ankle depends on the clinical and radiologic stage at which the diagnosis is made.

At the prefracture stage, with clinical symptoms and normal X-rays, relative relief with crutches and partial weight-bearing maintains minimal mechanical stimulus. Signs of bone reconstruction appear rapidly.

If an "at-risk site" is involved (sesamoid bones, navicular bone, fifth metatarsal), non-weight-bearing is mandatory until swelling and tenderness have subsided. At the late fracture stage, when spontaneous consolidation seems possible, total relief from weight-bearing, without a cast, is prescribed for an average period of 45 days. If complications arise, whether pseudarthrosis of the navicular, displaced fracture of the fifth metatarsal or complete fracture of the sesamoid bone, the opinion of a surgeon should be sought. The surgeon should be informed of the relative fragility of the bone fragments, which makes osteosynthesis more problematic. A medial sesamoid bone will generally be excised.

Prevention

Knowledge of optimal conditions for the adaptation of bone to stress makes it possible to prevent this lesion appearing. Progressivity and variety in physical training are the two major principles.

The existence of latent forms, the minor clinical nature of the prefracture syndrome, and the frequent course towards spontaneous healing explain the apparent difficulty in diagnosis.

Recent prospective studies using the most efficient diagnostic methods, information of athletes or recruits and those who train them, rigorous physical examination, and routine scintigraphy and radiologic investigation demonstrate the high frequency of this maladaptation of bone to stress, which is probably underestimated by all those responsible for athletic and military training programs.

If these findings are borne in mind, it should be possible to avoid the occurrence of decompensation by fracture, which leads to considerable loss of time for men for whom physical activity is a major factor.

References

1. Aloia JF, Vaswanni A, Ellis K, Yuen K, Cohn SH (1985) A model for involutional bone loss. Lab Clin Med 106: 630-637
2. Baker J, Frankel VH, Burstein A (1972) Fatigue fractures: biomechanical considerations. J Bone Joint Surg 54 A: 1345-1346
3. Bernard J (1988) Pathologie d'adaptation de l'os à l'effort: douleurs osseuses d'effort et fracture de fatigue. Encycl Med Chir (Paris France), Appareil locomoteur, 15904 A, 10, 4
4. Bernard J, Mazières B, Blasco A, Zenoun A (1990) Study of intraosseous changes in seven patients with stress fracture. In: Arlet, Mazieres B (eds) Bone circulation and bone necrosis. Springer Verlag, Heidelberg, pp 267-272
5. Bilanin JE, Blancharms S, Russel-Cohen E (1989) Lower vertebral bone density in male long distance runners. Med Sci Sports Exerc 21: 66-70
6. Brudvig TJ, Gudger TD, Obermeyer L (1983) Stress fractures in 295 trainees: a one-year study of incidence as related to age, sex, and race. Milit Med 148: 666-667
7. Chamay A (1980) Les fractures de fatigue: clinique, biomécanique, histopathologie. Considération sur l'hypertrophie d'adaptation. Rev Med Suisse Romande 100: 855-861
8. Comas JM, Anne D, Charrot F, Telmon N, Benazet JF, Ribot C, Pouilles JM, Bernard J (1992) Ostéodensitométrie corps entier : étude de la composition corporelle de jeunes recrues souffrant de douleur osseuse et de fracture de fatigue. Med et Armées 20: 603-607
9. Daffner RH (1978) Stress fractures: current concepts. Skeletal Radiol 2: 221-229
10. Devas MB (1975) Stress fracture. Churchill Livingstone, Edinburgh
11. Dietzen CJ (1990) Great toe sesamoid injuries in the athlete. Orthop Rev 19: 966-972
12. Doury P, Pattin S, Granier R (1984) Données nouvelles sur "les fractures de fatigue". À propos d'une observation de fracture bilatérale de l'astragale. Intérêt de la scintigraphie osseuse dans le diagnostic des fractures de fatigue. Rev Rhum 51: 483-486
13. Drinkwater BL, Nilson K, Ott S, Chesnut Ch (1986) Bone mineral density after resumption of menses in amenorrheic athletes. JAMA 2: 256-280
14. Eisele SA, Sammarco GJ, (1993) Fatigue Fractures of the foot and ankle in the athlete. J Bone Joint Surg Am 75: 290-298
15. Engh CA, Robinson RA, Milgrom (1970) Stress fractures in children. Trauma 10: 532-540

16. Fernandez - Fairen M. (1983) Le complexe os-tendon-muscle considéré comme entité biomécanique (1983) Acta Orthop Belg 49: 13-29

17. Ford LT, Gilula LA (1977) Stress fracture of the middle metatarsals following the Keller operation. J Bone Joint Surg (Am) 59: 117

18. Frankel VH (1978) Editorial comment. Am J Sports Med 6: 396

19. Frost HM (1987) Bone mass and the mechanostat: a proposal. Anat Rec 219: 1-9

20. Giladi M, Milgrom C, Simkin A, Stein M, Kashtan H, Margulies J, Rand N, Chisin R, Steinberg R, Aharonson Z, Kedem R, Frankel VH (1987) Stress fractures and tibial bone width. A risk factor of bone. J Surg 9B: 326-329

21. Greaney RB, Gerber FH, Laughlin RI, Kmet JP, Metz CD, Kilcheski TS, Rao BR, Silverman (1983) Distribution and natural history of stress fractures in US. Marine recruits. Radiology 146: 339-346

22. Ha KJ, Hahn SH, Chung M, Yang BK,Yi SR (1991) A clinical study of stress fractures in sports activities. Orthopedic Surg 14: 1089-1095

23. Johnson LC, Strafford HT, Geis RW (1963) Histogenesis of stress fractures. J Bone Joint Surg (Am) 45 A: 1542

24. Lanyon LE, Rubin CT (1983) Regulation of bone mass in response to physical activity. In: Discon A, Russel RGG, Stamp TCB (eds) Osteoporosis, a multidisciplinary problem. London Royal Society of Medicine. International congress séries 55: 51-56

25. Lechevalier D, Magnin J, Eulry F (1994) Huit fractures par insuffisance osseuse des têtes métatarsiennes. Med Chir Pied 10: 40-43

26. Li G, Zhang S, Chen G, Wang A (1985) Radiographic and histologic analyses of stress fracture in rabbit tibias. Am J Sports Med 13: 285-294

27. Markovic V, Kostial K, Simonivoc I, Buzina R, Brodrec A, Nordin B (1979) Bone status and fracture rates in two region of Yugolsavia. Am J Clin Nutr 32: 540-549

28. Mc Bryde J (1988) Stress fracture in runner. In: D'Ambrosia, Drez D (eds) Running injuries. Slack, New Jersey, pp 43-82

29. Meurman KOA (1981) Less common stress fractures in the foot. Br J Radiol 54, 637 1-7

30. Micheli LJ, Sohn RS, Solomon R (1985) Stress fractures of the second metatarsal involving Lisfranc's joint in ballet dancers. A new overuse injury of the foot. J Bone Joint Surg 67A: 1372-1375

31. Milgrom C, Giladi M, Stein M, Kashtan H, Margulies JY, Chisin R, Steinberg R, Aharonson (1990) Stress fractures in military recruits. A prospective study showing an unusually high incidence. Ann Intern Med 113: 754-759

32. Myburgh KH, Hutchins J, Fataar AB, Hough SF, Noakes TD (1990) Low bone density is an etiologic factor for stress fractures in athletes. Ann Intern Med 113: 754-759

33. Orava S, Jormakka E, Hulklo A (1981) Stress fractures in young athletes. Arch Orthop Trauma Surg 98: 271-274

34. Orcel Ph, Prier A, Crouzet J, Kaplan G (1987) Fissures et fractures spontanées des membres inférieurs chez des ostéoporotiques traités par fluorure de sodium. Nouv Presse Med 16: 571-575

35. Pauzat JE (1887) De la périostite ostéoplastique des métatarsiens à la suite des marches. Arch Med Pharm milit 10: 337-367

36. Politzer WS, Anderson JJB (1989) Ethnic and genetic differences in bone mass: a review with a hereditary vs environmental perspective. Am J Clin Nutr 50: 1244-1259

37. Pouilles JM, Bernard J, Tremollieres F, Louvet JP, Ribot C (1989). Femoral bone density in young male adults with stress fractures. Bone 10: 105-108

38. Protzman RR, Griffs CG (1977) Stress fractures in men and women undergoing military training. J Bone Joint Surg (Am.) 59 A: 825

39. Rabischong P, Avril J (1965) Rôle biomécanique des poutres composites os-muscles. Rev Chir Orthop 51: 437-458

40. Torg JS, Pavlov H, Cooley LH, Bryant MH, Arnoczky SP, Bergfeld J, Hunter LY (1982) Stress fractures of the tarsal navicular. A retrospective review of twenty one cases. J Bone Joint Surg 64A: 700-712

41. Yokoe K, Mannoji T (1986) Stress fracture of the proximal phalanx of the great toe. A report of three cases. Am J Sports Med 14: 240-242

42. Zwas S, Elkanovitch R, Frank G (1987) Interpretation and classification of bone scintigraphic findings in stress fractures. Nucl Med 28: 452-457

27.

Sprains of the ankle

J Rodineau and P Thoreux

Introduction

The ankle and foot have a two-fold function: a static function in weight-bearing and a dynamic function in propulsion.

The talocrural joint consists of the tibio-fibular mortice and the wedge of the talus. This is a hinge joint with only one degree of freedom, in the sagittal plane. It has a single working axis, slightly oblique backwards and outwards, permitting only movements of dorsiflexion (or flexion) and plantarflexion (or extension).

The joint is a very congruent one. Its congruence is ensured passively by the lateral ligaments, and actively by the periarticular muscles. The lateral collateral ligament (LCL) consists of 3 bands. The anterior talofibular ligament (ATFL) extends from the anterior border of the lateral malleolus to the neck of the talus, following a horizontal course forwards and inwards. The calcaneofibular ligament (CFL) is attached to the tip of the lateral malleolus and passes downwards and backwards to end above and behind the peroneal trochlea on the lateral aspect of the calcaneus. The posterior talofibular ligament (PTFL) extends from the lateral malleolus to the posterior margin of the body of the talus following a horizontal course backwards and inwards. The medial collateral ligament (MCL) consists of two layers: the deep layer stretches obliquely downwards and inwards from the medial malleolus to the medial aspect of the talus and the superficial layer, or deltoid ligament, stretches from the tip of the medial malleolus to the medial aspect of the talus, the small apophysis of the calcaneus and the upper aspect of the navicular bone.

The lateral and medial collateral ligaments are the real structures containing the talocrural joint, whereas the articular capsule is very loose at its anterior and posterior parts.

A lesion of the lateral ligaments is always produced by indirect mechanisms and involves the LCL almost exclusively. This ligament is damaged during forced movements in varus, equino-varus or inversion of the foot, which may exert their effects on all three bundles, giving rise to sprains of increasing severity from before backwards. The anterior bundle is the first to be involved, often associated with a lesion of the anterior capsule. The severity of the sprain is increased by rupture of the middle band (CFL), an isolated lesion which is possible but infrequent. Rupture of the posterior band is more rarely found, but may occur in combination with that of the anterior and middle bundles, or separately in a mechanism of forced dorsiflexion. A lesion of the MCL alone is rare and occurs most often in the context of a fracture of the lateral malleolus, when it is the equivalent of a fracture of the medial malleolus. The anterior capsule may be injured in a movement of forced plantarflexion and the lesion may trespass laterally on the ATFL and the anterior part of the deltoid ligament, producing an anterior sprain of the ankle. It may be associated with a rupture of the anterior tibiofibular ligament (ATFL) and a lesion of the superior talonavicular ligament.

The congruence of the talocrural articulation is also ensured by the collective action of the periarticular muscles: extensor digitorum longus, extensor hallucis longus and tibialis anterior on the anterior aspect; the peroneus longus and brevis on the lateral aspect; the tibialis posterior and flexor digitorum longus on the medial aspect; the triceps surae at the posterior aspect. Stabilization in the sagittal plane is ensured by the anterior muscle group, notably the tibialis anterior, and the posterior muscle group, especially the triceps surae. Stabilization in the frontal plane is dependent mainly on the peroneus brevis, which ensures lateral stability, and by the tibialis posterior, which ensures medial stability. The peroneus brevis produces recoil and ascension of the medial arch by direct traction; it activates all the mechanisms of eversion. The tibialis posterior acts by using the navicular bone as a patella; it activates all the mechanisms of inversion. A lesion of these muscles, especially of the lateral stabilizers, whether of neurologic, truncal, radicular or traumatic origin - rupture, dislocation or subluxation of the terminal tendon - is indicated by ankle instability, quite apart from any ligamentous laxity. Recognition of such lesions in the global context of ankle instability is therefore absolutely essential to the proper conduct of treatment.

From the anatomic and physiologic aspects, the talocrural articulation is closely linked to the subtalar and medio-tarsal articulations. This implies that a lesion of the talocrural joint may often be associated with a concomitant lesion of one or other of these articulations, especially during inversion mechanisms, which combine varus in the frontal plane, adduction in the horizontal plane, and equinus in the sagittal plane. It is therefore necessary to investigate these in every indirect injury of the ankle in order to establish a complete lesional diagnosis. This is the more necessary since these articulations, especially the calcaneocuboid articulation, may be damaged apart from any involvement of the talocrural joint, giving rise to problems of differential diagnosis which are the more important since their treatment is quite specific .

● Lateral ankle sprains

Lateral ankle sprains are very common in athletics and present a number of problems in diagnosis and treatment. The three main errors are the following:
• to class under the same heading lesions as different as a simple ligamentous stretching or a complete rupture of the entire lateral capsuloligamentous layer;
• to confuse a sprain of the ankle with other injuries such as a fracture of the dome of the talus, disloca-

tion of the peroneal tendons, or avulsion of the styloid process of the 5th metatarsal;
• to institute an all-purpose treatment, independent of the mildness or severity of the ligamentous lesions.

These three traps may be avoided by a triple precaution:
• careful questioning of the injured patient,
• meticulous examination,
• radiographic assessment guided by the clinical findings.

Interrogational data

These are a source of information of cardinal importance.

The conditions in which an ankle sprain may occur are extremely varied, ranging from a simple stumble in walking to landing from a jump. Too strict a parallel should not be drawn between the severity of the injury and the presumed gravity of the lesion.

Perception of crepitus or a feeling of a tear are good evidence of a severe lesion.

The painful reactions which accompany and follow a lateral sprain vary in intensity. During the accident it is quite usual to feel pain, but the course of this pain may give useful information. Usually, the initial pain is followed by some degree of relative comfort, and then, some hours later, by the reappearance of painful tension. In ligamentous ruptures the course of events may assume two aspects: either progressively increasing pain, or quite marked freedom from pain subsequent to the severe initial pain, uncomplicated by the delayed development of painful phenomena.

Swelling which develops within a few minutes in front of and below the malleolus constitutes the most reliable evidence of a severe lesion. This sign indicates at least a tear of the ATFL and part of the anterior capsule (AC). In a sprain of moderate severity, ecchymosis rarely appears before 24 hours and remains localized. In severe forms it appears much earlier and rapidly reaches the forefoot and lower leg. Periarticular swelling, which occurs at a variable period after the injury and reaches a maximum in 36-48 hours, does not seem to be, at least in itself, a good criterion of severity.

The degree of functional impairment may sometimes vary in parallel with the severity of the lesion, but is far from always being strictly proportional. In fact, once past the initial phase, the functional handicap experienced by the injured person may be moderate in some severe sprains and more marked in some milder sprains.

Physical examination

Clinical examination is of considerable importance and its value should not be underestimated, nor its difficulty.

Inspection includes checking for an abnormal position of the foot, swelling and bruising.

Palpation aims to detect any anterolateral capsuloligamentous dehiscence, which is formal evidence of a severe lesion.

Study of mobility relates to the tibiotarsal, subtalar and mediotarsal interspaces. It is performed passively, noting for each joint and movement if there is any limitation and to what degree, pain and its location.

Resisted muscular contraction is studied systematically. In lateral sprains, resisted contraction of the peroneal is most valuable as in some cases it will provoke pain indicative of a lesion of their sheath and also avoid missing a peroneal tendon dislocation or an avulsion of the styloid process of the 5th metatarsal.

A search for abnormal movements is essential in clinical examination, as the findings confirm ligamentous rupture. Tibiotalar laxity should be sought in two planes: frontal and sagittal.

In the frontal plane the evidence of this instability is:
• tibiotalar gaping, as evidenced by:
  -increased varus of the hindfoot compared with the opposite side,
  - perception of a talofibular sulcus when the foot is in forced inversion, a test made preferably with the patient prone and the knee flexed to 90°,
• ballottement, or talar "clunk", obtained by subluxating the talus inward and then restoring it to its original position. This sign must be sought with the foot in slight plantarflexion. It is by far the best evidence of instability in the frontal plane, since it indicates abutment of the supero-lateral border of the talar dome against the medial aspect of the lateral malleolus and therefore, in most cases, a ligamentous rupture.

In the sagittal plane, an attempt is made to demonstrate an anterior talar drawer sign during different maneuvers which are made with the knee more or less flexed and the foot at a right angle or in plantarflexion. The object is to demonstrate any anterolateral instability, either by producing advancement of the foot beneath the leg or by obtaining backward movement of the leg in relation to the foot. Different techniques have been suggested by:
• Landeros, who performs this maneuver with the knee flexed to about 60° and the foot at right angles. One hand grasps the heel and pulls it forward at a right angle while the other fixes the leg. The maneuver is positive when anterior displacement of the foot is felt;
• Castaing: the knee being slightly flexed, the foot is placed in some 15° of plantarflexion. The leg is held with one hand while the other pulls on the forefoot. When this maneuver is positive, contact with the talar dome is felt under the fingers or there is the impression that the lateral malleolus has shifted backwards;
• we ourselves consider that the best method consists of wedging the patient's heel on a hard surface with the knee flexed to around 50-60°, and then thrusting the leg backwards; this movement may sometimes be accompanied by creaking or crepitus.

Clinical examination is completed by a search for tender points. The attachments of the three bands of the LCL, the peroneal sheath, the capsule and ligaments of the calcaneocuboid articulation and the base of the 5th metatarsal are all palpated in succession.

Imaging

This must include the standard radiographs and, for some authors, films in forced positions, with the two-fold aim of not missing a bony lesion and of assessing the severity of the ligamentous involvement.

Standard films

These are made almost routinely but some authors question if they are really essential, particularly when the clinical examination suggests only a mild sprain. However, not to perform them seems unwise in an emergency setting, since they show not only fractures but also associated bony avulsions, and provide an assessment of the state of the ankle at the time, so as to distinguish between the effects of a recent lesion and its possible sequelae. This last point is essential in avoiding possible medicolegal litigation if there are painful sequelae. Besides the classical frontal and lateral views (which must be compared with those of the opposite side in children so as not to miss a lesion of the growth-plate), two supplementary films must be routinely made: a frontal view in internal rotation of the forefoot, which displays the lateral interspaces and identifies the talar dome, and an oblique lateral view of the tarsus which demonstrates avulsions at the lateral malleolus, the lateral process of the talus, the rostrum of the calcaneus, the cuboid and even the base of the 5h metatarsal. These four views reliably exclude any associated bony injury.

Films in forced positions

The importance of these films lies in confirming the parallel claimed by some authors between the severity of the displacement of the talus and the number of damaged ligaments. At the ankle, the dynamic films most often performed are the anterior talar drawer, which is increased by injury of the ATFL, and forced varus, which studies the anterior and middle ligaments. These films are usually made in comparison with the opposite side.

Ultrasound

This technique is rarely used and reported, though this method of imaging seems the most logical. The superficial topography of the ligaments allows the use of high-frequency probes possessing a very considerable degree of spatial resolution, and a direct view of the ligaments is available. In pathologic cases, its use is facilitated by the development of a periligamentous edema or hypoechogenic articular swelling, allowing better definition of the hyperechogenic outlines of the different ligamentous structures.

Ultrasound allows a relatively rapid overall assessment of the different medial and lateral structures, but also shows indirect signs of lesions at the tibiofibular, talonavicular, midtarsal and subtalar joints (hypoechogenic lesion opposite the sinus tarsi). The bony outlines are also studied, as well as the adjacent tendinous structures. In particular, the dynamic specificity of ultrasound may be useful in detecting a reducible dislocation of the peroneal tendons, and even of the tibialis posterior tendon. The structures at the posterior intersection are also well located.

A relaxed appearance of the ligaments, an important sign of rupture, may be visualized by successively putting the different articular compartments under tension. In acute episodes the ligamentous lesions are classified in three stages: edema of their attachments (mild sprain), partial rupture (-moderate sprain), and complete rupture with loss of ligamentous tension (severe sprain). There are also bony avulsions and periosteal stripping.

Ultrasound allows correct evaluation of the severity of the sprain and the visualization of associated lesions.

Treatment

This is based on the severity of the lesions, but also on the age of the patient, his personality, sporting and/or professional activities, and his motivation.

Treatment of mild sprains

Cryotherapy is an effective method. The application of an ice-pack is made as soon as possible after the accident and is often renewed during the first two days.

Massage may be used in different ways: effleurage and gliding pressure after the first hours and deep transverse friction after 2-3 days.

The application of a compression bandage allows reduction of the periarticular swelling and proves very efficacious.

Anti-inflammatory agents are useful and should be prescribed for 4-5 days.

Physiotherapy seems to be of uncertain usefulness in mild sprains.

Plaster immobilization is not justified. It does not seem to promote regression of the edema and incurs unnecessary risks.

Overall, the treatment that appears most effective consists of cooling the joint, application of a compression bandage and the prescription of anti-inflammatory drugs. This produces rapid regression of the vasomotor disturbance and painful phenomena and restoration of function within a short period.

Treatment of moderate sprains

This may be effected in four different ways:
• functional treatment, based on the avoidance of immobilization and a rapid return to activity. This

may be divided into two stages. The first stage (24-72 hours) consists of the following measures: ice-packs, compression bandage, avoidance of weight-bearing, use of sticks for walking, elevation of the lower limb during rest. The recovery stage is begun by active mobilization of the ankle when pain has diminished. Resumption of weight-bearing is allowed very soon. Then specific exercises against manual resistance are performed. Lastly, treatment is directed to rehabilitation exercises: pedaling on an exercise bicycle, jumping on the spot and jogging on even ground;
• conservative treatment with a plaster or resinated cast is a reasonable method of management but it must be applied early, extend from the base of the toes to just below the knee, keep the ankle at a right angle, and be left on for 3-4 weeks. In some cases, it can be replaced or substituted by a stabilizing appliance;
• treatment by supple containment is based on the use of a supporting bandage, preferably adhesive, or by strapping, which allows early resumption of walking;
• a prefabricated stabilizing appliance (orthoses) would seem to be an excellent compromise between functional treatment and strict immobilization. Different appliances can be used:
  - the Aircast splint is a removable pneumatic splint, consisting of two lateral shells whose inner apects carry pneumatic pads made of two compartments. These pneumatic pads are previously filled with air and it is not usually necessary to readjust the padding. However, the pneumatic pads can be regulated by means of a one-way valve which allows adaptation to each patient so as to exert a varying degree of compression on the tissues. The two lateral shells are joined by an adjustable heel-strap which accommodates the splint to the size of the heel. Closure is made with two Velcro bands. The splint should be worn in a lace-up shoe or trainer. Once adjusted, the pneumatic splint effectively limits movements of varus and valgus of the hindfoot and has little or no influence on plantarflexion.
  - The Gelcast appliance is similar in conception. It consists of two molded lateral shells, covered internally with silicone gel components which make lateral containment comfortable. Closure is by two straps. It should be worn over a moderately thick sock of non-synthetic material and in a lace-up shoe of trainer type. There has been no scientific report on the value of this appliance in the treatment of recent sprains of the ankle.
  - Sober's ankle appliance is a foam anklet reinforced by two lateral plastic shells, with a an adjustable heel band. Closure is made with Velcro.

  - The Malléoloc ankle stabilizing appliance consist of a sheet of thermoplastic material which starts from the anterior region of the fibula (at the junction of its middle and lower thirds), descends in front of the lateral malleolus, passes under the sole of the foot in front of the calcaneus, and reascends behind the medial malleolus to the posteromedial part of the tibia (junction of middle and lower thirds). A synthetic polyethylene material lines the inner aspect of this sheet and ensures protection and comfort. The sheet is held around the ankle by means of straps fixed by self-sealing closures. This spirally-shaped appliance molds the tibiotarsal mortice, limits varus and leaves the forefoot and posterior half of the heel free.

  Treatment with these removable appliances is important because of its numerous advantages. In practice, it ensures almost certain cure, without subsequent residual gapping or ankle stiffness. Rapid self-rehabilitation with early weight-bearing, a reduced number of rehabilitation sessions, as well as a shortened duration of prophylactic anticoagulant treatment are obtained. It allows a substantial reduction of time off work as well as an earlier resumption of athletic activity and thus contributes to limiting health costs.

Treatment of severe sprains

Prolonged immobilization in a walking plaster cast was for long the only treatment. Nowadays, it is increasingly rare for these types of injuries to be treated surgically. Treatment with a plaster or resinated cast combines simplicity, absence of risks, fewer complications and a rapid resumption of social and professional life. Surgical repair ensures perfect stabilization of the articulation and offers a guarantee of resumption of sport.

Non-operative treatment is based on three important factors:
• it must be undertaken early;
• weight-bearing can be allowed as soon as the cast is set and dry;
• immobilization must extend for at least 6 weeks.

Surgical treatment finds its best justification in the extent of the lesions found at operation, but the very small number of cases of chronic instability causing major functional handicap or requiring surgical stabilization does not argue in favor of reparative surgery for ankle sprains. After surgical repair, the period of immobilization is 6 weeks in a plaster or resinated boot. Weight-bearing is allowed at the end of two weeks. Rehabilitation is begun after removal of the cast and differs in no way from the rehabilitation of recent sprains.

● Anterior ankle sprains

Anterior ankle sprains are rare and often missed lesions.

Pathologic anatomy

The anterior capsule of the talocrural joint is relatively lax and is not completely tightened in forced plantarflexion. It plays little part in limiting this movement, which is effected mainly by the lateral ligamentous structures and by the shape of the bony components. Section of the anterior capsule has little effect on the stability of the talocrural joint, and in particular causes little or no anterior subluxation of the talus. The true restraints are more lateral; the ATFL and the anterior border of the MCL.

Injuries in forced plantarflexion of the ankle are rare. However, they are found in some circumstances. The skier who falls backwards, the footballer who kicks violently into the ground are examples. In these cases the more posterior structures are respected, but, there is a lesion of the anterior capsule which may extend laterally into the anterior talofibular ligament and the anterior part of the deltoid ligament. There may be an associated rupture of the anterior inferior tibiofibular ligament, as well as involvement of the superior talonavicular ligament.

Clinical assessment

A feeling of crepitus or the sensation of a tear and the character of the initial pain should be noted. This last is often intense and gradually dies away after a few days. The ankle quite rapidly becomes swollen, without the maximum swelling being lateral. There is no submalleolar hematoma. After several days the functional impairment has moderated and the patient can walk without any feeling of instability; it all amounts to a swollen and bruised but not very painful ankle.

The clinical examination shows that there is no frontal instability and no lateral or medial tender points, but on the other hand there are anterior tender points. The most suggestive feature is pain during forced plantarflexion and an anterior talar drawer sign.

Radiographic assessment

This may reveal two bony lesions: a small avulsion at the neck of the talus and a fracture of the posterior tubercle of the talus, but both lesions are inconstant.

Dynamic radiographs are made in comparison with the opposite side:
• the films in forced varus are normal,
• the films when eliciting the anterior drawer sign may show a shift of 10-15 mm,
• the lateral view in forced plantarflexion reveals forward and downward displacement of the talus with an anterior tibiotalar gap.

Treatment

If the sprain is mild, and when all that is left is pain on movement localized to the anterior part of the ankle, treatment is based on ice packs, possibly followed by physiotherapy. A simple appliance, simply for the pain, may be used for 4-5 days.

For cases of moderately severe sprain, with a drawer sign of less than 1-12 mm or a bony avulsion at the neck of the talus, treatment is conservative by immobilization with a walking plaster or resinated cast for 4 weeks.

Surgery is indicated only for severe lesions The anterior capsulo-ligamentous lesion often forms part of a more important picture of lateral ligamentous rupture The different lesions must be surgically repaired and in particular the anterior capsule.

● Medial ankle sprains

Although rare, and denied by some, lesions of the medial collateral ligament (MCL) do exist in isolation, without fracture of the lateral malleolus, without lesions of the inferior and anterior tibiofibular ligaments and without involvement of the fibula.

Pathologic anatomy

The thick firm medial collateral ligament has the shape of a fibrous fan. It consists of two layers: a superficial layer or deltoid ligament and a deep layer, which are firmly fastened to the medial malleolus and whose fibers diverge to gain attachment to the calcaneus, talus and inferior calcaneonavicular ligament.

The lesional mechanism is a movement of forced eversion, in which pronation markedly exceeds abduction and leads to an internal opening-up of the joint. Certain features may promote this isolated lesion of the MCL: excessive valgus of the hindfoot and pronation of the foot more limited than supination, causing more rapid increase in tension on the medial aspect.

Clinical assessment

As for lateral lesions, different degrees of severity may be observed, depending on the number of bundles damaged.

On interrogation, the patient describes very intense pain at the moment of injury. A feeling of cracking is often noted. On the other hand, there is hardly ever any immediate swelling. For a short period after the accident resumption of weight-bearing is usually possible, and even athletic activity may sometimes be continued. Physical examination shows bruising at the medial malleolus, spreading downwards and inwards and often invading the medial arch of the foot. Palpation demonstrates tender points at the MCL and should always include the anterior and inferior tibiofibular ligaments, lateral malleolus and neck of the fibula. Passive movement of the hindfoot exacerbates the medial pain during valgus strain, but sometimes just as much during a varus movement. The search for abnormal movements is very difficult and in the conscious state it is virtually impossible to demonstrate any increase in calcanean valgus or an anterior talar drawer sign in a recently injured ankle.

Radiographic assessment

Every injured ankle with medial bruising should have a standard radiographic assessment, including frontal and lateral views of the ankle. Further, if palpation reveals tenderness over the fibula, a radiograph of the entire leg should be requested in case there is a Maisonneuve fracture.

In some cases, the radiographs will reveal a small avulsion at the medial malleolus or at the medial border of the talus. They may also demonstrate a diastasis between the talus and medial malleolus, evidence of incarceration of the MCL.

Dynamic radiographs are sometimes made for comparison with the injured ankle:
• the films in forced varus are normal,
• the films when eliciting the anterior drawer sign may be positive,
• the films in forced valgus may show outward tilting of the talus and a medial gap of a few degrees in cases of severe sprain.

Treatment

This varies in relation to the severity of the lesion and of the physical and functional signs.

In mild sprains, treatment combines strapping or an adhesive bandage with immediate rehabilitation. Progress is rapidly favorable in all cases.

For moderately severe sprains, characterized by formal clinical evidence of a lesion of the MCL and radiographs which do not show any tibiotalar gap, treatment is based on relative immobilization by a supporting adhesive bandage, or strict immobilization in a plaster or resinated cast for 3-4 weeks.

For severe sprains, as evidenced clinically or proved by dynamic radiographs, treatment is usually by strict immobilization for 6 weeks. Surgical treatment is not justified unless, in rare cases, there is a major bony avulsion at the tip of the medial malleolus, or when there is incarceration of the MCL with medial talomalleolar diastasis.

Rehabilitation of ankle sprains

Whether the sprain is lateral, medial or anterior, once the initial phase of treatment is over some problems may persist: periarticular swelling, pain, ankle stiffness and decreased articular stability.

Countering residual edema

The most effective method is the application of a support bandage at an even pressure, applied in the morning before rising. At the beginning, this is only removed at the moment of getting into bed, then increasingly early in the day. Also used are various forms of massage, such as effleurage and gliding pressure. Physical treatments such as ionization and ultrasound can also be used.

Countering painful phenomena

Physical agents may be used: low-frequency currents, ultrasound, etc. Massage by deep transverse friction made at right angles to the direction of the fibers for ten minutes has some value and is given at a rate of 3 sessions a week. A beneficial effect may be expected from the 3rd or 4th session, but 6-8 sessions will probably be required for a satisfactory outcome. Local injections of corticosteroids at the attachments and course of the painful ligaments prove very effective.

Improving the range of movement

The problem arises at the talocrural joint, but also at the subtalar and to a lesser degree the midtarsal joints. The methods used to improve mobility vary with the joint. At the talocrural joint every technique may be used: active and passive mobilization, positioning, etc. At the subtalar joint, passive manual mobilization is used almost exclusively. At the midtarsal joint, only passive movements performed after fixing the hindfoot will allow improvement of the range of movement.

Restoration of full function

After a sprain of the ankle, not a few patients retain a feeling of instability which is not remedied by classical methods of rehabilitation. We must seek to redesign movement programs to obtain proprioceptive reafferentation of the articulation.

The method comprises:
• exercises to identify the movement induced: these are performed in the seated position, with the eyes closed, so that the patient may concentrate on perception of the different characteristics of the movement induced: direction, range, speed. The sole of the foot rests on a skate, an unstable platform, or a balloon or cushion, moved by the therapist The movements are initially performed in only one degree of freedom and rythmically; then they are made in an "anarchic" manner, both in space and time. To ensure that the induced movement is correctly perceived by the patient, he may be asked to imitate it synchronously on the opposite side.

During the early sessions the patient seems to perceive only movements that are rapid or of wide range. When the proprioceptive capacities attain their optimal expression, the patient is capable of identifying any movement "imperceptibly" induced by the therapist, by immediately adopting a mirror attitude with the healthy foot;
• exercises to realert proprioception in weight-bearing: at the start of rehabilitation the muscles, particularly the peronei, are stressed by brief stretching and the patient must learn to respond by a conscious muscular contraction. In the next stage, the patient practices reacting more and more quickly to a varus movement imposed on the hindfoot. Progress is based on rapid application of the stimulus and immediacy of the response;
• weight-bearing exercises: the patient takes weight on the injured side, protected in some cases by a support bandage or an ankle stabilizer. The therapist unbalances him by thrusting against the leg, and the patient learns to react as quickly as possible to the imbalance so created.
• exercises on unstable (tilting) platforms: at the start of rehabilitation these are made with weight-bearing on two platforms. The patient learns to steady the platforms in equilibrium, then to mobilize them by simple movements of the ankle. Subsequently, he learns to balance himself on the platform, first on both feet and then on one. At the end of the course the patient should be capable of walking along an unstable plane.

28.

Ankle sprain sequelae
(excluding reflex sympathetic algodystrophy)

M Bonnin

Simple ankle sprain is a lesion of the lateral ligamentous complex. It is the injury most commonly met with in sports, in daily life or at work. It generally occurs during a movement in equinovarus, more rarely in talus varus.

The incidence of ankle sprains is estimated at 1 per 10,000 persons per day [77] and young subjects aged between 15 and 35 years are mainly affected [9]. Overall, ankle sprains represent from 9.7% [39] to 18% [31, 94] of sports injuries. This frequence varies according to the sport, ranging from 0.5% in swimming to 20% in basketball and 50% in football [39, 77].

Sequelae may persist in spite of appropriate treatment: Smith observed sequelae in 50% of cases in athletes, affecting performance in 15% [94]. The symptoms are varied: pain, instability, sometimes simply a feeling of the ankle giving way, residual edema, crepitus and locking.

Management of these patients is difficult for several reasons:
• The initial injury has often been neglected and the mechanism forgotten. Lateral ligamentous complex sprain is then difficult to diagnose retrospectively and all the other types of injuries of the ankle have to be considered.
• In many ankle disorders following minor injury, the injury is merely a factor precipitating the failure of compensatory mechanisms. When an athlete consults for "ankle sprain sequelae", in 27% of cases an overuse disorder is in fact involved. This proportion may reach 70% in cycling, 40% in skating and 35% in running and dancing [39]. The physician

must therefore have a clear understanding of the actual movement carried out by the patient in his or her sport.
• Even if the initial injury was a true sprain of the lateral ligamentous complex, the ligamentous or bony sequelae can be multiple, so the symptoms must be analyzed in detail.
• There is no routine connection between (objective) laxity and (subjective) instability. This discordance can be explained by the difficulty of demonstrating subtalar and talar rotational laxity and by the fact that the instability is not necessarily related to abnormal joint laxity (fibular tendon lesions, defective proprioception, tibiofibular syndesmosis injuries, cartilaginous lesions).

A wide range of causes may thus underlie chronic ankle pain after sprain (table 28.1). Diagnosis is based on rigorous analysis of the history: injury mechanism, type and intensity of sport practiced, level of activity at which discomfort appears. The clinical examination must be precise and exhaustive. The ankle lends itself readily to clinical examination so it is generally possible to have a good idea of the diagnosis at this stage.

A complete set of radiographs must be routinely obtained in all cases of chronic ankle pain, including anteroposterior and lateral weight-bearing views and dynamic views in forced varus and anterior drawer of both limbs for comparison. Oblique views may be useful in certain cases.

Supplementary examinations should be considered when the basic investigations are normal and when pain persists after three to six months of

Table 28.1. Pathology of chronic post-traumatic ankle lesions

Complications of the ligamentous tear
Talocrural laxity
Subtalar laxity
Anterolateral impingement
Sinus tarsi syndrome
Syndesmotic tear
Traumatic lesions (other than ligamentous)
Osteochondral lesions of the talar dome
Tendinopathies:
- tibialis posterior tendon
- fibularis longus and brevis
Occult fractures
Decompensation of a long-standing condition
Congenital tarsal fusion
Os trigonum
Anterior impingement with tibio-talar osteophytosis
Tarsal tunnel syndrome
Inadequate rehabilitation
Reflex sympathetic algodystrophy

medical treatment and rehabilitation. CT and joint scan are invaluable if a bony lesion is suspected. Magnetic resonance imaging (MRI) is preferable for a soft tissue lesion. Technetium bone scan is extremely sensitive but lacks specificity and does not allow very precise localization of the area involved.

Arthroscopy of the talocrural joint gives a good view of the tibial and talar cartilage. It provides an adequate view of the anterior talofibular ligament and the deep bundle of the deltoid ligament. It can reveal tibiotalar laxity, tear of the anterior talofibular ligament, synovitis, anterolateral impingement or chondral lesions which are not detected by imaging methods.

Arthroscopy of the subtalar joint makes it possible to examine the posterior subtalar joint, the calcaneofibular ligament and the talocalcanear interosseous ligament and to detect subtalar laxity. If all other investigations are negative, and only then, arthroscopy may be performed with the aim of diagnosis. The diagnostic strategy is summarized in Table 28.2.

● Laxity of the talocrural joint

This is the principal sequel of serious ankle sprains. Instability is the predominant symptom.

Biomechanics

The lateral ligamentous complex of the talocrural joint is made up of three bands (Chapter 1):

• The anterior talofibular ligament (ATFL) is a capsular thickening. Its average length is 24.8 mm and its width 7.2 mm. It inserts into the anterior edge of the lateral malleolus just at the limit of the articular cartilage. The talar insertion lies on the articular surface of the lateral aspect of the talus. The ATFL courses obliquely and medially at an angle of 45° [16, 88]. It is not isometric and the tension in its fibers progressively increases during plantarflexion. It limits internal rotation, varus movement and anterior shift of the talus [26, 52, 73, 82, 95].

• The calcaneofibular (CFL) ligament stabilizes two joints, the talocrural joint and the subtalar joint. It is a thickening of the inner aspect of the fibular tendon sheath. Its average length is 36 mm and width 5 mm. When the foot is in neutral position, the CFL runs obliquely downwards and backwards at an angle of 130° to the fibula. It inserts into the anterior edge of the lateral malleolus 8.5 mm above its tip. Its calcaneal insertion is located 13 mm from the posterior subtalar joint [16, 88]. Tension is maximal in dorsiflexion and progressively decreases in plantarflexion. It limits external rotation and also talar and calcaneal varus movement. It also helps to limit anterior talar shift when the ankle is dorsiflexed [15]; experimental section of the CFL associated with ATFL section increases anterior shift of the talus by 14% to 30% as compared with ATFL section alone.

• The posterior talofibular ligament (PTFL) has received less attention. Its length is 24 mm and its width 6 mm. It runs from the posterior aspect of the lateral malleolus, 10 mm above its tip, to the extraarticular part of the posterior aspect of the talus. Tension in this ligament is minimal in a neutral position and increases in dorsi- and plantarflexion [16, 26].

The stability of the talocrural joint depends on this complex of three ligaments, but also on its own geometry and the weight of the subject. As the talus is wider anteriorly than posteriorly, dorsiflexion increases the intrinsic stability of the joint, both in anterior shift and in varus or internal rotation [52]. Overall, in a weight-bearing ankle, internal rotation is limited mainly by the anterior talofibular ligament (56% of the resistance), then by the deltoid ligament (30%). The other ligaments play only a minor role.

External rotation is limited by the calcaneofibular ligament (65% of the resistance), then by the

Table 28.2. Strategy in diagnosis and treatment of chronic post-traumatic ankle pain (OCLTD = osteochondral lesions of the talar dome; ATFL = anterior tibiofibular ligament)

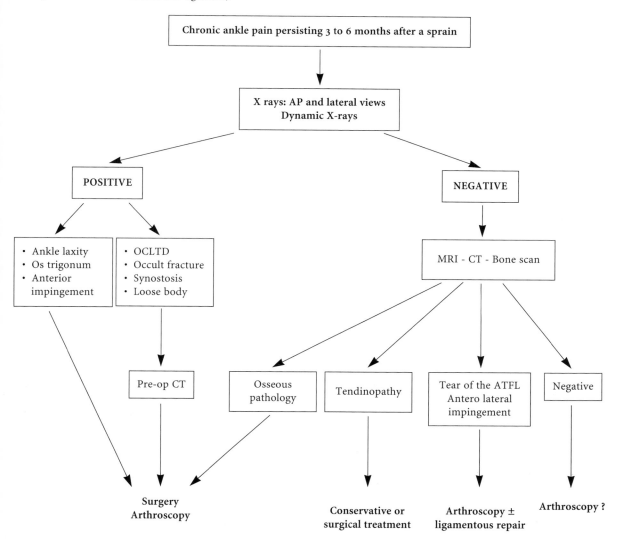

posterior talofibular ligament [98]. Inversion is limited above all by the inherent geometry of the joint, then by the anterior talofibular and calcaneo-fibular ligaments, the first predominating when the ankle is in plantarflexion and the second when the ankle is in neutral position or in dorsiflexion.

Diagnosis

Instability is the predominant functional sign, with recurrent sprains and a sensation of the ankle giving way when walking, generally on rough ground but sometimes even on level ground. Both clinical and paraclinical examinations should demonstrate objective talocrural laxity. After a course of several years, pain may become predominant with progressive disappearance of instability.

Laxity can be assessed by two basic clinical tests:

• The anterior drawer test is carried out with the patient supine and relaxed. The examiner holds the tibia with one hand, grasps the heel in the palm of the other hand and draws the foot forward. The test is carried out in a neutral position or in 10° of equinus [52, 59]. The difference in range between the injured and the opposite ankle is the important criterion. This test principally evaluates the ATFL, which is the main ligament limiting anterior shift of the talus.

• Forced varus is carried out by applying a movement combining varus and medial shift grasping the heel in the palm of one hand and immobilizing the tibia firmly in the other. This test assesses the degree of calcaneo-varus movement. Abnormal laxity is characterized by excessive varus movement of the calcaneus as compared with the other foot and by a "talar impact" when the hindfoot is brought back to its original position. This is mainly a test of the CFL, and to a lesser extent of the ATFL.

Dynamic radiographs can be obtained during both these tests in order to demonstrate the degree of laxity (fig. 28.1):

• In an anteroposterior view in forced varus, laxity is evaluated by measuring the tibiotalar angle, which is the angle between the lower edge of the distal end of the tibia and the upper edge of the body of the talus.

• In a lateral view, anterior shift of the talus is measured by the tibiotalar distance, a line from the poste-rior margin of the tibia to the center of the talar pulley.

These dynamic views can be obtained carrying out the tests manually or with a mechanical device, the latter having the advantage of reproducibility [49]. Views in active varus appear to be more sensitive than views in passive varus [79].

Dynamic views are sometimes difficult to analyze because the thresholds of abnormal values are not agreed. Physiologic laxity does exist and the tibiotalar angle can range from 0° to 23° [86] in asymptomatic subjects and the anterior drawer can be 5 mm [18, 19] or even 8 mm [62]. Comparative views of the other ankle are always necessary.

For Sauser, a tibiotalar angle greater than 10° is a sign of ligamentous injury in 90% of cases [89]. For Karlsson, an angle greater than 9° or a difference of more than 3° identifies ligamentous damage with 90% sensitivity and specificity [55]. Regarding anterior translation of the talus and depending on the authors, the abnormal thresholds are 4 mm [42],

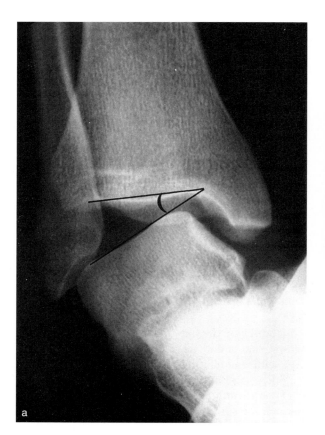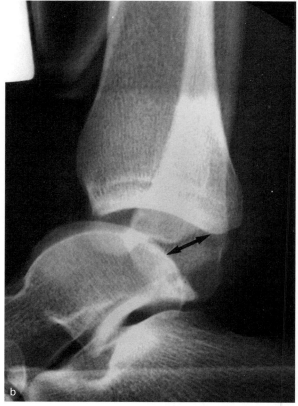

Fig. 28.1. Dynamic radiographs: **a** Talar tilt in forced varus on AP view. **b** Anterior drawer sign on lateral view

5 mm [51], 5 mm [18, 19], 9 mm [62], 10 mm [55] or a difference of 3 mm between the two ankles [55].

In MRI, the ATF is seen on axial sections in 100% of cases; the CFL is more difficult to locate and is visible in only 81% of cases [5]. Chronic lesions of these ligaments appear as ligamentous thickening and irregularity. Nonvisualization of the CFL cannot be considered a sign of its rupture [69, 83].

Treatment

In the treatment of talocrural laxity, conservative measures should always be attempted first, associating proprioceptive retraining, exercises to strengthen the fibular muscles and wearing of a protective orthotic device during sporting activity. If properly conducted treatment fails, surgery may be considered. Two types of surgical technique can be practiced:

• Ligament repairs involving the fibularis brevis tendon, in whole or part, are widely used. Numerous technical variants have been described. The various series of the literature report good or excellent results in 79 to 85% of cases [20, 22, 32, 33, 96, 103]. Nevertheless, these methods can be criticized on some points: sacrifice of a very powerful, active stabilizer of the ankle, difficulty of achieving correct tension during the transplant because of the absence of isometry [27], narrow margin of maneuver between residual laxity and iatrogenic rigidity of the subtalar joint.

• Direct repair of the ruptured ligaments was proposed as early as 1966 [7, 14]. The procedure consists of resection of fibrotic scar tissue and overlapping suture of the lateral edges or direct transosseous ligamentous reattachment to the lateral malleolus [30, 54]. Technical variants to strengthen the suture have been described using the periosteum [85] or the inferior extensor retinaculum [44, 92].

Results in the various series are encouraging with 80 to 96% of good or excellent results [23, 30, 44, 54, 85, 92]. These techniques have the advantage of anatomic repair, limiting the risk of residual stiffness and sparing the active stabilizers of the ankle. Their main disadvantage is the difficulty of finding serviceable ligament stumps in ankles with longstanding laxity.

Some authors propose combining ligament repair with osteotomy of the calcaneus to correct any excessive hindfoot varus [72].

Subtalar laxity

The role of subtalar laxity in ankle instability was emphasized in 1962 by Rubin and Witten [87], in 1968 by Laurin [62] and in 1977 by Brantigan [12]. Subtalar laxity was found to be associated with tibiotalar laxity in 30% of ankles operated on for chronic laxity [22, 54].

Most ankle sprains occur in a movement of equinovarus. The ATFL ligament is affected first and the CFL secondarily; subtalar laxity thus occurs in association with talocrural laxity. In varus trauma with the ankle dorsiflexed or in neutral position, the ATFL is relaxed and the first ligament to be affected is the CFL (fig. 28.2). Subtalar laxity may thus occur in isolation. Meyer [68], in a series of 40 recent ankle sprains, found 15 combined lesions of the ATFL and the CFL, and 6 cases of CFL lesions without ATFL lesions.

Biomechanics

The stability of the subtalar joint depends on several ligaments:

• The calcaneofibular ligament is the first element which limits varus motion of the calcaneus [56]. Isolated section of this ligament results in a gaping in the subtalar joint of 2.5° in dorsiflexion and 5° in plantarflexion, which is an increase of 25% to 50% over the normal range. The gap observed on radiographs is 5 mm [48].

• The lateral talocalcaneal ligament is a slender band parallel to the CFL. It inserts into the lateral talar process and runs obliquely downwards and backwards to insert on the lateral aspect of the calcaneus. It is sometimes fused with the CFL [88].

• The talocalcaneal interosseous ligament is situated in the sinus tarsi. It consists of three bands:

- a posterior band which is simply a thickening of the capsule of the posterior subtalar joint;

- an anterolateral band, or cervical ligament. This is the strongest of the three. It runs obliquely forwards, upwards and inwards to reach the lower aspect of the neck of the talus. If it alone is sectioned, a gap of 1.7° opens in forced varus (an increase of 14% over the normal range) [58];

- a medial band which forms a flat, fibrous band located frontally, running upwards and medially towards the lower aspect of the talar neck. Its section increases the talocalcanear gap by 1.8° (an increase of 16%) [58].

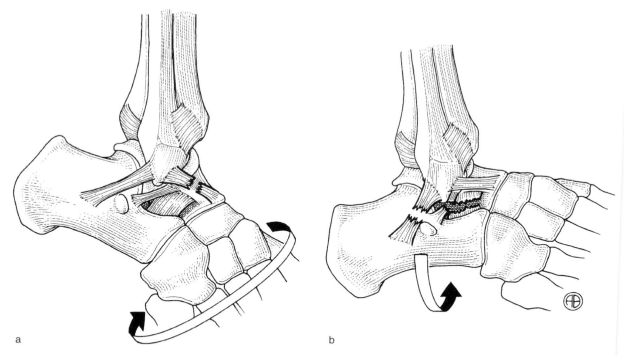

a   b

Fig. 28.2. a Equinovarus trauma: the first ligaments to be sprained is the ATFL. b Varus trauma in dorsiflexed or neutral position: the CFL and interosseous ligament are the first to be sprained.
(modified from Meyer, JM. with permission)

However, section of the talocalcaneal interosseous ligament only results in significant subtalar laxity if the CFL is also divided [48].

Clinical features

When subtalar laxity is associated with talocrural laxity, it raises no particular clinical problem but must be taken into account in surgical technique [54, 55]. Difficulties arise in the case of isolated subtalar laxity without talocrural laxity and with normal dynamic views. The main symptom remains instability.

More rarely, pain predominates, and some authors relate the sinus tarsi syndrome to this subtalar laxity. On clinical examination, laxity may be suspected if the calcaneus tilts excessively in forced varus.

There is no ancillary investigation which confirms the existence of subtalar laxity:
• Dynamic views (fig. 28.3): forced varus with an oblique view at 40° for good visualization of the posterior subtalar joint, described by Broden [13], has been widely assessed: some authors [24, 62]

consider that any loss of parallelism of the joint facets is a sign of laxity. Others require the presence of a gap of more than 5 mm [48]. However, Harper [45] demonstrated a subtalar gap in 12 of 13 asymptomatic patients and concluded that this technique was not reliable.

Moreover, the value of these dynamic views is debatable because they seek to reveal abnormal gaping of the subtalar joint, whereas during the course of a surgical procedure subtalar laxity is shown more often by excessive gliding than by excessive separation [24].

The lateral anterior drawer view will sometimes demonstrate displacement in the posterior subtalar joint.
• Arthrography of the subtalar joint coupled with CT can confirm CFL rupture by showing opacification of the fibular tendon sheath. This is frequently found in the first few hours after a sprain but the breach is rapidly filled by fibrosis and this investigation loses all sensitivity in chronic laxity.
• MRI seeks to demonstrate the lesion itself. It allows direct observation of the CFL and of the strands of the talocalcanear interosseous ligament (83). However, the CFL is not constantly seen and signs of

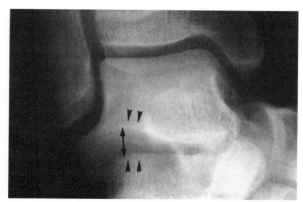

Fig. 28.3. Gaping of the subtalar joint in Broden's dynamic view in forced varus

rupture are still poorly characterized. This investigation even has a false-positive rate of 12% [70]. The talocalcaneal interosseous ligament is always well depicted, as well as post-traumatic anomalies such as edema and irregularities.

To sum up, subtalar laxity remains an indistinct entity. It should be suspected if the ankle is unstable and sometimes painful but with normal dynamic views; but at the present time no investigation, with the exception of arthroscopy, can give a totally reliable diagnosis.

Treatment

Various therapeutic problems may arise:
• When talocrural and subtalar laxity are associated, the difficulty is to recognize the CFL lesion and to treat it correctly. In direct suture, better results are obtained by routine repair of both the ATFL and CFL than by repair of the ATFL alone [54].
• In isolated subtalar laxity, the main problem is one of diagnosis and it may sometimes be necessary to decide on surgery if there is major instability with no objective signs of laxity. Technically, all ligamentous repairs using the fibularis brevis tendon effectively correct subtalar laxity [24, 90].

Anterolateral impingement

This diagnosis is made in a patient in whom pain is almost the only sequel, several months after an "ordinary" ankle sprain.

Pathophysiology

The ATFL and anterior capsular avulsion have healed imperfectly. This leads to chronic inflammation with anterolateral fibrosis which fills the talofibular groove of the ankle. Painful impingement on the lateral edge of the talar dome progressively develops.

This entity was described some years ago: it is the "internal derangement of the talofibular joint" of Wolin [104], the "chronic sprain" of Rodineau [84], or the "anterolateral impingement" of Ferkel [34].

The role of the antero-inferior tibiofibular ligament has been emphasized [2]; it impinges on the talar dome during anterior drawer movements in minor laxity, becomes hypertrophic and causes chronic anterolateral pain.

Clinical features

The principal symptom is pain with lateral premalleolar swelling, persisting several months after a sprain. Pain only appears on effort and makes any sporting activity impossible. More rarely, the patient may complain of the ankle giving way.

On examination, a painful lateral premalleolar swelling is found. Laxity is not found on clinical examination nor in dynamic views. CT and radionuclide bone scan show no anomaly. MRI may be useful in diagnosis by revealing fibrotic tissue filling the talofibular angle [69].

Only arthroscopy will give a definitive diagnosis. It reveals anterolateral fibrosis filling the talofibular groove, scarring of the ATFL, synovial hypertrophy, lateral cartilaginous lesions of the talar dome, and sometimes impingement on the lower band of the antero-inferior tibiofibular ligament.

Treatment consists of arthroscopic resection of all fibrotic tissue, anterolateral synovectomy and regularization of the lower band of the antero-inferior tibiofibular ligament [34, 64, 66].

Osteochondral lesions of the talar dome

This is a very common lesion which must be given systematic consideration in all cases of chronic ankle pain [11]. Since the first detailed description in 1922 [53], various names have been used: osteochondral

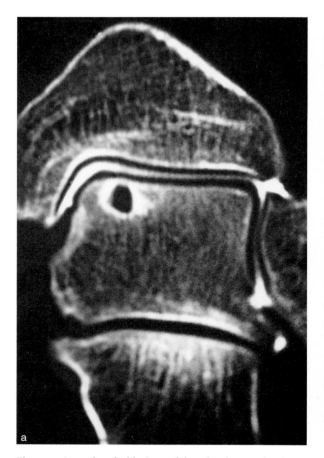 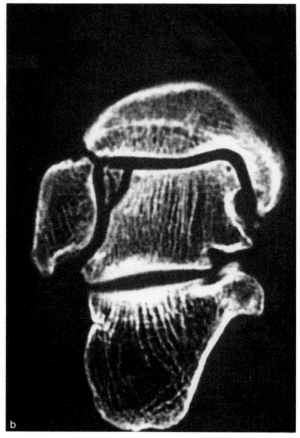

Fig. 28.4. Osteochondral lesions of the talar dome: **a** localized necrosis, **b** traumatic recent lesion

fracture, transchondral fracture, osteochondritis dissecans. These reflect the uncertainty as to its pathophysiology. While, for most authors, these lesions are always of traumatic origin [6, 41], for others they invariably arise from degenerative changes [17]. Lateral lesions appear to be almost always traumatic whereas medial lesions can only be linked with a genuine injury in 50% of cases [40, 60].

Berndt and Harty [6] in 1959 proposed a four-grade radiographic classification system. Since CT and MRI have become widely used, localized necrosis of the talus with intact overlying subchondral bone has been described (fig. 28.4a). The relationship between this particular type of lesion and classic lesions is debated: for some authors, the former represent a specific evolution of classic lesions [1, 63], while for others they constitute the initial stage [35]. Lastly, some consider that they are totally different and unconnected lesions [60]. Other classifications based on the CT or arthroscopic appearances have been described (table 28.3) [35, 80].

Generally speaking, lesions of the medial angle of the talar dome are posterior, deep and show little displacement. Lateral lesions are anterior and often displaced. Medial lesions seem to be slightly more frequent than lateral lesions. The apparent frequency of these lesions has increased due to the development of imaging methods: they are found in 57% to 81% of investigations of chronic ankle pain after sprain [35, 36].

Diagnosis is based on demonstration of the bone lesion. As plain radiographs are inadequate, further investigations must be pursued when pain persists after ankle injury.

Technetium-99m bone scan is extremely sensitive and always reveals increased uptake which precisely indicates the site of injury in 67% of cases [1], but in 33% it is diffuse throughout the ankle. CT

Table 28.3. Classification of osteochondritis of the talus

Radiographic classification of Berndt and Harty [6]
Grade I: localized area of compression
Grade II: fragment partially detached
Grade III: fragment free but remaining in the crater
Grade IV: fragment displaced, crater empty

CT classification of Ferkel [35]
Grade I: cavitary lesion with intact roof
Grade II: lesion extending to the surface
Grade III: open lesion with fragment in place
Grade IV: open lesion with fragment displaced

Arthroscopic classification of Pritsch et al [80]
Grade I: intact cartilage
Grade II: softened cartilage, depressed but intact
Grade III: open lesion of the cartilage

or MRI can then be more precisely targeted on the area of increased radionuclide activity.

Axial and coronal CT sections should be obtained. The lesion can be positively diagnosed and localized with precision, which is of great help in directing the surgical procedure. Arthrography coupled with CT makes it possible to differentiate between an open or a closed lesion. It is the investigation of choice when an osteochondral lesion is visible in plain radiographs (fig. 28.4b).

MRI is the most sensitive investigation. In the early stages, it reveals localized signal anomalies before any evidence on CT scan [1]. At a later stage, it gives a clear picture of the lesion, though in less morphologic detail than CT. Because of its great sensitivity, particularly in STIR (short T1 inversion recovery) sequences, MRI tends to supplant radionuclide bone scan and should be carried out first when plain radiographs are normal.

Treatment

• Relief from weight-bearing with joint-strengthening exercises for six weeks aims to initiate new blood supply to the lesion. This is a logical course if the hypothesis of a microtraumatic or degenerative origin of the lesion is retained, in particular in the young subject. Good results have been obtained with this simple treatment [4, 40, 78, 93].

• Surgical treatment routinely includes loose body removal, curettage and drilling of the cavity so that the defect can be colonized by healthy bone. Several technical questions may arise:

- should the fragment be secured or not? In recent lesions, a large fragment can be replaced using a fixation screw, absorbable pins [60], or biologic glue [61]. In chronic lesions, the bony fragment is necrotic and should preferably be resected;

- should the defect be grafted or not? Some authors propose inserting grafts of spongy bone in the cavity [60]. This is only a possibility if the defect is large, in particular in localized necrosis of the talus;

- which surgical approach should be chosen? The development of arthroscopy, and in particular the possibilities of joint distraction, have modified the indications during recent years. Lateral lesions are almost always anterior, and so easily approached by arthroscopy. Anteromedial lesions are rare. They can be treated by arthroscopy with the help of intra-articular distraction. Medial lesions involving the summit or posterior part of the talar dome, which are more frequent, are difficult to reach by arthroscopy, even with the help of a distractor. In such cases, it seems preferable to use an open technique, either by medial malleolar osteotomy or a medial retromalleolar approach [3, 63]. Some authors are in favor of an arthroscopic approach to these postero-medial lesions, using a posterior approach if necessary or drilling a tunnel in the distal end of the tibia [35, 36, 37].

Tibiofibular syndesmosis injuries

Syndesmotic sprains involve one or several of the following structures: the anterior tibiofibular ligament (ATIF), the posterior tibiofibular ligament (PTIF), the interosseous ligament and the interosseous membrane. The frequency of such lesions varies in the literature, ranging from 1% [50] to 10% [21] of ankle injuries. Functional recovery after such injuries is slow [11] and chronic pain may persist [56].

Anatomy and biomechanics

• The ATIF courses obliquely between the anterolateral tuberosity of the distal tibial epiphysis and the anterior edge of the lateral malleolus. It runs at an oblique angle of 45° to the distal end of the tibia. It measures 20 mm wide and 20 to 30 mm long [81, 88]. A separate lower band has been described [2].

• The PTIF consists of two bands: a thick superficial band runs obliquely between the posterolateral tuberosity of the tibia and the posterior edge of the lateral malleolus. It measures 30 mm long and 20 mm wide. The deep band is anterior to the superficial band. It inserts into the posteromedial part of the tibia and runs transversely to the posterior edge of the lateral malleolus. It forms a lip which prolongs the articular surface of the tibia and is visualized by an interarticular approach.

• The interosseous ligament joins the tibia to the fibula at a point 10 to 20 mm above the distal end of the tibia.

The tibiofibular syndesmosis allows a certain degree of motion. In movements of flexion and extension, the intramalleolar distance increases by 1.5 mm [25]. The main ligament providing stability is the ATIF, section of which results in a diastasis of 4 mm [8] which may increase to 10 mm if there is an associated lesion of the interosseous ligament.

Two mechanisms have been recognized as the cause of injury: forced external rotation [38, 50, 81] and forced dorsiflexion [50]. Two sports are particularly risky: skiing and football [11, 38].

Clinical features

If the patient is seen at an early stage, a careful examination will easily make it possible to distinguish between syndesmosis injury and a simple sprain: different mechanism, pain located only over the syndesmosis, pain on forced external rotation of the foot or when the tibia and fibula are compressed at midcalf level (squeeze test).

In general, the patient is seen secondarily for persistent ankle pain after a trauma which has been labeled "sprain". Diagnosis is then based on retrospective analysis of the mechanism and on clinical examination: no laxity, no tendon damage, pain over the syndesmosis, external rotation and squeeze test sometimes positive.

Plain radiographs may reveal calcification of the syndesmosis and the interosseous membrane [38, 100]. These images appear three to six months after the sprain and allow a reliable retrospective diagnosis (fig. 28.5a). The existence of a tibiofibular diastasis is rare in syndesmotic sprains. It may be sought for by obtaining dynamic views in external rotation and forced valgus. The radiographic criteria for diastasis are the existence of a clear tibiofibular gap of more than 6 mm in an anteroposterior view and a tibiofibular overlap of less than 1 mm in a mortice view [46] (fig. 28.5b).

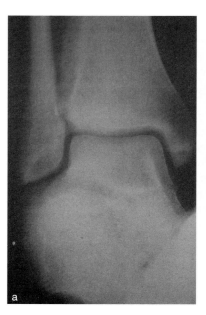 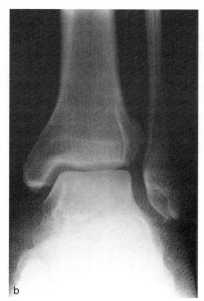 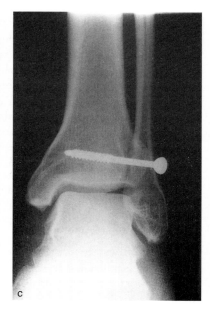

Fig. 28.5. Lesions of the tibiofibular syndesmosis. **a** Calcified deposits in the interosseous membrane 6 months after sprain of the syndesmosis; **b** tibiofibular diastasis after a recent syndesmotic sprain (X-ray through cast); **c** same patient after surgical reduction and screwing

Radionuclide bone scan may be useful by showing localized increased uptake by the syndesmosis. Calcification of the interosseous membrane or tibiofibular diastasis may be visible on CT scan. MRI for chronic ankle pain reveals syndesmotic lesions in 7% of cases [29], with thickening and irregularity of the ATIF and sometimes of the interosseous membrane. However, nonvisualization of the ATIF should not be considered abnormal.

At the stage of chronic pain, **treatment** is difficult. In most cases there is a gradual improvement and conservative treatment is sufficient. If a particularly hazardous sport such as skiing is practiced or if diastasis persists, surgical intervention may be necessary. This may consist of simple debridement of the syndesmosis with ligament repair and insertion of a temporary screw [24] (28.5b). Sometimes tibiofibular ligamentoplasty may be required [28, 84] or even tibiofibular arthrodesis [56].

Sinus tarsi syndrome

This clinical entity was defined by O'Connor in 1958 [74]. Lateral pain with instability and a sensation of the ankle giving way persist after an inversion injury, without clinical or radiographic laxity. Several authors [67, 99, 102] have linked this syndrome to partial lesions of the talocalcaneal interosseous ligament, assimilating it to minimal subtalar laxity.

Certain histologic studies have revealed neuromas in fibrotic scar tissue within the sinus tarsi [67]. Because of the difficulty of demonstrating subtalar laxity, it is still not easy to distinguish between a simple fibrotic lesion of the talocalcaneal interosseous ligament without laxity, and true subtalar laxity.

The symptoms consist of lateral sub- and premalleolar pain on walking, particularly on uneven ground. The patient often relates this problem to an untreated or inadequately treated ankle sprain. Clinical examination shows tenderness in a very limited area at the lateral orifice of the sinus tarsi. No talocrural or subtalar laxity is observed.

Simple and dynamic radiographs are normal. Arthrography of the subtalar joint may show a pool of contrast material at the sinus tarsi [67]. However, this investigation has fallen into disuse since the advent of MRI, which gives a detailed picture of lesions of the talocalcaneal interosseous ligament or of fibrotic scar tissue in the sinus. As we have seen, because of uncertainty as to evaluation of the calcaneofibular ligament, this investigation cannot differentiate between simple fibrotic scar tissue and true subtalar laxity.

Treatment

If possible, conservative methods should initially be attempted, consisting of up to 3 corticosteroid injections, proprioceptive rehabilitation and the use of an ankle brace. If there is no response, surgical curettage of the sinus tarsi may be considered. The series of the literature, taken together, report 96 cases treated surgically with 66 excellent results, 24 good results and 6 failures [24].

Occult fractures

Certain occult fractures which are not recognized at the time of the initial injury may be the source of chronic pain. These occult fractures are all the more misleading as they occur during an injury in equinovarus. Two sites are particularly common:

• **Fractures of the lateral process of the talus**, which represent 24% of fractures of the body of the talus. They are produced by a movement of varus and dorsiflexion of the hindfoot, and sometimes by external rotation [47]. Initial symptoms are very similar to those of a common sprain and the fracture line is poorly visible in the emergency radiographs. The injury is often missed and diagnosed only at the stage of chronic ankle pain. Fracture can generally be suspected on plain radiographs but CT scan is the key examination, evaluating the size of the fragment and its position in relation to the subtalar joint (fig. 28.6). At a late stage, the treatment is surgical removal of the fragment.

• **Fractures of the beak of the calcaneus**: their incidence is poorly estimated as many are missed. They represent 3 to 23% of calcaneal fractures. The most frequent mechanism is an injury in equinovarus, with avulsion of the calcaneal insertion of the bifurcate ligament.

The symptoms and mechanism are the same as those of the common sprain; the initial radiographs are often considered to be normal and the fracture goes unrecognized. The diagnosis is made later when there is chronic ankle pain. It is based on plain

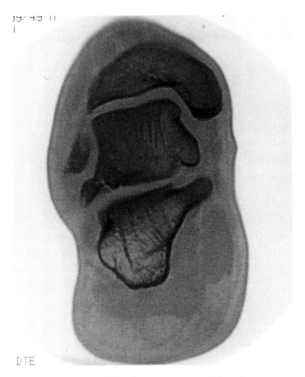

Fig. 28.6. Fracture of the lateral process of the talus

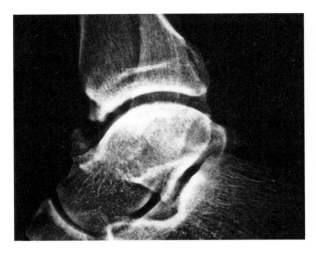

Fig. 28.7. Anterior tibiotalar osteophytes

oblique radiographs and CT scan is rarely necessary. At the stage of chronic pain, treatment consists of surgical removal of the ununited bony fragment but the results are often mediocre.

Anterior impingement syndrome

The development of osteophytes on the front of the distal end of the tibia and on the talar neck may lead to chronic pain and ankle stiffness in the athlete. The first description of this disorder was that of Morris [71] in 1943; then McMurray [65] in 1950 popularized the term "footballer's ankle". As all sports subjecting the ankle to repeated microtrauma can be incriminated, the term of "anterior impingement syndrome" is gradually being adopted. Such spurs are observed in 45% of football players and in 59% of dancers [75, 97]. They are due to repeated movements in extreme plantar- or dorsiflexion.

The diagnosis is usually made in an athlete aged over thirty who complains of anterior pain and restricted dorsiflexion of the ankle towards the end of a game. Free intra-articular spur fragments are sometimes responsible for ankle locking or sharp stabs of pain. The athlete may sometimes connect the pain with a recent ankle injury. Pain, and never instability, is the essential complaint.

Lateral radiographs show osteophytes on the anterior border of the distal end of the tibia and on the talar neck. Four radiographic stages have been described [91] (fig. 28.7). Osteophytes can develop anterior to the medial and lateral malleoli and there may be detached fragments within the joint. They generally accumulate in the anterior recess or in the submalleolar regions.

Initially, treatment should always be conservative: heel inserts, corticosteroid injections. If this fails, surgical resection of the spurs gives good results. Their precise location should be defined preoperatively, by CT scan if necessary, as it is sometimes difficult to locate all spurs and loose bodies during the procedure.

Surgery can be done as an open procedure or under arthroscopy [91].

Pathology of the posterolateral talar tuberosity

The posterior aspect of the talus has two tubercles: the small posteromedial tubercle, and the posterolateral tubercle, which is generally larger. These two tubercles bound a fibro-osseous tunnel which

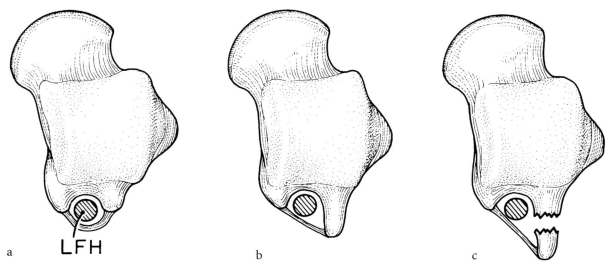

Fig. 28.8. Different aspects of the posterolateral tubercle of the talus: **a** usual aspect; **b** long tail of the talus (trigonal process); **c** os trigonum. LFH: flexor hallucis longus

contains the flexor hallucis longus tendon (FHL). The lateral tubercle can have several anatomic forms [81]:
• It may be small, as is usually the case (fig. 28.8a).
• It may be prolonged by an accessory ossicle which is completely separate: the os trigonum. This sesamoid bone is attached to the tuberosity by fibrous or fibrocartilaginous tissue. The incidence of the os trigonum varies from 2.7% to 7.7% according to the series [88]. It is bilateral in 50% of cases (fig. 28.8b).
• This accessory ossicle is sometimes fused with the posterolateral tubercle: it is the "long tail" of the talus or the trigonal or posterior process (fig. 28.8c). This process may be injured in two ways [101]:
• **After acute trauma:** forced plantarflexion of the ankle or a direct impact (rugby tackle) can cause true fracture of the process or rupture of the fibrous attachments of the os trigonum.
• **After minor trauma:** some sports in which the ankle is repeatedly in extreme plantarflexion lead to posterior impingement between the os trigonum on the one hand and the tibia and calcaneus on the other. This is the case of ballet dancers in "en pointe" and "demi-pointe" positions [43].

In both these situations, the patient complains of chronic posterolateral pain which increases when running, jumping or walking downstairs. Walking on tiptoe is painful.

When there is associated FHL tendon injury, pain may irradiate posteriorly from the medial malleolus. On examination, pain is localized behind the fibular tendons and in front of the calcaneal tendon. The fibular tendons are not painful on effort. Forced passive plantarflexion of the ankle produces sharp pain. Increased pain on medial retromalleolar pressure and on movement of the great toe indicates associated FHL injury.

Plain lateral radiographs show the os trigonum, but there is no formal criterion which makes it possible to differentiate between a true fracture of the posterolateral talar tubercle and a damaged os trigonum.

If the os trigonum is damaged or fractured, radionuclide bone scan [76] reveals focal increased uptake. If pain persists despite conservative treatment, surgical excision of the bony fragment is necessary. The posterolateral approach is technically simpler but there is a risk of damage to the sural nerve. The posteromedial approach makes it possible to free the FHL if there is associated tenosynovitis, but care must be taken to locate the posterior tibial neurovascular pedicle. This approach endangers the medial calcaneal nerve.

References

1. Anderson IF, Crichton KJ, Grattan-Smith T, Cooper RA, Brazier D (1989) Osteochondral fractures of the dome of the talus. J Bone Joint Surg (Am) 71A: 1143-1152
2. Basset FH, Gates HS, Billys JB, Morris HB, Nikolaou PK (1990) Talar impingement by the antero inferior

tibio fibular ligament: A cause of chronic pain in the ankle after inversion sprain. J Bone Joint Surg (Am) 72A: 55-58

3. Basset FH, Billys JB, Gates HS (1993) A simple surgical approach to the postero-medial ankle. Am J Sports Med 21: 144-146

4. Bauer M, Jonsson K, Linden B (1987) Osteochondritis dissecans of the ankle: A 20 years follow-up study. J Bone Joint Surg (Br) 69B: 93-96

5. Beltran J, Munchow AM, Khabirih (1990) Ligaments of the lateral aspect of the ankle and sinus tarsi: An MR imaging study. Radiology 177: 455-458

6. Berndt L, Harty M (1959) Transchondral fractures (osteochondritis dissecans of the talus). J Bone Joint Surg (Am) 41: 988-1020

7. Blanchet A (1971) Les réfections ligamentaires immédiates dans les entorses externes de la tibio-tarsienne. Lyon Chir 67: 139-140

8. Bonnin JG (1970) Injuries to the ankle. Darien, Conn, Hafner 147-185

9. Boruta PM, Bishop JO, Braly WG, Tullos HS (1990) Acute lateral ankle ligament injuries: a literature review. Foot Ankle 11: 107-113

10. Bosien WR, Staples OS, Russel SW (1955) Residual disability following acute ankle sprains. J Bone Joint Surg (Am) 37A: 1237-1243

11. Boytim MJ, Fisher DA, Neumann L (1991) Syndesmotic ankle sprains. Am J Sports Med 19: 294-298

12. Brantigan JW, Pedegana LR, Lippert FG (1977) Instability of the subtalar joint: Diagnosis by stress tomography in three cases. J Bone Joint Surg (Am) 59A: 321-324

13. Broden B (1949) Roentgen examination of the subtaloid joint in fractures of the calcaneus. Acta Radiol 31: 85-91

14. Brostrom L (1966) Sprained ankles: Treatment and prognosis in recent ligament ruptures. Acta Chir Scand 132: 537-550

15. Buculu C, Thomas KA, Halvorson TL, Cook SD (1991) Biomechanical evaluation of the anterior drawer test: The contribution of the lataral ankle ligaments. Foot Ankle 11: 389-393

16. Burks RT, Morgan J (1994) Anatomy of the lateral ankle ligaments. Am J Sports Med 22: 72-77

17. Campbell CJ, Ranawat CS (1966) Osteochondritis dissecans: The question of etiology. J Trauma 6: 201-219

18. Castaing J (1968) Les entorses de cheville. Conférences d'enseignement de la SOFCOT. Expansion Scientifique Française, Paris, pp 23-41

19. Castaing J, Delplace J (1972) Entorses de cheville : intérêt de l'étude de la stabilité dans le plan sagittal pour le diagnostic de gravité. Rev Chir Orthop 58: 51-63

20. Castaing J, Delplace J, Dien F (1975) Instabilité chronique externe de la cheville. Rev Chir Orthop 61 (suppl II): 167-174

21. Cedell C (1967) Supination outward rotation injuries of the ankle. A clinical and roentgenological study with special reference to the operative treatment. Acta Orthop Scand (suppl 110): 1-148

22. Chrisman OD, Snook GA (1969) Reconstruction of lateral ligament tears of the ankle: An experimental study and clinical evaluation of seven patients treated by a new modification of the elmslie procedure. J Bone Joint Surg (Am) 51A: 904-912

23. Christel P, Witvoet J, Jaulin Ph (1988) Traitement chirurgical des instabilités tibio-tarsiennes chroniques chez le sportif par rétention trans-osseuse du plan capsulo-ligamentaire externe. Journal de Traumatologie du Sport 5: 177-184

24. Clanton TO, Schon LC (1993) Athletic injuries to the soft tissues of the foot and ankle-Subtalar sprains. In: Mann RA, Coughlin MJ (eds) Surgery and the Foot and Ankle. Mosby, St Louis, pp 1153-1165

25. Close JR (1956) Some applications of the functional anatomy of the ankle joint. J Bone Joint Surg (Am) 38A: 761-781

26. Coville MR, Marder RA, Boyle JJ, Zarin S B (1990) Strain measurement in lateral ankle ligaments. Am J Sports Med 18: 196-200

27. Coville MR, Marder RA, Zarin S B (1992) Reconstruction of the lateral ankle ligaments: A biomechanical analysis. Am J Sports Med 20: 594-600

28. Delplace J (1974) Que peut-on proposer aux instabilités de la cheville ? Ann Med Phys 17: 338-357

29. Denhartog B, Cardone BW, Johnson JE, et al (1991) The role of magnetic resonance imaging in evaluating chronic ankle pain after sprain. American Orthopedic Foot and Ankle Society Meeting, Boston, July 27

30. Duquennoy A, Letendard J, Loock Ph (1980) Remise en tension ligamentaire externe dans les instabilités chroniques de la cheville. Rev Chir Orthop 66: 311-316

31. Eiff MP, Smith AT, Smith GE (1994) Early mobilisation versus immobilisation in the treatment of lateral ankle sprains. Am J Sports Med 22: 83-88

32. Elmslie RC (1934) Recurrent subluxatious of the ankle joint. Ann Surg 100: 364-367

33. Evans DL (1953) Recurrent instability of the ankle: A method of surgical treatment. J Royal Soc Med 46: 343-344

34. Ferkel RD, Karzel RP, Delpizzo W, Friedman MJ, Fisher SP (1991) Arthroscopic treatment of antero-lateral impingement of the ankle. Am J Sports Med 19: 440-446

35. Ferkel RD (1993) Arthroscopy of the ankle and foot. In: Mann RA, Coughlin MJ (eds) Surgery of the Foot and Ankle, 6th edn. Mosby, St Louis, pp 1277-1310

36. Ferkel RD, Scranton PE (1993) Current concepts review: Arthroscopy of the ankle and foot. J Bone Joint Surg (Am) 75A: 1233-1242

37. Flick AB, Gould N (1985) Osteochondritis dissecans of the talus (transchondral fractures of the talus): Review of the literature and new surgical approach for medial dome lesions. Foot Ankle 5: 165-185

38. Fritschy D (1989) An unusual ankle injury in top skiers. Am J Sports Med 17: 282-286

39. Garrick JG, Requa RK (1988) The epidemiology of foot ankle injuries in sports. Clin Sports Med 7: 29-37

40. Gérard Y, Bernier JM, Ameil M (1989) Lésions ostéochondrales de la poulie astragalienne. Rev Chir Orthop 75: 466-478

41. Girardier J (1982) Les fractures ostéochondrales du dôme astragalien. Thèse de Médecine, Lyon, n°200

42. Gould N, Seligson D, Glassman J (1980) Early and late repair of lateral ligaments of the ankle. Foot Ankle 1: 84-89

43. Hamilton WG (1982) Stenosing tenosynovitis of the flexor hallucis longus tendon and posterior impingement upon the os trigonum in ballet dancers. Foot Ankle 3: 74-80

44. Hamilton WG, Thompson FM, Snow SW (1993) The modified Brostrom procedure for lateral ankle instability. Foot Ankle 14: 2-7

45. Harper MC (1992) Stress radiographs in the diagnosis of lateral instability of the ankle and mind foot. Foot Ankle 13: 435-438

46. Harper MC (1993) An anatomic and radiographic investigation of the tibio fibular clear space. Foot Ankle 14: 455-458

47. Hawkins LG (1965) Fracture of the lateral process of the talus. J Bone Joint Surg (Am) 47A: 1170-1175

48. Heiman AE, Braly WG, Bishop JO, Noble PC, Tullos HS (1990) An anatomic study of subtalar instability. Foot Ankle 10: 224-228

49. Hintermann B, Holzach P, Matter P (1990) Die radiologische funktionsprüfung bei der fibularen band läsion Eine kritische analyse und klinische studic. Schweiz Ztschr Sport Med 38: 79-85

50. Hopkinson WJ, St Pierre P, Ryan B, Wheeler JH (1990) Syndesmosis sprains in the ankle. Foot Ankle 10: 325-330

51. Jaivin JS, Ferkel RD (1994) Ankle and foot injuries. In: Fu FH, Stone DA (eds) Sports Injuries, Mechanisms, Prevention, Treatment. Williams & Wilkins, Baltimore, pp 977-1000

52. Johnson EE, Markolf KL (1983) The contribution of the anterior talofibular ligament to ankle laxity. J Bone Joint Surg (Am) 65A: 81-88

53. Kappis M (1922) Weitere Beitrage zur traumatisch mechanischen Entstehung der "spontanen" knorpel-ablösungen (Sogen Osteochrondritis Dissecans). Deutsch Z Chir 171: 13-29

54. Karlsson J, Bergsten T, Lansinger O, Peterson L (1988) Reconstruction of the lateral ligaments of the ankle for chronic lateral instability. J Bone Joint Surg (Am) 70A: 581-588

55. Karlsson J, Lansinger O (1990) Lateral instability of the ankle joint. Clin Orthop 276: 253-261

56. Katznelson A, Lin E, Militiano J (1984) Ruptures of the ligaments about the tibio fibular syndesmosis. Injury 15: 170-172

57. KjaersgaardAndersen P, Wethelund JO, Nielsen S (1987) Lateral talocalcaneal instability following section of the calcaneo fibular ligament: Kinesiologic study. Foot Ankle 7: 355-361

58. Kjaersgaard Andersen P, Wethelund JO, Helmig P, Soballe K (1988) The stabilizing effect of the ligamentous structures in the sinus and canalis tarsi on movements in the hind foot: An experimental study. Am J Sports Med 16: 512-516

59. Kjaersgaard Andersen P, Frich LH, Madsen F, Helmig P, Sogard P, Sojbjerg JO (1989) Instability of the hind foot after lesion of the lateral ankle ligaments: Investigations of the anterior drawer and adduction maneuvers in autopsy specimens. Clin Orthop 266: 170-179

60. Kouvalchouk JF, Schneider-Maunoury G, Rodineau J Paszkowski A, Watin Augouard L (1990) Les lésions ostéochondrales du dôme astragalien avec nécrose partielle ; leur traitement chirurgical par curetage et comblement. Rev Chir Orthop 76: 480-489

61. Kriestensen G, Lind T, Lavard P, Olsen PA (1990) Case report: Fracture stage 4 of the lateral talar dome treated arthrocopically using biofix for fixation. Arthroscopy 6: 242-244

62. Laurin CA, Ouellet R, St Jacques R (1968) Talar and subtalar tilt: An experimental investigation. Can J Surg 11: 270-279

63. Loomer R, Fischer C, Lloyd-Smith R, Sisler J, Cooney T (1993) Osteochondral lesions of the talus. Am J Sports Med 21: 13-19

64. Martin DF, Curl WW, Baker CL (1989) Arthroscopic treatment of chronic synovitis of the ankle. Arthroscopy 5: 110-114

65. Mac Murray TP (1950) Footballer's ankle. J Bone Joint Surg 32B: 68-69

66. Meislin RJ, Rose DJ, Parisien JS, Springer S (1993) Arthroscopic treatment of synovial impingement of the ankle. Am J Sports Med 21: 186-189

67. Meyer JM, Lagier R (1977) Post traumatic sinus tarsi syndrom: An anatomical and radiological study. Acta Orthop Scand 48: 121-128

68. Meyer JM, Garcia J, Hoffmeyer P, Fritschy D (1986) The subtalar sprain: A roentgenographic study. Clin Orthop 226: 169-173

69. Mink JH (1992) Ligaments of the ankle. In: Deutsch AL, Mink JH, Kerr R (eds) MRI of the foot and Ankle. Raven Press, New York, pp 173-197

70. Mitchell JR, Shereff MJ, Erickson S, Timins M (1994) Abnormal MRI scans of the ankle in asymptomatic individuals. American Orthopaedic Foot and Ankle Society, Coeur d'Alène, Idaho, 1994, June 30-July 3

71. Morris LH (1943) Athlete's ankle in proceedings of the British orthopaedic association. J Bone Joint Surg 25: 220

72. Morscher E, Hefti F, Baumann JU (1986) Kombinierte lateralere bandplastik und calcaneusosteotomie bei der rezidivierenden distorsio ped is. Orthopäde 15: 461-465

73. Nigg BM, Skarvan G, Franck CB, Yeadon MR (1990) Elongation and forces of ankle ligaments in a physiological range of motion. Foot Ankle 11: 30-40

74. O'Connor D (1958) Sinus tarsi syndrome: A clinical entity. J Bone Joint Surg (Am) 40A: 720

75. O'Donoghue DH (1966) Chondral and osteochondral fractures. J Trauma 6: 469

76. Paulos LE, Johnson CL, Noyes FR (1983) Posterior compartment fractures of the ankle: A commonly missed athletic injury. Am J Sports Med 11: 439-443

77. Peters JW, Trevino SG, Renstrom PA (1991) Chronic lateral ankle instabiliy. Foot Ankle 12: 182-191

78. Pettine KA, Morrey BF (1987) Osteochondral fractures of the talus: A long term follow-up. J Bone Joint Surg (Br) 69B: 89-92

79. Peyre M, Eladan G, Kouadio V, Rodineau J (1993) L'autovarus: Une technique d'exploration des instabilités externes de cheville. 3èmes Journées d'Imagerie OstéoArticulaire de la Salpétrière L'imagerie pratique du mollet, de la cheville et du pied (8 et 9 octobre 1993)

80. Pritsh M, Horoschovski H, Farine I (1986) Arthroscopic treatment of osteochondral lesions of the talus. J Bone Joint Surg (Am) 68: 862-865

81. Rasmussen O (1985) Stability of the ankle joint: Analysis of the function and traumatology of the ankle ligaments. Acta Orthop Scand (suppl 211): 1-75

82. Renstrom P, Wertz M, Incavo S, Pope M, Ostgaard HC, Arms S, Haugh L (1988) Strain in the lateral ligaments of the ankle. Foot Ankle 9: 59-63

83. Rijke AM, Goitz HT, Mac Cue FC, Dee PM (1993) Magnetic resonnance imaging of injury to the lateral ankle ligaments. Am J Sports Med 21: 528-534

84. Rodineau J (1978) La cheville. Laboratoires Besins Iscovesco, Paris

85. Roy-Camille R, Saillant G, Gagna G, Benazet JP, Feray Ch (1986) Les laxités externes chroniques de cheville-cure chirurgicale par une ligamentoplastie au périoste. Rev chir Orthop 72: 121-126

86. Rubin G, Witten M (1960) The talar tilt ankle and the fibular collateral ligaments: A method for the determination of talar tilt. J Bone Joint Surg (Am) 42A: 311-326

87. Rubin G, Witten M (1962) The subtalar joint and the symptom of turning over the ankle: A new method of evaluation utilizing tomography. Am J Orthop 4: 16-19

88. Sarrafian SK (1983) Anatomy of the Foot and Ankle: Descriptive, Topographic, Functional Syndesmology. Lippincott, Philadelphia, pp 159-217

89. Sauser DD, Nelson RC, Laurine MH (1983) Acute injuries of the lateral ligaments of the ankle comparison of stress radiography and arthrography. Radiology 148: 653-657

90. Schon LC, Clanton TO, Baxter D (1991) Reconstruction for subtalar instability: A review. Foot Ankle 11: 319-325

91. Scranton PE, Mac Dermott JE (1992) Anterior tibiotalar spurs: A comparison of open varsus arthroscopic debridement. Foot Ankle 13: 125-129

92. Segal Ph, Dehoux E, Deprey F, Nickel SE (1991) Le traitement chrirugical des laxités externes chroniques de la cheville par ligamentoplastie au frondiforme. J Trauma Sport 8: 24-27

93. Shea MP, Manoli A (1993) Osteochondral lesions of the talar dome. Foot Ankle 14: 48-55

94. Smith RW, Reischl SF (1986) Treatment of ankle sprains in young athletes. Am J Sports Med 14: 465-471

95. Smith RW, Reischl SF (1988) The influence of dorsiflexion in the treatment of severe ankle sprains: An anatomical study. Foot Ankle 9: 28-33

96. Snook GA, Chrisman OD, Wilson TC (1985) Long term results of the Chrisman-Snook operation for reconstruction of the lateral ligaments of the ankle. J Bone Joint Surg (Am) 67A: 1-7

97. Stoller SM (1984) A comparative study of the frequency of anterior impingement exostosis of the ankle in dancer and non dancer. Foot Ankle 4: 201

98. Stormont DM, Morrey BF, Kai-Nan AN, Cass JR (1985) Stability of the loaded ankle: Relation between articular restraint and primary and secondary static restraints. Am J Sports Med 13: 295-300

99. Taillard W, Meyer JM, Garcia J (1981) The sinus tarsi syndrome. Int Orthop 5: 117-130

100. Taylor DC, Englehard T DL, Basset FH (1992) Syndesmosis sprains of the ankle: The influence of heterotopic ossification. Am J Sport Med 20: 146-150

101. Veazey BL, Heckman JD, Galindo MJ, Mac Ganity PL (1992) Excision of uninited fractures of the posterior process of the talus: A treatment for chronic posterior ankle pain. Foot Ankle 13: 453-457

102. Vidal J, Fassio B, Buscayret C (1974) Instabilité externe de la cheville: Importance de l'articulation sous-astragalienne. Nouvelle technique de réparation. Rev Chir Orthop 60: 635-642

103. Watson-Jones R (1962) Fractures and joint injuries, 4th edn. Williams & Wilkins, Baltimore, pp 821-823

104. Wolin I, Glassman F, Sideman S (1950) Internal derangement of the talofibular compartment of the ankle. Surg Gynecol Obstet 91: 193-200

29.

Current concepts in the treatment of acute and chronic lateral ankle instability

WG Hamilton

The sprained ankle is the most common injury in sports that involve running and jumping. Eighty to ninety percent of these sprains involve the lateral ligament complex [7]. Treatment of these injuries in the past has been somewhat controversial [14]. There is common agreement regarding the initial treatment of the acute injury: "Rest, Ice, Compression and Elevation", followed by a rehabilitation program that stresses fibular strengthening and proprioceptive exercises while the ankle is protected by taping, aircast or bracing [12]. Controversy begins when we consider the question of when does one recommend surgery, and if so, which operation? The purpose of this article is to discuss the rationale involved in the decision-making process, and to review the basic anatomy and concepts leading to these decisions.

Ligament injuries (sprains) are customarily graded as: Grade I - a mild stretch with no instability, grade II - a partial tear with some instability, and grade III - a complete tear with gross instability (O'Donoghue) [12]. In order to apply this system to the lateral ankle specifically, a brief review of the anatomy is necessary.

Inman [11] in his excellent monograph drew analogies between the medial knee and the lateral ankle, noting that both structures are conical; that the anterior talofibular ligament was analogous to the anterior cruciate ligament, the calcaneofibular ligament to the medial collateral ligament and the posterior talofibular ligament to the posterior cruciate ligament (table 29.1). He also pointed out that the talar dome is shaped like the segment of a cone with its apex on the medial side of the ankle and its base on the lateral side. In addition, the sides of the segment are not parallel, but converge front to back so that the anterior width of the talus is wider

Table 29.1. Inman's analogies [11]

Ankle	Knee
Anterior talofibular lig.	Anterior cruciate lig.
Calcaneofibular lig.	Medial collateral lig.
Posterior talofibular lig.	Posterior cruciate lig.

than the posterior width (in solid geometry, this shape is called a "frustum"). This configuration results in a compact, stable ligamentous complex on the medial side, the deltoid ligament, but three distinct, separate, and less stable ligaments on the more expanded lateral side. These three ligaments, the anterior talofibular (ATFL), the calcaneofibular (CFL) and posterior talofibular (PTFL), radiate outward from the lateral malleolus like the spokes of a wheel, forward, downward and backward. He also noted that the angle between the ATFL and CFL is highly variable, usually between 100-135°, adding to the potential instability found in lateral ankle anatomy (In the knee, the cone is reversed, the medial knee being the base of the cone).

The order in which the ligaments tear depends upon the position of the ankle and foot when the inversion stress is applied. In running sports this is almost always in some degree of equinus or plantar-flexion, and in this position the ATFL is in a more vertical position and under tension, so that it is usually injured first. If the stress continues, the CFL tears next (see fig. 28.2). Also, this is why ankle sprains almost always occur with the loading or unloading phase of gait. The ankle ligaments are not actually necessary when the ankle is loaded. Stormont [16] found that, in the loaded condition,

Table 29.2. Working classification of acute ankle sprains

Severity	Injury	Phusical findings (drawer sign)	X-ray findings
Grade I	Partial tear ATFL	Negative	Normal talar tilt and drawer
Grade II	Torn ATFL Intact CFL	+ ++	Moderate talar tilt and drawer
Grade III	Torn ATFL Torn CFL	+++ (Grossly unstable)	Marked talar tilt and drawer

ATFL: Anterior talofibular ligament; CFL: Calcaneofibular ligament
Drawer sign (normal 4-5 mm)   + = Slightly greater than normal side
                                   ++ = Definitely greater than normal
                                   +++ = Grossly positive (>15°)

80% of ankle stability comes from the bony congruity of the joint, so in this position the ankle is stable even when all the ligaments are sectioned.

Although some authors have reported injuries to the PTFL, I have never found this ligament to be involved in ordinary ankle sprains and do not believe that such an injury exists. On rare occasions the CFL can be torn and the ATFL spared. This can happen when the ankle is in dorsiflexion at the time that inversion occurs, e.g., when a patient steps into a pothole so that the ankle dorsiflexes and then inverts when the heel hits the bottom of the hole. I have seen several cases of an isolated tear of the CFL, but ATFL followed by CFL tears are by far the most common. We use an injury classification based upon O'Donoghue's [12] that correlates well with the anatomic injury, the drawer sign on physical examination and the X-ray findings (table 29.2).

Over the years I have placed increasing emphasis on the drawer sign rather than the talar tilt X-ray. Others (Cox et al) [5] have questioned the reliability of the stress X-ray, due to normal variation in uninjured ankles, reproducibility (amount of force applied, position of the ankle at the time of stress application, use of local anesthesia, etc.), history of prior sprains, and the subtalar component of the instability. (The CFL is a major stabilizer of the subtalar joint and when it is torn, as in third degree sprains, there is always a subtalar component to the instability). This subtalar factor can sometimes be seen on a Broden stress X-ray, but this is somewhat difficult to perform (see fig. 28.3).

Most Grade I and II instabilities will do well with conservative treatment when there is no "hidden injury" that will cause the ankle to remain sympto-

Table 29.3. The "sprained ankle that won't heal"

* Unrecognized residual fibular weakness (probably the most common cause)
* Rotatory and/or subtalar instability
* Partial tear of the anterior tibiofibular ligament - the "high" ankle sprain
* Osteochondral fracture of the dome
* Avulsion fracture at the tip of the fibula
* Lateral process fracture of the talus
* Posterior process fracture of the talus ("Shepherd's fracture")
* Fracture of the anterior process of the talus
* Fibular tendon pathology of the talus (rents or splits)

matic after the sprain has healed. The "sprained ankle that won't heal" can be a diagnostic dilemma for the clinician (table 29.3).

Little controversy exists in the treatment of Grade I and II ankle injuries. There is almost universal agreement that early active use and rehabilitation are the treatments of choice [1, 4, 5, 9, 12]. However, the treatment of acute third degree sprains remains controversial. Traditionally, there have been three choices: 1) early active use with protection and rehabilitation, 2) cast immobilization (some authors favor immobilization in dorsiflexion to bring the ends of the ATFL close together [15], and 3) primary surgical repair. In the "old days" there was more hesitation to make a surgical rather than a nonsurgical decision because the procedures used to reconstruct chronically unstable ankles were difficult and involved [14]. Since the advent of the modified Brostrom operation good results are relatively easy to obtain later if the ankle remains symptomatic.

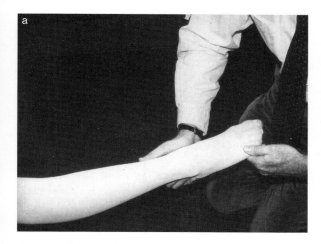
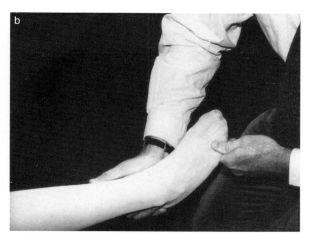

Fig. 29.1. Clinical evaluation of fibular strength. **a** A well conditioned athelete is able to resist to the varus force. **b** The fibulars are weak if the physician can push the foot into varus

This, and the fact that most studies now report an 80 to 90% success rate with non-operative methods [14], have all but eliminated the indications for primary repair of third degree ankle sprains.

There are, however, a few exceptions. One is the professional ballet dancer [9]. Fortunately, third degree ankle sprains are quite rare in dancers. Grade I and II sprains are by far the most common injury. On the rare occasion that a Grade III sprain does occur, operative repair might be considered for the following reasons:
• Unlike basketball players, dancers usually cannot dance with a Grade II sprain, so they will be "out" for three to six weeks, sometimes longer.
• Primary surgical repair (using the modified Brostrom) is very easy, with little associated morbidity. It is performed under local anesthesia, as an out-patient.
• They heal very well. Most surgically treated third degree sprains look better at six weeks post injury than second degree sprains treated non-operatively.
• Finally, it will take about three months to see if the ankle will work. If it doesn't, they will have to undergo an operative procedure, and that will take another three months. So there is a chance that they could miss six months out of a professional career that is not that long to begin with. With surgery, they are more certain to return at the earlier time.

Of course, the surgeon should discuss the two alternatives, along with their benefits and risks, with the patient. The final decision is a mutual one. The ultimate outcome fortunately is in the range of 75% to 100% success, regardless of whether the treatment is operative or non-operative. The difference is in the time lost to their career.

Regardless of the method of treatment, adequate physical therapy and proper rehabilitation are necessary to restore normal use following injury. Restoration of full fibular strength is essential. My preferred method is progressive resisted exercises (PREs) in the fully plantarflexed position [9]. Residual fibular weakness is a commonly unrecognized condition in dancers [9] and can cause a myriad of obscure symptoms such as unexplained swelling and discomfort, or poor timing with rapid movements. Any athlete complaining of these symptoms should be checked for weak fibulars. This is done by having them place their foot in full plantarflexion, (the "tendu" position for dancers), and asking them to hold this position against varus and then valgus stress. A well-conditioned athlete should be able to resist as much force as one can manually apply to the foot in this position. If you can push the foot into varus, the fibulars are weak and should be rehabilitated (fig. 29.1). The uninjured side can be checked for comparison if necessary. Weakness usually means that the fibulars have not been adequately rehabilitated, or they have been exercising in the neutral position rather than full plantarflexion. (Cybex and other exercise machines are not very good for ankle rehabilitation because the ankle cannot be placed in full plantarflexion). I use a home exercise program over the end of a sofa or couch with the dancers on their side using a weight bag in full plantarflexion. Abduction exercises are performed with the ankle supported so that it can only move

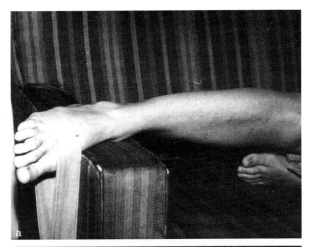

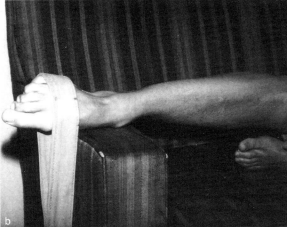

Fig. 29.2. Home rehabilitation for reinforcement of the fibulars. **a** Relaxed ankle. **b** Abduction exercise

for functional difficulties and not simply on the basis of a drawer sign or a positive stress X-ray. There are many professional athletes and dancers working quite well with loose ankles that are not symptomatic enough to warrant surgical repair.

The modified Brostrom procedure for symptomatic lateral ankle instability

Lennart Brostrom [2] in 1966 described an anatomic repair of the attenuated ATF and CF ligaments for correction of chronic lateral instability. They were shortened to their physiologic lengths and sutured at their anatomic locations, thus preserving a full range of motion. The operation depends on the fact that the ATF ligament lies within the capsule of the lateral ankle, similar to the glenohumeral ligaments of the shoulder. It is there, but it has been stretched and attenuated. The operation simply restores the original anatomy by shortening the lax ligaments. Brostrom reported 58 excellent or good results out of 60 cases. The procedure was very effective for dealing with laxity in the ATF ligament, but was less successful in correcting problems with CF laxity and subtalar instability.

In 1980 Nathaniel Gould [8] added his modification to the Brostrom operation: at the end of the procedure, the lateral portion of the extensor retinaculum is mobilized and sutured to the tip of the lateral malleolus over the repaired ligaments. This accomplishes 3 things: 1) it reinforces the repair, 2) it limits inversion, the position of danger for re-injury, 3) most importantly, it helps correct the subtalar component of the instability. (The CF ligament is an important stabilizer of the subtalar joint and when it is injured, as in most third degree sprains, there is usually a combination of tibiotalar and subtalar instabilities) (fig. 29.3).

upward in valgus and the patient can relax the ankle in between lifts (fig. 29.2). They lift 1.5 kg, 25 times slowly, morning and evening, increasing the weight in the bag by 1.5 kg each week to a total of 7.5 kg. When they can lift 7.5 kg slowly times they are adequately rehabilitated. I have never seen this method fail to restore normal fibular strength. The symptoms do not always disappear, and if they don't you have to look elsewhere for the cause (often a bone scan).

Secondary or delayed ankle ligament reconstruction may be necessary in an athlete but it should only be considered after full fibular strength has been obtained (see above) and the athlete is still unable to perform. In turning athletes, (e.g., dancers, skaters, gymnasts, etc.) often the problem is rotatory instability rather than varus instability. It must be emphasized that reconstruction should be done only

Indications

• Chronic lateral ankle instability, unresponsive to conservative therapy.
• Acute third degree sprains in selected professional or high performance athletes who need full range of motion and preservation of fibular function.

Contraindications

• Usual surgical precautions: circulation, infection, etc.

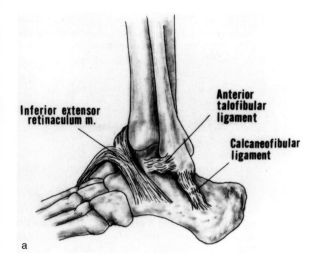

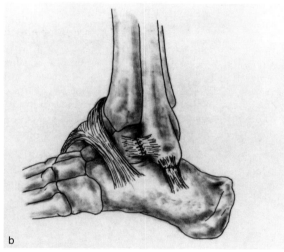

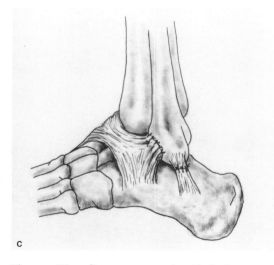

Fig. 29.3. Direct ligamentous repair with the Broström-Gould technique. **a** Attenuated ATFL and CFL. **b** Direct repair. **c** Reinforcement with the extensor retinaculum

• Neurologic weakness of the fibular muscles.

• Insufficient rehabilitation. The most common cause of "rolling over" in the ankle is not instability, but residual fibular weakness. Many athletes with positive stress films will not need surgery if their peroneals are strong.

• The heavy athlete who does not need both stability and motion. In these cases, one should consider supplementing the repair with an Evans type procedure using half of the fibularis brevis tendon.

• Fixed heel varus: a calcaneal osteotomy should be performed along with the reconstruction in these cases.

The operation is performed as an outpatient with general or spinal anesthesia in the lateral decubitus position, with a thigh tourniquet over cast padding. A short incision follows the anterior border of the distal fibula to the fibular tendons. The lateral portion of the extensor retinaculum is identified (running transversely over the distal portion of the capsule and ATF) and mobilized for attachment later.

A capsular incision is made, leaving a cuff on the fibula. The ATF ligament is usually seen as a thickening in this capsule. The CF ligament is identified deep to the tendons of the fibular muscles and is also divided, leaving a stump on the tip of the fibula for reattachment after the ligament has been shortened. The capsule and ligaments are then shortened to their normal length and sutured to their anatomic locations with permanent sutures. The extensor retinaculum is then pulled up over the tip of the fibula and sutured there with chromic catgut. The ankle is then checked for stability and taken through a full range of motion. A subcuticular closure is performed with an absorbable suture and steri-strips. The ankle is placed in anterior-posterior plaster splints and the patient discharged non-weight-bearing, on crutches.

Postoperative regimen: at 5-7 days post-op, a short leg cast or walking boot is applied for 3-4 weeks. At 4 weeks post-op, the cast is removed and the ankle is protected with an aircast. Physical therapy and swimming are begun. Inversion is avoided. Running and jumping are allowed at 7-8 weeks and full activities when the fibular muscles are strong, at 8-10 weeks.

I feel strongly that the tendon of the fibularis brevis muscle should never be used for ankle reconstruction in a professional dancer for two reasons. First, the fibularis brevis is too important as a support tendon for dancing on full pointe to be sacrificed. Second, it is not necessary to use it. I have had excellent results using the Brostrom repair as described by Gould [8]. In 50 professional dancers and athletes, this technique has not failed to give an excellent result with full range of motion and strength. A 15 year follow-up of my first case does not reveal any stretching of the repaired ligaments in spite of several re-injuries.

References

1. Boruta PM, Bishop JO, Braly WG, et al (1990) Acute lateral ligament injuries: a litterature review. Foot Ankle 11: 107-113
2. Brostrom L (1966) Sprained Ankles VI. Surgical treatment of "chronic" ligament ruptures. Acta Chir Scand 132: 551-565
3. Broden B (1949) Roentgen examination of the subtaloid joint in fractures of the calcaneus. Acta Radiol 31: 85-91
4. Clanton TO, Schon LC (1993) Athletic injuries to the foot and ankle. In: Mann RA, Coughlin MJ (eds) Surgery of the Foot and Ankle. Mosby, St Louis, pp 1095-1224
5. Cox J, Brand R (1977) Evaluation and treatment of lateral ankle sprains. Phys Sports Med 5: 51-55
6. Cox J (1985) How to prevent chronic ankle instability. J Musculoskel Med: 66-75
7. Garrick JG (1977) The frequency of injury, mechanism of injury and epidemiology and ankle sprains. Am J Sports Med 5: 241-242
8. Gould N, Seligson D, Glassman J (1980) Early and late repair of the lateral ligament of the ankle. Foot Ankle 1: 84-89
9. Hamilton WG (1982) Sprained ankles in ballet dancers. Foot Ankle 3: 99-102
10. Hamilton WG, Thompson FM, Snow SW (1993) The modified Brostrom procedure for chronic lateral ankle instability. Foot Ankle 14: 1-7
11. Inman V (1976) The joints of the ankle. Williams & Wilkins, Baltimore
12. O'Donoghue DH (1976) Treatment of injuries to athletes. WB Saunders, Philadelphia
13. Peters W, Trevino SG, Renstrom PA (1991) Chronic ankle instability. Foot Ankle 12: 182-191
14. St Pierre R, Allman F, Basset F (1982) A review of lateral ankle ligamentous reconstructions. Foot Ankle 3: 114-123
15. Smith RW, Reischel S (1988) The influence of dorsiflexion in the treatment of severe ankle sprains. Foot Ankle 9: 28-33
16. Stormont DM, Morry BF, An K, et al (1991) Stability of the loaded ankle. Relation between articular restraint and primary static restraints. Am J Sports Med 19: 583-587

30.

Bone tumors, dystrophies and rare bone lesions of the foot

M Bouvier

● Bone tumors [3, 9, 13, 17, 39, 41, 51, 56]

Bone tumors, benign or malignant, primary or secondary, are only rarely found in the feet. This low incidence, generally reckoned to be under 1%, gives rise to risks of error in diagnosis as well as delaying the necessary investigations and subsequent decisions regarding treatment.

Standard radiographs remain essential, but are not sufficient for diagnosis except for typical aspects of a very limited number of bone tumors [exostosis, chondroma, idiopathic cyst]. Bone scintigraphy, computed totography (CT) and magnetic resonance imaging (MRI) are all very often valuable aids in diagnosis and treatment. Scintigraphy measures the activity of the lesion and confirms the normal form of the rest of the skeleton. CT is currently the most used supplementary examination; it shows the presence of intratumoral calcification [cartilaginous tumors] or fluid [idiopathic cyst or aneurysmal cyst] and indicates possible extension to the soft parts [malignant tumors]. This examination may not provide a formal etiologic diagnosis, but allows surgery to be planned together with any preceding or accompanying biopsy. MRI, more effective than CT for soft tissues, can prove a useful additional imaging technique in difficult cases. Histologic examination remains essential to diagnosis in almost every case.

Benign tumors represent three-quarters of the cases of bone tumors of the foot. Osteoid osteoma is the commonest, followed by aneurysmal cyst and chondroma. The hindfoot is affected in around 60% of cases, the forefoot [metatarsus and phalanges] in 30% and the tarsus in 10%. Lytic appearances predominate in the calcaneus [idiopathic cyst, aneurysmal cyst, giant-cell tumor, chondroblastoma], whereas the denser or mixed aspects are most often seen in the talus [osteoid osteoma, osteoblastoma]. Cartilaginous tumors [exostosis, fibromyxoid chondroma] are most often seen in the forefoot. Among primary malignant tumors, Ewing's sarcoma is the most frequent, followed by chondrosarcoma and osteosarcoma; the hindfoot, especially the calcaneus, is most frequently affected. However, Ewing's sarcoma and chondrosarcoma seem to affect the calcaneus and the phalanges equally often. Secondary malignant tumors are really quite rare, but are a possibility to be kept in mind.

● Cystic lesions which simulate tumors [11]

Idiopathic cyst [20, 21, 26, 48]

Described by Virchow in 1877, the idiopathic cyst has a predilection for two locations, the upper ends of the humerus and femur, but among other locations, the calcaneus has a special place. It has also been observed in the talus, metatarsus and phalanges. Nonetheless, no more than 5% of cases affect the foot.

The lesion occurs during the first two decades of life. It is often asymptomatic and its discovery a matter of chance. Pathologic fractures, occurring frequently in the long bones, are rarer in the calcaneus.

The radiographic appearance is generally pathognomonic. Presenting a trapezoidal form, the cyst is located in the area of low trabeculation under the growth plate. The anterior cortex is vertical, whereas the posterior outline tends to follow the profile of the bone. The periphery is well defined by a marginal sclerosis, but the center is totally lacking in bony structure. Nevertheless, an idiopathic cyst must not be confused with images of metaphyseal rarefaction, often on both sides, which are a physiologic feature both in adults and children.

The usual therapeutic approach is one of caution, although local injections of corticosteroids have been tried. Only in the case of complicated fractures can surgery involving a bone graft be justified. Recovery occurs in all cases.

Aneurysmal cyst [28, 38, 45]

Described as a distinct entity by Lichtenstein in 1942, an aneurysmal cyst is most frequently located in the metaphyseal region of the long bones and in the posterior arch of the vertebrae, but it can be found in any bone, especially in the foot, where Ruiter ascribes it a frequency of around 10% of all cases. Its location there can be varied: the calcaneus, talus, metatarsus and, in exceptional cases, the tarsus and phalanges.

The lesion is generally found in the young, under the age of 20. There may be some recollection

of an injury during the months preceding discovery. The pain, usually localized, may be discovered by palpation and is often accompanied by swelling with an increase in local warmth and redness of the skin. The occurrence of a pathologic fracture may also be revelatory.

Standard radiographs show an area of osteolysis crossed by dividing septa to give a multilocular appearance (fig. 30.1a). The development of the lesion is often eccentric and asymmetric. The cortex may be destroyed but the lesion remains restricted by the periosteum, which it displaces and which is visualized by newly-formed bone on its deep aspect.

Among supplementary examinations, scintigraphic hyperfixation provides very precise location. Arteriography objectivizes the vascular character of the tumor (fig. 30.1b). CT is the examination of choice: it indicates the limits of the lesion and allows assessment of the periosteal shell, sometimes so fine that its continuity escapes standard radiologic examination. It confirms that the content is non-mineralized and may show up fluid levels located in cystic formations. MRI gives virtually identical information (figs. 30.1c, d).

Treatment is by surgery. Curettage and packing may in certain cases be supplemented by cryosurgery, but cannot rule out recurrence. It may therefore be preferable to perform resection, which is

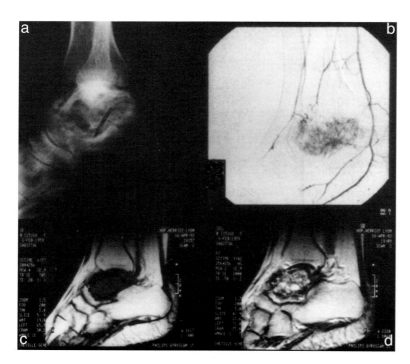

Fig. 30.1. Aneurysmal cyst of the talus. **a** Lateral radiograph of ankle: ballooned cystic lacunar lesion. **b** Selective digitized arteriography, heterogeneous "lumpy" contrast projecting on talus. **c** MRI T1: pathologic hyposignal affecting entire talus with thickening of cortex and periosteum. **d** MRI T2: mixed tissue and fluid hypersignal, "cystic" and "septate"

necessary in any case when extension will not permit curettage. Radiotherapy is effective but may cause sarcomatous degeneration, which excludes its use for the feet.

Tumors with exclusive or predominant bone differentiation

Osteoid osteoma [2, 4, 12, 23, 29, 36, 53]

Described by Jaffe in 1935, osteoid osteoma is a benign osteoblastic tumor composed of fibrous tissue with atypical osteoid bony tissue. According to data collected by us in 1979, the skeleton of the foot is affected in 10% of cases, occupying third place after cases occurring in the lower and upper limbs, and ahead of the spine. A predominance among men was found, and the lesion was most frequent between the ages of 10 and 30. There was some recollection of previous traumatism, but it was difficult to establish whether this precipitated or merely revealed the lesion.

Any bone in the foot may be affected, the talus most often, followed by the toes, calcaneus, tarsus and metatarsals. In every case the lesion was revealed by a painful syndrome. The pain is usually fixed and persistent, with nocturnal paroxysms which can usually be calmed by anti-inflammatory drugs, especially aspirin. On examination, there is normally tenderness at a precise site corresponding to the lesion. Local swelling is sometimes seen, especially of the toes, where hypertrophy accompanied by clubbing of an individual digit is the norm, but osteoid osteoma of the foot may quite frequently present a deceptive appearance: intermittent pain of a neuralgic nature, wasting of the leg muscles, or even pseudo-inflammatory manifestations located in the soft parts if the lesion has affected one of the superficial bones (metatarsals and especially phalanges), or if it is para-articular location, simu-

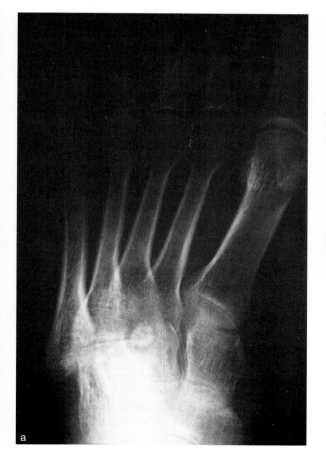

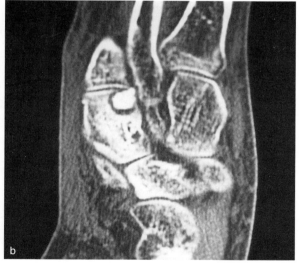

Fig. 30.2. Osteoid osteoma of second cuneiform appearing as a dense, rounded image on plain radiograph (**a**) with a classical rosette appearance on CT (**b**) (Courtesy of Pr. G. Llorca)

lating monoarthritis with inflammatory features and sometimes giving an appearance of nonspecific synovitis at synovial biopsy.

In standard radiographs osteoid osteoma normally appears as a clear area surrounded by a denser halo, or like a rosette if the center of the nidus is calcified (figs. 30.2a, b), but this appearance, in the feet as at other sites, is inconstant. When the lesion is located within the spongy tissue, it may remain invisible for a longer or shorter time, because of the absence of any sclerotic reaction. The lesion may also elude detection if it is located in the cortex and is concealed by the extent of perifocal sclerosis. There may be confusion with a patchy algodystrophy or a stress fracture. When the osteoid osteoma affects the neck of the talus, it may appear in various forms, indicating its superficial location and tendency to develop outside the bone: the image is of a notch in the cortex, with a periosteal reaction or calcification of the soft parts at this level indicating the location of the nidus outside the bone; at most, it may resemble an exostosis. Exceptional cases have been reported of a regional osteoporosis of the foot or premature fusion of the growth-plate in children.

When there is no radiographic evidence, or when the images are difficult to interpret, supplementary investigations become important. Bone scintigraphy gives a very precise location prior to any radiographic changes and enables CT to be correctly centered. As an element in diagnosis, scanography gives access to regions which are difficult to explore using conventional methods and allows analysis of deceptive or atypical forms. When the nidus is of sufficient size, the injection of an iodized bolus or an angioscanner may reveal its hypervascularity. Moreover, CT is useful pre-operatively in precise determination of the resection necessary, and post-operatively, to confirm adequate excision of the nidus. MRI is often not as effective as the scanner in showing the nidus and may give falsely sinister images by emphasizing the edematous reaction, to the extent that bone scintigraphy followed by use of CT remains at the core of diagnostic technique.

Treatment is of course by surgery. It consists of an en bloc excision of the lesion, the only way to avoid recurrence and to ensure complete and definitive recovery. Where location is difficult, standard radiographic techniques may be supplemented by bone scintigraphy at the preoperative stage.

Osteoblastoma

Osteoblastoma [46] is a very rare benign tumor whose differentiated osteoblastic cells produce osteoid material. It was described by Jaffe and Lichtenstein in 1956. It differs from osteoid osteoma in its size, greater than 3 cm, less marked reactive sclerosis and different histologic picture. However, as with osteoid osteoma, it occurs predominantly in males and especially between the ages of 10 and 30. It shows a marked predilection for the posterior arch of the vertebrae, then - in decreasing order - the pelvis, long bones of the limbs and foot, where it shows a particular affinity for the talus and calcaneus. It is evidenced by varyingly severe pain, less than that of osteoid osteoma, localized and of gradual onset. If the lesion is superficial there may be swelling; pathologic fracture is rare.

The radiographic appearance is often not very specific. The osteoblastoma appears as a rounded focus of osteolysis whose boundaries, sometimes marked by a moderate reactive osteosclerosis, are not always well-defined. Speckled opacities, indicative of the quality and maturation of the osteoid, may exist within the tumor. The appearance of the cortex may be similar to that found in aneurysmal cysts. In the tarsus, the tumor is normally located on the dorsal aspect of the anterior part of the talus, or may present as an expansive lesion, well-defined but extending to the soft parts at some distance from the bone. CT and MRI are indispensable in determining the limits of the tumor. Angiography, if used, will show up its intense vascularization.

The histologic diagnosis from osteosarcoma remains difficult in certain cases. Treatment is surgical and consists of resection of the tumor. Recurrence is possible but rare. Radiotherapy [around 40 Gy] is effective but reserved for vertebral lesions, particularly since sarcomas have been reported to develop in irradiated osteoblastomas.

Osteosarcoma

Osteosarcoma [17] is the commonest primary malignant bone tumor after plasmocytoma. It consists of mesenchymal cells which tend to differentiate into osteoblasts. If we except the exceptional secondary forms developing in pre-existing bony lesions, notably Paget's disease, osteosarcoma occurs mainly between the ages of 10 and 25. In the overwhelming majority of cases it is located at a metaphysis of one of the long bones; the foot represents only around 1% of cases.

The pain is often severe, associated with a hard or resistant swelling covered by taut red skin with local warmth and an increased collateral circulation. Pathologic fracture is rare at the outset. Development is rapid. Standard radiographs often combine zones of sclerosis and osteolysis. The periosteal reaction is accompanied by invasion of the soft parts, the extent of which can be assessed by CT and MRI.

Chemotherapy has transformed the prognosis. Administered pre-operatively, it increases the possibility of conservative surgery; post-operatively, it controls the otherwise very high percentage of pulmonary metastases.

Tumors with exclusive or predominant cartilaginous differentiation

Exostoses

Exostoses or osteochondromas may be solitary or multiple. The latter form a particular group known as "exostotic disease" (multiple exostoses), which is a genetic disorder.

Solitary exostoses
[22, 24, 25, 43, 54]

Formed of bone and covered with a cartilaginous cap, from which the lesion has developed, the solitary exostosis is the commonest of the benign tumors affecting the skeleton. It is found especially at the active metaphyses of the long bones but can develop in any bone with enchondral ossification. It is however relatively rare in the foot, where it is generally located on a tubular metatarsal or phalangeal bone. The distal phalanges may be affected and subungual lesions are classical but usually post-traumatic.

Diagnosis is generally made in patients under the age of 20 who notice swelling and find it difficult to put their shoes on, with an occasionally calcified bursitis and, in exceptional cases, a post-traumatic fracture.

Radiography shows up the bony part of the exostosis whereas CT and MRI display the cartilaginous covering. The radiologic appearance is generally typical, comparable in all respects to that of exostoses affecting the metaphyses of the long bones. The outlines are clear, but showing the base of implantation - whether sessile or pedicled - may require several different views. Areas of calcification may be seen within the lesion.

Surgical resection of the exostosis may be required, either because of the discomfort caused or because a rapid increase in size arouses fears (despite its rarity) of malignant degeneration.

Exostotic disease
(multiple exostoses) [8]

So called by Léry in 1925, exostotic disease is a chondrodystrophy occurring much less frequently than solitary exostosis. In this case the exostoses are generally multiple and relatively symmetric. They affect the active metaphyses of the long bones in particular, but all bones preformed in cartilage are susceptible. The skeleton of the foot is often affected, especially the metatarsals and phalanges.

Diagnosis is generally made at an early stage from the hereditary context and the concomitant deformity, with shortening of the affected bones. Examination of the foot reveals one or more palpable and visible swellings, frequently associated with a valgus due to asymmetric growth of the leg bones. Radiography shows the characteristic image of the exostosis and the shortening of the metatarsal or phalanx on which it is located.

The malignant degeneration of an exostosis, which frequently occurs in the trunk and proximal parts of the limbs, is rare in the foot, so much so that resection is only required for mechanical handicap.

Chondromas

Chondromas [9, 52], like exostoses, may be solitary or multiple. In the latter case they constitute a genuine chondrodysplasia, usually designated by the term enchondromatosis.

Solitary chondroma

This is generally found within the bone (enchondroma), more rarely between the bone and the periosteum (juxtacortical chondroma).

Enchondroma

This is quite common, representing 12% of benign bone tumors, and begins to develop in childhood, although diagnosis may be made at any age as it can often remain asymptomatic for an indefinite period. Nonetheless, when located in a superficial bone, it may become evident through swelling or a pathologic fracture.

More than half of all enchondromas are observed in the tubular bones of the hands but they may also be seen in the femur, humerus, tibia, fibula and the tubular bones of the foot. Their growth is slow and they generally remain small. They present a typical radiographic image of a round or ovoid lacuna, central or peripheral, tending to be expansive but respecting the contours of the bone, either homogeneous or containing scattered microcalcifications (figs. 30.3).

Malignant degeneration, a frequent occurrence in the long bones and limb girdles, is very rare in the hands and feet. Enchondroma of the foot does not need treatment unless it causes repeated fractures necessitating curettage with bone grafting. Recurrence, though recorded, is very rare.

Juxtacortical chondroma

This is a rare variety of chondroma which may affect the foot. It manifests itself as a hard, almost painless swelling. Radiologic examination may show only a slight excavation of the cortex with an osteosclerotic border. The presence of small foci of calcification within the lesion is, here too, of great diagnostic importance. In some cases a juxtacortical chondroma may grow to a considerable size and require block excision.

Multiple chondromas or enchondromatosis

Much rarer than the solitary chondroma and lacking any hereditary-familial features, enchondromatosis is characterized by the presence of multiple enchondromas associated with deformation and shortening of the long bones. The bones most frequently affected are, after the hand, the tubular bones of the foot, the femur, leg bones, pelvis, humerus and the bones of the forearm. The bones of the carpus and tarsus are not affected. Radiologically, the metatarsals and phalanges are full of lacunae, and are shortened and widened with a thinned cortex. The appearance of the foot is therefore very similar to that of the hand. Although it frequently occurs elsewhere, sarcomatous transformation takes place neither in the hand nor the foot.

Chondrosarcoma [27]

A malignant cartilaginous tumor which can be primary or secondary, chondrosarcoma occurs at a relatively advanced age. It develops either from the

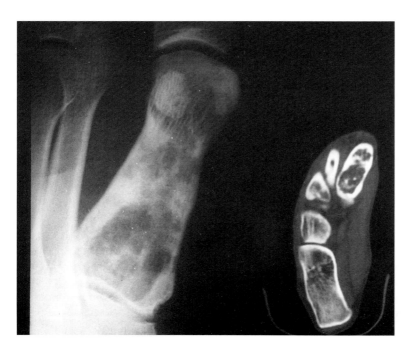

Fig. 30.3. Chondroma of first metatarsal: 3/4 oblique radiograph of first ray (*left*) and horizontal section by CT (*right*) osteolysis of first metatarsal respecting bony cortices: spotty central calcifications, highly indicative of chondroma

interior of the bone (central chondrosarcoma) or from an exostosis (peripheral chondrosarcoma). Lesions of the hands and feet are exceptional. Its fairly slow development may lead to delayed diagnosis. The histology is often difficult to interpret, to such an extent that the clinical and especially the radiologic findings become particularly important, whether it is a question of progressive osteolysis by a central chondrosarcoma or of the opaque foci typical of a peripheral chondrosarcoma. Treatment is exclusively by surgery and offers very good chances of recovery since metastases are rare and late in developing.

Benign chondroblastoma [9, 52]

The benign chondroblastoma is a tumor with an epiphyseal or apophyseal site, occurring between the ages of 10 and 25. The most frequent locations are in the humerus, tibia and femur, but the bones of the foot, notably the calcaneus and talus, are among the classic sites.

The pain is generally moderate and can continue for months if not years, or be elicited by injury. Swelling may be observed in superficial forms. Radiography reveals an area of radiolucency which is eccentric, rounded or lobular with sharp outlines and the frequent presence of small calcified particles. Confusion with a simple cyst in the calcaneus is possible. The cortex may be ballooned by the tumor. The sclerosed margins may be partially or entirely absent, raising questions as to the benign nature of the tumor. Its dimensions are often modest, no greater than 1 or 2 cm, but there are expansive cases which may invade the joints and adjacent bone. Bone scintigraphy shows an unimpressive hyperfixation. CT and MRI, far more useful, sensitively detect the intratumoral calcification and determine the extent of the lesion.

Treatment is by surgery with careful curettage of the lesion, supplemented if necessary by a bone graft or the insertion of acrylic cement. Local recurrence is possible. There is no malignant degeneration except for radiotherapy-induced sarcoma, whose treatment is altogether different.

Chondromyxoid fibroma [1, 16]

Chondromyxoid fibroma is the least frequent of the cartilaginous tumors. It is especially found between the ages of 10 and 30 and in 80% of cases is sited at the metaphyses of the long bones. Extension to the epiphysis is possible after ossification of the growth plate. The foot skeleton is not spared, especially as regards the calcaneus and the metatarsals. It is sometimes revealed by moderate and intermittent pain or by swelling, but incidental discovery is common. Radiographically, it appears as a rounded or oval area of osteolysis with polycyclic contours and a dense peripheral border, frequently eccentric, ballooning and narrowing the cortex. Spotty calcification may be observed. The bony expansion may be fusiform.

Cure is usual after simple surgical curettage, sometimes supplemented by a bone graft, but some practitioners admit the possibility of recurrence and even of malignant transformation.

Giant-cell tumor [14, 19, 30, 31]

Although they show a particular predilection for the epiphyses of the knee and the lower extremity of the radius, giant-cell tumors may occur in other locations, especially the pelvis and sacrum. They represent from 5 to 8% of primary tumors of the foot. Any foot bone may be affected: calcaneus, talus, navicular, cuboid, cuneiform, metatarsals or phalanges. Diagnosis is generally made during the third or fourth decade of life. Pain is usual and generally mechanical in origin. It is accompanied by dysfunction and often by swelling, sometimes large, and an inflamed appearance with increased local warmth and redness of the skin. Pathologic fractures are not exceptional.

X-rays show an osteolytic lesion, occasionally with dividing septa. The appearance is ballooned and tends to be asymmetric (fig. 30.4). There is no periosteal reaction or invasion of the soft parts, hence the importance of CT and MRI in this context.

Treatment by curettage and packing has been improved by the use of cryotherapy and acrylic cement, but does not rule out recurrence. Resection - whether optional or inevitable - is therefore more widely indicated in the foot than at other sites, especially when the metatarsals or phalanges are affected and above all when the form is potentially malignant.

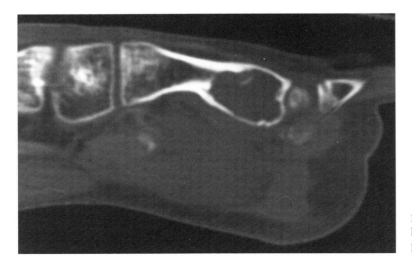

Fig. 30.4. Giant-cell tumor appearing as a large osteolytic area ballooning the distal part of the first metatarsal

Vascular tumors

Angioma or hemangioma [37]

A well-known bone lesion, often remaining asymptomatic throughout life, the angioma or hemangioma has a predilection for the body of the vertebra where it usually gives the pathognomonic appearance of a striated vertebra. A honeycombed appearance is most frequent in the skeleton of the limbs, but location in the foot is in any case exceptional.

Angiosarcoma or hemangioendothelioma [7, 32]

These are rare tumors which can be seen at all ages, most frequently situated in the metaphysis or diaphysis of the long bones of the limbs. Out of 66 cases, five lesions in the foot were reported by Campanacci and Ruggieri [11]. Pain may be accompanied by swelling. The radiographic appearance is that of an osteolysis, sometimes aggressive with obliteration of the cortices; only its possibly multicentric character suggests the diagnosis. The prognosis remains grave despite treatment combining surgery, radiotherapy and chemotherapy.

Lipoma

A benign tumor, consisting of adipocytes of medullary origin, lipoma is among the rarest of primary bone tumors (Rhodes). When located in the foot it shows a predilection for the calcaneus (fig. 30.5). Apt to be asymptomatic, it may nevertheless produce a painful swelling of the heel. Radiographic expression is lytic with a cystic appearance, sometimes expansile with a thin but intact cortex. CT and MRI, by assessing the density of the bone tissue, help distinguish a lipoma from solitary and aneurysmal cysts, provided any calcification within the lesion is not too extensive. The prognosis is excellent. Nevertheless, treatment by curettage and packing must take into account not just the functional handicap, but also the proximity of the subtalar joint with the risk of intra-articular fracture. Lesions of the tubular bones of the foot are exceptional.

Bone marrow tumors

Ewing's sarcoma [10, 35]

Ewing's sarcoma is a tumor with small round cells whose nature is yet to be established and which remains classified by Dahlin and Unni as one of those tumors whose histogenesis is still unknown. Its greatest frequency occurs between the ages of 10 and 20, with a marked predilection for the metaphyseal and diaphyseal regions of the long bones and for the skeleton of the trunk. However it may sometimes be observed in the foot, with a frequency recently reported by Campanacci and Ruggieri as 13 cases out of 409 [10]. It may be found in the tarsus, metatarsals and more rarely in the phalanges.

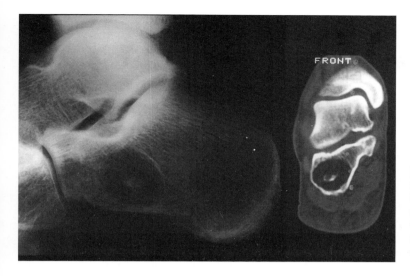

Fig. 30.5. Intraosseous lipoma of calcaneus. Calcaneus in lateral view: radiolucent image involving calcaneus, clearly defined, with central calcification (*left*). Coronal section by CT; the fatty density confirms the diagnosis of lipoma. The characteristic central calcification is clearly visible (*right*)

Attention is generally drawn to it by a painful swelling which grows rapidly in size, accompanied by deterioration of the general state of health involving fever, weight-loss, anemia and an increase in the erythrocyte sedimentation rate. Standard radiographs show an essentially osteolytic image which may however be accompanied by a reactive ossification of the periosteum. Its extension within the bone and especially its invasion of the soft parts is best shown by CT and MRI. Scintigraphy is useful for determining extension in the affected bone and especially for detecting the possible presence of other skeletal lesions. Biopsy is indispensable for diagnosis and must be read by an expert histologist as confusion is possible with several other pathologic bone processes.

Spontaneous development is generally rapid, with frequent visceral (notably pulmonary) or skeletal dissemination. Polychemotherapy has however considerably increased the period of survival. It is used both pre- and postoperatively. It is an essential partner to surgery, whose effectiveness is increased in this disease if the lesion is suitable for amputation. Radiotherapy is not as important for the foot as for other bone sites; the combination of polychemotherapy and surgery gives some hope of a favorable prognosis in the long term.

Solitary plasmocytoma of the bone
[5, 34, 39, 49, 50, 51, 55]

Solitary plasmocytoma of the bone is a rare tumor affecting men in particular, often before the age of 50. It is located especially in the vertebral column, pelvis and long bones. Lesions in the distal extremities, notably the feet, are rare. Pain, frequently nocturnal, is the usual presenting feature. A tumor in the foot is often palpable, as for other superficial lesions. Pathologic fracture is possible.

Standard radiographs supplemented by modern imaging procedures usually show an appearance of localized osteolysis with sharp boundaries, but with no sclerotic peripheral reaction. An image similar to a giant-cell tumor with a ballooned trabeculated appearance may be observed. Laboratory evidence is absent or minor. Acceleration of the sedimentation rate and the presence of monoclonal gammapathy are very irregular. The myelogram is by definition normal. There is no anemia or change in renal function or any disturbance of calcium and phosphorus metabolism. Bone scintigraphy confirms the pathologic and progressive nature of the radiologic image and confirms that it is a solitary lesion, although the inconstancy and unobtrusiveness of the hyperfixation of certain plasmocytic lesions are known and invite circumspect interpretation. Aspiration or surgical biopsy is the only way to determine the plasmocytic nature of the lesion.

Treatment is based on surgical excision with supplementary radiotherapy (40 to 60 Gy). Disappearance of the monoclonal component, where it exists, is a good prognostic factor. Local recurrences are rare, but transformation into multiple myeloma, sometimes late, is always a concern. This requires chemotherapy, which is not justified for solitary bone plasmocytoma.

Distal metastases [6, 18, 39, 44]

Very frequent in the axial skeleton, bony metastases are rare, indeed exceptional, beyond the elbow and knee. We have personally recorded in 252 cases the following distribution: forearm = 39 cases, hand = 85 cases, leg = 78 cases, foot = 50 cases. In the 50 cases affecting the skeleton of the foot, the primary cancer responsible was as follows: uterus = 13 cases, breast = 12 cases, lungs = 9 cases, kidney = 6 cases, digestive tract = 4 cases. Other sites of origin, notably prostatic, were very rare. The frequency of uterine cancer, notably of the cervix, is very unusual here. The lesion generally affects the tarsus. It is mostly solitary and only forms part of a generalized metastatic dissemination in the bones, except in cases of mammary origin. Though revelatory in rare cases, it normally appears in parallel with a progressive resumption of activity in the primary tumor.

Pain is the main signal but the existence of a swelling is frequent, given the superficial nature of the affected bones. The bone tumor may take on an inflamed, pseudo-arthritic appearance, with local redness and heat. The radiographic appearance is almost always osteolytic and marked by a loss of substance affecting a bone in either part or whole (figs. 30.6 & 30.7). Osteolysis occurs progressively, and is often difficult to perceive initially, but leads to secondary rupture of the cortex which can be detected by CT and MRI, whereas bone scintigraphy is primarily concerned as the main indicator of extension to the rest of the skeleton. There is a fairly frequent occurrence of "satellite" osteoporosis affecting the bony segments immediately above and below and which simulates an idiopathic algodystrophy. The rarity of metastases in the foot necessitates histologic confirmation as a general rule.

The distal site of the metastasis modifies treatment only slightly. Radiotherapy is the basic treatment, alleviating the pain, stabilizing and often

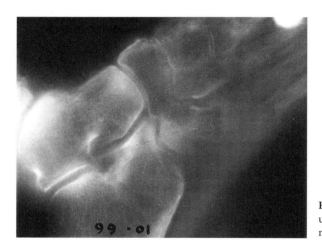

Fig. 30.6. Metastasis of medio-tarsus secondary to cancer of the uterus: zone of osteolysis affecting the navicular, cuboid and middle cuneiform bones

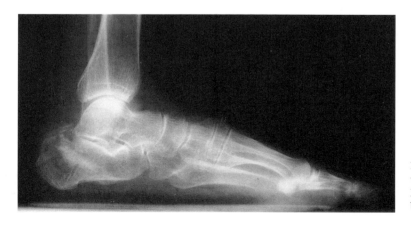

Fig. 30.7. Lateral radiograph: pathologic fracture of calcaneus through metastasis of an ENT cancer surgically treated one year before

densifying the radiologic images. Hormone therapy has the same indications as in standard locations. Surgical excision has only a minor role. It may however be used when an isolated metastasis is detected and the primary tumor is cured locally or is itself accessible to surgical treatment. Secondary amputation following radiotherapy and local recurrence enabled us to observe a genuine recovery at a follow-up of more than 15 years in a navicular metastasis of uterine origin, but generally speaking a distal site does not alter the gravity of the prognosis.

Bone dystrophies [39, 52]

Paget's disease

Its location in the foot bones is quite frequent with a particular affinity for the calcaneus. Rarely solitary, this location is almost always within the framework of a case of multifocal Paget's disease. Its clinical expression is as a diffuse or plantar heel pain, sometimes with an increase in the volume of the heel region making it difficult to put shoes on. Simple radiographs provide diagnosis by showing the combination of osseous hypertrophy of either the entire calcaneus or only its posterior portion, with modeling of structure of fuzzy or fibrillary type. This affection may give rise to a posterior subtalar arthrosis with beak-shaped osteophytes. A lesion of the navicular bone, which is much rarer, is normally of fibrillary structure. Osteosclerosis may be observed in the metatarsals and phalanges and a broadening of the diaphysis with cortico-medullary dedifferentiation. Wearing of a supple support for the heel may be added to the general treatment [calcitonin, diphosphonates] in the case of heel pain. Anti-inflammatory radiotherapy is formally contra-indicated, given the risk of sarcomatous transformation.

Fibrous dysplasia

Histologically characterized by an invasion of the medullary cavity by fibrous tissue, this is a congenital disease which is relatively frequent, especially in its monostotic form. In the limbs, the frequency of location diminishes from attachment to extremity, to the extent that the foot, like the hand, is rarely affected, and only appears in the most extensive

cases. The tarsus is generally spared. On the other hand a metatarsal ray may be affected, the radiographic signs being a broadening of the diaphysis, deformation and remodeling of the bony framework, with cavities and narrowing of the cortex. Cystic forms are rare.

Rare bone lesions [39, 52]

Constitutional osteopetroses

These are genetic diseases characterized by an abnormal sclerosis of bone, general or local, uniform or otherwise.

The osteopetrosis called "marble bone disease" by Albers-Schönberg appears as a diffuse sclerosis of the skeleton. Alternating light and dark bands give the bone a characteristic appearance. The broadening of the long bone metaphyses into the shape of a bludgeon or golf club is also characteristic. The medullary channel may narrow until it disappears altogether. The early form, with recessive transmission, is serious because of its hematologic effects, whereas the development of the later forms, with dominant transmission, is mainly indicated by fractures, compression of the cranial nerves and osteitis of the jaws of dental origin. The tarsal nuclei show variable densities: homogeneous, centered or surrounded by a lucent image. These aspects may appear in adults as images of "a hole in the bone" or "a bone within the bone". Sclerosis in the metatarsals and phalanges predominates at the epiphyses, but fractures are usually of the diaphyses.

Pyknodysostosis is a disease with autosomal recessive transmission involving a deficiency in stature, short limbs, dysmorphism - especially of the cranio-facial area, generalized osteosclerosis and fragility of the bones. All the bones are abnormally dense but without remodeling. The hands and feet are short with malformed nails. There is hypoplasia or osteolysis of the distal phalanges with fraying of the terminal tufts. Fractures occur mainly in the diaphyses of the metatarsals. The combination of bone sclerosis with dysmorphism permits straightforward diagnosis.

Osteopoikilosis is a dominant hereditary affection with no clinical expression, usually characterized by a scattering of small oval or rounded islets of sclerosis, giving the affected bone segments a mottled appearance. Distribution is symmetric. The most numerous patches appear at the distal extremities of the limbs, in the skeleton of the hands and feet. The striated form described by Voorhoeve is much rarer.

Melorheostosis is a rare affection whose genetic origin is a moot point. It is characterized by a ribbon-like sclerosis of the bone, typically localized to one limb where it spreads as if flowing from one end to the other on its lateral or medial aspect. Small bones, especially in the feet, are often completely sclerotic. The tarsus, metatarsus and phalanges may be affected. The affection may provoke pain, unequal limb length and walking difficulties.

Genetic bone diseases with excessive bone transparency

We will only mention here Lobstein's disease (osteopsathyrosis) which is the late form of an osteogenesis imperfecta. It is a familial and hereditary disorder characterized by abnormal bone fragility with multiple fractures, generally appearing in childhood. Associated with the bone fragility are blue scleros and deafness. The bones are abnormally transparent with very thin cortices. The deformations which they usually suffer are the result of fractures as much as their lack of resistance. In the feet the tarsus has a fibrillary structure but the metatarsal shafts are the seat of a paradoxical skeletal sclerosis.

References

1. Alchermes LS, Rusnack T, Alachermes LA (1984) Chondromyxoïd fibroma. A rare benign bone tumor. J Am Podiatry Assoc 74: 363-367
2. Assoun J, De Haldat F, Richardi G, Billey T, Dromer C, Fournie B, Bonnevialle P, Railhac JJ (1993) Imagerie par résonance magnétique des ostéomes ostéoïdes. Rev Rhum 60: 28-36
3. Atlas Radiologique (1974) Les tumeurs osseuses. Comité néerlandais. Maloine, Paris
4. Bakst R, Janigian J (1987) Osteoïd osteoma of the talus. A case report and literature review. J Am Podiatry Assoc 77: 512-516
5. Bataille R. Sany J (1981) Solitary myeloma: clinical and prognostic features of a review of 114 cases. Cancer 48: 845
6. Bouvier M, Lejeune E, Robillard J, Colombani R (1970) Les métastases osseuses distales. Revue lyonnaise de Médecine 19: 811-844
7. Bundeus WD Jr, Brighton CT (1965) Malignant hémangioendotheliomas of bone. Report of two cases and review of the literature. J Bone Joint Surg 762: 47
8. Bresnahan PJ., Morris DK (1988) Multiple cartilaginous exostosis. J Am Podiatry Assoc 78: 532-535
9. Campanacci M, Ruggieri P (1992) Tumeurs osseuses à histogenèse cartilagineuse. Encycl Med Chir (Paris, France), Appareil locomoteur 14030-C10
10. Campanacci M, Ruggieri P (1993) Sarcome d'Ewing. Encycl Med Chir (Paris, France), Appareil locomoteur 14030-D40
11. Campanacci M, Ruggieri P (1993) Lésions pseudotumorales. Encycl Med Chir (Paris, France). Appareil locomoteur 14030-K10
12. Carfagni A, Moreschini O, Billi A (1990) The importance of clinial semiotics and instrumental investigations in the diagnosis and surgical treatment of osteoid osteoma: a report of 6 cases. Ital J Orthop Traumatol 16: 25-37
13. Casadei R, Ferraro A, Ferruzzi A, Biagini R, Ruggieri P (1991) Tumori ossei del piede: epidemiologia e diagnosi. Chir Organi Mov 76: 47-62
14. Charisse Dunn E, Mauro G, Cohen R (1992) Giant-cell tumor of the intermediate cuneiform. A case report. J Am Podiatry Assoc 82: 208-211
15. Chesi V, Lennortz KJ (1975) A case of sarcoma of the talus giving the radiographic apperence of a "cyst". Z Orthop 1027: 113
16. Crisafulli JA, Adams D, Sakhuja R (1990) Chondromyxoid fibroma of a metatarsal. J Foot Surg 29: 164-168
17. Dahlin DC, Unni K (1986) Bone tumors. General aspects and data on 8542 cases. Charles C. Thomas, Springfield
18. Desmanet E, Amrani M, Fievez R, Six Ch (1991) Les acrométastases. À propos de deux cas. Revue de la littérature. Ann Chir Main 10: 154-157
19. Dunn EC, Mauro G, Cohen R (1992) Giant-cell tumor of the intermediate cuneiform. A case report. J Am Podiatry Assoc 8: 208-211
20. Epstein J, Wertheimer SJ (1984) Unicameral bone cyst of the calcaneous. Literature review and case studies. J Am Podiatry Assoc 74: 76-79
21. Frankel SL, Chioros PG, Sidlow CJ (1988) Steroïd injection of a unicameral bone cyst of the calcaneus: literature review and 2 cases. J Foot Surg 27: 60
22. Freedman DJ., Luzzi A, Piccioti J (1987) Solitary osteochondroma of the distal phalanx. A case report. J Am Podiatry Assoc 77: 615-617
23. Freiberger RH, Lottman BS, Helpern M, Thomson TC (1959) Osteoïd osteoma: a report on 80 cases. Am J Roentgenol 82: 194-205
24. Greenberg D, Lenet MD, Sherman M (1983) A large osteochondroma of the third toe. J Am Podiatry Assoc 73: 208-211
25. Greger G, Catanzariti (1992) Osteochondroma: review of the literature and case report. J Foot Surg 31: 298-300
26. Grumbine NA, Clark GD (1986) Unicameral bone cyst in the calcaneus with pathologic fracture. A literature review and case report. J Am Podiatr Assoc 76: 96-99
27. Joseph R, Stones G., Klein DE., Cavuoto JW (1987) Chondrosarcoma of the foot. J Am Podiatr Assoc 77: 223-227

28. Kashuk KB, Hanft JR, Schabler JA, Kado KE, Wolosky BD (1990) Anevrysmal bone cyst of the cuboid. J Am Podiatr Med Assoc 80: 558-594

29. Kent K Wu (1991) Osteoid osteoma of the foot. J Foot Surg 30: 190-194

30. Kent K Wu (1992) Giant-cell tumor of the foot. J Foot Surg 31: 414-419

31. Khanna AK, Sharma SV, Kumar M (1990) A large metatarsal gian-cell tumor. Acta Orthop Scand 61: 271-272

32. Khiyami A, Green LK, Gyorkey F, Landou G (1991) Primary angiosarcoma of the cuboidal bone: a case report. Diagn Cytopathol 7: 520-523

33. Khurana JS, Mayo-Smith W, Kattapuram SV (1990) Subtalar arthralgia caused by juxta articular osteoid osteoma. Clin Orthop 252: 205-208

34. Lasker JC, Lane M (1991) Solitary myeloma of the talus bone. Cancer 68: 202-205

35. Leeson MC, Smith MJ (1989) Ewing's sarcoma fo the foot. Foot Ankle lo: 147-151

36. Lejeune E, Dejour H, Bouvier M, Llorca G, Andre-Fouet A (1979) Ostéome ostéoïde du pied. À propos de 4 observations personnelles. Rev Rhum 46: 711-717

37. Lidholm SV, Lindbone A, Spjut HJ (1961) Multiple capillary hemangiomas of bones of the foot. Acat Pathol Microbiol Scand 51: 9

38. Montagne J, Chevrot A, Galmiche JM (1980) Atlas de Radiologie du Pied. Masson, Paris

39. Mc Namara G, Beheshti F, Saunders TG., Glubo SM (1982) Aneurysmal bone cyst of a metatarsel. A case report and review of the literature. J Am Podiatr Assoc 72: 356-360

40. Newcott EP (1987) A solitary plasmocytoma in the foot. J Am Podiatr Assoc 77: 187-190

41. Nicholas A, Grumbine DPM, Gregory DC (1986) Unicameral bone cyst in the calcaneus with pathologic facture. A literature review and case report. J Am Podiatr Assoc 76: 96-99

42. Rajesh Makashir, Chauhan S, Kapoor Ravi, Mandal AK (1991) Primary tumors of small bones: a clinico-pathological and radiological study. Indian J Pathol Microbiol 34: 30-38

43. Rosen James S (1983) Solitary osteochondroma of the metatarsal. J Am Podiatr Assoc 73: 261-262

44. Rosen A, Halperin N, Halevi A, et al (1985) A rare metastasis from breast adenocarcinoma to the big toe. Orthoped Rev 14: 428

45. Ruiter OJ, Van Rijsell TG, Van Der Velde EA (1977) Aneurysmal bone cysts: a clinicopathological study of 105 cases. Cancer 39: 2231

46. Semer LC, Fleming WC, Drossner B, Levin R (1990) Osteoblastoma of the distal phalanx of the hallux. J Foot Surg 29: 357-360

47. Shaderr AF, Schwartzenfeld SA (1989) Osteoid osteoma: report of a case. J Foot Surg 28: 438-441

48. Smith RW, Smith CF (1974) Solitary unicameral bone cyst of the calcaneus. J Bone Joint Surg 56A: 49

49. Snapper I, Kahn A (1971) Myelomatosis: fundamentals and clinical features. University Park Press, Baltimore, pp 179-267

50. Sprinkle RLB, Santangelo L, De Ugarte R (1988) Solitary plasmocytoma of bone in the calcaneus. J Am Podiatr Assoc 78: 636-642

51. Todd IDH (1965) Treatment of solitary plasmocytoma. Clin Radiol 16: 395

52. Trial R (1969) Os. Pathologie générale. Masson, Paris

53. Vicens JL, Aubspin D, Buchon R, Schoenenberger P, Flageat J (1990) Intérêt de la tomodensitométrie dans les ostéomes ostéoïdes. Sem Hop Paris 66: 909-913

54. Warren MG, Reid JM (1982) Osteochondroma of the first metatarsal bone. A case report. J Am Podiatr Assoc 72: 469-470

55. Wiltshaw E (1976) The natural history of extramedullary plasmocytoma and its relationship to solitary myeloma of bone and myelomatosis. Medicine 55: 217

56. Wold LE, Unni KK, Beahout JW, Ivius JC, Bruckman JE, Dahlin DC (1982) Hemangioendothelial sarcoma of the bone. Am J Surg Pathol 6: 59-70

57. Yeager KK, Mitchell LM, Sartoris DJ(1991) Diagnostic imaging approach to bone tumors of the foot. J Foot Surg 30: 197-208

Additional references

Rhodes RD, Page JC (1993) Intraosseous lipoma of the os calcis. J Am Podiatr Med Assoc 83: 288-292

31.

Overuse syndromes of the foot during running

M Bouysset, E Noël and M Bonnin

Injuries of the foot and ankle during running occur in 30 to 50% of cases [7, 19, 22]. A single incident is rarely the cause; in the great majority of cases repeated micro-traumatisms during athletic activity must be incriminated, usually in an endurance sport activity. The concentration of stresses in some areas produces lesions which finally create an overuse pathology [15]. The following text is restricted to a discussion of some general notions about the factors which provoke this pathology.

Several anatomic structures may be concerned (tendons, bursae, muscles, aponeuroses, ligaments, capsules, nerves, cartilage, bones); several pathologic features may be associated [5, 7, 15, 19, 31, 32, 36]; bone involvement with stress fractures is dealt with another chapter.

It is known that physical activity provokes histologic and biochemical changes in the tendons, whose capacity to adapt to external stress varies with the nature and intensity of the activity. The functioning of this process appears more efficient when adaptation is gradual; tendon lesions may appear when the increase of effort is abrupt [12, 17, 18]. This example emphasizes the value of progressive training, which helps to compensate for certain forms of imbalance [5].

The treatment of the overuse pathologies must eliminate the causal disturbances, i.e., a lower level of activity must be practiced to allow recovery. For a runner, this may extend from a slight reduction of training distance to a non- weight-bearing situation. To keep up acceptable physical activity during treatment, the patient may practice substitution sports which do not add to the existing stresses [14, 15, 39].

● Etiology

The factors provoking the appearance of overuse pathology may be innocuous in everyday life but are manifested after a certain threshold of physical activity.

Intrinsic factors
[8, 13, 14, 15, 17]

The foot, but also the upper joints of the lower limb, may be affected by anatomic or functional anomalies [5]. These intrinsic factors have various consequences with the type of sport [27, 36]; their treatment will attempt to restore function as nearly as possible to normal and after the symptoms may disappear [13, 15].

Malalignment syndromes

• **Hindfoot hyperpronation** seems to be involved in around 56% of cases in runners [16, 19]. During walking or running, at the moment of heel strike the foot is slightly supinated and then rapidly pronates under load [4, 29, 40]. During this transition from supination to pronation, a variable amount of stress is absorbed by the structures supporting the foot. Any constraint which is opposed to the harmonious distribution of the ground reaction forces may focus these forces at one point, where a local secondary lesion may appear [5, 21]. Hyperpronation increases internal rotation of the tibia and leads to fatigue of the support structures of the foot; stretching of the midfoot and subsequent stresses on the plantar aponeurosis and plantar muscles. Though stresses may have no consequences during normal walking, during running the ground reaction forces reach two or three times the body weight; pathologic involvement of the support structures of the foot may then appear, involving bones or soft parts or both [14, 19, 24, 36]. Hence the role of overweight in the development of overstrain pathology.

• **The cavo-varus foot** has too high an instep and above all is too rigid. The normal pronation is lost, the ground reaction forces are insufficiently absorbed, and the foot cannot adapt to the ground surface [4, 21]. The repetition and the increased intensity of the microtraumatisms lead to various lesions: metatarsalgia, calcaneal tendinopathy and painful heel syndromes [4, 19, 20, 21, 31].

• **Other malalignments** in the transverse plane are often more difficult to analyze. Rotational disturbances of the hip, particularly excessive anteversion, frequently seem to be incriminated. They modify the value of the angle of gait; the latter is defined by the direction of progression of the body and the axis of the foot at heel strike, and seems to vary according to the person and the type of sport; when it is greater, the tendency to hyperpronation increases with the consequences described before [5, 33, 37]. In the lower limb as a whole, disturbances compensatory to torsions and frontal malalignment may be associated with overuse injuries. James describes the "miserable malalignment" which includes excessive anteversion of the femoral neck, patellar deviation with lateral subluxation, external torsion of the tibia in its proximal part, genu varum and subtalar joint hyperpronation [16].

Limb-length discrepancy

Limb-length discrepancy is common in the lower limbs. It provokes an asymmetry in joint function and may explain overuse injuries.

Two sorts of limb-length discrepancy may be described [1, 2, 3, 36, 38]:

• Structural limb-length discrepancy is an anatomic shortening between the femoral head and the talocrural mortice, without biomechanical disorders. Many affections may produce this shortening: unequal development, sequelae of fractures, or diseases like poliomyelitis and osteomyelitis. During running, the longer leg has a prolonged stance phase; as the pace increases, support becomes increasingly monopodal, subjecting the longer limb to increased stress for a longer period of time; the subtalar joint of the longer limb hyperpronates and reciprocally the subtalar joint of the shorter limb supinates [3]. Other stresses affect the ankles, knees, hips and lumbar spine.

• Functional limb-length discrepancy is due to altered mechanics of the lower limb: the joints function asymmetrically and a shortening of the limb appears during motion on weight-bearing. The asymmetry of calcaneal valgus is an example; for some authors, when the difference in calcaneal pronation during weight-bearing at midstance between the two feet is 3 degrees or more, a functional limb discrepancy will exist [2, 3]. During the practice of a sport malalignment increases because, on the one hand, the body weight is on a single foot and, on the other, ground reactions forces may increase greatly. However, if clinical assessment is made in the well-balanced bipodal position the deformations do not appear, or are less obvious. This emphasizes the value of clinical evaluation in conditions as near as possible to the sport practiced [36]. Such abnormalities with functional asymmetry of the lower limbs may be observed at the hips and knees. Subotnick emphasizes the possible combination of structural and functional limb length discrepancy [38].

The evaluation of this functional asymmetry of the lower limbs concerns not only the practitioner and patient, but also the entourage of the sport team who can observe whether the equipment has been modified.

• The clinical methods of studying limb-length discrepancy are various, always approximate, and subject to criticism [30]. The direct method with a tape measure from the anterior superior iliac spine to the medial malleolus can be inaccurate for several reasons: unilateral deviation of the long axis of the limbs (e.g., genu varum or valgum), difficulty in finding the landmarks (worse if the patient is obese), pelvic obliquity, joint stiffness and finally asymmetric thigh circumference. Variations of this direct method include measuring from the anterior superior iliac spine to the lateral malleolus and from the umbilicus or xiphoid process to the medial malleolus; these are unreliable: the xiphoid is often difficult to palpate and the umbilicus is often oblique [2, 3]. For some authors, measuring from the anterior superior iliac spine to the medial malleolus is acceptable [4].

Many authors advocate indirect methods [2]. The clinical assessment of limb length discrepancy must commonly be done with the patient standing in stable balance, in conditions as near as possible to those of the functional activity of the sport; this is particularly important since running is done in alternating monopodal weight-bearing. Several distances from the ground are evaluated: from the iliac crests, the anteriorsuperior iliac spines and the great trochanters. The level of the gluteal folds is also a useful landmark.

With the patient standing in relaxed calcaneal position, the iliac crests are palpated with the flat of the hands which are directed backwards and parallel to the ground. The anterior superior iliac spines are palpated with the thumbs which are directly opposite one another and parallel to the supporting surface. For the great trochanters the hands are parallel to the supporting surface and the flat of the hand palpates the trochanter [2].
• Imaging is usually considered to be the reference for diagnosis.

Pelvic radiography in the standing position measures the difference of level between the top of the femoral heads; this method used in good conditions remains acceptable for most cases, though an asymmetric pelvis is not detected. Teleradiography of the whole of the lower limbs, made at 2.50 m distance, includes the hips and ankles; a satisfactory measurement is possible and sometimes the cause of the malformation is observed [25]. The patient, in the weight-bearing and balanced position, must be assessed in conditions as near as possible to his sporting activity. Particularly when the feet are side by side and parallel, therefore in supination, or when the hips or knees are flexed during the procedure, this cannot be the case. Comparison of the clinical and X-ray findings is all the more important.

In general, orthoradiography and computed tomography are the most accurate methods if performed on the supine subject, but this does not approximate to the conditions of sports activity and mistakes in positioning such as allowing hip or knee flexion are sources of mistakes.

The evaluation of limb-length discrepancy therefore appears difficult because many mistakes may be made during measurement and every procedure is prone to error. In the majority of individuals, the discrepancy is usually insignificant (about 1 cm at maturity) and in most cases easily compensated.

Muscle weakness

Muscle weakness or imbalance may generate intrinsic overuse injuries [8, 14, 15, 17, 36]. The muscle produces energy but also is an attenuator of forces in the body; it absorbs the forces of weight-bearing. Deterioration in muscle function gives rise to modified movements. In such circumstances the runner has a shorter, less supple, jerkier stride and may even drag his heels. This impairment in muscle function can overstrain and damage bones, ligaments and tendons. The limitation of talocrural dorsiflexion secondary to stiffness of the posterior muscular chains of the calf is a frequent example.

Other factors

In the forefoot many anomalies can be described. Disturbances are possible in the usual gait: restricted dorsiflexion of the hallux provokes overstrain of the posterior muscular chains, particularly at the calcaneal tendon.

The different morphotypes of the toes, or of the metatarsal bones, are another example: a longer hallux favors microtraumatisms of the first metatarsophalangeal joint when the shoes are too short and in cross-country skiing; a longer second metatarsal bone favors lesions of the second metatarsophalangeal joint at the end of gait, particularly when the sole of a running shoe is too supple. The combination of forefoot disturbances and previously described factors produces various disorders: Morton's metatarsalgia, bursitis between adjacent metatarsal heads, metatarsal stress fractures and sesamoid lesions.[6]. All these injuries occur more in sports stressing the anterior propelling triangle of the foot, for instance in sprint conditions [6, 27].

Extrinsic factors [5, 10, 15, 17]

These include:
• **Technical conditions** due to the type of sport [27, 37] but the style of practice of the sport also plays a part. For James, training errors provoke overuse involvement in 60% of cases [16]: increasing the running distance, the frequency of running periods and the intensity of exertion too quickly; too often repeated alternation between fast and slow running; inadequacy or omission of warming-up or stretching [4, 5, 11, 12, 13, 30, 35, 36]. Abrupt change of the type

of terrain without gradual adaptation during training is also a factor which is often observed.

• **Environmental conditions** mainly include running surfaces, but also atmospheric conditions (cold or heat, rain) [23, 34]. The various characteristics of the ground play an important role (wet or dry grass, sand, macadam, hard courts); thus macadam, a hard surface, exploits to the maximum the shock-absorbing capacities of the foot, whereas a soft sandy surface greatly strains the tendons of the flexor and extensor muscles of the ankle, especially the triceps surae muscle. Other characteristics of the ground can be cited: uphill running, which requires increased dorsiflexion of the ankle; downhill running, which requires increased plantarflexion of the ankle; a cambered surface, running on a transverse gradient in one direction only, with one leg on a lower level than the other causes a common functional lower limb discrepancy with secondary symptoms, i.e., the "short leg syndrome" which is easy to treat since all that is needed is to alternate the direction of running [38].

• **Improper equipment** plays an important role in the appearance of overuse injuries, especially when this equipment is unsuitable (wearing rope-soled sandals for instance). Poor footwear may create altered mechanics and thus a functional limb length discrepancy; this is the case with asymmetric wear and deformation of a running shoe.

The most adequate shoe varies from one sport to another since each sport has its particular stresses. The running shoe (fig. 31.1) must include a well-padded tongue which protects the dorsum side of the foot from rubbing; a firm and non-traumatizing heel counter which maintains the hindfoot in good position; a molded pad to protect the calcaneal tendon from microtraumatisms; a flared and sufficiently high heel which increases stability, facilitates the development of the gait, and protects the heel with shock absorbing materials (foam, etc.) [21]; notched soles which allow a better grip of the ground; a rounded and sufficiently high toe-cap (3.5 cm minimum) which allows better protection of the toes; upward curve of the anterior part of the sole,

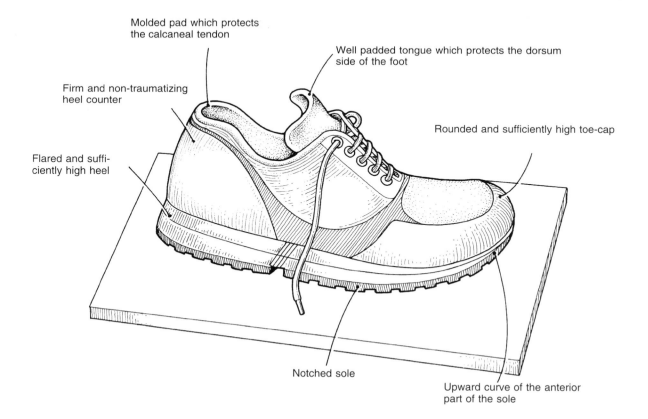

Fig. 31.1. Desirable characteristics of the running shoe

which facilitates the running cycle. Such a shoe is not appropriate for sports which involve frequent and sudden pronation and supination movements of the foot, like football, because the high heel of the running shoe increases the risk of ankle instability (fig. 31.1) [4, 10, 28]. For every sportsman and for every sport (even for different technical demands like training or competition) there is an ideal shoe; all the individual physiologic parameters cannot be evaluated, therefore when the sportsman has found a suitable shoe, he should be wary of changing the pattern.

Modification of the characteristics of the equipment during the sports activity is very important to consider: for instance, the initial shock absorption capability of a running shoe decreases by 30% or more after 500 miles (800 km) of running [9, 28]. In the same way, when the back of a running shoe is put out of shape by hyperpronation, overuse syndromes are more likely.

When lesions secondary to anatomic or biomechanical changes appear, the wearing of plantar insoles is indicated. Nevertheless, their prescription must be cautious [5, 36]; the body may compensate in a number of ways for runners and consequently no symptoms appear; however the wearing of insoles may reveal secondary problems in an asymptomatic individual with previously compensated anomalies and the symptoms that arise are then due to the use of these supports [3, 5].

● Conclusion

Overuse syndromes include very different pathologic features. Appropriate treatment necessitates a good knowledge of the etiologic factors.

References

1. Amico (D') JC, Dinowitz H, Polchaninoff M (1985) Limb Length Discrepancy: an Electrodynographic Analysis. J Am Podiatr Med Assoc 75: 639-643
2. Blake R, Ferguson H (1992) Limb Length Discrepancies. J Am Podiatr Med Assoc 82: 33-38
3. Blustein SM, D'Amico JC (1985) Limb Length Discrepancy, Identification, Clinical Significance and Management. J Am Podiatr Med Assoc 75: 200-206
4. Brody M (1981) La pathologie du jogging. Clinical symposia. Ciba
5. Clancy WG Jr (1980) Symposium. Runner's injuries (part 1). Am J Sports Med 8: 137-144
6. Claustre J (1984) Les syndromes de surmenage du pied du sportif. In: Claustre J, Bénézis C, Simon L (eds) Le pied en pratique sportive. Masson, Paris, pp 105-116
7. Clement DB, Taunton JE, Smart GW, Mc Nicol KL (1981) A Survey of Overuse Running Injuries. The Physician and Sports Medicine 9: 47-59
8. Clement DB, Taunton JE, Smart GW (1984) Achilles Tendinitis and Peritendinitis. Etiology and Treatment. Am J Sports Med 12: 179-184
9. Cook SD, Kester MA, Brunet ME, Haddad RJ Jr (1985) Biomechanics of Running Shoe Performance. Clin Sports Med 4: 619-626
10. Drez D, MD (1980) Running footwear. Examination of the Training Shoe, the Foot, and Functional Orthotic Devices. Am J Sports Med 8: 140-144
11. Elliott B, Ackland T (1981) Biomechanical Effects of Fatigue on 10,000 Meter Running Technique. Research Quarterly For Exercise and Sport 52: 160-166
12. Fyfe I, Stanish WD (1992) The Use of Eccentric Training and Stretching in the Treatment and Prevention of Tendon Injuries. Clin Sports Med 11: 601-624
13. Galloway MT, Jokl P, Dayton OW (1992) Achilles Tendon Overuse Injuries. Clin Sports Med 11: 771-782
14. Greenfield B (1990) Evaluation of Overuse Syndromes. In: Donatelli R (ed). Biomechanics of the Foot and Ankle. F.A Davis Company, Philadelphia, pp 153-170
15. Herring SA, Nilson KL (1987) Introduction to Overuse Injuries. Clin Sports Med 6: 225-239
16. James SL, Bates BT, Osternig LR (1978) Injuries to Runners. Am J Sports Med 6: 40-50
17. Järvinen M (1992) Epidemiology of Tendon Injuries in Sports. Clin Sports Med 11: 493-504
18. Leadbetter WB (1992) Cell-Matrix Response in Tendon Injury. Clin Sports Med 11: 533-578
19. Lutter L (1980) Injuries in the Runner and Jogger. Minnesota Medical: 45-51
20. Lutter DL (1982) Running Athlete in Office Practice. Foot Ankle 3: 53-59
21. Lutter DL (1984) La talalgie de l'athlète. In: Claustre J, Bénézis C, Simon L (eds). Le pied en Pratique Sportive. Monographies de Podologie 5. Masson, Paris, pp 117-122
22. Mac Bryde (1989) Stress Fracture in Runner. In: D'Ambrosia RD, Drez D Jr (eds) Prevention and treatment of running injuries, 2nd edn. Slack, New Jersey, p 49
23. Macera C, Pate RR, Powell KE, Jackson KL, Kendrick JS, Craven TE (1991) Predicted Lower-Extremity Injuries among Habitual Runners. In: Kominsky (ed) Yearbook of Podiatric Medicine & Surgery. Mosby, Saint Louis, pp 35-36
24. Mann RA (1982) Biomechanics of Running. In: Mack RP (ed). American Academy of Orthopedic Surgeons. Symposium on the Foot and Leg in Running Sports. Mosby, Saint-Louis, pp 1-29

25. Masse P (1981) Inégalités de Longueur des Membres Inférieurs. In: Grossiord A, Held JP (eds) Médecine de rééducation. Flammarion Médecine Sciences, Paris, pp 650-665

26. Mondenard (De) JP (1989) Technopathies du cyclisme. Ciba-Geigy

27. Moyen B Les Syndromes d'Hyperutilisation du Pied Sportif. Encycl Med Chir, Appareil Locomoteur, suppl. 14-999

28. Perlmann P (1990) Podiatric Sports Medicine. In: LA Levy (ed) Principles and Practice of Podiatric Medicine. Churchill Livingstone, Edinburgh, pp 647-666

29. Phillips RD (1990) Biomechanics of the Lower Limb. In: LA. Levy (ed) Principles and Practice of Podiatric Medicine. Churchill Livingstone, Edinburgh, pp 39-106

30. Roy S, Irvin R (1983) Sports Medicine: Prevention, Evaluation, Management, and Rehabilitation. Prentice-Hall, Englewood Cliffs, New-Jersey, pp 426-427

31. Saillant G, Rodineau J, Thoreux P, Roy-Camille R (1991) La Tendinite d'Achille. Rev Prat (Paris) 18: 1644-1649

32. Salathe Jr EP, Arangio GA, Salathe EP (1990) The Foot as a Shock Absorber. J Biomechanics 23: 655-659

33. Sgarlato TE (1971) A Compendium of Podiatric Biomechanics. College of Podiatric Medicine, San Francisco, California

34. Smith WB (1980) Environmental Factors in Running. Am J Sports Med 8: 138-140

35. Stanish W (1989) Neurophysiology of Stretching. In: D'Ambrosia RD, Drez D Jr (eds) Prevention and treatment of runnning injuries, 2nd edn. Slack, New Jersey, pp 209-219

36. Subotnick S (1978) Biomechanics of Running. Medicine Sports 12: 169-173

37. Subotnick S (1979) Variations in Angles of Gait in Running. The Physician and Sports Medicine 7: 110-115

38. Subotnick S (1981) Limb length discrepancies of the lower extremity (the short leg syndrome). J Orthop Sports Phys Ther 3: 11

39. Subotnick S, Sisney P (1986) Treatment of Achilles Tendinopathy in the Athlete. J Am Podiatr Med Assoc 76: 552-557

40. Wu KK (1990) Foot Orthoses, Sport Shoes and Sports medicine. In: WU KK (ed). Foot Orthoses: principles and clinical applications. Williams and Wilkins, Baltimore, pp 29-47

Additional references

Deutsch AL, Mink JH, Kerr R (1992) MRI of the foot and ankle. Raven Press, New York, pp 67-197 & 281-312

Tomaro JE, Burdett RG, Chadran AM (1996) Subtalar joint motion and the relationship to lower extremity overuse injuries. J Am Podiatr Med Assoc 86: 427-432

32.

Foot orthoses

*D Acker, M Bouysset, G Guaydier-Souquières,
D Vial and F Lapeyre-Gros*
*with the help in making the orthoses of Mr Kieffert,
Mr Lavigne, Mr Menou and Mr Gérard*

Introduction

Foot orthoses aim at:
• correcting static and dynamic disorders of the foot [20],
• relieving painful overloaded areas by distributing bearing forces harmoniously,
• protecting and preventing trophic risks,
• accommodating fixed lesions,
• stimulating anatomic parts of the foot.

Foot orthoses must not induce traumas or allergies. Their indications are sometimes different from one school of thought to another, and their fabrication may vary depending on the different specialists (physicians and technicians) involved. They are widely used and in most cases must be considered as a treatment in themselves. Their use is invaluable in the treatment of foot diseases; nevertheless, their effectiveness is still to be objectively demonstrated because it depends entirely on the patient's satisfaction and the physician's visual assessment. Consequently, a close collaboration and the exchange of experience between all the specialists involved are absolutely necessary [3].

There are many possibilities of design and adaptation, thus the orthoses can always be carefully adapted to a particular case. Manufacturing foot orthoses may be considered as a real art and many mass-produced orthoses, without individual adjustment, may be unsuitable. In theory, convenient footwear should be adapted to the orthosis, otherwise it may decrease or even cancel its effectiveness. Commercially available shoes are sometimes not wide enough to contain a specially designed orthosis. Therefore the indication for special shoes, custom-made or not, proves necessary. Orthotic inserts (wedge, Thomas bar, etc.) may also be added to the outsole of a mass-produced shoe and thus complete the treatment [45]. Clinical data are the major reference for the indication and design of foot orthoses. In most cases, these data alone prove to be sufficient for the indication, prescription and fabrication of orthoses.

Different types of orthoses

Foot orthoses are usually classified in several categories:
• corrective orthoses: these aim at correcting reversible static disorders,
• accommodation orthoses: these are palliative and relieve fixed deformities by being closely fitted to the foot,
• stimulatory orthoses: these aim at activating the muscles, tendons and ligaments of the foot. Their main indication is for hypermobile flatfoot in children [27],
• preventive orthoses: they are useful in static disorders with known trophic risks, in the case of neuropathy or arteriopathy, and sometimes in some cases of inflammatory rheumatism. They distribute the stresses and avoid over-pressure in some areas.

There are many other classifications [20, 31, 45]. Corrective or stimulatory orthoses are preferably used as often as possible, and accommodation orthoses are generally reserved for irreducible deformities. Nevertheless, it must be emphasized that a single classification is much too simple for the biomechanical complexity of the foot. Indeed, each case has its own characteristics and there is no such thing as a standard orthosis for each type of disorder.

Materials [19, 25]

Three types of materials are used.
• Leather and leatherwork derived from animal hides with different tanning methods chosen according to various criteria: age, corpulence, species of animal, etc. They may be replaced by synthetic materials with equal qualities of comfort and solidity.
• Glues.
• Materials composing orthotic inserts. The association of these materials can be compared to a jigsaw puzzle horizontally - different elements are fitted together in order to obtain a determined biomechanical effect - and to a stratification vertically.

Leather, leatherwork and synthetic materials are used for basic support and cover.
• Basic support (also called primary sole)
    - The most flexible parts of leathers (generally derived from cow-hide: belly, shoulder;
    - synthetic materials: "synderms" ("chipboard-like" reconstitution of natural material);
    - foams (artificial material) that will provide shock-absorption at the level of weight-bearing areas.
• Cover
    - Leatherwork: the most commonly used are derived from pigskin, goatskin, lambskin, horse-skin, etc., and also chamois leather. Leather and leatherwork are obtained through complex and diversified tanning methods.
    - Synthetic materials: textile (bouclé fabric, extensible in both directions in order to avoid creases). These are convenient in cases of acrohyperhydrosis or skin fragility.

It must be emphasized that the covering material is not compulsory in the fabrication of molded orthoses because it might reduce their effectiveness, but the basic support remains essential in the specifications given for their fabrication (see below: legislation).

Two types of glues are used.
• Strong adhesion ("neoprene-like") glues for sticking:
    - the layers of materials that compose the orthotic insert (providing good homogeneity and further adjustment of the insert);

- inserts and basic support, because they must be perfectly interdependent.
• Medium adhesion glues for sticking leatherwork or synthetic material on the orthosis (cover). Neoprene glue would not be suitable because it might harden the leatherwork and it would not allow peeling-off for further adjustments.

Components of orthotic inserts
They may offer different qualities. In order to choose one among the components, the characteristics of the material and its final use are assessed: weight, density, shock-absorbing capacity, fragility, and reducibility deformation (possibility to regain the original shape). Other criteria are also taken into account: baromolding or thermomolding, thermoforming, thermowelding, cutting and polishing. Some thermoformed materials provide shape reversibility (possibility to modify the shape by thermoforming it again), unlike expanded or other materials (polyurethane resins, carbon fibers, etc.). Reinforcements may also be added to the orthosis, they may be of wood veneer, resin or other materials. The choice of the most appropriate material is based more on experience than on the physicochemical properties of products. These products may be cork, chipboard cork, latex-derived cork with variable flexibility, variable-density foams (made of latex, polyethylene, polyurethane).

Composition of the orthosis

To compose the orthosis the practitioner chooses among the different available materials the ones that seem better adapted to each case, depending on the therapeutic effect aimed at, the use the patient will have of it - sex, weight, occupation, etc. - but also depending on the type of orthosis that will finally be chosen (standard or molded).
• In the case of a standard orthosis, different inserts will be assembled together and stuck to the bases;
• for a molded orthosis, a block (molded replica of the foot) will be shaped and adjusted to the foot.

The latter kinds of orthoses include the following:
• thermoformed orthoses, molded on the foot either directly or in the shoe in a weight-bearing position. Materials are softened in an oven and then applied under the foot. Heat also welds together the different components without using glue, in the case of materials that can be worked at low temperatures.

Another technique provides the possibility to mold them under vacuum.

Thermoforming may also be used on a rigid cast corresponding to the plantar side of the foot. This cast, called the positive, is made by pouring plaster or polyurethane resin into a negative cast obtained by molding the foot with plaster bandages for example.

• Molded orthoses may also be manufactured in polyurethane resin (a material obtained from a chemical reaction, by mixing two liquid components), either directly on the foot and progressively set in a weight-bearing position or by vacuum suction. The elasticity of these orthoses depends on the proportion of their components, but they do not provide shape reversibility. All molded orthoses are convenient because they provide comfort and relieve medioplantar contractures. They may receive standard inserts to obtain correction or stimulation of the foot.

Clinical assessment before prescribing foot orthoses

Firstly the patient's age must be taken into account, as well as the type of his or her disease. Two cases are possible:

• either the location in the foot of a systemic or regional disease with consequences on osteoarticular structures, like inflammatory rheumatism or impaired deep sensibility and vascularization in certain diseases with neurotrophic lesions (diabetes, ulceromutilating acropathy, spina bifida, Hansen's disease, nerve-trunk trauma) or sequelae of cerebrovascular disease and in arteriopathy;

• or statodynamic disorders [13, 14], which are situated in the foot; they are generally less progressive and therefore have fewer consequences at the functional, trophic and bone levels. When the disease and its possible course are known, it is easier to avoid mistakes. Thus, a rigid rheumatoid foot with destruction of the metatarsophalangeal joints must not be treated with orthoses which aim at stimulating a foot that, in this case, cannot respond.

Other factors also taken into account in the design of foot orthoses have already been described: the patient's age, weight and particularities. For example, in the case of athletes, the particular physical demands of the sport must be taken into account

- the side of the take-off foot, landing method, direction of the curve during the race, ground surface, type of shoe [7, 31, 37]. Similarly, job requirements which are very variable, must be acknowledged - axes of the lower limbs during work, the wearing of specific shoes for work, dampness or heat of the floor.

Clinical examination

The clinical examination [4, 7, 8, 20, 22, 45] is indispensable for the indication of foot orthoses. At the end of the examination, the movements in space and time of bone segments should be understood in order to locate the necessary orthotic insets precisely, whether they will be used to correct or to accommodate a lesion [20].

In practice, the orthosis can be designed from a plantar footprint on paper (podogram) obtained with a podograph; this document may be kept for records and compared to subsequent documents.

In addition to the items described in the previous chapters, several points are studied with special care:

• The wear and tear of the shoe resulting from pressures on the heel, shank, sole, insole and upper part of the shoe. The disfigurements of the patient's shoes give clues about the biomechanical constraints of the foot. For example a dynamic varus may sometimes be only clinically suspected, whereas it is confirmed by the wear and tear and the twisting of the shoe base (visible on the shank-piece and sole), not only by the wear and tear of the heel.

• The study of the heel axis and orientation of the midfoot is necessary but not sufficient.

• Dynamic items should also be investigated if possible: while the patient is standing on one foot, the position of the head and neck is changed (neutral position, head in the axis of the body); while the patient is walking on the same spot he or she is asked to lift his or her knees forward, this may reveal an imbalance; the patient is also observed while walking barefooted and then with shoes on in order to reveal biomechanical abnormalities.

The clinical examination takes into account:

• Dynamic axial modifications of the medial column (talus, navicular bone, medial cuneiform bone, first metatarsal bone): tarsal instability with jerking movements, in varus-supination and in valgus-pronation, muscular contractions and clawtoes resulting from instability, hallux erectus. In an immobile patient, a calcaneovalgus may hide violent jerking movements in varus which are observed when the patient is walking.

• The possibilities of reducing deformities with the foot in weight-bearing and in neutral position are recorded, as well as the mobility or stiffness of proximal and distal joints. In valgus flatfoot pronation with eversion of the hindfoot, different tests are possible: reduction test of the calcaneovalgus by asking the patient to stand on tiptoe, external rotation of the leg, dorsiflexion of the hallux. When there is a varus with supination and inversion: reduction test by placing inserts under the calcaneus, the cuboid bone, the lateral metatarsal bone and its head, and even under the fifth toe. When there is a hallux valgus: location and strength of flexor muscles, assessment of manual reducibility.

The different levels of the lower limbs (gluteal area, knee, leg, ankle and foot) have an influence on each other: any alteration at one level may have consequences on the others [22]. Leg axes and hip rotations are evaluated, as well as the angle of gait: when the latter is important, there can be over-pressure and even flattening of the midtarsus; on the contrary, when the angle of gait is low that can provoke varus disorders. Conversely, a static disorder of the foot may entail and maintain knee pain (especially a patellofemoral pain syndrome) [22], tendinopathy (gluteus medius, adductors) or low back pain.

Prescription

The prescription is written as follows: "custom-made foot orthoses including from back to front.." and then the different orthotic inserts are listed (the prescription may also be different for each foot). A drawing with top view and cross and longitudinal sections of the orthosis allows a better cooperation with the orthotist. The shape and physicomechanical properties of the inserts are also detailed. It is very difficult, except for the accommodation of limb-length discrepancies - which is made progressively, particularly in athletes - to give millimeter - precise measurements. Later adjustments of the orthosis [4, 18, 41] must always be possible and they are made according to the patient's observations or after the control examination. This control examination, which is indispensable, is carried out at short or long-term depending on the disease: at very short-term if the feet are affected by neuropathy or arteriopathy, or after about six weeks in the case of mechanical disorders. Some authors use temporary

orthoses [41], which make it possible to check the good location of inserts (over-pressures are revealed by the changes of aspect and crushing of the material) and observe a difference in symptomatology and gait during the control examination.

Examples of foot orthoses

The following paragraphs only give a few examples, which tackle general ideas about the design of foot orthoses.

Metatarsalgia [17]

This results from a support disorder at the forefoot with general or localized over-pressure. It is controlled by locating orthotic inserts behind, under

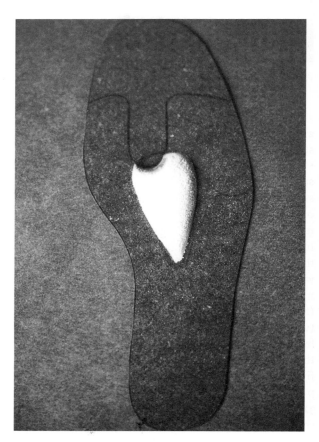

Fig. 32.1. Bulge behind median metatarsal heads with a hollow to decrease the pressure under the second metatarsal head

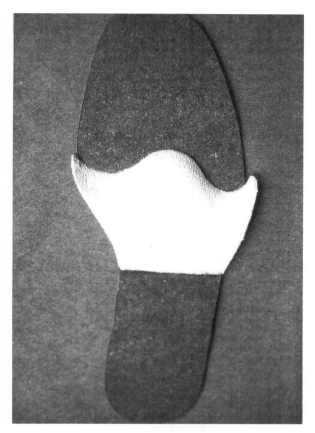

Fig. 32.2. Bar behind metatarsal heads with a median bulge

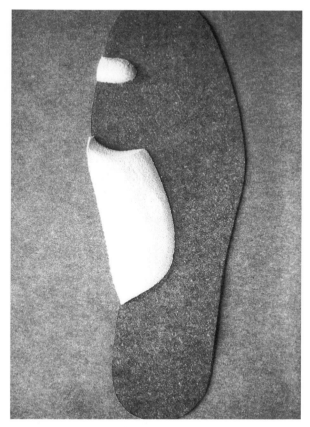

Fig. 32.3. Medial arch support situated mainly under the first metatarsal with a small support under the first phalanx of the hallux

and in front of the metatarsal heads (retrocapital, subcapital and antecapital metatarsal inserts).

• Retrocapital inserts raise the metatarsal heads and stop at the metatarsal necks. The median retrocapital support (fig. 32.1) is the simplest example: it consists of a raise behind the median metatarsal heads that may be placed depending on the metatarsal ray involved. The more limited and narrow the insert, the more it tightens the metatarsus; the higher it is, with an abrupt anterior limit, the more it sets the metatarsophalangeal joint in plantar flexion. A notch (fig. 32.1) made in the anterior retrocapital support (whose anterior limit extends beyond the neck), and facing the second metatarsal head provides relief to this head in cases of functional insufficiency of the first articular chain (hallux valgus, metatarsus primus adductus). The retrocapital bar (figs. 32.2 & 32.6) raises all the metatarsal heads backwards; its shape may modify the statics of the forefoot:

    - when it is flat and uniform it tends to spread the forefoot;

    - a bulge on the median area makes the metatarsus narrower and relieves the median heads, all the more so if it is high and abrupt in its front part;

    - lateral grooves for the first and fifth metatarsals, which are thus lowered, are indicated in the case of anterior flat foot [11];

    - lastly, a metatarsal bar provides stabilization at the frontal level and prevents varus disorders [11].

• Inserts situated under and in front of the metatarsal heads may be added to the inserts described above, on each side of one or several metatarsal heads. The empty space thus created may provide a relieving empty area with varying length, which may include the first phalanx. The inserts last mentioned seem to be indicated more in fixed metatarsophalangeal deformities. They tend to maintain the metatarsophalangeal joint in dorsiflexion and are more effective in the last phase of gait. However, their adaptation raises problems of the size of the orthosis, which increases the risks of rubbing between the forefoot and the shoe.

In the particular case of metatarsalgia related to sesamoid bone disease (over-pressure due to cavus, atrophy of plantar soft tissue or Renander's disease), a retrosesamoid insert with an anterior limit of varying abruptness is indicated. For example half an arch, which reaches the limit just in front of the metatarsal head (fig. 32.3), is the most bulky kind of retrosesamoid insert; it can raise the first metatarsal but its inversion effect will have to be checked.

Finally, the practitioner gives his advice about footwear: even if well-designed, an orthosis worn in a shoe with too high heels and a too narrow heel base will scarcely reach its goal.

Varus pes cavus

A neurologic examination is carried out before prescribing the orthosis. The standard orthosis include:

• a retrocapital bar that raises the metatarsal heads, distributes stresses better and stabilizes the forefoot. This insert modifies the spread of the metatarsus depending on its precise location, shape and density. The other inserts that may compose it have the same role: a medial bulge, an empty area on each side of the foot for the first and fifth metatarsals, lateral and medial flanges to stabilize them. The design of retrocapital bars varies according to authors:

- for some, short "active" bars are generally used in children, medium-sized bars in adults and long bars especially in the elderly [11]. The slope of the bar may be ascending towards the back, thus creating an oblique surface that corresponds to the surface and inclination of metatarsal shafts [24].

- For others, in severe cavus, when standard bars fail and do not eliminate metatarsalgia or trophic disorders, the medial and lateral arches are blocked from the necks to the anterior or intermediate tarsus by a raise behind the metatarsal heads (they are thus better relieved). Raising provides support, correction and stability to the foot. This effect will also depend on the shape, dimensions and density of inserts.

In pes cavus, it is important to assess the indication and dimensions of a heel lift. Indeed, the triceps surae muscle, the calcaneal tendon and the plantar aponeurosis must be relaxed according to two parameters: the decreasing degree of dorsiflexion of the talocrural joint related to the cavus on the one hand, and the height of the lift under the heel of the shoe on the other. Pes cavus essentially presents the risk of instability which occurs with the presence of a permanent or dynamic varus hindfoot. Posterior orthotic inserts must respond to the instability and sometimes to extreme tensions developing from the calcaneus to the toes. A neutral heel insert with a cup shape, i.e., without pronating or supinating effects, will stabilize the hindfoot. Depending on the data resulting from the biomechanical analysis, the heel cup may induce pronation by being higher laterally (lateral side) or by its double density - firm laterally and flexible medially [12].

Instability with varus tendency may also be controlled by a pronating wedge (lateral post), or a pronating strap (laterally situated on the orthosis) of varying length: a full-length strap from the heel to the lateral toes or to the necks of the fourth and fifth metatarsals, or a medium-sized strap from the cuboid bone to the neck of the metatarsals. In some cases, the pronating insert includes a subcuboidal, ovoid-shaped insert that may be replaced by a local insert resembling a hemisphere (the effect on fibular muscles is supposed to be more stimulating) [1, 2].

Very often, the tarsal instability of pes cavus induces not only varus and supination disorders, but also jerking movements in varus or valgus. In this case, some authors use a heel cup of particular shape, which controls jerking movements, and add stimulating inserts that provide very subtle adjustments at midfoot level (subnavicular and subcuboid spheres).

Lastly, in pes cavus, achillo-bursitis resulting from rubbing between the shoe and the vertical calcaneus may be observed. In addition to advice from the practitioner about adequate footwear, this rubbing may be resolved by prolonging the orthosis with a posterior heel, part of which protects the bursitis and is excavated at the level of the bursitis if necessary.

Hallux rigidus

Arthrosis of the first metatarsophalangeal joint results in stiffness in dorsiflexion; orthotic inserts must decrease stresses and over-pressure at this level. To reach this goal, an anterior hemisphere is used (medial arch located mainly under the first metatarsal), with a basal reinforcement made of resin, very narrow and rather rigid extending from the pulp of the hallux to the heel. Others add a reinforcement under the first phalanx of the hallux [12,

28]. The volume of the hemisphere must not induce rubbing between the upper part of the shoe and the bulge caused by a possible exostosis of the first metatarsal head.

Pain and stiffness caused by hallux rigidus and by the orthotic inserts described above sometimes set the foot in a varus position of mechanical origin or to avoid pain. Therefore control by a posterolateral insert may be necessary, its characteristics are chosen in order not to localize the pressure too much on the medial side at the first metatarsophalangeal arthrotic joint.

Hallux valgus

The treatment of hallux valgus is mainly surgical but orthoses may have a palliative action, mainly at the beginning of the deformity. Obviously, the shoe must be adapted. The design of the orthosis takes into account the metatarsus, primus adductus, its reducibility, the severity of the exostosis and the instability of the medial articular chain.

A medial flange can be used (facing the medial side of the first metatarsal) with varying length.

Then, if the footwear allows, an extremely narrow median retrocapital support is added. This retrocapital support also protects the second metatarsophalangeal joint from pressures related to the functional insufficiency of the first ray.

Lastly, a very narrow retrosesamoid insert supplements the actions of the previous structures when the hallux valgus is reducible.

These three inserts have two goals: blocking the first articular chain, and acting on the muscles that stabilize it.

The participation of a varus or valgus during gait in the genesis of metatarsus varus of the first metatarsal and phalangeal valgus must be assessed. This observation leads one to prescribe a corrective insert for this dynamic varus or valgus. Other authors prefer using a retrocapital support behind the metatarsophalangeal joints with a bulge and flanges on its sides (first and fifth metatarsals) particularly at the medial side [11].

Flatfoot [6, 12, 32, 33, 34]

Static flatfoot in adults

The medial arch is depressed, collapsed or even inverted, and there is a pronation of the hindfoot. The head of the talus and the navicular bone are depressed and the first metatarsal becomes horizontal. Flattened forefoot, a result of the previous deformity, seems constant. Articular stiffness progressively appears and the deformity will not be very reducible or not at all. The degree of reducibility determines the shape of the medial orthotic insert facing the medial osteoarticular column (talus-navicular - medial cuneiform-metatarsal).

To obtain support and prevent painful stretching of the foot in a weight-bearing position, a medial arch with varying flexibility or firmness and possibly a reinforcement under the navicular bone are used. In extreme cases, with inversion of the medial arch, some authors recommend a localized relieving hollow under the navicular bone or the head of the talus (over-pressure areas). Others recommend thermoformed orthoses. A median retrocapital support contains the over-pressure on the median metatarsal heads. At the heel level, a supinating insert ("medial post") attempts to stabilize the hindfoot. The shoe must maintain the foot axes in a position as near as possible to the physiologic position of the foot. The shoe must necessarily include excellent quality counters and a solid shank-piece.

Hypermobile flatfoot in children
[6, 7, 11, 23, 26, 28, 33, 34, 38, 43, 44]

The standard detorsional orthosis (functioning like a helix) may be used: a posterior supinating wedge ("medial post") aims at reducing the calcaneovalgus and an anterior pronating wedge controls the supination of the forefoot [29]. In children, proprioceptive orthoses are increasingly used nowadays. In theory, the foot analyses the perception of the insert when it comes into contact with the ground, then the mechanical actions necessary for mobilization of the various bone segments and for the modification of position during action. A good indication depends on the response to the previous stimulation given by the inserts that compose the orthosis.

In practice, a supinating wedge reduces constraints in valgus and avoids hyperpronation. An anterocapital wedge under the first metatarsal head and the hallux activates the flexor hallucis muscles, which play an anti-valgus role, and stimulates fibular muscles (fig. 32.4). A median retrocapital support may also be added [28].

There are other ideas for children's flatfoot orthoses. For example, some authors use a bulge

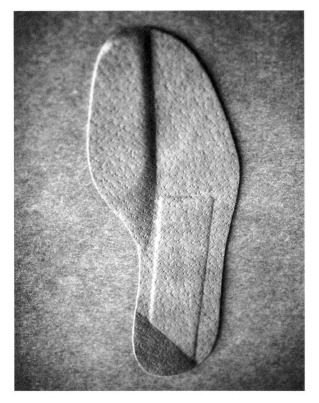

Fig. 32.4. Medial post- and anterocapital wedge under the first metatarsal head

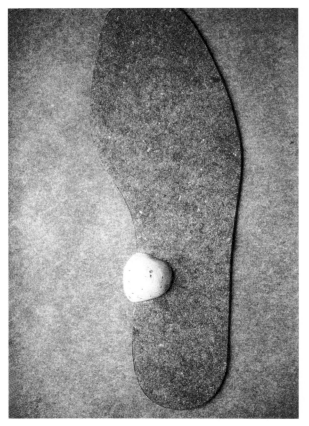

Fig. 32.5. Ball under the navicular bone

under the navicular bone (fig. 32.5) whose precise location and firmness (nearly nociceptive as in Spitzy's orthosis) combats the flattening of the medial column [21, 39, 40]. This device does not require any particular footwear (like a counter, high upper or reinforced shank-piece) and stimulates the muscles at the level of the medial arch. The concept seems very satisfactory, but Spitzy's soles sometimes entail tolerance problems.

The treatment of hypermobile flatfoot shows how much the design and purpose of foot orthoses can vary. Several types of orthoses have already been described but there are other types: heel orthoses with a shell shape attempt to maintain the calcaneus in the axis in order to reequilibrate the foot; the soles used by the University of California are another example [16].

To end this section, the results presented by Meary indicate that in 100 cases of flatfoot occurring in childhood, 65 are reduced spontaneously (with or without soles), 30 will remain flat but well tolerated, five will remain very flat and of these three will require surgical treatment. However, many authors

think that in the absence of reliable prognostic criteria, children with hypermobile flatfoot must be equipped with orthoses [23]. The physician faced with a painful foot must investigate for a synostosis of the tarsus before prescribing foot orthoses. Of course, the treatment also includes advice from the practitioner about footwear and adapted physiotherapy.

Talalgia [16, 30, 31] (see chapter 22)

The orthosis takes into account overstrain of the triceps surae muscle, calcaneal tendon and plantar aponeurosis. In every case, a heel lift is provided, it can be mass-produced and commercially available [29] or more elaborate and adapted individually to the biomechanical requirements of the tarsus and forefoot of each patient. Many "anti-shock", "shock-absorption" or "anti-vibration" materials are available to absorb and distribute ground-reaction forces.

In acute plantar talalgia, the heel orthosis may include either an excavation under the painful area that corresponds to the site of the posteromedial calcaneal apophysis, or an area (that replaces the excavation) made of very soft material. The other parts of the heel orthosis are also soft, but firmer. It is often beneficial to add a medial arch support to reduce stress on the medial arch (plantar aponeurosis and short plantar muscles).

Rheumatoid arthritis

[10, 15, 42, 43, 45]

This destructive and deforming disease requires careful monitoring of the foot; its progress leads to modification of the orthoses, which have two aims:
• to relieve pain and possible existing trophic disorders,

• to avoid increasing a deformity [15, 42].

These two aims are difficult to achieve; the foot must not be constrained, which would provoke pain, but it must be maintained in a good position. The orthosis will attempt to correct deforming tendencies and particularly existing static disorders, but will avoid any trauma. The least bad result seems to obtain ankylosis of the foot in a functionally acceptable position [9, 42]. If metatarsalgia is developing in an inflammatory forefoot, a retrocapital support is indicated (figs. 32.1, 32.2 & 32.6).

Orthoses with median excavations under the metatarsal heads relieve the forefoot but maintain the deformity which, little by little, will become fixed. Such a purely palliative solution, which is better accepted by the patient and therefore easier to implement for the physician, will sometimes have harmful consequences. Thus, an irreducible stiffened flat forefoot can be created, which will have its own complications. Therefore, excavations are only indicated in cases with severe deterioration of the metatarsophalangeal joints and fixed deformities and in cases where surgery is impossible. The aim of orthoses is then only palliative.

The collapse and dislocation of the tarsus, often appearing insidiously, are particularly disabling at an advanced stage. Therefore the orthosis must be prescribed very early on when the deformity can still be controlled. Plantar support must be sufficiently firm to be effective [42, 43]. However, skin atrophy and wasting of the plantar soft tissues often induce tolerance problems locally. Thermoformed orthoses can be of help in this case

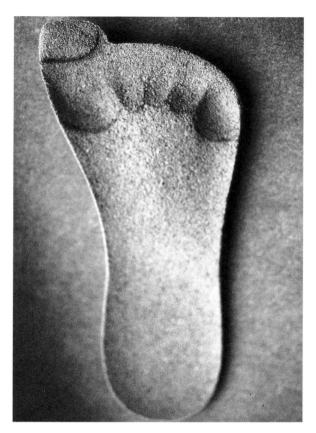

Fig. 32.6. Bar (support) behind metatarsal heads with five relieving area

but their design and fabrication must be precisely adapted.

If the deformities of the foot are fixed, and in the absence of indications for surgery or if surgery is not possible, the orthosis attempts to relieve by using palliative (and therefore non-corrective) flexible or semi-flexible materials.

The volume variations in size of the rheumatoid foot in the different stages of evolution and the bulk of the orthosis sometimes make it difficult to wear commercially available standard shoes. A specially adapted mass-produced shoe therefore proves necessary:
• a mass-produced therapeutic shoe for permanent use

• or another range of material, for temporary use, some models of which are available at present.

Eventually a custom-made shoe will be necessary to attempt to correct a deformity or provide appropriate footwear when all the possibilities previously listed have proved to be unsuitable.

Neurotrophic feet

In the treatment of decompensated neurotrophic feet with foot orthoses, orthotic inserts are as corrective and preventive as possible if skin and osteoarticular fragility due to neuropathy and/or vascular disorders are not too severe. Their aim is to eliminate localized over-pressure that could possibly provoke perforating ulcers of the foot. The design of these orthoses is described in the chapter on the diabetic foot.

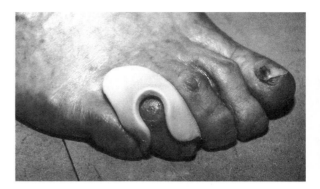

Fig. 32.7. Toe-orthosis for dorsal corn of the fourth toe

Toe orthoses

Toe orthoses are made of silicone elastomere (fig. 32.7). They essentially aim at avoiding rubbing between the toes and the shoe or between the toes themselves (protective toe orthoses). Some authors think they have a preventive action and can reduce deformities.

They are indicated in painful disorders at toe level, which are related to hyperkeratosis under the forefoot, dorsal callosities or callosities between the toes. They can be made on the toe in the neutral or semi-weight-bearing (sitting) position, by surrounding the toe with silicone and adding and adjusting layers outside the frictional area. The layers of materials are intended to receive pressures when the shoe is worn. Toe orthoses may also be manufactured by injecting elastomere into the spaces between the toes, the foot being in a weight-bearing position and the toes maintained in the corrected position. They must be particularly carefully finished. The effectiveness and tolerance of toe orthoses depend on the know-how of the practitioner. They may supplement the therapeutic action of foot orthoses.

Legislation regarding foot orthoses in France in 1998

The renewal period is one year for an adult and six months for a child up to fifteen years. The total guarantee related to the fabrication, finishing and quality of the product (excluding normal wear and tear) lasts six months from the definitive delivery onwards.

In 1998, partial reimbursement amounted to FF 90 per orthosis, and varied according to the size. For a molded foot orthosis, manufactured by molding the foot in a weight-bearing position and reserved for disabling rheumatoid and neurotrophic conditions, the reimbursement amounted to about FF 170 per orthosis. This amount does not cover the whole of the sum paid by the patient.

The following devices are not reimbursed:
• mass-produced soles,
• proprioceptive soles with ascending action by magnetic stimulation,
• heel socks,
• toe orthoses.

It is compulsory for the prescribing physician to write a particular prescription, including all the indications for a correct application. This prescription is submitted to a preliminary review and reimbursement will be effective only if the orthosis is delivered by an authorized orthotist in the conditions described by the regulations.

Conclusion

Foot orthoses are an important therapeutic tool in the treatment of foot pathology mainly for foot disorders but also for disorders affecting higher parts of the lower extremities (ankle, leg, knees, pelvis, spine) or even the entire body [35, 36, 37].

Their indications and designs may vary from one school of thought to another, but only the therapeutic result needs to be taken into account ultimately; the orthosis must provide a function as close as possible to physiologic mechanics and suppress pain.

References

1. Acker D, Menou P (1993) Valgus-varus du pied : traitement orthétique de l'instabilité du tarse, de ses conséquences loco-régionales et à distance par des billes sous-cuboïdiennes et sous-scaphoïdiennes. Actualités podologiques (le podologue) 72: 12-13

2. Acker D, Retton R (1987) Intérêt de la stabilisation du tarse dans certaines algies jambières à prédominance antéro-externe pseudo-vasculaires. Société Française de Phlébologie 40: 265-273

3. Acker D, Sedel L (1989) Indication des orthèses plantaires: réalisation, réglage et adaptation sont infinis et définissent un véritable artisanat d'art. Rev Prat (Paris) 61: 1245-1250

4. Blake R, Ferguson H (1992) Limb Length Discrepancies. J Am Podiatr Med Assoc 82: 33-38

5. Blake RL, Ferguson H (1992) Extrinsic rearfoot posts. J Am Podiatr Med Assoc 82: 202-207

6. Bordelon RL (1983) Hypermobile flatfoot in chidren. Clin Orthop 18: 7-14

7. Bordelon RL (1989) Orthotic shoes and braces. Orthop Clin North Am 20: 751-757

8. Bordelon RL (1990) Clinical assessment of the foot. In: Donatelli R, Wolf SL (eds) The biomechanics of foot and ankle. FA Davies, Philadelphia, pp 85-97

9. Bouysset M, Tebib J, Noël E, Nemoz C, Schnepp J, Ducarme D, Bouvier M (1992) Le métatarse rhumatoïde: évolution originale du premier métatarsien. Rev Rhum Mal Osteoartic 59: 408-412

10. Braun S (1983) Les orthèses plantaires du pied rhumatoïde. In: Claustre J, Simon L (eds) Le pied en pratique rhumatologique. Masson, Paris, pp 203-208

11. Braun S (1995) Orthèses plantaires et métatarsalgies mécaniques. Rhumatologie 47: 95-102

12. Braun S, Panahi F (1978) Les orthèses plantaires. Rev Prat (Paris) suppl 28: 1213

13. Braun S, Panahi F (1978) Les assises plantaires anormales et pathologiques. Rev Prat (Paris) 28: 1071

14. Braun S, Panahi F (1978) L'assise plantaire dite normale. Rev Prat (Paris) 27

15. Budiman-Mak K, Conrad K, Roach J, Moore X, Lertratanakul A, Koch J, Skossy C, Froolich N, Joyce-Clark (1993) Can foot orthoses prevent deformity in rheumatoid arthritis? American College of Rheumatology, San Antonio nov. 7-11

16. Campbell JW, Inman VT (1974) Treatment of plantar fasciitis and calcaneal spurs with the UC-BL shoe insert. Clin Orthop 103: 57-62

17. Carret JP, Schnepp J (1982) Les métatarsalgies statiques. In: Claustre J, Simon L (eds) Troubles congénitaux et statiques du pied. Orthèses plantaires. Monographie de podologie 1. Masson, Paris, p 224

18. Clancy WG Jr, MD (1980) Symposium. Runner's injuries (part one). Am J Sports Med 8: 137-144

19. Claustre J, Olie L (1982) Orthèses plantaires et matériaux utilisables et techniques. I: Claustre J, Simon L (eds) Troubles congénitaux et statiques du pied. Orthèses plantaires. Monographies de podologie 2. Masson, Paris, p 203

20. Donatelli R, Wooden M (1990) Biomechanical orthotics. In: Donatelli R, Wolf SL (eds) The biomechanics of foot and ankle. FA Davis , Philadelphia, pp 193-216

21. Doncker (De) E, Kowalski C (1976) Cinésiologie et rééducation du pied. Masson, Paris

22. Eng JJ, Pierrynowski MR (1993) Evaluation of soft foot orthotics in the treatment of patellofemoral pain syndrome. Phys Ther 73: 62-70

23. Froin-Dencausse M,Denis A (1982) Orthèses plantaires et pied plat valgus souple de l'enfant. In: Claustre J, Simon L (eds) Troubles congénitaux et statiques du pied. Orthèses plantaires. Monographie de podologie 2. Masson, Paris, p 208

24. Goldcher A (1989) Orthèses plantaires de répartition des charges et pathologies de surcharge. De la théorie à la pratique. Med Chir Pied 5: 134-143

25. Henderson WH, Campbell JWardossian WH, Campbell JW (1967) the UC-BL shoe insert: casting and fabrication. Biomechanics Laboratory of the University of California

26. Helfet AJ (1956) A new way of treating flat feet in children. Lancet 1: 262-264

27. Lavigne A, Braun S (1982) Orthèses de stimulation ou de rééducation. In: Claustre J, Simon L (eds) Troubles congénitaux et statiques du pied. Orthèses plantaires. Monographie de podologie 2. Masson, Paris, p 211

28. Lelièvre J (1971) Pathologie du pied. Masson, Paris, p 430-450

29. Levitz S, Dykyj D (1990) Improvement in the design of visco-elastic heel orthoses: a clinical study. J Am Podiatr Med Assoc 12: 653-656

30. Mann RA, Baxter DE, Lutter LD (1981) Running symposium. Foot Ankle 1: 190-224

31. Meary R (1967) Le pied creux essentiel. Rev Clin Orthop 53: 389

32. Meary R (1969) Symposium sur le pied plat. Annales d'Orthopédie 1: 57

33. Mereday C. Dolan CME. Lusskin R (1972) Evaluation of the University of California Biomechanics Laboratory Shoe insert in "flexible" pes planus. Clin Orthop 82: 45-58

34. Niederecker K (1959) Der Platt fuss. Ferdinand Fuke, Stuttgart

35. Okubo J, Watanabe I, Baron JB (1980) Study on influences of the plantar mechano receptors on body way. Agressologie 21 D: 61-70

36. Okubo J. Watanabe I, Takkya JB (1979) Influence of foot position and visual field condition in the examination for quilibrism function and way of the center of gravity in normal persons. Agressologie 20: 127-132

37. Rossi W (1982) The shoe counter and the foot. Footwear and the podiatrist. J Am Podiatr Assoc 72: 326-327

38. Seringe R (1990) Les pieds plats. Revue de Médecine Pratique 41: 1

39. Spitzy H (1904) Der pes planus? Z Orthop 12: 777-797

40. Subotnick SI, Sisney P (1986) Treatment of Achilles tendinopathy in the athlete. J Am Podiatr Med Assoc 76: 552-557

41. Tillmann K (1979) The rheumatoid foot. Georg Thieme, Stuttgart, pp 98-100

42. Vainio K (1956) The rheumatoid foot. A clinical study with pathological and roentgenological comments. Ann Chir Gynaecol 45 (suppl1): 19-34

43. Wenger DR, Mauldin D, Speck G, Morgan D, Lieber RL (1989) Correctives shoes and inserts as treatment for flexible flatfoot in infants and children. J Bone Joint Surg 71A: 800-810

44. Wooden MJ (1990) Biomechanical evaluation for functional orthotics. In: Donatelli R and Wolf SL (eds) The biomechanics of foot and ankle. FA Davies company, Philadelphia, pp 131-147

45. Wu KK (1990) Foot orthoses. Williams and Wilkins, Baltimore, pp 71-78 & 328-333

Références additionnelles

Autrusson MC (1994) Orthoplastie, orthomyxie. Encycl Med Chir (Paris) Kinésithérapie-Rééducation Fonctionnelle, 26-161, A10, 2 p

Jourdain R, Cazalet C (1994) Techniques récentes pour la réalisatoin des semelles orthopédiques. Encycl Med Chir (Paris) Kinésithérapie-Rééducation Fonctionnelle, 26-161, A10, 5 p

Kieffert P (1985) Les orthèses d'orteil. In: Claustre J, Simon L (eds) Pathologie des orteils. Masson, Paris

Lavigne A (1985) Les orthèses d'orteil. Résultats cliniques. In: Claustre J, Simon L (eds) Pathologie des orteils. Masson, Paris

Levy LA, Hetherington VJ (1990) Principles and Practice of Podiatric Medicine. Churchill Livingstone, New York

Whitney AK, Whitney KA (1990) Padding and Taping Therapy. In: Levy LA, Hetherington VJ (eds) Principles and Practice of Podiatric Medicine. Churchill Livingstone, New York

33.
General ideas about footwear

F Lapeyre-Gros and T Serpollet

History

Throughout history various types of footwear have been used depending on social classes: wooden clogs were reserved for the underprivileged people whereas the well-off wore leather shoes or satin court shoes. The shoe, which was hand-crafted until the end of the 19th century and meant to protect the foot, has always been influenced by the vagaries of fashion and has often been curiously unphysiological. Indeed in the Middle Ages, the length of spiked shoes could reach 75 cm! and in France, in 1368 a decree forbade the lower classes to wear them, which led to the invention of excessively large shoes - "bear's paws"!

The right and left shoes were undifferentiated until 1822 when a distinction appeared in Philadelphia, but it turned out to be a failure. It was only after the end of the American Civil War, in 1865 that this strange distinction was accepted. It later developed in Europe; however, French Carmelite nuns continued to wear two identical shoes until about the 1940s! The weight of shoes was sometimes particularly excessive, for example the pair of combat shoes worn by soldiers used to weigh more than 3 kg!

The industrial revolution gave rise to present fabrication techniques: standard sizes; comfort (new materials including rubber); specialization of shoes (town shoes, evening shoes, sport shoes, army shoes, etc.). It was quickly realized that each continent had its own particular shape of foot. For example, in Japan the army decided to stop using the traditional but obsolete sandals and wear Western boots instead, but the project was abandoned because the feet of the Japanese could not fit into the boots.

The shoe has its own history and its specific peculiarities; it is closely related to fashion and often highly symbolic, though it must in theory be adapted to the foot. It is made around a last, which is defined by different characteristics: dimensions, morphology, instep, and especially the specific fitting properties of the model that will be made. A specific last, created for a specific foot, cannot be used to manufacture two different models.

The shoe (fig. 33.1)

(see figure and chapter 34)

This is composed of two distinct parts: the upper part and the sole. The upper covers the foot entirely, except for the plantar surface. After the creation of a model by a fashion designer, in order to make the shoe several patterns will be assembled to form the upper part. These patterns are called the quarters and the back strap at the back, and the vamp and tongue at the front. The upper comprises the cover and the lining:
• the lining is in contact with the foot. It is made of leatherwork (pig, goat, etc.), often of textile fiber and is frequently omitted in low-cost products,
• the cover is in contact with the external environment, it protects and isolates the foot. It is also made of leatherwork, but from different animal hides (kid, box-calf, peccary, crocodile, etc.). Textile and synthetic materials are also used, especially for sport or leisure shoes.

When the shoe is made according to traditional methods, the upper must include reinforcements,

UPPER PART

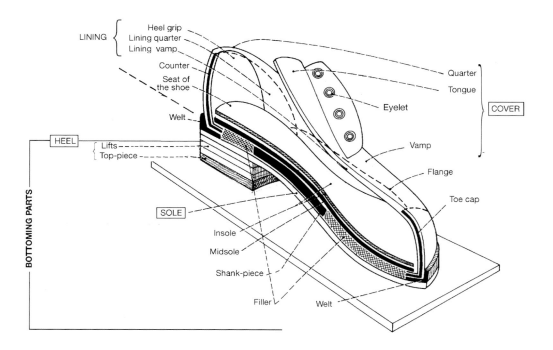

Fig. 33.1. Traditional man's shoe

which are fitted between the cover and the lining during the assembly phase of the fabrication:
• the counter covers all the hindfoot and has two roles: on the one hand it prevents the collapse of the back of the shoe, and on the other it supports the soft parts of the hindfoot, which tend to be compressed in weight-bearing. The counter is made of shoulder leather (very resistant and rigid) or synthetic materials.
• The two flanges, which are rarely used in mass-production, are located on each side of the shoe and extend from the counter to the toe cap. They are traditionally made in the same materials as the cover and constitute a flexible reinforcement, which supports the spread of the metatarsus in weight-bearing.
• The toe cap is located at the front of the upper, under the vamp. It is now made of synthetic materials to the exclusion of leather (belly). It is less rigid than the counter and aims at protecting the toes and maintaining the shape of the shoe.

The bottom part of the shoe bears the weight of the body and supports the foot at the level of the plantar surface by protecting and insulating it. It is composed of two parts: the sole and the heel.

• The sole is composed of several layers:
- the insole, which is directly in contact with the foot, must be permeable to absorb sweating. Generally, it is made of the same leatherwork as the lining;
- the midsole, which is in soft leather or synthetic material, is also permeable and located under the insole. It is stuck or stitched to the upper;
- the shank-piece, which is in wood or metal, supports the midfoot (instep of the foot) between the heel and the forefoot (it stops at the back of the metatarsal heads);
- the filler, which is in cork or leather, fills the empty space created by the shank-piece. With its absorbing components it reinforces the permeability and comfort of the insole and midsole;
- the sole itself, also called the outsole (fig. 33.1), which is made of leather or synthetic material, must be flexible to provide flexion at the metatarsophalangeal joints. It must also be resistant because it is in direct contact with the ground. The outsole is stuck or stitched to the shoe. Beside economic reasons, sticking makes the shoe lighter and more flexible, whereas stitching provides higher rigidity and better resistance.

• The heel may be made of leather, wood, plastic, cork, etc. Its height is imposed by the shank pitch of the last: a significant modification of the height of the heel may result in a modification of the shank pitch, which could have disadvantages. The heel of the shoe has an important role in the statics of the foot. The size of the surface in contact with the ground is extremely variable and uniquely depends on the designer's imagination: a minimal surface in contact with the ground in the case of high heels or a maximal surface in the case of wedge heels. The heel is stuck or nailed to the shoe in different ways: added to the sole (wooden or plastic heels), included in the sole (mountain shoes), or is inserted between the outsole and the insole (wedge heels).

Basic requirements of proper shoes

To play its role perfectly a shoe must do the following activities:
• cover the foot without constraining it or without losing its shape during gait,
• be easily put on and removed, while staying on the foot without constricting it,
• respect the size variations of the foot in a weight-bearing position and during all the phases of gait,
• allow for perspiration and not impede the arterial and venous circulation,
• provide for the physiologic role of the different foot joints,
• reinforce the dynamic and static equilibrium of the foot.

Covering the foot

This function requires careful choice of materials and their cuts. Materials must be soft, easily exten-sible in the direction needed, and must regain their original shapes almost entirely. Leather has this property provided it is cut according to a certain method for the fabrication of the upper. For leather-work, this possibility of extension is called "stretch". Textile materials also have extension qualities, but their elasticity is inferior. The maximum extension must be located transversally at the level of the meta-tarsophalangeal joints.

Ease of putting on and removal, while staying on the foot

• In the case of shoes with a low upper, which hold to the foot only if fastened with a lace, Velcro strap, strap and buckle or zipper, two additional condi-tions are required: on the one hand, the AB distance must always be smaller than the AC distance; and on the other, as the shoe does not cover the malleoli, in order to prevent gaping the last must always be hollowed along the BD line (fig. 33.2).
• To keep the shoe on the foot when there is no shoe closure (pumps), the submalleolar cavity must be accentuated and at the level of the metatarsophalan-geal joints the shoe girth must be reduced. Thus the same last cannot be used to build two models with different designs (fig. 33.3).
• Ankle boots (fig. 33.4) cover the malleoli and, unlike the previous example, the building of the last exactly duplicates the measurement of the foot.
• Boots may be difficult to put on. This difficulty is resolved by using soft materials for the upper (fig. 33.5) or by adding a zipper to the quarters.

Respect for the size variations of the foot

These variations affect both the length and width of the foot. During gait, the foot slides towards the

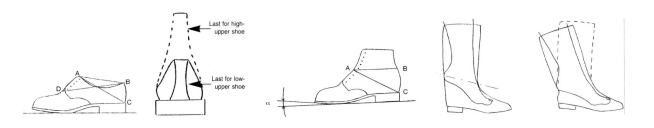

Fig. 33.2   Fig. 33.3   Fig. 33.4   Fig. 33.5

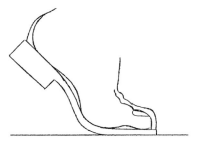

Fig. 33.6

front of the shoe, so that the shoe must always be longer than the foot (fig. 33.6), and the metatarsus spreads, which increases the surface in contact with the ground. The shoe must respect certain areas: width and girth (both measurements must be taken into account) at the level of the metatarsophalangeal joints, girth of the instep, perimalleolar girth, insertion of the calcaneal tendon. Conversely, the shoe will constrain other parts of the foot for cosmetic reasons.

Allowance for perspiration and freedom of circulation

The shoe must not constrict the vascular network of the instep. During walking and efforts, the local temperature rises and causes perspiration, which must be evacuated. Consequently materials must, as much as possible, be permeable to sweat and impermeable to external elements.

Allowance for unrolling of the step

The shoe must bend during the unrolling phase of gait. To facilitate unrolling, the tip of the last is raised (toe-spring) (fig. 33.4), with an alpha angle between 6 and 15°. The toe-spring varies depending on the rigidity of the sole, the mobility of the talocrural joint (in a boot the toe-spring is higher than in a low-upper shoe), the use of the shoe (jogging), the surface on which it will be worn (the more flat and even the surface, the less a toe spring is necessary because there are fewer risks of collision with something on the ground); and lastly, its height is in inverse proportion to the height of the shank pitch.

Contribution to the static and dynamic equilibrium of the foot

The shoe must play its support role by respecting the curve of the plantar surface and the stretch of

support areas in a weight-bearing position, but without being too loose and being closely interdependent with the foot during movements. It is important to check the wear and tear of the heel and sole, which may be at the origin of unnecessary disequilibrium disorders.

The last (fig. 33.7)

The last is the template around which the shoe is built. Traditionally the last was made of wood but today plastic is increasingly used. The last does not duplicate the deformities of the foot in order not to be detrimental to the appearance of the shoe. However it must:
• resemble the shape of the foot,
• take into account the deformations of the foot during walking or running,
• keep up with fashion (high heel, pointed toe-cap, etc.),
• respect the shape of the model to be made (pumps, boots, etc.).

Fashion has much influence on the building of a last, so that the shape of the foot is not the only preoccupation of manufacturers. It is therefore necessary to assess the size of the last by taking into account the prerequisites mentioned above. As the last is a complex form, an alternation of concavities and convexities, three measurements are taken:
• the length of the foot: distance between the posterior extremity of the heel and the anterior extremity of the longest toe;

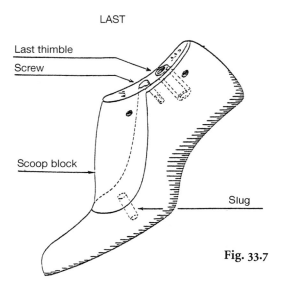

Fig. 33.7

• the width of the foot: corresponding to the maximum width of the foot on the plantar surface;
• the ball girth of the foot: measurement of the perimeter of the foot at the metatarsophalangeal joints.

The values obtained for these three measurements vary according to growth but also considerably from one individual to another (differences of morphology: Latin feet, Anglo-Saxon feet, etc.).

Thus a system of sizes proves to be absolutely necessary.

The different units of measurement

Due to differences of morphology and the lack of consultation, several countries have implemented their own sizes.
• The French system (Paris point): for a "normal" foot, the interval between two successive sizes is taken as 5 mm at ball girth; and according to the shape of the French foot, this corresponds to a 2/3 cm increase in shoe length, i.e. 6.66 mm.
Thus for a size 40 the shoe will have the following dimensions: length: 40 × 6.66 = 266.4 mm; girth: 40 × 5 = 200 mm. This shoe will be size 40 and girth 0. For wider feet, up to girth 6, the measurement system is the same: for a last of size 40, girth 4, the length is 40 × 6.66 = 266.4 mm, and the girth is (40 + 4) × 5 = 220 mm.
• The English system: is based on the inch (25.4 mm). The English unit is equal to a third of an inch, i.e. 8.46 mm. This unit of measurement is longer than the French unit, and is supposed to correspond better to the morphology of Anglo-Saxon feet. For simplification reasons, the English have created two scales:

- one is numbered from 0 to 13 and is reserved for children, it corresponds to the sizes between 16 and 32 in the French system;
- the other, numbered from 1 to 13, is reserved for adults (between sizes 33 and 48 in the French system).
• American sizes: there are two scales, one for children from 0 to 14 and an adult scale from 2 to 11. In France, where the American unit is frequently used, the French size can be obtained by adding 33 to the American size: size 3 is roughly equivalent to size 36 in France.
• The Brannock scale (named after the inventor of a device that determines size depending on the length and girth of the foot) is mainly used in Great Britain

and in the United States. It is based on the English system but with a size difference of 1 and 3/4: size 5 in England corresponds to sizes 6.5 or 7 on the Brannock scale.
• Germany: a new measurement system reserved for children has been implemented in Germany: AKA 64. This system is based on the observation that, unlike in adults, in children the relation between the length and girth of the foot is not constant. In practice, with this new system shoes are longer and narrower than in the old system.

Because existing systems were so different, complex and imprecise, international studies have led to the creation of the "Mondopoint". The unit used to determine the length and girth of the foot is the millimeter. Precise statistical analyses have assessed the necessary length interval between two sizes; the interval adopted is 5 mm, and sometimes 7.5 mm for certain shoes (boots, laced boots, etc.). However, due to the diversity of feet all over the world and variations of growth in children, no criterion has been retained for the increase in girth, for which only one study has been carried out for men's town shoes.

Different types of shoes: advantages and drawbacks

• Open-instep shoes: all the shoes that reveal the instep entirely, i.e. pumps, flats, and other shoes partially leaving the instep free and possibly including a strap and buckle, an elastic band or a Velcro strap (one-bar shoe, instep-tie shoe). These shoes leave the instep totally free and are very cosmetic, but they need to be very tight at the forefoot and submalleolar area to hold on to the foot and they often have very high heels.
• Low-upper shoes - Bluchers, Oxford shoes, moccasins, loafers, sport shoes - cover the instep, hold on to the foot and are not too tight (except moccasins, which cling to the foot tightly). Closure methods - laces, Velcro straps, zippers - cover the instep entirely and these shoes are very easy to put on (except moccasins and Oxford shoes however). This type of shoes includes many pattern combinations, for example moccasin-style Bluchers, etc. (fig. 33.8).
• High-upper shoes cover the foot and ankle entirely. They are similar to low-upper shoes, and they include balmorals, laced boots, ankle-boots and boots. They hold to the foot perfectly without tightening it. They are easy to put on, except boots.

The weight born by a foot over several kilometers each day averages out at several hundred tons, and the distance covered in an individual's life amounts to several dozens of thousands of kilometers (more than once around the world). It is therefore particularly crucial to find the right shoe.

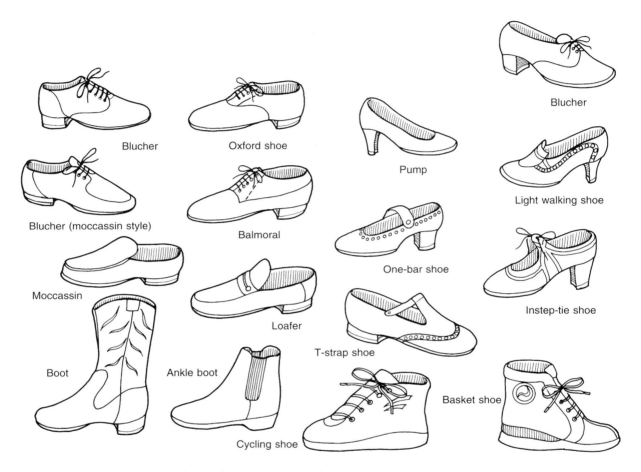

Fig. 33.8. Main types of high shoes (drawing F Lapeyre)

34.

The orthopedic shoe

F Lapeyre-Gros and F Gaillard
With the technical support of Patrick Vernay,
technician at the Centre d'Appareillage de Lyon
(Lyon's Orthopedic Institution)

The "orthopedic shoe", as it is traditionally called, or the "custom-made therapeutic shoe" for foot disorders remains a therapeutic entity that is very versatile in its different parts. Consequently, it must be well-known and prescribed advisedly and explicitly if it is to be as effective as more active and well-managed treatment. It acts as a prosthesis for the foot, i.e., it may, on the one hand, comfortably support, correct or replace a deformed foot or, on the other, compensate for leg-length discrepancy or replace part of an amputated foot. Nevertheless, it is also visibly worn and has an esthetic role to play, and pedorthists have made considerable efforts in this field to satisfy their customers.

The different parts of the orthopedic shoe will allow us to examine its main therapeutic indications.

● The different parts of the orthopedic shoe and manufacturing principles

The shoe is custom-made or molded, and is composed of:
• the inner orthosis (or orthotic cork sole), not present in a normal shoe and used as a basis for manufacturing the shoe, which is constructed around this cork sole,
• the upper and support pieces,
• the outsole.

The inner orthosis (or orthotic cork sole)

As its former name suggests, this was originally made of cork, but now it is more generally made of synthetic material and comprises, if necessary, correcting or supporting elements, which provide good coaptation between the foot to be equipped (represented by a wooden replica designed according to the shape of the foot, or by plaster or resin casts) and the insole. The use of synthetic materials is justified by their lighter weight and greater firmness. Moreover, these new materials, thanks to their properties, provide a wide range of therapeutic possibilities. These materials include:
• thermosetting polyurethane resins, with varying densities according to formulation (polyol + isocyanate mix),
• thermoplastic foams derived from polyethylene (TP foam) or ethyl-vinyl-acetate (EVA), widely used in podology (static or skin disorders),
• elements made of silicone elastomere, shock-absorbing and anti-vibration materials which are very useful when the disorder (osteoarthritic lesions of the legs, disc disorder, talocrural arthrodesis) requires such treatment,
• non-thermoplastic foams, used only to accommodate marked discrepancies (shortening, irreducible talipes equinus).

The upper and support pieces

The upper is made from a pattern whose technique has greatly changed since the once usual kraft paper;

a paraffin plate, and thermoforming PVC film are now used. It is composed of two lateral quarters at the back, and in front it includes a vamp prolonged by a tongue on the instep.

The upper comprises a leather lining (pigskin, goatskin) and outer leatherwork made of boxcalf, kid or rough calf. The choice of leatherwork is made according to the pathology of the foot (requirement for flexibility or resistance) and the use of the shoe (patient's age, way of life, environment, etc.). The upper is, in addition to its esthetic role (extremely large and/or wide foot for example), the corrective or replacement element for the statics or function of the foot. Consequently it will be ankle-high whenever necessary (the reasons must be explained to the patient in order to gain acceptance) and may be reinforced with basic elements fitted between the lining and the skin, except for elevators, which are fitted inside or outside the shoe.

These elements may be:
• a toe-cap, also made of leather or thermoplastic material which protects the toes and may be replaced, if the shoes are worn at work, by a steel toe-cap (similar to those of safety shoes),
• flanges, pieces of leather designed to make the upper rigid between the toe-cap and the counter, which create a continuum between these two elements. Depending on the patient to be equipped, they may incorporate the following therapeutic components:
• extended supports, also called counters, that may be unilateral or bilateral, and set either vertically or horizontally. They are made of molded leather, of varying thickness, or thermoplastic material (a polycarbolactone resin) with varying thickness according to the support to be given to the foot, or of cellulose material with the addition of acetone.

A spring steel support may be set at the back of the upper and prolonged by a whole-length steel sole, which creates a lever effect. In this case, and also whenever a lever effect is required for good mechanical advantage, the upper must be rather high.
• Unilateral or bilateral corset, sometimes associated with upstanding supports and foot elevators.
• Foam padding, sometimes necessary for good skin tolerance of the aforementioned elements.
• Elastic foot lifters are set either outside or inside the upper and are generally designed to compensate for muscle deficiencies.
• Accessory elements may be added to the upper with therapeutic, cosmetic or ergonomic objectives:

- zipper, velcro strap, or buckle,
- outer or inner correcting lateral strap (antisupination or antipronation lever effect),
- elastic bands (on a low upper, in order to don the shoe more easily with a long handled-shoehorn in the case of osteoarthritis of the hip for example),
- protective pieces set on the sides, back or anterior end of the shoe (in the case of walking disorders causing abnormal wear and tear of part of the shoe).

The sole

The sole comprises various elements (insole, outsole, heel) that make up the bottom part of the shoe.
• The insole, which is made of highly resistant shoulder leather, is fixed to the inner orthosis before constructing the upper. A steel or thermoplastic material shank-piece is glued under the insole, then leather or cork offcuts are stuck onto it. The shank piece may be replaced by a whole or half-length steel sole to reduce sagittal mobility of the joints of the foot. In order to improve the statics of the shoe, the sole may be made wider by sticking or sewing a welt around the upper. Similarly, in order to facilitate the stance phase, a Thomas bar which allows rolling of the foot during gait may be stuck under the insole. Lastly, a medial or lateral wedge which promotes supination or pronation may improve the statics of the forefoot.
• The outsole, stuck or sewn underneath, is made of processed leather that provides a high resistance or of microcellular or solid rubber derivatives.
• The heel, made of leather, wood, or rubber material, may also carry corrective elements: medial or lateral heel wedges, with varying medial or lateral length. They make it possible to correct the axis of the hindfoot or improve the statics of the foot.

● Indications

It is only after a complete examination of the patient, including the shoes, mode of walking, mobility and requirements as well as examination of the feet, leg, pelvic balance and articulations that it is possible to prescribe orthopedic shoes. This prescription has not only an esthetic aim but must treat a disorder and take its place among all other available forms of treatment, other equipment and other shoes. Thanks to its precise role and perfect adaptability to a

Table 34.1.

Goals	Means
Support • malformation or deformity of the foot inducing difficulties in wearing shoes, or static disorders • joint laxity • painful joint movements (ankle, foot) • skin fragility, weight-bearing stresses on painful areas	• molded inner orthosis, may be very inclusive • custom-made or molded shoe • adaptation of the sole: medially or laterally broadened heel • supports (molded counters) • corseting of the upper • molded supports (counters) • sole with varying rigidity + shank-piece with varying length towards the ball of the foot • improvement of the stance phase (roller-bar) • seamless upper • upper padding (complete or partial) • special closure methods • foam or plastazote sole (thermomolded if necessary) • inner orthosis • adaptation of the orthosis by drilling holes, adding elements with varying density foams
Correction (for reducible deformities) • static foot disorders (calcaneovalgus or calcaneovarus) • deviation of the forefoot • improvement of weight-bearing stress distribution and abnormal foot positions (reducible clawtoes)	• inner orthosis (wedges, straps with pronation supination effects • T-strap (to control a talipes varus for example) • corset • height of upper • long counter extended towards the first metatarsal head • corrective inner orthosis: retrocapital metatarsal pad or bar • arch support • molded inner orthosis
Replacement • stance phase disorder • deficiency of lever muscles • partially reducible equinus	• toe-raising spring • roller bar or inner orthosis • height of upper • upstanding supports • corset • posterior steel support + steel sole (lever effect) • unilateral or crossed foot elevators (unilateral to enhance pronation or supination effect) • height of upper • supports • corset • adapted inner orthosis if necessary
Equalization • shortening • irreducible or poorly reducible equinus • amputation	• raised inner orthosis with accurate compensation for the forefoot and hindfoot • raised inner orthosis • taking into account the other shoe • higher counters (to support the foot laterally despite the thickness of the orthosis) • high upper, if made necessary by orthosis thickness • if distal amputation: low-upper shoe possible • otherwise sufficient upper height • toe-filler (cosmetic) • orthosis with padded stiffened tongue in the case of short stump (+ contralateral equalizing orthosis to facilitate stance phase) • metatarsal pad on inner orthosis • special shoe devices (that can sometimes be inserted into commercially available shoes)

specific disorder (all its different parts have one and the same exact therapeutic goal), the shoe occupies an important place amongst the aids at our disposal. Consequently, it is important to be well acquainted with all its possibilities and limitations.

Indications are summarized in table 34.1.

Rheumatologists and the orthopedic shoe

A rheumatologist rarely has to equip amputated or neurogenic feet, but is sometimes faced with a prescription for leg-length discrepancy; the usual requirement is to treat rheumatoid feet or marked static disorders. Even more than in other conditions, the custom-made shoe must not only be adapted in order to gain the patient's acceptance but also be attractive and light. This implies a close collaboration between patient, physician and pedorthist in the light of their respective aims and abilities. The cosmetic aspect is cardinal for rheumatoid feet; the patient can choose shoes from models exposed, a photograph or a catalogue. Lightness implies the use of adapted modern materials, and a low upper if possible, made of kid for example.

For rheumatoid feet, requirements are as follows: good support, relief of painful joints and creation of a stabilizing support that prevents static disorders induced by joint disorders, as much as possible The insole acts as a correcting element,

makes it possible to relieve plantar pressure and often accommodates the atrophy of plantar soft tissues.

The prescription must be precise as regards the role of the shoe, its shape, the height of the upper, the leatherwork, the closure method, the insole, and possible inserts. In France, the prescription is filled according to two processes depending on its origin. If it comes from a general practitioner, a consultation is organized at the appliance center ("centre d'appareillage") in order to design the most suitable equipment. If the prescription comes from a rheumatologist, an orthopedic surgeon or a specialist in physical medicine, consultation at the centre d'appareillage is optional. Consequently the prescribing physician, in this case the rheumatologist, is not only responsible for the prescription, but must also check if the shoes are comfortable and well adapted. Thus, after the patient has received the shoes, a consultation is organized to check their effectiveness and correct possible disorders. When the shoes are satisfactory, a second pair of shoes may be ordered. This is authorized only in the first year.

In conclusion, it is necessary to be well acquainted with the wide range of prescriptions for custom-made shoes for foot disorders. These shoes are expensive - FF 3,500 to FF 4,300 for one pair - and part of the price is payable by the patients, but insurance companies often share the cost. Well-prescribed, well-adapted, as attractive and as light as possible, they can be very useful for patients disadvantaged in their comfort and ambulation.

Index

Acromegaly 108
Aircast splint 283
Algodystrophies 149-156
   clinical forms 152-153
   " cold " phase 149, 151
   " hot " phase 149, 151
   imaging 50, 151, 152
   risk of definitive sequellae 151
   scintigraphy 65, 152
   sesamoids 204
Amputation
   diabetes 92, 97, 98
   of second ray 224
Amyotrophy 175
Analgesics 154
Anatomy 1-14, 179, 247
   of first ray 183
   imaging
      CT 32-38
      MRI 32, 38-45
   metatarsals 22, 209
Angioma 316
Angiosarcoma 316
Angle(s)
   Boehler 's 22
   cavus 22, 177
   Distal Articular Set 188
   flat foot 22
   forefoot 22
   hallux adductus 22
   intermetatarsal 22, 210
   medial arch 22, 25, 161, 178
   M1P1 22
   proximal phalangeal articular 188
   radiographic 21
   tibiotalar 178
   see also Pitch
Ankle
   appliances 283
   deformations 249
   infection 87
   instability, treatment 303-308
   pain 62
   sprains 279-286
   see also Joint, talocrural
Ankylosis 131
   in rheumatoid foot 119, 124

   of tarsus 112, 117, 140
Anterior drawer test 19
Anterior talar drawer sign 281, 284
Anteversion, excessive 324
Antibiogram 96
Antibiotherapy 88, 89, 101
Anticoagulant treatment 101
Antigen, HLA B27 62, 135, 136
Antispasmodic agents 72
Aponeurectomy, plantar posterior
   180
Aponeurosis, plantar 10, 233
   imaging 47, 54
   rupture 235
   windlass mechanism 17
Arch
   medial, angle 22, 25, 161, 178
   plantar, physiology 234
Arteriography, in diabetes 96
Arteriopathy, in diabetes 92, 97, 101
Artery
   fibular 11
   anterior tibial 11, 15
   posterior tibial 11
Arthritis
   imaging 47
   reactive 135, 143
   rheumatoid 111-127
   septic 85-90
      chronic 89
   of sesamoids 205
   talocrural 119
   of tarsus 112
Arthrodesis 59, 131
   ankle joint 132
   cuneometatarsal 194
   double 169
   evaluation by scintigraphy 59
   interphalangeal 223
   metatarsophalangeal 131, 194, 201,
      208
   osteotomy 179
   partial 167
   subtalar and midtarsal 169, 181,
      251
   triple 75, 82
Arthrography with CT 29, 63, 64

Arthropathies
   erosive 119
   metabolic 105-109
   neuropathic 67
Arthroplasty 131, 223
Arthrorises 75
Arthrosis 208
   of center of rotation 165
   hallux 187
   midtarsal 65
   sesamoids 205
   subtalar 250
Aspiration of joint 62, 85, 87
   see also Synovial fluid
Atonic foot 115
Axis
   of ankle joint 18
   of calcaneus 24
   diaphysial 178
   talometatarsal, malalignment 157,
      161, 162
   of talus 24, 178
   tarsometatarsophalangeal, mal-
      alignment 160

Bacteriologic diagnosis 85
Bar, of orthoses
   retrocapital 333, 337
   Thomas 329, 348
Bauer's toe 141
Biopsy-arthroscopy of the ankle 65,
   86
Block, regional sympathetic 154
Blockade, chemical 74
Bone(s) 2
   accessory 1, 6
      navicular 250
   anomalies, surgery 167
   cuboid 1, 247, 252
      fracture 49
   cuneiforms 1, 183, 247
   densitometry 271
   dystrophies 319
   erosion *see* Erosion
   intermetatarsal 6, 187
   navicular 1
      accessory 6, 250

fracture 48, 273
pathology, CT 47
secondary calcaneal 7
sesamoids 1, 203
    fractures 273
    pathology 203-206
spur 163
sustentacular 7
tibial 6
tumors 309-321
Vesalian 7
see also names of different bones
Brachymetatarsus 218
Buniectomy 192, 208
Bunion 207
see also Exostoses
Bursae, 12, 227
    intercapito-metatarsal 14, 227
Bursitis 117, 120, 139
    lateral, of 5th metatarsal head 220
    preachilles 237
    reactive 187
    retrocalcaneal 236, 241
        painful 138

Calcaneal
    canal 12
    pitch 22, 178
    spurs 120
        false 138
    valgus 24, 112, 161
    varus 177
Calcaneocavus foot 70
Calcaneus 2
    deviation, measurement 24
    fracture 237, 273, 297
    Haglund's deformity 144, 243
    pronation 158
    tuberosity 1, 158, 233
Calcitonin 154
Calcium pyrophosphate deposition
        disease 107
Callosities 219
    round forefoot 216
    subcuboid 181
Callus, bone 271
Capsulotomy 213
Cartilage of hallux, lesions 195
Cauda equina root lesions 176
Cavus foot see Pes cavus
Cerebral
    lesions 81
    palsy 80
Charcot's disease 68, 94
Charcot-Marie-Tooth's disease 75,
        78, 175

Chiropodal care 97, 122
Chondroblastoma 315
Chondrocalcinosis 107, 205
Chondroma 313, 315
Chondrosarcoma 314
Clawing of toes
    neuropathic foot 70
    pathogenesis 221
    pes cavus 174, 177, 181
    rheumatoid foot 113, 117, 222
    swan-neck deformities 117, 224
    total 223
    treatment 79, 223
        reduction 179
Clinodactyly 224
Clubbing of a digit 311
Condylectomy 217
Corticosteroids injection 122, 123,
        239, 251
CPPD 107
Cryotherapy 282, 315
Crystal arthropathies 87, 105-107,
        205
CT 27-56, 63
    arthrography 29, 63, 64
    tenography 29, 63
    versus MRI 46
Cyst
    aneurysmal 310
    idiopathic 309

Deformities
    1st ray 183-202
    forefoot 69, 113, 116
    hindfoot 69, 112, 117
    midfoot 69
    of toes 113, 224
    see also Clawing of toes, Foot
Degenerative spinocerebellar
        diseases 176
Dejerine-Sottas disease 76, 175
Diabetes 86, 91-104
Diastasis, tibiofibular 296
Dislocation, 47
    of fibular tendons 255
    of tibialis posterior tendon 252
DMAA 190
Drainage 88
Dysplasia
    hereditary areflexic 175
    fibrous 59, 319
Dystrophies
    bone 319
    muscular progressive 175
    onychomycotic 93

Edema 15, 49, 165, 285, 315
    algodystrophy 150
    rheumatoid foot 115
Ehlers-Danlos disease 111, 157
Electromyography 65, 71, 75, 261
Electrotherapy 73
Emission tomographic 59
Enchondroma 314
Enchondromatosis 314
Enthesitis 135
Entrapment neuropathies 65, 236,
        259-268
Equinus foot 70, 76, 178, 216
Ergotherapy 121
Erosion, bone
    gout 106
    rheumatoid arthritis 119
    spondylarthropathies 138
Eversion, forefoot 16, 17
Ewing's sarcoma 316
Examination
    auxiliary investigations 61-65
    clinical 15-20, 61, 93, 211, 222
        of diabetic foot 93
    neurologic 71
Exostosis 187, 313
    calcaneal spur 235, 236
    see also Bunion
Exostotic disease 313

Fasciitis, chronic 235
Fibroma, chondromyxoid 315
Fibula 2
    fracture 274
Fibular neck syndrome 265
Flange, shoe 342, 348
Fluoroquinolones 242, 244
Foot
    anterior round 216
    ataxic 67
    atavistic 186, 210
    atonic 115
    calcaneal 209
    calcaneocavus 70, 77
        paralytic 77
    cavus 112, 173-182
        anterior 173, 179, 181
        mixed 173, 181
        neuropathic 78, 175, 181
        orthoses 178, 334
        posterior 173, 179, 181
        rheumatoid 112
        treatment 178
        tripod 173
        varus 173, 324, 334
    cavo-varus 324

central neuropathic 79
Charcot's 94
drop 79
equinus 70, 76, 178, 216
index plus minus 210
neurodegenerative 78
neuropathic 67-84
morphotypes 184, 190, 210
flail 76
flat
    orthoses 166, 335
    talus neonatal 198
    treatment 166, 170
    valgus 157-171, 186
paralytic 77
paraplegic
    flaccid 76, 79
    spastic 79
prints 331
    pes cavus 177
rheumatoid 111-127
    orthoses 122, 337
    and septic arthritis 87
    sesamoid lesions 205
    treatment 121, 129-133
Footwear 341-346
    diabetes 99, 100
    hallux valgus 186
    neuropathic foot 73
    orthopedic shoe 347-350
    rheumatoid foot 111, 122
    running shoes 326
    types of shoes 346
    units of measurements 345
Forefoot
    abduction 249
        measurement 162
    deformities
        neuropathic foot 69
        rheumatoid foot 113-116
        round 216
        in spondylarthropathies 139
    hyperlaxity 192
    lateral deviation 115
    morphotypes 184
    round 216
    splaying 113
    static pathology 209-226
    triangular, rheumatoid 115, 116, 210
    valgus 16
    varus 16
Formula
    digital 184, 190, 210
    metatarsal 184, 186

Fracture(s)
    by bone insufficiency 274
    imaging 47-49, 271
    multifocal 274
    occult 47, 297
    repair, radiography 271
    stress 273, 269-277
        metatarsals 273
        metatarsal heads 214
        navicular bone 273
        rheumatoid foot 121
    scintigraphy 58, 271
    sesamoids 204
Fragile chromosome X, syndrome 157
Freiberg's disease 214, 215, 229
Friedreich's ataxia 79
Fusion(s)
    of the 1st MP joint 208
    calcaneonavicular 169
    tarsal 157-171

Gadolinium 32
Gait
    clinical examination 19
    physiology 184, 209, 234
    reeducation 144
    rheumatoid arthritis 121
    role of sesamoids 203
    supination of forefoot 199
Gangrenous lesions 92
Gaping
    subtalar joint 293
    tibiotalar 281
Gelcast appliance 283
Gout 61, 105-107
    bone erosion 106
    heel pain 237
    pseudo-, sesamoids 205

Hallomegaly 186, 195, 207
    shortening of proximal phalanx 192, 195, 201, 207
Hallux
    canoe-shaped 200
    cartilage lesions 195
    dolorosus 200, 201
    interphalangeal 187
    limitus 200
    rigidus 117, 199-202, 245
        orthoses 334
    valgus 183-198
        rheumatoid foot 113, 116
        orthoses 335
        role of shoes 186

Heel
    clinical examination 17
    fat pad, thinning 236
    pain, 61
        acute, 236, 237
        of mechanical origin 233-240
        orthoses 238, 244, 336
        plantar rheumatoid 120
        spondylarthropathies 137, 143
Hemangioendothelioma 316
Hemiplegy 81
Hemochromatosis 108
Hindfoot, deformities
    hyperpronation 323
    neuropathic foot 69
    rheumatoid foot 112, 117
    spondylarthropathies 137
Hydrotherapy 144, 155
Hydroxyapatite crystals arthropathy 107
Hyperkeratose 94, 97
    intractable, plantar 219
Hyperlipidemia 108
Hyperostosis 237
Hyperpronation 241
    of hindfoot 323
Hyperurucemia 105, 106

Impingement syndrome 47, 121
    anterior 298
    antero-lateral 293
Implants, cartilage lesions 195
Infections 85-90, 205
    diabetes 93
    scintigraphy 58, 85, 96
Inflammation and algodystrophy, treatment 143
Innervation of the foot 11
Instability of the ankle 286, 288
    chronic 303
Insufficiency of first ray 210
Intercapitometatarsal space 12
Inversion, forefoot 16, 17

Joint(s)
    calcaneocuboidal 5
    cuneometatarsal 183
        stiffness 207
    interphalangeal 6, 17
    metatarsophalangeal 6, 17, 203, 207
        hallux 183, 187, 199
        stiffness 195
        subluxation 117
    metatarsosesamoid 6
    protection 121

range of motion 16, 18, 286
subtalar 5, 17
    gaping 293
    laxity 291
talocrural 2, 17
    laxity 288
    radiography 24
    range of motion 18
    see also Ankle
talonavicular 5
tarsometatarsal 2, 6, 17
transverse of tarsus 2, 16, 17
see also specific pathologies

Kagger's clear preachillean triangle
    244
Keratoderma palmaris and plantaris
    141
Köhler's disease 214

Laboratory tests 62
Last, of shoe 344
Lateral deviation of toes 114
Latex test 62
Laxity
    subtalar 291
    talocrural 288, 291
    tibiotalar 281, 288
Ledderhose's disease 151, 238
Lelièvre parabola 184, 190, 210
Lengthening
    of calcaneal tendon 74, 181
    of extensor muscles 223
Leukonychia 93
Ligament
    anterior cruciate 303
    anterior talofibular 18, 279, 303
        partial tear 304
    anterior talonavicular 18
    anterior tibiofibular 3, 279, 292,
        295
    calcaneofibular 5, 18, 279, 290-
        292, 303
    cervical 291
    clinical examination 18
    deep transverse metatarsal 14,
        227
    deltoid 4, 18, 279, 288
    direct repair 291, 307
    dorsal calcaneocuboid 5
    examination 18
    glenoid 6, 203
    interosseous talocalcaneal 4, 5,
        54, 291, 292
    inferior calcaneocuboid 5
    inferior calcaneonavicular 5

injuries 303
    imaging 52
intersesamoid 203
lateral calcaneonavicular 5
lateral collateral 3, 52, 279
    lesions 52, 287
lateral glenosesamoid 185
lateral talocalcaneal 291
lesions imaging 52
medial calcaneocuboid 5
medial collateral 4, 52, 279
medial tibiocalcaneal 5
posterior talofibular 279, 289, 303
posterior tibiofibular 3, 295
repairs 291
ruptures, imaging 47, 50
superior talonavicular 5
tear, complications 288
transverse metatarsal 203, 227
Ligamentoplasty 307, 291
Ligamentous repair 291, 307
Limb-length discrepancy 324
Limp, intermittent 94
Line of Meary 22
Lipoma, bone 316
Lobstein's disease 320
Loose bodies imaging 47, 50
Luxation 48
    of 1st phalanx 210
    imaging 48, 52
    metatarsophalangeal 208
    metatarsosesamoidal 207
    of sesamoids 185, 203

Malalignment syndromes 323
Malleoloc appliance 283
Marfan's disease 157
Massage 90, 122
    sprains of ankle 282
Meary's method 24
Medial pain syndrome, valgus flat
    foot 164-165
Melorheostosis 320
Metabolic arthropathies 105-109
Metastases, bone 318
Metatarsal head(s)
    fifth
        lateral bursitis 220
        and rheumatoid arthritis 115
        and spondylarthropathies 140
    fracture 214
    necrosis 214
Metatarsalgy 211, 216
    acute 61, 219
    foot orthoses 332
    Morton's see Morton's syndrome

postoperative 196
spondylarthropathy 139
transfer 218
Metatarsals 1
    1st, varus 188
    bone erosion 116
    insufficiency 218
    morphotype 209
    pitch 22, 209
    protrusion distance 209-21
    splaying 113
    stress fracture 273
Metatarsectomy 181, 179
Metatarsus
    adductus 207
    varus of 1st ray 113, 186, 207, 210
Microangiopathy 92
Midfoot 2
    infections 87
    neuropathic foot 69
Morton's syndrome 54, 217, 227-230,
    259
    imaging 54
    recurrent 230
    surgical evaluation 231
MRI 27-56, 63
    versus CT 46
Muscles (s) 16
    abductor digiti minimi 10, 16, 233
    abductor hallucis 9, 184, 233
    abductor hallucis brevis 13
    adductor hallucis 10, 16, 185
    dorsal interosseous 10, 16, 227
    dorsiflexor, weakness 68
    dysfunction
        hallux valgus 185
        pes cavus 174
    extensor digitorum brevis 9
    extensor digitorum longus 8, 16
    extensor hallucis longus 7, 16, 185
    fibularis brevis 16, 253
    fibularis digiti quinti 252
    fibularis longus 8, 16, 297
        tendinopathies 253
    fibularis quartus 252
    fibularis tertius 7, 253
    flexor digitorum brevis 9, 16, 233
    flexor digitorum longus 8, 16
    flexor hallucis brevis 9, 16, 185
    flexor hallucis longus 9, 184, 185
        tendinopathies 256
    function 16
    gastrocnemius 9
    intrinsic 9, 16, 183
        atrophy 78
    lumbricals 14, 16, 222

plantar flexor weakness 68
plantar interosseous 10, 16
quadratus plantae 9, 16
soleus 9
tibialis anterior 7
    tendinopathies 256
tibialis posterior 8, 13, 16, 158, 247
    tendinopathies 247
triceps surae 9, 16
    overuse 242
Mycosis, and diabetes 93, 100
Myopathy 175

Nail
    ingrowing, and diabetes 99
    mycosis 93
    psoriasic 141
Necrosis see Osteonecrosis
Nerve(s)
    to abductor digiti minimi
        muscle, compression 236,
        262
    deep fibular 11
        compression 265
    digital
        compression 259
        plantar 14, 227
    distribution in the foot 260
    lateral plantar 13, 233, 259
        compression 263
    medial calcaneal, compression
        234, 259
    medial plantar 13
        compression 263
    saphenous 11
        compression 265
    sensory 233
    superficial fibular 11, 291
        compression 263, 265
    sural 11
        compression 266
    tibial 11, 13, 233
        compression 262
Neuro-ablative surgery 74
Neuro-arthropathy 95
Neurolysis 74, 265
Neuropathy 67-84
    central neuropathic foot 79
    diabetes 92, 95
        treatment 101
    neurodegenerative foot 78
    peripheral neuropathic foot 75
    pes cavus 175
    see also Foot, neuropathic
Neurotomies 74

Nodules 241, 243
    rheumatoid foot 120
        subcutaneous 121

Onycholysis 141
Onychomycotic dystrophy 93
Orthopedic shoe 347-350
Orthoses 329, 340
    ankle appliance 283
    clawed toes 223
    diabetic foot 99
    flat foot 166, 335
    hallux rigidus 334
    hallux valgus 335
    of heel 238, 245
    inner, orthopedic shoes 347
    legislation 338
    materials 330
    Morton's syndrome 230
    neuropathic foot 73
    pes cavus 178
        varus 334
    plantar 332-338
    rheumatoid foot 122, 129, 337
    round forefoot 217
    spondylarthropathies 144
    talalgy 336
    of toes 99, 122, 178, 338
    types 329
Os trigonum 6, 288, 299
Osteitis
    heel pain 238
    imaging 50, 47
Osteoblastoma 312
Osteochondral lesions of talar
        dome 49, 293-295
Osteochondritis 214
    imaging 47, 58
Osteochondroma 313
Osteogenesis imperfecta 320
Osteoid osteoma 311
    heel pain 237
    scintigraphy 59
Osteolysis 312
Osteomyelitis 96
    imaging 50
    of sesamoids 205
Osteonecrosis
    imaging 47, 50
    scintigraphy 58
    sesamoids 204
    of talus 50, 294
Osteopenia 151
Osteopetrosis 319
Osteophytes, anterior tibiotalar 298
Osteophytosis 119

Osteopoikilosis 319
Osteoporosis, and fractures 237, 274
Osteosarcoma 312
Osteotomy (ies) 74, 130, 201
    basimetatarsal 193, 201, 213
    bipolar 193
    of calcaneus 77, 169, 179, 181
        elevation 218
    of 1st cuneiform 194
    diaphysial 193, 196
    distal 193
    Dwyer's 77, 167, 169
    Gauthier's 196, 223
    hallux rigidus 201
    hallux valgus 192-194
    inverted-V 179
    metatarsal 179, 192, 196, 208, 217,
        223
    pes cavus 179
    phalangeal 195
    for 1st ray 192
    for 2nd ray 213
    Scarf 194
    Weil's 214, 218, 223
    see also Surgical techniques
Overcorrections, hallux valgus 198
Overloading, lateral plantar 219
Overloading, plantar 219
Overuse syndromes during running
        323-328
Oxalate crystals 107

Pachyonycchia 141
Paget's disease 319
    heel pain 238
    bone scintigraphy 59
Pain
    on accessory navicular bone 251
    acute, gout 105
    chronic of ankle 289
    flat foot 164-165
    hallux valgus 187
    pes planovalgus 165
    retromalleolar 253
    strategy in diagnosis 64
    tendinopathy 242
        extrinsic fibular tendons 255
        lateral metatarsal 219
    see also Metatarsalgia, Talalgia
Pain, medial, syndrome, valgus flat
        foot 164-165
Painful os peroneum syndrome 255
Parkinson's disease 79
PASA 190
Peritendinitis 241, 243

Pes
  cavus see Foot, cavus
  planovalgus 112, 118
  planus see Foot, flat
Phalanx 1
  1st, fracture 274
  hallux 183
    deviation 188
    shortening 192, 195, 207
  valgus 207
Physiotherapy 144
  neuropathic foot 72
Pitch
  calcaneal 22-23, 178
  metatarsal 22, 209
  talar 22-23
Plantar
  aponeurosis see Aponeurosis,
    plantar
  pad 211
  plate, overstretching 210,
    222
Plasmocytoma of bone 317
Poliomyelitis 76, 77
  anterior, pes cavus 176
Pronation 17
Prostheses
  hallux rigidus 201
  hallux valgus 194
  of rheumatoid joints 132
  Swanson's 194
Pseudarthrosis 59, 276
  of metatarsals 218
Pseudogout 107
Psoriasis 141, 142, 237
Pustulosis palmaris and plantaris
  141
Pyknodysostosis 319

Quintus varus 220, 224

Radiography 21-25, 62
  algodystrophy 151
  angles 22, 178
  flat foot and tarsal fusions 161
  in forced position, sprains 282,
    284, 285
  hallux valgus 188
  pes cavus 177
  rheumatoid arthritis 116, 118
  views 21, 24, 204
    in weight-bearing 22
Range of motion, joint 18, 286
  active 16
  passive 16

Ray
  first
    insufficiency 210, 212
    pathology 183-202
  second, syndrome 210, 212
Reeducation 72
  round forefoot 217
  sprains 283, 285
  flat foot 166
Reiter's syndrome de 135, 237
Renander's disease 204
Resection, tarsometatarsal 179
Retinaculum
  inferior of fibular muscles 13
  extensor 7, 12
  flexor 12, 13, 259
Rhizotomy, sectorial posterior 74
Rheumatoid foot see Foot,
    rheumatoid
Riley-Day disease 76
Rose-Waaler test 62
Rupture(s)
  of calcaneal tendon 51, 241, 243,
    245
  ligamentous 47, 50, 280
  of plantar aponeurosis 235
  of tendon of tibialis posterior
    muscle 62, 165, 170, 248

Sarcoma, Ewing's 316
Sciatic
  neurotmesis 76
  root, lesion 237
Scintigraphy 57-60, 63, 152, 271
  infections 58, 85, 96
Sclerosis, fracture repair 271, 274
Second ray syndrome 210, 212
Sesamoid bones
  anatomy 2, 183, 203
  disorders 203-206
  sling 183
    displacement 190
    reentering 192
  translocation 185
Sever's disease 236
Shoes see Footwear
Short leg syndrome 326
Shortening of phalanx of hallux 192,
    195, 207
Sign
  daylight 116
  Johnson's too many toes 249, 250
  Lasègue's toe 228
  Mulder's 228
  podal of Lachmann 211
  of split target 49

Siliconitis 201
Sinus tarsi 5
  syndrome 288, 292, 297
Sober ankle appliance 283
Sole 342, 348
  orthotic cork 347
  orthopedic shoe 348
Spina bifida 77
Split lesions
  of fibularis brevis tendon 253
  imaging 47, 52
Spondylarthropathies 135-147, 237
  classifications 136
  sesamoid 205
Spondylitis, ankylosing 61
Sprains of the ankle 279-286
  "chronic" 293
  classification 304
  imaging 281, 284
  sequelae 287-302
  treatment 282, 284
Spur, calcaneal 236
Stark-Kaeser scapulofibular
    amyotrophy 175
Subluxation
  imaging 52
  metatarsophalangeal joints 117
  proximal phalanges 113
Subtalar laxity 291
Sudeck's atrophy 90
Supination 17
  forefoot 161
  resisted 249
Supraductus of 2nd toe 224
Surgical technique(s) 74
  Brostom-Gould's 306, 307
  Dwyer's 77, 167, 169
  Judet's 167, 169
  Gauthier's 216, 223,230
  Girdlestone 262, 263
  Green's 167, 213, 223
  Grice's 167, 169
  de Keller-Brandes-Lelièvre 194,
    196, 201, 212, 227
  Kidner's 251
  ligamentous repair 307
  Mayo 212
  Mc Bride's 192
  neuroablative 74
  see also Osteotomies
Sustentaculum tali 2, 13, 247
Synchondroses 163
  imaging 50, 164
Syndesmosis, tibiofibular
  clinical examination 18
  lesions 295

Synostosis
  calcaneonavicular 159, 162
  fibrous 163
  imaging 47, 50
  talocalcaneal 159, 162
  tarsal 65, 157-171, 288
Synovectomies 130
Synovial fluid
  aspiration 62, 85-87
  in gouty arthritis 106
  hydroxyapatite crystals 107
  oxalate crystals 107
  urate crystals 106
Synovitis 111, 135

Tailor's bunion 220
Talalgy see Heel Pain
Talar beak 163
Talus 1
  angles of inclination and
      declination 158
  dome, osteochondral lesions 49,
      293
    classification 294
  domed 163
  fracture of lateral process
      297
  necrosis 50
  postero-lateral tuberosity,
      pathology 298
  stress fracture 273
Tarsal
  ankylosis 112, 117, 140
  arthritis 112
  synostoses 157-171, 288
  tunnel syndrome 120, 238, 259,
      288
Tarsectomy 75
  anterior 179, 181
  midtarsal 179, 181
Tendinopathies 52, 164
  ankle 247-258
  calcaneal 241-245
  fibularis brevis, split lesions of
      253
  fibularis muscles 252
    longus 253
  flexor hallucis longus 256
  rheumatoid foot 118
  see also Tendon
Tendinosis 241, 243

Tendon(s)
  Achilles see calcaneal
  of anterior tibialis muscle,
      pathology 256, 303
  calcaneal 12
    imaging 47, 51
    lengthening 74, 81, 167, 181
    painful 138
    rupture 51, 241, 245
    short 159
    tendinopathy 241-246
  fibular, pathology 252-256
  of fibularis brevis m., elongation
      167
  of flexor hallucis longus,
      pathology 256
  of posterior tibialis muscle 247-
      252
    dislocation 252
    dysfunction, classifications
        249
    flat foot 159
    ruptures 62, 165, 170, 248
    vascularisation 248
  ruptures 165, 169, 248
    imaging 47, 51, 52
    repair 130, 245
  transfer 74, 167, 169, 251
    Girdlestone's technique 223
  transplantation, pes cavus 179
  see also Tendinopathies
Tenography with CT 29, 63
Tenosynovectomies 130
Tenosynovitis 140, 164
  imaging 47, 51
  retromalleolar 112
  rheumatoid 118
Thévenard's disease 76
Thompson's disease 244
Thyroid acropachy 108
Tibia 2, 6
  fracture 274
Toe(s)
  amputation 98
  Bauer's 141
  clawed see Clawing of toes
    pathogenesis 221
    total 223
  deformations 142, 221
    clinodactyly 224
    contracted 142
    lateral deviation 114

  rheumatoid foot 113
  sausage-like 137, 139, 142
  swan-neck 222
  digital formula 184
  examination 17
  fifth, of rheumatoid foot 115, 116
  second, supradductus 224
  too many, sign 249, 250
Toe-cap, shoes 348
Tophaceous gout 106
Tumors
  bone 47, 309-321
  bone-marrow 316
  giant-cell 315
  imaging 51, 54
  scintigraphy 59
  vascular 316
Tunnel
  fibular 13
  tarsal 13
    syndrome 120, 238, 259

Ulcers, plantar 67, 80, 86, 93, 94
Ultrasonography 63
Uric acid, gout 106
Uricemia 62, 106

Valgus
  hindfoot 19, 158
    flat foot 112
  calcaneal 24, 112, 161
  flat foot 112, 157-171
  hallux 183-198
  metatarso-phalangeal of 1st ray
      189
Varus 17
  1st metatarsal 188
  equino- 292
Vascularisation of the foot 11
Volkmann's syndrome 175

Wart, plantar 219, 238
Web space 227
Wedge, orthoses
  Berthet's 329, 348
  pronating 334
  supinating 335
Wilson's disease 108

Xanthomata, intratendinous 108
Xanthomatous infiltration,
      calcaneal tendon 243

Maquette et mise en page : Michelle Pradel

Imprimé en France, à Niort,
par Soulisse et Cassegrain
en avril 1998

Dépôt légal : mai 1998
N° d'impression : 3694